Pediatric Musculoskeletal Physical Diagnosis:

A Video-Enhanced Guide

Pediatric Musculoskeletal Physical Diagnosis:

A Video-Enhanced Guide

Editors

Kenneth Noonan, MD, MHCDS
Associate Professor
Department of Orthopaedics
University of Wisconsin School of Medicine and Public Health
Madison, Wisconsin

Mininder Kocher, MD, MPH
Chief, Division of Sports Medicine
Professor of Orthopedic Surgery, Harvard Medical School
Boston Children's Hospital
Boston, Massachusetts

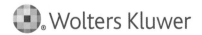

Philadelphia • Baltimore • New York • London
Buenos Aires • Hong Kong • Sydney • Tokyo

Acquisitions Editor: Brian Brown
Development Editor: Sean McGuire
Editorial Coordinator: David Murphy
Marketing Manager: Phyllis Hitner
Production Project Manager: Bridgett Dougherty
Design Coordinator: Stephen Druding
Artist/Illustrator: Rob Flewell
Manufacturing Coordinator: Beth Welsh
Prepress Vendor: TNQ Technologies

9 8 7 6 5 4 3 2 1

Printed in China

Library of Congress Cataloging-in-Publication Data

ISBN-13: 978-1-975109-27-1

Cataloging in Publication data available on request from publisher.

---

shop.lww.com

How often do you hear: "Children are not just small adults"?

This multimedia textbook, *Pediatric Musculoskeletal Physical Diagnosis: A Video-Enhanced Guide* will become the gold standard; demonstrating to the student of musculoskeletal medicine why this statement is so true. The book also explains why understanding a child's growth and development is so important in order to make an accurate assessment of their condition.

World-renowned pediatric orthopedic surgeons Drs. Noonan and Kocher have combined the knowledge of like-minded, caring, skilled clinicians to give their thoughts on how to undertake a musculoskeletal history and examination of the child and adolescent. These two editors have a passion for education, and they have crafted this book as an educational resource for anyone caring for children with musculoskeletal disorders. As you read this book, you will realize this isn't the type of information you find on the internet. This is a book full of "words of wisdom" from experienced clinicians who have spent their lifetime listening and carefully examining the musculoskeletal systems in children and adolescents. The emphasis of this book is on the assessment and decision-making for the child, not the "incision." There are many didactic textbooks and atlases on "how to treat"; however, this book addresses the importance of the patient (family)/doctor relationship, the art of taking an accurate history, and how the careful examination can often give you a diagnosis before any imaging or investigations.

Many of the authors have been taught by the doyens of orthopedic surgery in the art of history and examination. In my pediatric fellowship at the University of Iowa, I was mentored by Drs. Ponseti, Weinstein, and Deitz and other members of that department on the importance of developing the trust of the patient and their extended family, and really understanding their musculoskeletal condition and its natural history before even contemplating any intervention. I observed simple examination techniques that saved unnecessary and expensive further investigations. For example, the late Dr. Deitz would ask a patient to walk upright on their knees to assess hip flexion contractures—no need for gait analysis!

Mentally and physically every child is so different. We couldn't get a more heterogeneous species. The clinician really has to be skilful in understanding the child, their family, and caregivers who accompany them in order to get an accurate history of the symptoms. This can be challenging at times and Chapter 3: Pearls and Pitfalls of the Pediatric Musculoskeletal Examination does an outstanding job in highlighting how to cope with this.

One of the worrying aspects of looking after a child with a musculoskeletal disorder is potentially missing a serious diagnosis. In our busy clinics, we see such a range of conditions from a mild limp or intoeing to aggressive malignant bone tumors. The clinician therefore needs a stepwise system to cope with these variables, and following the guidelines in this book will certainly help you with this.

The history and physical examination is such an important component for the evaluation of children with musculoskeletal conditions. Inaccurate diagnosis based on the wrong findings can lead to missed diagnosis or, equally important, could lead to inappropriate referrals, thus resulting in patient and parental anxiety and the wasteful use of healthcare resources.

Previous authors have written outstanding textbooks covering similar topics with emphasis more on adult musculoskeletal conditions. Hoppenfeld's *Physical Examination of the Spine and Extremities* has been a landmark publication for decades. Apley's *System of Orthopaedics and Fractures* first published in 1959 emphasized the importance of the "systemic gathering of information" from history through to special investigations. The authors introduced the simple but effective "look, feel, move" concept to the physical examination. Although these and other publications have been around for so many years, history taking and physical examination seems to have become a lost art.

Pediatric Musculoskeletal Physical Diagnosis: A Video-Enhanced Guide is revitalizing this art. It is also available as an e-book and available on handheld devices. In this way, the art of the musculoskeletal examination will be continually updated and never lost. It is so integral to the optimal care of children.

- Haemish Crawford, MD
Auckland New Zealand

Alexandre Arkader, MD
Pediatric Orthopedics & Orthopedic Oncology
The Children's Hospital of Philadelphia
Associate Professor of Orthopedic Surgery
Perelman School of Medicine at University of
Pennsylvania
Philadelphia, Pennsylvania

Joshua M. Abzug, MD
Associate Professor
Departments of Orthopedics and Pediatrics
University of Maryland School of Medicine
Director, University of Maryland Brachial Plexus Practice
Director of Pediatric Orthopedics, University of
Maryland Medical Center
Deputy Surgeon-in-Chief, University of Maryland
Children's Hospital
Director and Founder, Camp Open Arms
Baltimore, Maryland

Naomi Brown, MD
Pediatric and Adolescent Sports Medicine
The Children's Hospital of Philadelphia
Assistant Professor of Clinical Pediatrics
Perelman School of Medicine at University of
Pennsylvania
Philadelphia, Pennsylvania

Pablo Castañeda, MD
The Elly and Steven Hammerman Professor of
Orthopaedic Surgery
NYU Grossman School of Medicine
Division Chief, Pediatric Orthopaedic Surgery
NYU Langone Health / Hassenfeld Children's Hospital
New York, New York

Roger Cornwall, MD, FAOA
Professor
Divisions of Orthopedic Surgery and Developmental
Biology
University of Cincinnati College of Medicine
Cincinnati Children's Hospital Medical Center
Cincinnati, Ohio

Aristides I. Cruz Jr, MD, MBA
Assistant Professor
Department of Orthopaedic Surgery
Warren Alpert Medical School of Brown University
Providence, Rhode Island

Craig Eberson, MD
Associate Professor and Chief, Pediatric Orthopedics
and Scoliosis Service
Director, Brown University Orthopaedic Residency
Program
The Warren Alpert School of Medicine at Brown
University
Rhode Island Hospital/Hasbro Children's Hospital
Providence, Rhode Island

Eric W. Edmonds, MD, FAOA
Director of Orthopaedic Research
Director of 360 Sports Medicine
Rady Children's Hospital San Diego
Professor of Clinical Orthopedic Surgery
University of California San Diego
San Diego, California

Ron El-Hawary, MD, MSc, FRCS(C)
Professor
Department of Surgery
IWK Health Center
Dalhousie University
Halifax, Nova Scotia, Canada

Martin Herman, MD
Professor of Orthopedic Surgery and Pediatrics
Drexel University College of Medicine
Section Chief of Orthopedic Surgery
St. Christopher's Hospital for Children
Philadelphia, Pennsylvania

Benton E. Heyworth, MD
Department of Orthopedics, Division of Sports Medicine
Boston Children's Hospital
Assistant Professor of Orthopedic Surgery
Harvard Medical School
Boston, Massachusetts

Danielle A. Hogarth, BS
Medical Doctorate Candidate
University of Virginia
Charlottesville, Virginia

Pooya Hosseinzadeh, MD
Assistant Professor, Department of Orthopedic Sugery
Washington University School of Medicine
St. Louis Children's Hospital
St. Louis, Missouri

Dr. Andrew Howard, MD, FRCSC, MSc
Associate Professor
Departments of Surgery & Health Policy, Management
    & Evaluation
University of Toronto
Ontario, Canada

Christopher A. Iobst, MD, FAOA
Director, Center for Limb Lengthening and
    Reconstruction
Clinical Associate Professor, Orthopaedic Surgery
The Ohio State University, College of Medicine
Nationwide Children's Hospital
Columbus, Ohio

James G. Jarvis, MD, FRCSC
Professor of Surgery
University of Ottawa
Children's Hospital of Eastern Ontario
Ottawa, Ontario, Canada

Samuel Johnson, BS
School of Medicine
Vanderbilt University Medical Center
Nashville, Tennessee

Megan E. Johnson, MD
Assistant Professor of Orthopaedic Surgery
Monroe Carell Jr. Children's Hospital at Vanderbilt/
    Vanderbilt University Medical Center
Nashville, Tennessee

Robert M. Kay, MD
Professor of Orthopaedic Surgery
Keck School of Medicine of the University of Southern
    California
Vice Chief
Children's Orthopaedic Center
Children's Hospital Los Angeles
Los Angeles, California

Derek M. Kelly, MD
Pediatric Orthopedic and Spinal Deformity Surgeon
Professor of Orthopedic Surgery
University of Tennessee - Campbell Clinic Department
    of Orthopedic Surgery
Memphis, Tennessee

Joseph G. Khoury, MD
Shriners Healthcare for Children – Florida
Associate Professor
Department of Orthopedic Surgery
University of South Florida
Tampa, Florida

Dennis E. Kramer, MD
Boston Childrens Hospital
Assistant Professor of Orthopaedic Surgery
Harvard Medical School
Boston, Massachusetts

Karen L. Lakin, MD, MSPH, FAAP
Assistant Professor
Department of Pediatrics
University of Tennessee Health Science Center
Memphis, Tennessee

A. Noelle Larson, MD
Professor
Department of Orthopedic Surgery
Mayo Clinic
Rochester, Minnesota

Raymond W. Liu, MD
Victor M. Goldberg Professor, Pediatric Orthopaedics
Rainbow Babies and Children's Hospital
Case Western Reserve University
Cleveland, Ohio

Stephanie N. Moore-Lotridge, PhD
Department of Orthopaedic Surgery
Vanderbilt University Medical Center
Nashville, Tennessee

Corina Martinez, DPT, ATC, LAT, PT, SCS
Physical Therapist
Duke Health
Durnham, North Carolina

**Christina L. Master, MD, FAAP, CAQSM,
FACSM**
Professor of Clinical Pediatrics
Perelman School of Medicine at the University of
    Pennsylvania
Co-Director, Minds Matter Concussion Program
Pediatric and Adolescent Sports Medicine, Division of
    Pediatric Orthopedics
Attending Physician, Care Network - Karabots Center
The Children's Hospital of Philadelphia
Philadelphia, Pennsylvania

Amy L. McIntosh, MD
Professor of Orthopedic Surgery
Texas Scottish Rite Hospital
Dallas, Texas

William P. Meehan III, MD
Director
Micheli Center for Sports Injury Prevention
Director of Research
Brain Injury Center
Boston Children's Hospital
Boston, Massachusetts

Matthew D. Milewski, MD
Pediatric Orthopaedics & Sports Medicine
Boston Children's Hospital
Assistant Professor of Orthopaedic Surgery
Harvard Medical School
Boston, Massachusetts

Ryan D. Muchow, MD
Department of Surgery
Kentucky Clinic
University of Kentucky
Lexington, Kentucky

Kishore Mulpuri, MHS, MSc, MBBS, FRCSC
Investigator, BC Children's Hospital
Pediatric Orthopaedic Surgeon, Department of
    Orthopaedic Surgery,
BC Children's Hospital
Vancouver, British Columbia, Canada

Tom F. Novacheck, MD
Professor of Orthopedic Surgery
University of Minnesota
Associate Medical Director of Integrated Care Services
Gillette Children's Specialty Healthcare
Saint Paul, Minnesota

Shital N. Parikh, MD
Professor of Orthopaedic surgery
University of Cincinnati School of Medicine
Co-director, Orthopaedic Sports Center
Cincinnati Children's Hospital Medical Center
Cincinnati, Ohio

Susan A. Rethlefsen, PT, DPT
Physical Therapist IV
Children's Orthopaedic Center
Children's Hospital Los Angeles
Los Angeles, California

Anthony I. Riccio, MD
Professor
Department of Orthopaedic Surgery
Texas Scottish Rite Hospital for Children
University of Texas Southwestern Medical Center
Dallas, Texas

Jonathan G. Schoenecker, MD, PhD
Jeffrey Mast Chair of Orthopaedic Trauma and Hip
    Surgery
Associate Professor
Department of Orthopaedic Surgery
Vanderbilt University Medical Center
Nashville, Tennessee

Benjamin Shore, MD, MPH, FRCSC
Associate Professor in Orthopaedic Surgery
Co-Director Cerebral Palsy and Spasticity Center
Program Director, Pediatric Orthopaedic Fellowship
Harvard Medical School
Boston Children's Hospital
Boston, Massachusetts

M. Wade Shrader, MD
Professor and Freeman Miller Endowed Chair of
    Cerebral Palsy
Department of Orthopedic Surgery and Pediatrics
Nemours A.I. duPont Hospital for Children
Sidney Kimmel Medical College, Thomas Jefferson
    University
Wilmington, Delaware

Eileen P. Storey, BA
Clinical Research Coordinator
Center for Injury Research and Prevention
The Children's Hospital of Philadelphia
Philadelphia, Pennsylvania

Vishwas R. Talwalkar, MD, FAAOS, FAAP
Professor, Orthopaedic Surgery and Pediatrics
Shriners Hospital for Children Medical Center
University of Kentucky
Lexington, Kentucky

Dr. Bryan Tompkins, MD
Staff Orthopedic Surgeon
Shriners Hospitals for Children
Spokane, Washington

Michael Wolf, MD
Assistant Professor of Orthopedic Surgery and
    Pediatrics
Drexel University College of Medicine
Section Chief of Orthopedic Surgery
St. Christopher's Hospital for Children
Philadelphia, Pennsylvania

Dan A. Zlotolow, MD, FAOA
Pediatric and Adult Upper Limb Surgeon
Shriners Hospitals for Children
Philadelphia Hand to Shoulder Center
Philadelphia, Pennsylvania
The Hospital for Special Surgery
New York, New York

Over the past century, there have been changes in the care of children afflicted with orthopedic conditions. Diagnosis of diseases such as tuberculosis and polio have come, and have largely gone away. In their wake are physical examination methods, treatments, and procedures that are now applied to other conditions with increased incidence such as cerebral palsy. Since the early 1960s, we have learned to appreciate the existence of nonaccidental trauma and how to look for it. Within the past three decades, we have witnessed changes in the frequency and incidence of athletic injury (acute and overuse) and traumatic conditions. Today's infectious agents, and how they physically affect children, are constantly changing as a result of immunizations and evolving pathogens.

There has also been an evolution in medical training. Today's primary providers of pediatric care are responsible for the broadening spectrum of children's health; as a result, there is less education on pediatric musculoskeletal medicine. This is unfortunate, as it has been estimated that 30% of a pediatrician's practice requires knowledge of musculoskeletal medicine. A rising unfamiliarity in pediatric musculoskeletal issues parallels an increase in unnecessary referrals to pediatric orthopedic specialists. This results in an increase in parental anxiety and burdens the healthcare system.

Orthopedic training has similarly changed; gone are the days where 20% of an orthopedic resident's training was spent with children. Our residents have less exposure to children, and deficiencies in their physical assessment of children have led us to depend upon expensive and sometimes unnecessary technology such as MRI, ultrasound, and CT scans for making a diagnosis.

What hasn't changed? Children still present with physical manifestations of hundreds of potential disorders noted by family and caregivers. Parents and providers are faced with determining what is a normal physical variant (bowlegs) and what is an orthopedic condition that requires referral (Blount disease) or is perhaps the initial presentation of a systemic disorder (rickets). In the pediatric orthopedic clinic, physical examination is still a critical part of the evaluation of a child with a musculoskeletal condition. A good examination can confirm normal development, identify disease, and guide cost-effective testing.

The purpose of this book is to demonstrate and guide the examination of a child's skeleton in order to make a diagnosis, and determine the next diagnostic steps and when to refer for evaluation. We now appreciate that children are not little adults, and thus, our approaches to their diagnosis are different, and the pearls and pitfalls for these evaluations are also different. We endeavor to present images, videos, and text that will help you examine a child. In writing this book, the authors share their experiences and what they learned about examining a child or adolescent from their professors and mentors. Those who taught us were clinicians who primarily used history, observation, and nuanced examination techniques to evaluate and treat children. Through this book, they continue to show us how.

Kenneth Noonan, MD, MHCDS
Mininder Kocher, MD, MPH

Chapter 1: Common Pediatric Orthopedic Nomenclature

Video 1.1. Ultrasound examination of the left hip in an infant. Ultrasound can be used as a diagnostic study and/or as an adjunct to physical examination.

Video 1.2. Digital Cobb angle measurement of the spine and visualization of the iliac wing apophysis to determine the Risser stage.

Video 1.3. Digital RVAD measurement of infantile scoliosis.

Chapter 2: Differences Between Pediatric and Adult Musculoskeletal Systems

Video 2.1. Bilateral radioulnar synostosis in a five-year-old boy. Video showing apparent motion due to generalized laxity of immaturity.

Video 2.2. Video showing testing for generalized ligamentous laxity.

Video 2.3. Video showing palpation over growth plate in suspected ligamentous injury.

Video 2.4. Immature gait, first steps in a one-year-old boy.

Chapter 3: Pearls and Pitfalls of the Pediatric Musculoskeletal Examination

Video 3.1. Infant brachial plexus examination.

Video 3.2. Examination on table toptabletop versus lap.

Video 3.3. Cerebral Palsy child walk versus run.

Chapter 4: Observational Gait Analysis and Correlation With Static Examination

Video 4.1. This is an 8-year-old female with cerebral palsy (CP) who functions at Gross Motor Function Classification System (GMFCS) level I. When running, she demonstrates decreased right arm swing and posturing. (Video with permission of the Children's Orthopaedic Center, Los Angeles.)

Video 4.2. Video of a Gower sign.

Video 4.3. Video of antalgic limp.

Video 4.4. This 12-year-old male has right hemiplegia and a dislocated hip. He walks with a Trendelenburg gait, with a trunk lean to the right in stance phase on the right. The right leg is also quite short functionally, and the right knee is very stiff in swing phase (since it does not need to bend to achieve adequate foot clearance). (Video with permission of the Children's Orthopaedic Center, Los Angeles.)

Video 4.5. This 22-year-old man has arthrogryposis and walks with many typical features of a short leg gait. On the long (left) leg, the knee is flexed, and he goes up on the toes on the short (right) leg. Pelvic obliquity is also evident. (Video with permission of the Children's Orthopaedic Center, Los Angeles.)

Video 4.6. An ambulatory male with Duchenne muscular dystrophy (DMD) demonstrates a typical DMD gait. Despite the evident pseudohypertrophy of the calves, the child is weak. The weak hip extensors result in anterior pelvic tilt and lumbar lordosis. The weak hip abductors necessitate lateral trunk lean in stance phase bilaterally. There is also a drop foot in swing on the left more than the right.

Video 4.7. An 11-year-old male with cerebral palsy (CP) (Gross Motor Function Classification System [GMFCS] II) walks with ataxia and also dystonic posturing of his extremities. His unsteadiness results in a significant increase in double-limb stance (usually 20% of the gait cycle) and a decrease in single-limb stance (usually 80%), compared to typical gait. (Video with permission of the Children's Orthopaedic Center, Los Angeles.)

Video 4.8. This 13-year-old male has cerebral palsy (CP) and functions at Gross Motor Function Classification System (GMFCS) level III. He previously underwent bilateral Achilles tendon lengthenings and now demonstrates calcaneal crouch gait, characterized by hip and knee flexion, and excessive ankle dorsiflexion. (Video with permission of the Children's Orthopaedic Center, Los Angeles.)

Video 4.9. This 6-year-old male with cerebral palsy (CP) (Gross Motor Function Classification System [GMFCS] III) demonstrates scissoring bilaterally. The scissoring results in marked narrowing of his base of support during gait. He also has a "jump" gait pattern (a type of crouch characterized by hip and knee flexion, along with ankle equinus). (Video with permission of the Children's Orthopaedic Center, Los Angeles.)

Video 4.10. This 17-year-old male with cerebral palsy (CP) (Gross Motor Function Classification System [GMFCS] II) is 10 years postoperative from bilateral hamstring and hip adductor lengthenings. There is left knee recurvatum (hyperextension) in stance phase, combined with a stiff left knee in swing phase. He demonstrates a plantar flexion–knee extension couple during gait, as the left ankle plantar flexion during stance moves the ground reaction force anteriorly, thus exacerbating the tendency to hyperextend the knee. (Video with permission of the Children's Orthopaedic Center, Los Angeles.)

Video 4.11. This 5-year-old female has a history of right peroneal nerve palsy, and resultant weakness and equinovarus foot deformity. Her drop foot in swing phase is evident, and she compensates with a steppage gait (rapid hip and knee flexion to compensate for the drop foot and facilitate foot clearance in swing phase). (Video with permission of the Children's Orthopaedic Center, Los Angeles.)

Video 4.12. This video shows the confusion test in an 8-year-old male (Gross Motor Function Classification System [GMFCS] I to II). When asked to selectively dorsiflex the ankle, the child is unable. When he flexes the hip, a mass action pattern is activated, and the tibialis anterior fires, dorsflexing the ankle. (Video with permission of the Children's Orthopaedic Center, Los Angeles.)

Chapter 5: Diagnostically Directed Examination for Neurological Disorders

Video 5.1. Stiff Knee Gait. When ambulating, this child walks with a stiff knee gait on the right side, secondary to rectus spasticity. She has diminished swing phase knee flexion and tends to abduct and externally rotate her foot in order to clear it in swing phase.

Video 5.2. Duncan Ely Test. This girl with spastic diplegia has a positive Duncan-Ely test. By flexing the knee rapidly, the hip will secondarily rise due to increasing contracture/spasticity in the rectus femoris tendon.

Video 5.3. Hemiplegic Gait. This boy with hemiplegia has an equinus gait and upper extremity posturing often seen when walking and running.

Video 5.4. Drop foot. This child with hemiplegia has a dropped foot on the left side. Accommodation to clear the foot during swing phase is noted with increasing hip and knee flexion in swing phase.

Video 5.5. Equinovarus foot. This boy with cerebral palsy has an equinovarus deformity of his right foot. During gait, he has a foot drop and must have his leg abducted in order to clear it in swing phase. The tight Achilles leads to equinus positioning and back knee gait in stance phase.

Video 5.6. Equinovarus foot. This hemiplegic boy has an equinovarus foot deformity marked by equinus positioning and fixed varus positioning in stance phase; likely due to spasticity/contracture of the posterior tibialis tendon.

Video 5.7. Confusion test. This young woman with hemiplegia has dynamic forefoot supination, secondary to spasticity of the anterior tibialis tendon. She is unable to dorsiflex her foot without flexing her hip and knee, demonstrating a positive confusion test.

Video 5.8. Upper Extremity. This boy with spastic hemiplegia has classic findings in the upper extremity including flexion, ulnar deviation, and decreased supination. He has difficulty with grip and is only able to actively extend his fingers with the wrist flexed.

Video 5.9. Fascioscapular humeral dystrophy. This boy with facioscapulohumeral dystrophy has difficulty with shoulder abduction. Winging of the scapula is noted.

Video 5.10. Child with Spinal Cord Tumor. This young boy has a spinal cord tumor documented in Figure 5.49. During play, he has difficulty walking and does not move his neck in order to see things. Torticollis can be one of the earliest physical examination features for spinal cord tumors of the cervical spine.

Video 5.11. Asymmetric Abdominal Reflexes. This child with a syrinx has asymmetric abdominal reflexes.

Chapter 6: Physical Examination for Unusual and Syndromic Conditions

Video 6.1. Valgus. This adolescent girl with MFS has genu valgum which is not symmetric and affects her ambulatory ability.

Video 6.2. Achon. This toddler with achondroplasia has genu varum with internal tibial torsion.

Video 15.3. Demonstration of the measurement of hip internal rotation and hip external rotation in a child with femoral anteversion.

Video 15.4. This child with external tibial torsion demonstrates out-toeing gait.

Video 15.5. Demonstration of limited hip internal rotation and increased hip external rotation consistent with external hip rotation contracture in an infant.

Video 15.6. Demonstration of foot position in a child with flatfoot and Achilles contracture. Although it is not the focus of this chapter, it is important to note that Achilles tightness should be assessed with the foot inverted to lock the midfoot which otherwise may mask the true tightness, then first with the knee extended to keep the gastrocnemius tight, and then with the knee flexed to relax the gastrocnemius. In this child the tight Achilles prevents full ankle dorsiflexion, requiring motion through the midfoot to allow the foot to fully dorsiflex. The axis of movement of the midfoot is different from the ankle, and out-toeing is created.

Video 15.7. An example of a patient with genu varum and a lateral thrust to their gait pattern. The tibia subluxes laterally on the femur during stance phase with each step. This is revealed as a momentary wobble (or thrust) at the knee during walking.

Video 15.8. A video demonstrating a patient walking with bilateral genu valgum. The valgus is worse on the left than the right. Note the medial femoral condyles bumping into each other during the gait cycle.

Video 15.9. Demonstration of the Ober test to check the flexibility of the iliotibial band.

Video 15.10. Patient walking with a leg length discrepancy. The right side is short causing the pelvis to tilt downwards on that side. Notice how the pelvis tilts back and forth with each stride.

Video 15.11. Demonstration of how to examine the leg lengths in the standing position. Blocks can be used to level the pelvis. If blocks are not available, books or magazines can be stacked under the short limb to determine the leg length discrepancy.

Video 15.12. Demonstration of how to examine the spine in a patient with a suspected leg length discrepancy. Sitting allows the spine to be examined without the influence of leg lengths on the spinal alignment.

Video 15.13. Demonstration of the supine examination of a patient with a suspected leg length discrepancy. Range of motion of the hips, knees, and ankles is tested. The Galeazzi test, knee heights, and foot sizes can be compared between the two limbs.

Video 15.14. Demonstration of the Galeazzi test to measure the femoral lengths. With the feet placed flat on the examination table and the knees flexed, the length of the tibia to the plantar aspect of the foot can also be compared between the two sides.

Video 15.15. Demonstration of the prone position examination to measure the femoral and tibia segments of each limb.

Video 15.16. Demonstration of the physical examination of the knee for a patient with a knee flexion contracture.

Video 15.17. Demonstration of the Lachman maneuver to test the stability of the anterior cruciate ligament (ACL). Notice the substantial anterior translation of the tibia on the femur in this patient with an incompetent ACL.

Video 15.18. Demonstration of the proper way to evaluate the flexibility of the gastrocnemius–soleus complex. Inverting the foot prevents inadvertent motion in the midfoot. Flexing the knee relaxes the gastrocnemius muscle because it crosses both the knee and ankle joints.

Chapter 16: Hip Disorders

Video 16.1. This video highlights general physical palpation for areas of tenderness.

Video 16.2. The Trendelenburg test will help identify hip abduction dysfunction as a result of gluteus medius weakness or altered hip mechanics.

Video 16.3. The Thomas test is helpful to identify hip flexion contractures that can be a result of muscle tightness (psoas or rectus femoris) hip joint contracture or bony dysplasia.

Video 16.4. Ober test: This test is helpful to diagnose iliotibial band tightness seen in patients with muscular dystrophy. More mild tightness can lead to hip and knee pain in normal athletes.

Video 16.5. Ortolani's test is also demonstrated here with the abduction and anteriorly directed force allowing the dislocated hip to reduce.

Video 16.6. The Galeazzi test for femoral shortening.

Video 16.7. This 20-month-old girl with a dislocated right hip walks with a short-limbed gait. Her foot is in equinus to accommodate the difference in length as a result of her dislocation. This is an example of a *functional* limb length discrepancy. Her femur is not anatomically short, but she has a joint problem (hip dislocation) that makes her *functionally* limb short.

Video 16.8. This video example demonstrates the ultrasound examination of the infant's hip.

Video 16.9. Drennan's sign is demonstrated in the left hip here with obligate external rotation as the hip is flexed. This is consistent with the diagnosis of slipped capital femoral epiphysis.

Video 16.10. Thirds test is a sensitive examination for identifying intra-articular pathology such as FAI or a labral tear.

Video 16.11. The sit-up test can be effective in identifying patients with a sports hernia.

Chapter 17: Chest and Shoulder Deformity

Video 17.1a and 17.1b. This adolescent male has limited shoulder abduction and scapular winging consistent with FSHD.

Video 17.2. This girl has cleidocranial dysplasia and absent clavicles.

Video 17.3. This boy has asymmetric scapular winging with limited shoulder abduction.

Video 17.4. From the back, this video demonstrates winging of the scapula with inability to abduct his shoulders.

Chapter 18: Pediatric Elbow and Forearm Conditions

Video 18.1. Clinical video of the palpation of the elbow examination assessing for any areas of tenderness, bony abnormalities, and/or fullness. (Courtesy of Joshua M. Abzug, MD.)

Video 18.2. Clinical video of a patient undergoing an upper extremity range of motion examination. (Courtesy of Joshua M. Abzug, MD.)

Video 18.3. Clinical video of the pivot-shift test utilized on a patient to determine the amount of ligamentous laxity and instability present about the elbow. Note that this test is best performed while the patient is under anesthesia. (Courtesy of Joshua M. Abzug, MD.)

Video 18.4. Clinical video of a patient undergoing a neurological exam following an iatrogenic ulnar nerve injury. (Courtesy of Joshua M. Abzug, MD.)

Video 18.5. Rotational osteotomy for forearm synostosis procedure. (Courtesy of Dan A. Zlotolow, MD.)

Video 18.6. This child has internal rotation contracture of the shoulder and whose hand and wrist appear pronated. Elbow release will not help unless humeral osteotomy is performed.

Chapter 19: Hand and Wrist Problems

Video 19.1. Watson test video legend: The Watson test for scapholunate ligament injury: pressure is placed with the thumb volarly on the distal pole of the scaphoid, and the wrist is passively radially deviated. A positive test is one that provokes dorsal wrist pain (even though no direct pressure is applied dorsally) or a palpable and painful clunk in the wrist when pressure is released.

Video 19.2. MCP ligament video: Assessing metacarpophalangeal (MCP) joint stability and integrity of the MCP collateral ligaments differs between the thumb and fingers. In the thumb, the MCP joint is stabilized by the volar plate when fully extended, so the MCP joint should be flexed 30° to assess the collateral ligaments. In the fingers, the collateral ligaments are slack in MCP extension and taut in MCP flexion, so the MCP joint should be flexed 90° before applying radial or ulnar deviation stress to assess the collateral ligaments.

Video 19.3. Dynamic volar prominence of the distal ulna due to distal radioulnar joint instability in the setting of a radius malunion (supination dissociation injury).

Video 19.4. Rotation through the radiocarpal joint in a child with complete radioulnar synostosis and no forearm rotation between the radius and ulna.

CONTENTS

Common Pediatric Orthopedic Nomenclature

Aristides I. Cruz Jr and Joseph G. Khoury

Nomenclature

Proper examination of the musculoskeletal system requires a fundamental knowledge of standard anatomic nomenclature. This understanding forms the basis of the physical examination and helps with developing a differential diagnosis. It also facilitates communication with other musculoskeletal caregivers when discussing pediatric orthopedic conditions.

Anatomic Descriptors

Terms such as *proximal/distal* and *medial/lateral* are relative terminologies with the core or midline of the body forming the basis of descriptive anatomic nomenclature (**Figure 1.1**). These descriptive terms are important when describing the extremities/appendages. *Proximal* structures are closer to the core of the body while *distal* structures are further away. *Medial* structures are closer to the midline and *lateral*

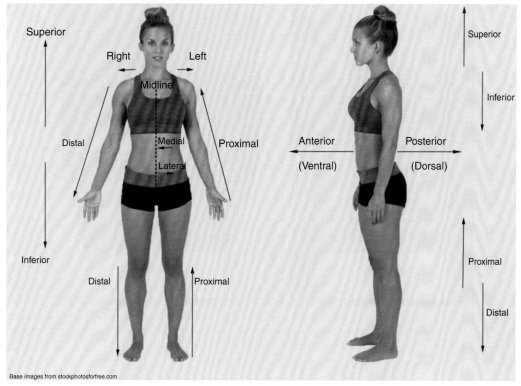

Base images from stockphotosforfree.com

FIGURE 1.1 Common terms used to describe anatomic relationships.

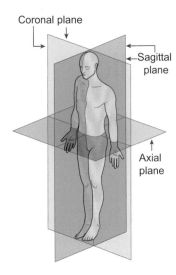

FIGURE 1.2 The representation of the human body demonstrates the three common planes often used to describe three-dimensional imaging.

structures are located away from the midline. Often times, the body can be additionally described in three-dimensional (3D) planes and this nomenclature is very common in radiological descriptions (**Figure 1.2**).

Joint or limb angulation can also be described in standard anatomic terms. Varus and valgus are terms that can be used to describe coronal plane limb alignment at the hindfoot and ankle, knee (**Figure 1.3**) and elbow. Typically, these terms are used to describe joint position in the coronal/frontal plane, *varus* is when the distal limb segment is pointed toward the midline and *valgus* is when it is pointed away from the midline. Normally, the hindfoot and ankle, knee and elbow are in some degree of valgus. Radiographically, these terms can also be used to describe deviations from normal alignment. For instance, the normal neck shaft angle of the proximal femur is about 135°. A hip can be said to be in relative valgus with a neck shaft angle greater than 145° and in relative varus with a neck shaft angle less than 130°.

Because the spine is itself a midline structure, it is divided into its anatomic segments when describing location—*cervical, thoracic, lumbar,* and *sacral. Scoliosis* is an abnormal curvature in the coronal/

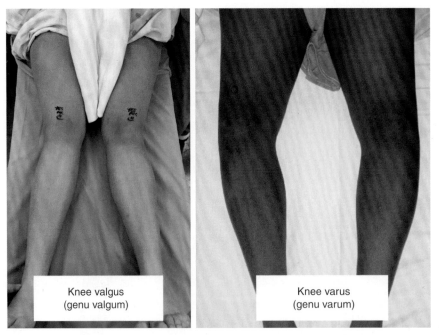

Knee valgus
(genu valgum)

Knee varus
(genu varum)

FIGURE 1.3 Examples of pathologic valgus and varus at the knee. Remember that the mature knee is normally in slight valgus (5°-9°). Relatively speaking, a knee with more than this (>9° of valgus) can be considered to have abnormal valgus, while a knee with less than 5° of valgus is considered in relative varus.

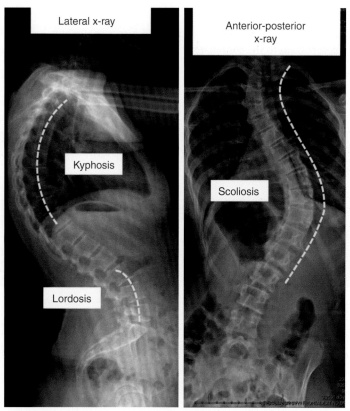

FIGURE 1.4 The normal spine has some degree of thoracic kyphosis and lumbar lordosis. The spine is normally straight in the coronal plane and any curvature greater than 10° is considered scoliosis.

frontal plane of greater than 10°. In the sagittal plane, the thoracic spine normally has a roundness of 20° to 40°, which is called *kyphosis*. In the lumbar spine, there is normally concavity of 30° to 50° and this is termed *lordosis*. In cases where the normal values are exceeded, the spine may be considered to be relatively kyphotic or lordotic (**Figure 1.4**).

The hands and feet also carry specific nomenclature conventions: *volar* and *plantar* refer to the palm of the hand and sole of the foot, respectively; the *dorsum* of the hand or foot refers to the opposite side of each.

Planes of Motion

It is useful to understand the planes of motion specific to each joint and illustrate common planes of motion for frequently examined appendages. Because different joints such as the shoulder can have multiple planes of motion, it is important to understand standard descriptors of joint motion relative to anatomic planes. *Flexion/extension* describes motion in the sagittal plane, *abduction/adduction* describes motion in the coronal plane, and *internal rotation/external rotation* describes motion in the transverse plane. For the forearm, rotation is termed *supination/pronation* and describes forearm rotation in the transverse plane. The same term can be used to describe forefoot position. One can quantitate the degree of joint movement with a measuring device such as a goniometer. Zero degrees is considered that point that the standing body is in in with hands at the sides. For example, a knee is fully extended at 0° and usually flexes to 140°; one would report knee motion of 0° to 140°. If the knee hyperextends 10° the motion is described as –10° to 140°.

Shoulder

Due to the extreme mobility of the shoulder, it can be difficult to quantify motion in the individual planes. In general, comparison to the contralateral side can illicit differences in abnormal motion.

1. *Flexion/extension* (**Figure 1.5**).

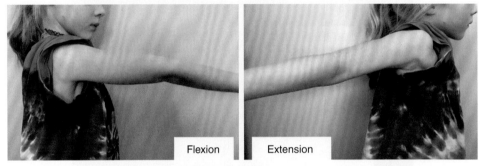

Flexion   Extension

FIGURE 1.5 Shoulder flexion (left panel) and extension (right panel).

2. *Abduction/adduction* (**Figure 1.6**).

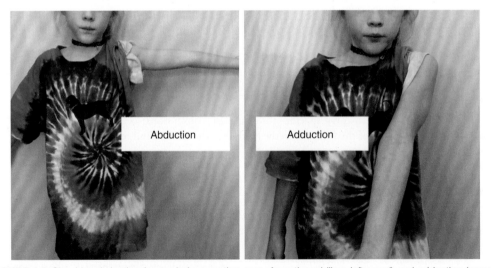

Abduction   Adduction

FIGURE 1.6 Shoulder abduction (coronal plane motion away from the midline; left panel) and adduction (coronal plane motion toward the midline; right panel).

3. ***Internal/external rotation*** (**Figure 1.7**).

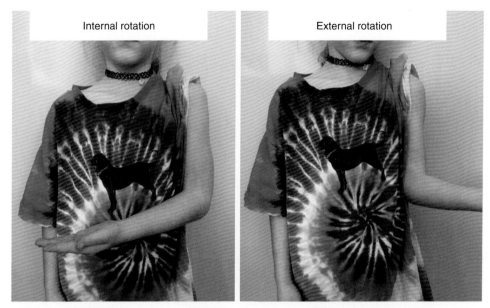

FIGURE 1.7 Shoulder internal rotation (left panel) and external rotation (right panel).

Elbow

1. ***Flexion/extension*** (**Figure 1.8**). Normal motion is from full extension (0°) with flexion to around 160°.

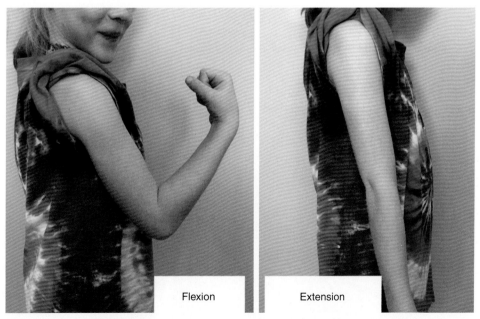

FIGURE 1.8 Elbow flexion (left panel) and extension (right panel).

Forearm

1. *Supination/pronation* (**Figure 1.9**). Normal motion: ≥80° of pronation and supination from the neutral position.

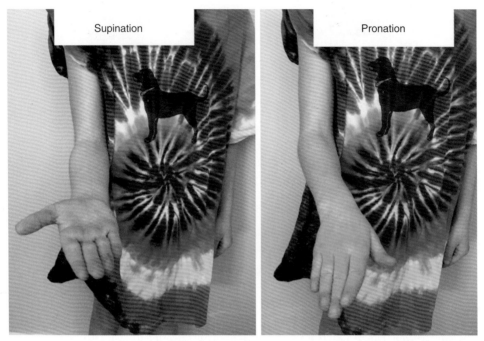

FIGURE 1.9 Forearm supination ("palm up," left panel) and pronation ("palm down," right panel).

Wrist

1. *Flexion/extension* (**Figure 1.10**). Normal motion: 75° of flexion and extension from the neutral position.

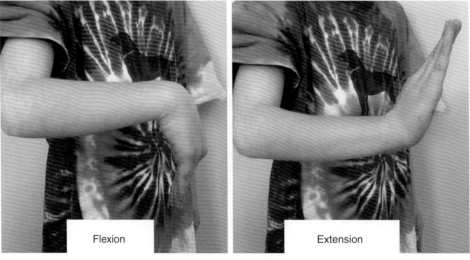

FIGURE 1.10 Wrist flexion (left panel) and extension (right panel).

2. **Ulnar deviation/radial deviation** (**Figure 1.11**). Normal motion: 20° to 30° in each direction from the neutral position.

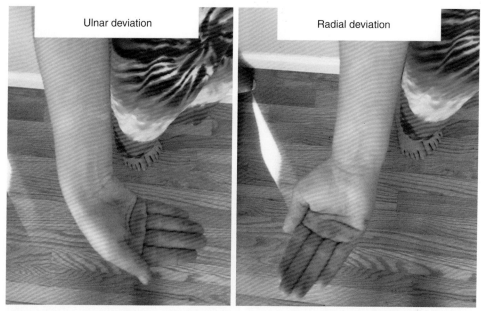

FIGURE 1.11 Ulnar deviation (coronal plane motion toward ulna; left panel) and radial deviation (coronal plane motion toward radius; right panel).

Finger

1. *Flexion/extension* (**Figure 1.12**). Normal finger motion at the distal interphalangeal (DIP) joint and the proximal interphalangeal (PIP) joint is from full extension (0°) with flexion to around 80°. Metacarpal phalangeal (MP) joint motion is from full extension (0°) with flexion to around 70°.

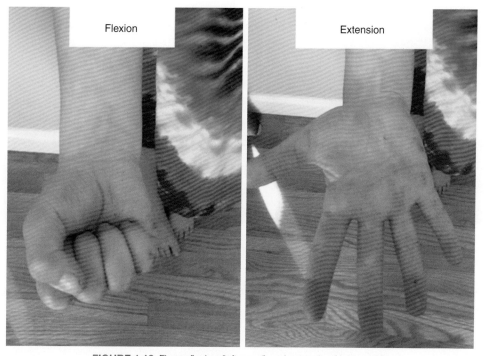

FIGURE 1.12 Finger flexion (left panel) and extension (right panel).

2. *Adduction/abduction* (**Figure 1.13**).

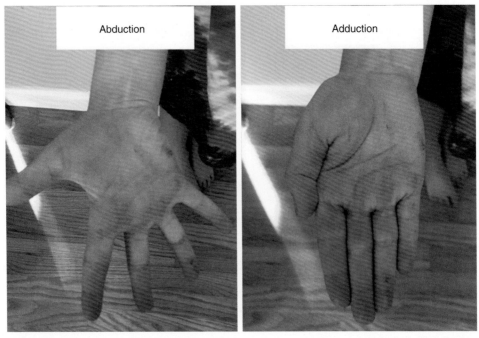

FIGURE 1.13 Finger abduction (coronal plane motion away from the midline; left panel) and adduction (coronal plane motion toward the midline; right panel).

Hip

1. *Flexion/extension* (**Figure 1.14**). Normal motion: 15° of extension to 120° of flexion.

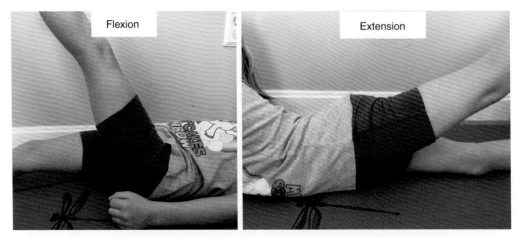

FIGURE 1.14 Hip flexion (left panel) and extension (right panel).

2. *Abduction/adduction* (**Figure 1.15**). Normal motion: 30° of adduction to 50° of abduction from the neutral position.

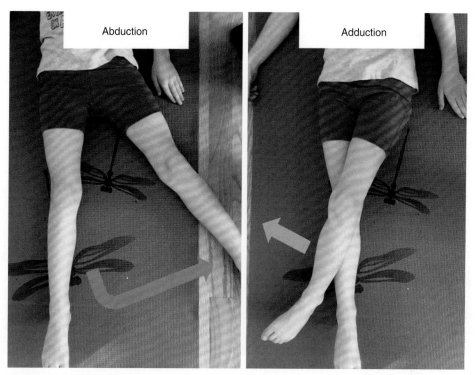

FIGURE 1.15 Hip abduction (coronal plane motion away from the midline; left panel) and adduction (coronal plane motion toward the midline; right panel).

3. *Internal/external rotation* (**Figure 1.16**). Hip internal and external rotation can be measured in the prone or supine (as shown here) position. The supine position is less frightening for toddlers who will have less anxiety if they can see the examiner. Prone measures of hip internal and external rotation are more accurate as the hip is extended and the hip capsule is usually at its normal tension. Due to anatomic differences in the proximal femoral hip geometry; there is a wide range of normal hip

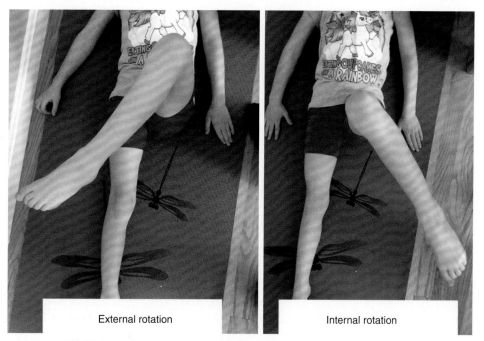

FIGURE 1.16 Hip internal rotation (right panel) and external rotation (left panel).

internal and external hip motion. Most normal children and adolescents have about 90° of total rotation. Thus if a child internally rotates 60°, one can expect about 30° of external rotation. Pathology is suspected if the measures are not symmetric from side to side.

Knee

1. *Flexion/extension* (**Figure 1.17**). Normal motion: full extension (0°) to 140° of flexion.

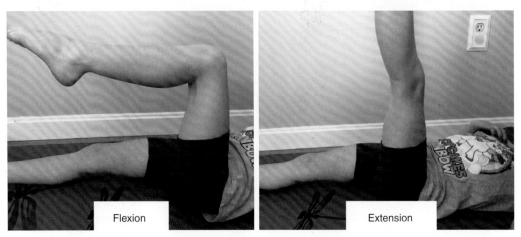

FIGURE 1.17 Knee flexion (left panel) and extension (right panel).

Ankle

1. *Dorsiflexion/plantarflexion* (**Figure 1.18**). Normal motion: 20° to 30° of dorsiflexion from neutral to 60° of plantar flexion from neutral.

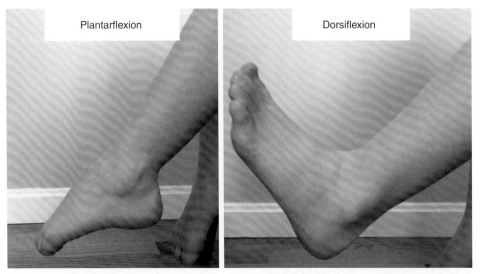

FIGURE 1.18 Ankle dorsiflexion (aka ankle extension; right panel) and plantar flexion (aka ankle flexion; left panel).

Foot

The foot is a complicated structure and several terms can be used to describe the position of the entire foot or, in some cases, the relationship of the forefoot to the midfoot or the forefoot to the hindfoot. For instance, the

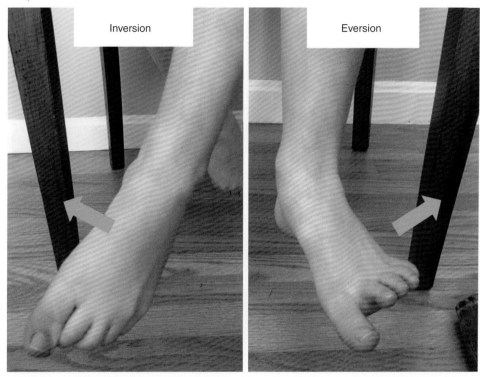

FIGURE 1.19 Foot inversion (sole of foot rotated toward the midline; left panel) and eversion (sole of foot rotated away from the midline; right panel).

foot is considered **inverted (inversion)** when the entire foot is rotated with the sole turned in toward the midline and **everted (eversion)** when the foot is rotated with the sole out away from the midline (**Figure 1.19**). The **adducted** foot is deviated medially and the **abducted** foot is deviated laterally (**Figure 1.20**). In metatarsus adductus, the term adductus refers to forefoot adduction relative to the midfoot. When the forefoot is

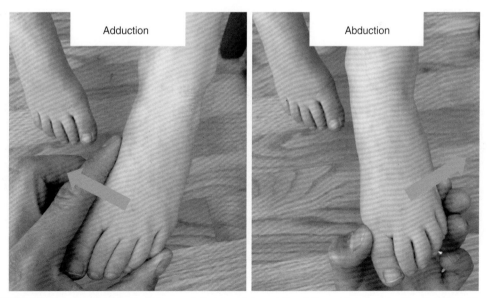

FIGURE 1.20 Foot adduction (deviation medially toward the midline; left panel) and abduction (deviation laterally away from the midline; right panel).

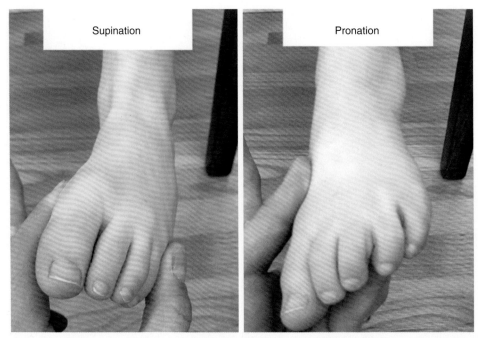

FIGURE 1.21 Forefoot supination (sole of foot rotated toward the midline; left panel) and pronation (sole of foot rotated way from the midline; right panel).

rotated up relative to the hindfoot, it is considered **supinated** and when the forefoot is rotated down relative to the hindfoot, it is considered **pronated** (**Figure 1.21**). The normal foot has a slight arch (**pes cavus**). Excessive cavus usually implies some pathology. While some pathologic conditions can present with flat feet, many normal and asymptomatic children can be completely flat (**pes planus**) (**Figure 1.22**). Finally, the hindfoot and ankle is normally in slight **valgus**; **varus** positioning is abnormal and implies some pathology (**Figure 1.23**).

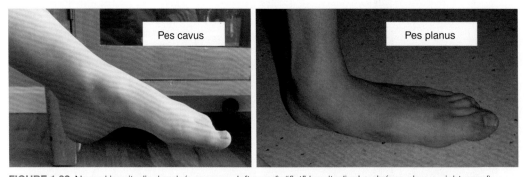

FIGURE 1.22 Normal longitudinal arch (pes cavus; left panel); "flat" longitudinal arch (pes planus; right panel).

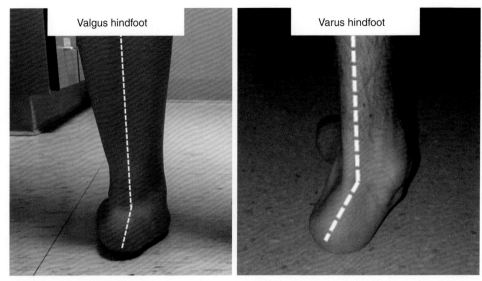

FIGURE 1.23 Posterior view of left ankle showing hindfoot valgus (left panel); posterior view of right ankle showing hindfoot varus (right panel).

Imaging Nomenclature

Growing Bone

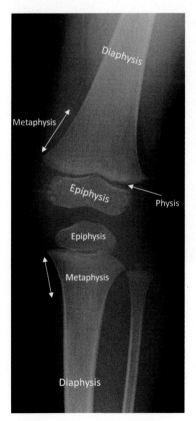

Physis, Epiphysis, Metaphysis, Diaphysis, and Apophysis

The anatomic nomenclature of the immature skeleton is centered around the *physis* or "growth plate" (**Figure 1.24**). Practitioners often interchange words to describe the growing cartilaginous disk; these include, the "growth plate," the "physis" and the "epiphyseal plate". There is no clear point on a long bone where metaphyseal bone transitions to diaphyseal bone; most practitioners speak of this area as the meta-diaphyseal junction. Growth plate or physeal fractures can be described according to the *Salter-Harris classification*. The classification is based on the location of the fracture's "exit" as it traverses the physis (**Figure 1.25**).

Commonly Symptomatic Apophyses

Besides the physis, bone growth also occurs at various *apophyses* (singular: apophysis). The *apophysis* is the site of a tendinous attachment, and in patients who are skeletally immature, pain can occur at these sites, usually as the result of overuse and excessive tension (red arrow) of the offending tendon which attaches at the apophysis. Common sites and diagnoses of "apophysitis" include:

- Tibial tubercle (*Osgood-Schlatter disease*) (**Figure 1.26**)
- Calcaneus (*Sever disease*) (**Figure 1.27**)
- Base fifth metatarsal (*Iselin disease*) (**Figure 1.28**)

FIGURE 1.24 Anterior-posterior left knee radiograph. Schematic of different named portions of the distal femur and proximal tibia.

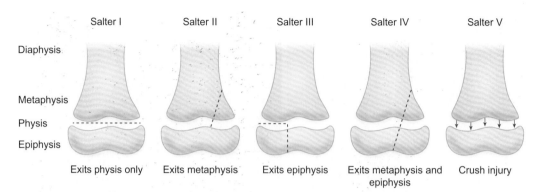

FIGURE 1.25 Schematic representation of end of long bone. Red dashed line represents the primary fracture line that involves the physis. By definition, this fracture line enters the physis and the Salter-Harris classification is based on where this primary fracture line exits.

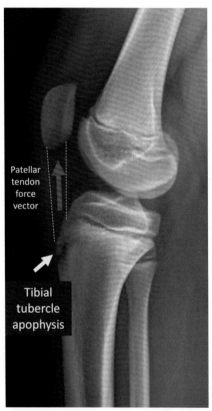

FIGURE 1.26 Lateral radiograph of a skeletally immature knee. Schematic representation of the pathophysiology underlying the Osgood-Schlatter disease.

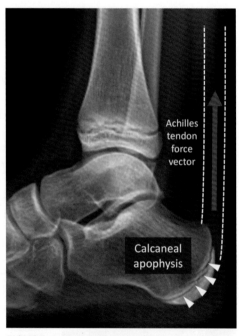

FIGURE 1.27 Lateral radiograph of a skeletally immature hindfoot. Schematic representation of the pathophysiology underlying the Sever disease.

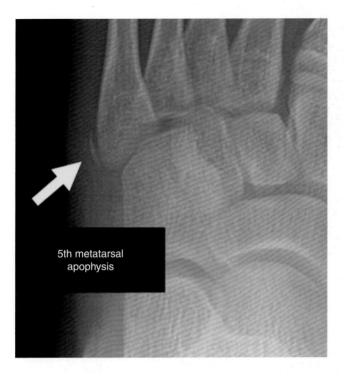

FIGURE 1.28 Radiograph of base of fifth metatarsal. If the patient had pain at this apophysis he or she would be classified as having Iselin disease.

Categories of Imaging

1. Plain radiography, are also referred to as "plain films". This includes two-dimensional images obtained by shooting x-rays through a body part. Tissues with higher density (such as bone) absorb more of the radiation and show up white on the image.
   a. "Weight-bearing" x-rays. Some body parts look very different if they are imaged when bearing weight. For example, someone with a flat foot may appear to have an arched foot on x-ray, unless it is taken when standing. Whenever possible, x-rays of the legs and spine should be ordered in the standing position.
   b. "Orthogonal view" (**Figure 1.29**). This refers to obtaining two images at right angles to one another. In most situations, the two views obtained are anteroposterior (AP) which means front to back and

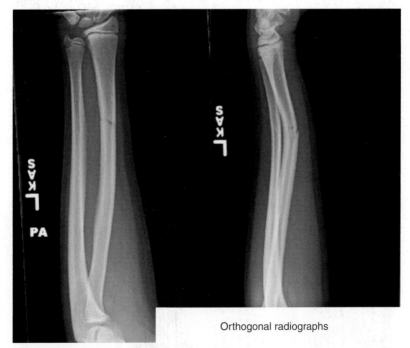

Orthogonal radiographs

FIGURE 1.29 Orthogonal anteroposterior (AP) and lateral radiographs of the forearm. This example illustrates the importance of obtaining orthogonal radiographs since the fracture angulation is appreciated on one view only.

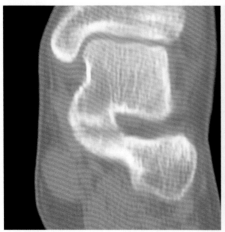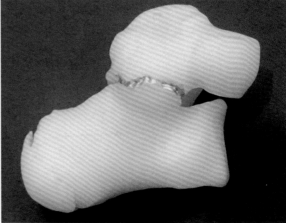

FIGURE 1.30 CT image (left panel) and 3D printed model (right panel) of a subtalar tarsal coalition.

lateral which is taken from the side. In general, a good rule of thumb is to get orthogonal radiographs of the bone under question as well as the joint above and below the pathology. Oblique images may be ordered which are taken at a 45° angle to the other views.

2. Cross-sectional imaging.
   a. Cross-sectional imaging is generally displayed in three dimensions; the axial or transverse plane (straight across the body), the sagittal plane dividing right to left, and the coronal plane dividing front to back. Planes are coronal, sagittal, and axial (**Figure 1.2**).
   b. *Computed tomography (CT)* is a cross-sectional study using radiation where the bones are whiter and show up best compared to soft tissues. Because CT uses ionizing radiation to obtain images, efforts are made to minimize its use in children. The images can be displayed in any plane of the body, but generally are displayed in the three planes described above. Today, CT data can be used to produce a virtual 3D model and can also be used to produce an actual model via 3D printers (**Figure 1.30**).
   c. *Magnetic resonance imaging (MRI)* (**Figure 1.31**). MRI images show soft structures (tendon, muscle, ligament, and fluid) much better than CT and are also generally displayed in the three planes described above.
3. *Ultrasound* can characterize anatomy by emitting sound waves and recording the "echo" the waves make when they bounce off structures of different density. This technology is gaining popularity as no radiation is needed (▶ **Video 1.1**).
4. *EOS* is an x-ray technology that greatly improves the quality and simplicity of obtaining long x-rays, such as scoliosis x-rays of the entire spine or long leg x-rays. The technology reduces parallax and radiation dose significantly by utilizing a moving slit emitter of radiation from both planes and detectors on opposite sides (**Figure 1.32**).

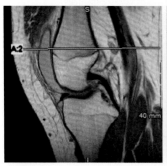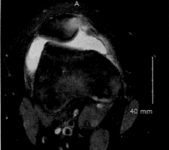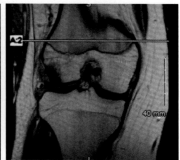

FIGURE 1.31 MRI images of the knee in the sagittal (left panel), transverse/axial (middle panel), and coronal (right panel) planes.

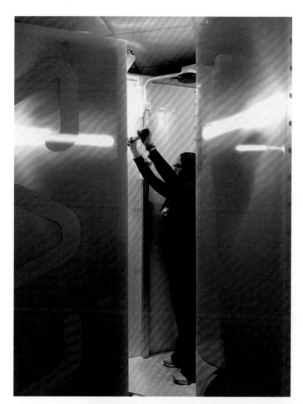

FIGURE 1.32 Patient in EOS machine which can be used to obtain long films of the spine or lower extremities. EOS uses a slit emitter of radiation which has been shown to reduce the amount of radiation exposure compared to conventional radiographs.

Common Radiographic Angles and Measurements

Spine

1. *Cobb angle* is the workhorse method for measuring the severity of a curve in either the frontal (to determine scoliosis) or lateral planes (to quantify kyphosis or lordosis). Prior to digital imaging, a ruler was needed to quantify the curve (**Figure 1.33**). It is measured by determining the angle between the vertebral end plate at the top of the most tilted vertebra and bottom of the most titled vertebra for each curve (▶ **Video 1.2**).

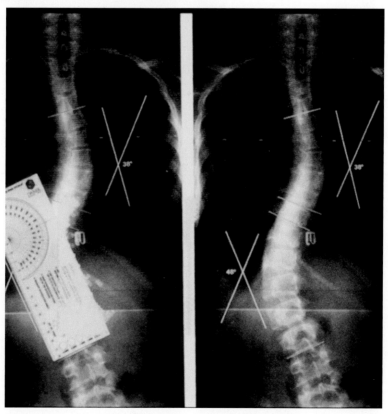

FIGURE 1.33 Cobb angle measurements of a scoliotic spine. Historically, manual measurement was performed on x-ray films utilizing a ruler/goniometer (left panel). Today's digital radiography has software tools that are easier to use.

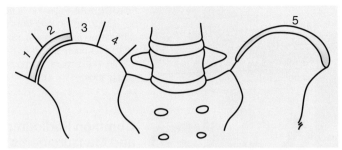

FIGURE 1.34 Schematic representation of Risser sign. The iliac crest is divided into four equal parts from lateral to medial. Stages I-IV represent ossification of the lateral-medial most quadrants, respectively. Stage V represents closure of the iliac wing apophysis and occurs at complete skeletal maturity.

2. *Risser sign* is one radiographic method of determining skeletal maturity and reflects the degree of ossification and fusion of the iliac wing apophysis (**Figure 1.34**; ▶ **Video 1.2**).
3. Bone age is another radiographic method of determining skeletal maturity and is determined by comparing the degree of maturation of the fingers and wrist with an atlas of standards for each age.
4. *RVAD* (**Figure 1.35**) (rib vertebral angle difference) is a method of measuring the difference of the angle of the ribs on either side of the apex vertebra of a curve in patients with infantile scoliosis. It is a predictor of progression, with RVAD >20° indicating a high (80%) likelihood of progression (▶ **Video 1.3**).

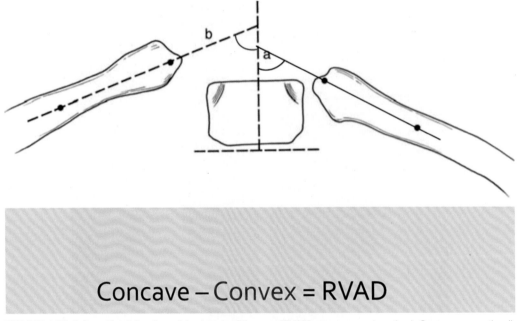

FIGURE 1.35 Schematic of the rib vertebral angle difference (RVAD) measurement method. One measures the rib vertebral angle (RVA) of the rib to the apical vertebral body on the concave side of the curve (a) and RVA on the convex side of the curve (b); the difference in the two RVAs is the RVAD.

Pelvis

Different radiographs can be taken of the pelvis. Examples include AP pelvis, frog lateral, abduction internal rotation (AIR), and cross-table lateral. The AP pelvis is taken either standing or lying down (supine) with knees pointing forward. The frog view is a common way to get a "lateral" view of both hips and is taken lying down with both hips flexed, externally rotated, and abducted. The AIR (aka Von Rosen) view is taken in abduction and internal rotation. It is designed to show how deeply a hip can reduce in the acetabulum. The cross-table lateral shows one hip at a time in a true lateral projection by flexing the other hip and shooting the image through the groin.

1. *Hilgenreiner line, Perkin line, sourcil, Shenton line, acetabular index, tear drop, and medial clear space.* These are common measurements made on an AP pelvis radiograph that are used to evaluate hip dysplasia. The Hilgenreiner line (**Figure 1.36**) is a horizontal line drawn through both triradiate cartilages, and the Perkin line is drawn perpendicular to that from the lateral edge of each acetabulum. These lines are used to identify hip displacement in children less than 4 to 6 months of age whose femoral heads have not yet developed radiographic ossification centers. When the medial aspect of the femoral neck (yellow arrow) is not in the low medial quadrant, (yellow arrow), the hip is displaced. The Shenton line (can be reliably used in children greater than 3 years of age) (**Figure 1.37**) is one line outlining the inferior surface of the superior pubic ramus and the inferior femoral neck; these two lines should appear to be part of the same arc in located hips. The acetabular index (**Figure 1.38**) is an angle between the Hilgenreiner line and the acetabulum and quantifies socket shape. The tear drop (**Figure 1.39**) is a shape on the medial side of the acetabulum indicating good formation of the acetabulum, and the "sourcil" (French for "eyebrow") refers to the roof of the acetabulum, which should take a slight downturn at its lateral edge like a human eyebrow. Triradiate cartilage (**Figure 1.40**) is noted only in an immature pelvis radiograph and is seen as a horizontal line in the acetabulum on the AP or frog lateral pelvis x-ray. It closes at the time of fastest growth in adolescence.

2. *Ultrasound measures* (**Figure 1.41**) depicts a coronal plane image of the hip with structures labeled. The upper (beta) angle represents the labral coverage, the alpha angle represents bony coverage, and the circle depicts the femoral head with the amount of head below the line representing femoral head coverage.

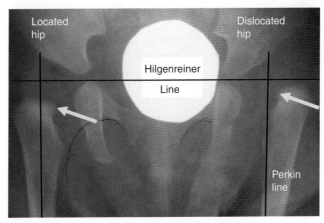

FIGURE 1.36 Anteroposterior (AP) pelvis radiograph showing the Hilgenreiner line (red line). The line is drawn as a horizontal line through the triradiate cartilages of both sides of the pelvis. The Perkin line (blue line) is drawn perpendicular to the Hilgenreiner line at the lateral edge of the acetabulum.

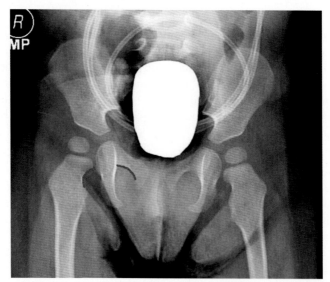

FIGURE 1.37 Anteroposterior (AP) pelvis radiograph showing the Shenton line which is drawn as a curve outlining the inferior surface of the superior pubic ramus and the inferior aspect of the femoral neck. This line should be a continuous line. A "break" in the Shenton line may represent hip subluxation/dislocation.

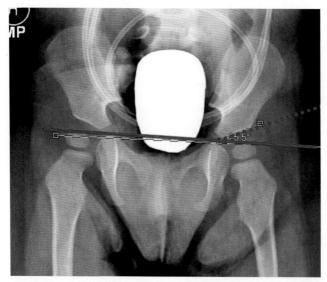

FIGURE 1.38 Anteroposterior (AP) pelvis radiograph showing measurement of the acetabular index, which helps quantify the acetabular shape.

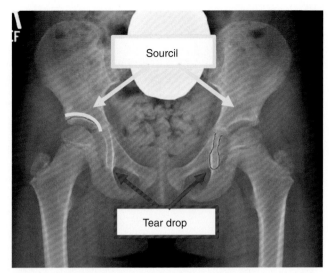

FIGURE 1.39 Anteroposterior (AP) pelvis radiograph schematic showing the outline of the acetabular "tear drop" (medial wall of the acetabulum; red line) and the acetabular "roof" or sourcil (yellow line).

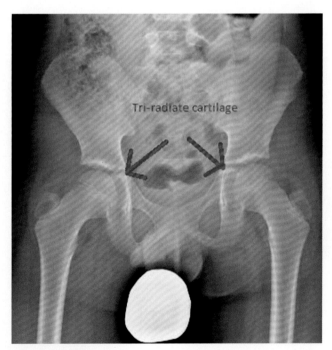

FIGURE 1.40 Anteroposterior (AP) pelvis radiograph of patient with "open" triradiate cartilage. The triradiate cartilage is the growth center where the three pelvic bones meet (ilium, ischium, and pubis) and eventually fuse at skeletal maturity.

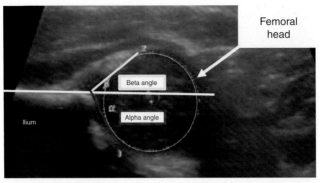

FIGURE 1.41 Hip ultrasound image (longitudinal axis).

Upper Extremity

1. *Radiocapitellar line, Baumann angle, anterior humeral line.* The radiocapitellar line (**Figure 1.42**) is a line drawn along the neck of the proximal radius and should transect the capitellum on ANY view of the elbow. Disruption indicates a radial head dislocation. The anterior humeral line (**Figure 1.42**) is drawn along the anterior cortex of the distal humerus on the lateral view and should at least touch the capitellum if not bisecting it. Disruption indicates a distal humerus fracture. The Baumann angle (**Figure 1.43**) is an angle between the long axis of the humerus and the capitellar physis. Normal should be 70° to 75°.

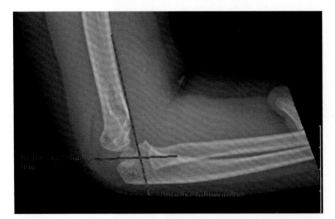

FIGURE 1.42 Lateral radiograph of an elbow depicting the radiocapitellar line and anterior humeral line which helps to assess the integrity of the radiocapitellar joint and amount of displacement of a distal humerus (most commonly supracondylar humerus) fracture, respectively.

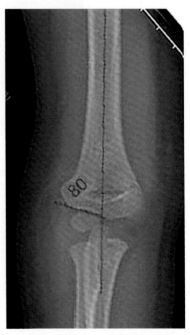

FIGURE 1.43 Anterior-posterior radiograph of the elbow depicting the Baumann angle. The normal value is 70°-75°.

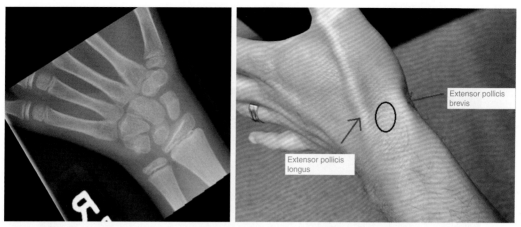

FIGURE 1.44 Scaphoid view of a right wrist (left panel) and clinical photo showing the anatomic snuffbox (right panel, black circle). The scaphoid view can be obtained when there is suspicion of a scaphoid fracture (eg, tenderness to palpation in the anatomic snuffbox).

2. *Scaphoid view* (**Figure 1.44**) is a PA (posteroanterior) view of the wrist taken in ulnar deviation to show the scaphoid bone without other bony overlap and also extends the bone to show it longer and better in plane. It is taken when there is suspicion of a scaphoid fracture as in, when there is tenderness in the anatomic snuff box.

Lower Extremity

1. *Orthoroentgenogram, scanogram.* These two similar techniques are used to judge leg length inequality. The scanogram images the hip, knee, and ankle with three separate exposures while the patient remains still, and a ruler is laid under the patient (**Figure 1.45**). Teleroentgenogram is a long x-ray of the entire lower limb with a ruler taken from at least 10 ft away (**Figure 1.46**).
2. *Mechanical axis, anatomic axis, LDFA, MPTA, MAD.* The mechanical axis of the lower extremity (**Figure 1.47**) is a line from the center of the hip to the center of the ankle, it usually passes in the center of the knee. The anatomic axis follows the shaft of the bone. Note, for the tibia, they are almost the same. The mechanical axis deviation (MAD) (**Figure 1.48**) is the distance between the middle of the knee joint and the mechanical axis of the limb (normal is 0). The mechanical lateral distal femoral angle (mLDFA) (**Figure 1.49**) is the angle between the mechanical axis of the femur and the end of the femoral condyles (normal 87°). The medial proximal tibial angle (MPTA) is the angle between the mechanical axis of the tibia and a line across the tibial plateau (normal 87°).
3. *Specialized knee radiographs: Sunrise/Merchant View, tunnel/notch view.* The Sunrise and Merchant views (**Figure 1.50**) are similar views taken over the top of a flexed knee designed to show the relationship between the patella (knee cap) and trochlea (groove in front of the femur). The tunnel and notch views (**Figure 1.51**) are essentially synonymous and are taken as a front (AP or PA) view of the knee with the knee flexed. This is designed to show pathology of the posterior articular surface of the femur, which may not be visible on an x-ray taken with the knee in extension.

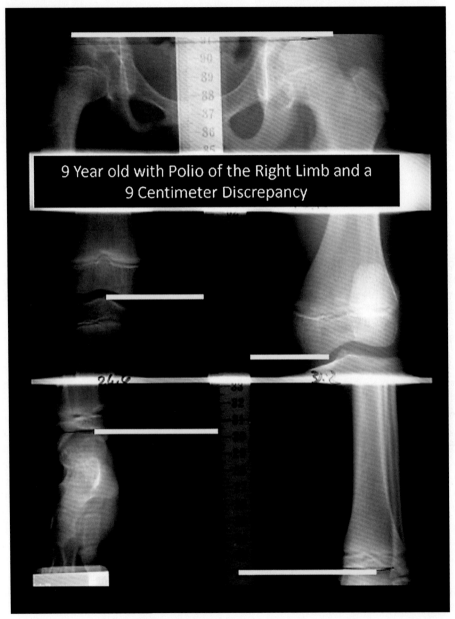

FIGURE 1.45 Scanogram of the lower extremities is taken with both hips, knees, and ankles on each x-ray image with an underlying ruler to measure potential leg length inequalities.

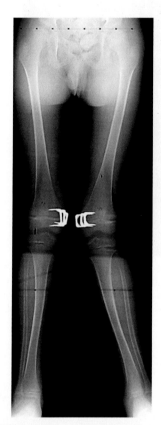

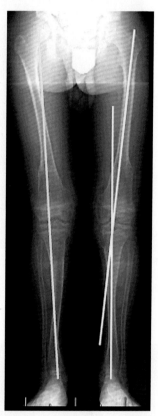

FIGURE 1.46 Teleroentgenogram is a radiograph of the entire lower limb taken on a large cassette which can be used to measure mechanical alignment and assess leg length inequalities.

FIGURE 1.47 Teleroentgenogram showing the mechanical axis (yellow line) and anatomic axis (normal is 5°-9°) of the femur and tibia (white lines). The anatomic angle is a line drawn along the shaft each of the bones. The mechanical axis is a line drawn from the center of the femoral head to the center of the talus, it normally passes in the center of the knee.

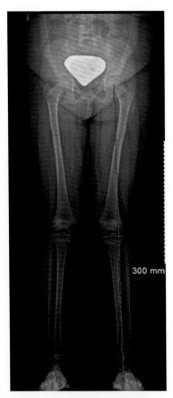

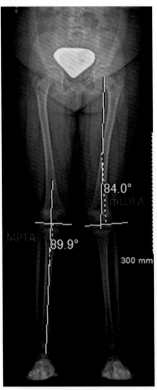

FIGURE 1.48 Teleroentgenogram showing the mechanical axis deviation of the left knee, which is the distance from the anatomic center of the knee joint to the mechanical axis at the knee joint.

FIGURE 1.49 Teleroentgenogram showing the mechanical lateral distal femoral angle (mLFDA) and the medial proximal tibial angle (MPTA). These measurements are used to assess the anatomic sources of genu varum or valgum to help guide treatment.

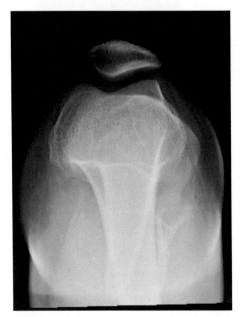

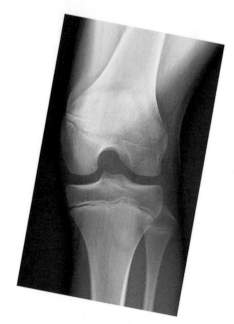

FIGURE 1.50 Sunrise or Merchant view of the knee is an axial/tangential view of the patellofemoral joint and is used to assess the relationship between the patella and the trochlear of the femur.

FIGURE 1.51 Tunnel/notch view of the knee is taken with the knee flexed about 45°. This view shows the intercondylar notch of the femur and also helps visualize the posterior aspect of the femoral condyles.

Foot and Ankle

1. *Meary angle and calcaneal pitch.* These are measured on the lateral, standing view of the foot; Meary angle (**Figure 1.52**) is drawn between the long axis of the talus and the first metatarsal. Normal is 0° (±10) with lower numbers indicating a depressed arch (planus) and higher numbers indicating a high arch (cavus). The calcaneal pitch (**Figure 1.53**) is also measured on the same view and represents an angle between the underside of the calcaneus (heel bone) and the floor. Normal ranges from 20° to 40°. Lower numbers suggest a tight Achilles tendon (equinus), and higher numbers suggest a weak Achilles tendon.
2. *Hallux valgus angle, IMA, and DMAA.* These measurements are all used in the assessment of a bunion (hallux valgus) (**Figure 1.54**). The hallux valgus angle is the angle of the actual bunion itself. The intermetatarsal angle (IMA) is the angle between the first and second metatarsal. The distal metatarsal articular angle (DMAA) is the angle between the articular surface at the end of the first metatarsal and the long axis of the bone.
3. *Harris view* (**Figure 1.55**) is an axial view of the calcaneus and can be used to quantify the hindfoot positioning (varus or valgus) as well as the integrity of the subtalar joint.

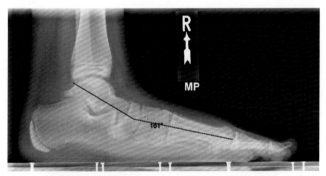

FIGURE 1.52 Lateral, weight-bearing radiograph of the foot depicting the Meary angle (measured between the long axis of the talus and first metatarsal). The Meary angle (normal 0°±10°) can be used to assess pes planus or pes cavus.

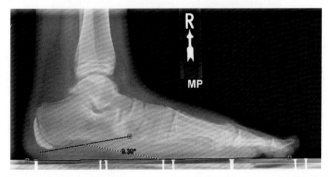

FIGURE 1.53 Lateral, weight-bearing radiograph of the foot depicting calcaneal pitch (measured as the angle between a line drawn along the plantar aspect of the calcaneus and the floor; normal 20°-40°).

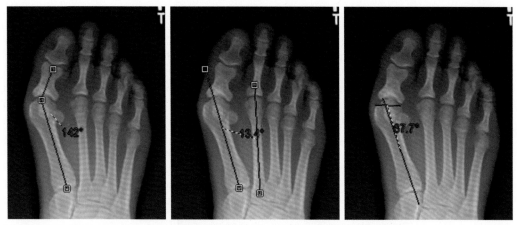

FIGURE 1.54 Anterior-posterior radiographs of the foot depicting three ways to assess hallux valgus (bunion). Hallux valgus angle (left panel) is the angle between the long axis of the first metatarsal and the proximal phalanx. The intermetatarsal angle (IMA) is the angle between the long axis of the first and second metatarsal. The distal metatarsal articular angle (DMAA) is the angle between the long axis of the first metatarsal and line drawn along the distal metatarsal articular surface.

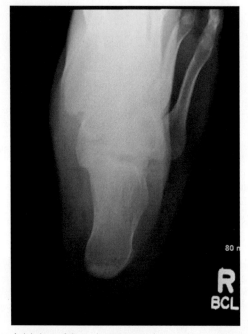

FIGURE 1.55 Harris heel view. Axial view of the calcaneus can be used to assess the hindfoot (eg, calcaneus fracture, hindfoot varus/valgus).

X-ray Findings

Subluxation, Dislocation

These terms can apply to any joint. Subluxation is when a joint is partially out of alignment, and dislocation is when the joint is completely out of alignment. **Figure 1.56** is an AP pelvis x-ray of a patient with cerebral palsy who has a subluxated hip on the left and a dislocated hip on the right.

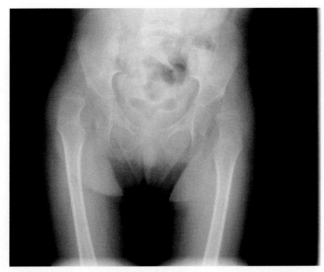

FIGURE 1.56 Anteroposterior (AP) pelvis radiograph depicting joint subluxation (left hip) and dislocation (right hip).

Lytic, Blastic, Destructive, Contained/Geographic, Cystic, Ground Glass, Stippled, Onion Skinning, Periosteal Elevation, Expansile, Cortical Thinning

These are terms used to describe the appearance of lesions of bone. Infections of bone and tumors of various kinds are known to produce these specific findings (**Figures 1.57-1.59**).

1. Lytic refers to lesions that appear to destroy the surrounding bone.
2. Blastic refers to lesions that appear to create bone (eg, osteosarcoma).
3. Contained or geographic lesions have clear boundaries on all sides.

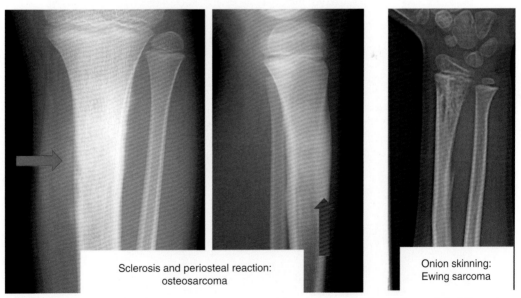

Sclerosis and periosteal reaction: osteosarcoma

Onion skinning: Ewing sarcoma

FIGURE 1.57 Anteroposterior (AP) and lateral radiographs of the proximal tibia (left, middle panel) depicting sclerosis of bone (red arrow) and periosteal reaction (blue arrow). AP radiograph of the wrist (right panel) depicting "onion skinning" of bone which can be seen in Ewing sarcoma.

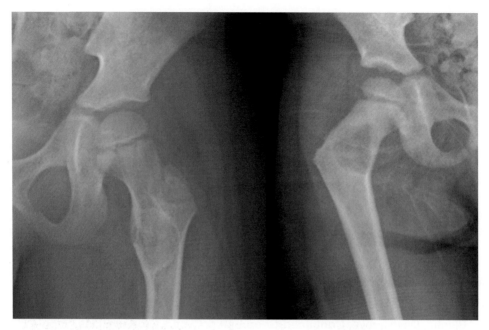

Ground glass:
fibrous dysplasia

Lytic lesion:
unicameral bone cyst

FIGURE 1.58 Anteroposterior (AP) radiograph of the hip (left panel) showing "ground glass" appearance of a bony lesion in the proximal femur. AP radiograph of the hip (right panel) showing "lytic" appearance of a bony lesion in the proximal femur.

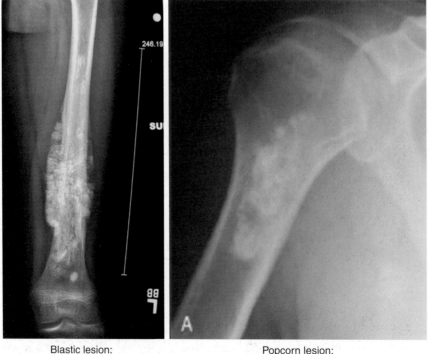

Blastic lesion:
osteosarcoma

Popcorn lesion:
enchondroma

FIGURE 1.59 Left, An AP femur film demonstrates blastic bone development (outside the normal confines of the bone) from this child with osteoblastic osteosarcoma. Right, An AP of the proximal humerus demonstrates increased density within the confines of the bone. Sometimes this popcorn appearance is seen in cartilaginous lesions.

4. Ground glass lesions have a smooth, opaque appearance (eg, fibrous dysplasia).
5. Stippling refers to small calcific elements within a lesion sometimes referred to as "popcorn" calcifications. Cartilage lesions commonly have this appearance (eg, enchondroma and chondrosarcoma).
6. Onion skinning refers to layers of bone applied to the outside surface of the bone. Commonly seen with osteosarcoma and Ewing sarcoma.
7. Periosteal elevation refers to a new outside layer of bone cortex seen when a lesion lifts off the periosteum (bone covering) and it continues to make bone. Seen with infection, healing fractures, and some tumors.
8. Expansile lesions increase the diameter of the bone.
9. Cortical thinning occurs when a lesion within the bone pushes against the inside of the cortex and thins the bone.

Callus

Callus is new bone formed around a healing fracture or osteotomy (**Figure 1.60**).

Dysplasia

The term dysplasia refers to something that is not the correct shape. For example, hip dysplasia describes any abnormality of the hip and can include hip dislocation, subluxation, or any radiographic measure of the socket or the femur that is outside the normal values (**Figure 1.56**). Genetic disorders resulting in globally abnormal bones are often referred to as "skeletal dysplasia." These can include achondroplasia (dwarfism) (**Figure 1.61**).

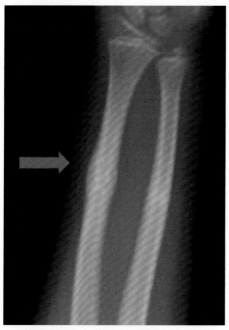

FIGURE 1.60 Anteroposterior (AP) radiograph of the forearm showing callus formation (blue arrow) after a radial shaft fracture.

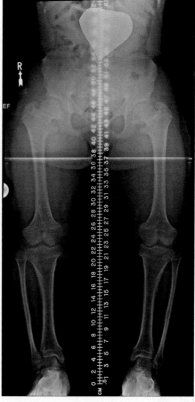

FIGURE 1.61 Teleroentgenogram of a patient with achondroplasia. Note the shortened appearance of the long bones, particularly the proximal femurs.

Fracture Terminology

Fracture Patterns

1. *Transverse, oblique, comminuted, spiral, torus/buckle, and greenstick.* These are common descriptions of fracture patterns that help describe an injury in addition to location and bone.
   a. Transverse fractures (**Figure 1.62**) are straight across the bone perpendicular to the long axis of the bone.
   b. Oblique fractures (**Figure 1.63**) are obliquely oriented with respect to the long axis of the bone.
   c. Comminuted fractures (**Figure 1.64**) are high-energy injuries that produce multiple fracture fragments.
   d. Spiral fractures (**Figure 1.65**) are the result of twisting injuries. A common example is the toddler fracture.
   e. Torus or buckle fractures (**Figure 1.66**) are very common in children due to the plasticity of their bones. These are incomplete fractures with buckling on the compression side of the bone.
   f. Greenstick fractures (**Figure 1.67**) are also incomplete fractures with failure on the tension side of the bone.

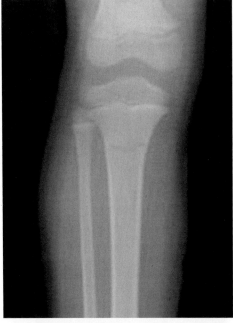

FIGURE 1.62 Anteroposterior (AP) radiograph of the proximal tibia showing a transverse fracture of the proximal tibia.

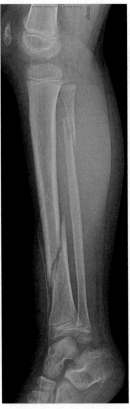

FIGURE 1.63 Lateral radiograph of the tibia showing oblique fracture of the tibia.

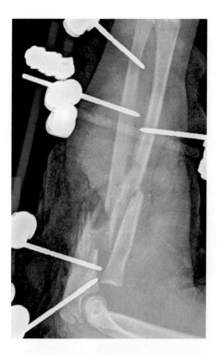

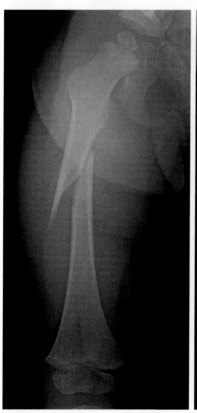

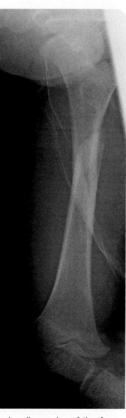

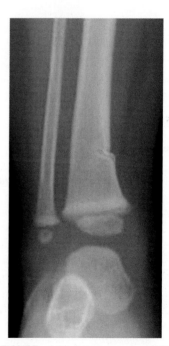

FIGURE 1.64 Lateral radiograph of the proximal forearm showing comminuted fractures of the proximal ulna and radius. The radiograph also shows external fixation pins placed in the radius and ulna.

FIGURE 1.66 Anteroposterior (AP) radiograph of the distal tibia/fibula showing a unicortical buckle fracture of the medial aspect of the distal tibia.

FIGURE 1.65 Anteroposterior (AP) and lateral radiographs of the femur showing a spiral fracture of the femoral shaft.

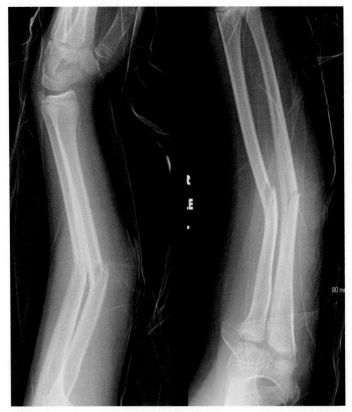

FIGURE 1.67 Two radiographic views of the forearm showing greenstick fractures of the radius and ulna. Greenstick fractures are incomplete fractures with one side of the bone's cortex remaining intact.

Fracture Alignment

1. ***Anatomic, displacement, angulation, reduced, and bayonet.*** These terms are used to describe the alignment of a fracture either before or after treatment. *Anatomic alignment* refers to perfect or normal alignment of the fracture. *Displacement* describes translation of the fracture fragments relative to one another and is often described in terms of percent of bone diameter and direction of displacement of the distal fragment. *Angulation* similarly describes the degree of angulation and is expressed as the direction of angulation of the distal segment relative to the proximal segment or the direction of angulation. *Reduced* describes the alignment of the fracture after it has been improved toward normal alignment. *Reduction* is the act of returning the bone to normal alignment and can be done open (with surgery) or closed (with manipulation). *Bayonet apposition* describes a situation where there is 100% displacement of a fracture with shortening so that the two segments are overlapped.
2. ***Remodeling.*** This describes the process of gradual return toward normal bone alignment and shape after a fracture has healed in a somewhat abnormal position. It is a process that favors youth and occurs more readily near rapidly growing physes (growth plates) and in the direction of motion of the nearby joint (**Figure 1.68**).

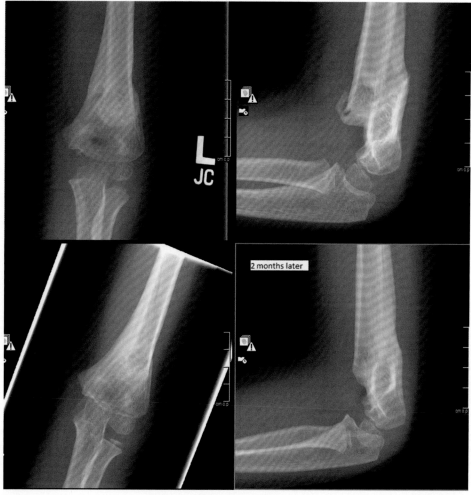

FIGURE 1.68 Remodeling the distal humerus after a supracondylar humerus fracture. The top panels show early remodeling after injury and the bottom panels show late remodeling.

⬤ *Nomenclature Related to Physical Examination*

Gait

The observation of gait is a very common portion of the pediatric orthopedic examination. It is done informally on most patients by systematic observation of gait in the hallway outside the examination room. Formal gait analysis can also be done on certain patients and is covered in more detail in Chapter 4.

Range of Motion

1. **AROM, PROM**. Active and passive range of motion. These terms are often used in the description of the physical examination and when writing physical therapy orders. Active describes the range of motion the joint can achieve under the patient's own control/power. Passive range of motion describes the range of motion the joint can achieve with the assistance of the examiner.

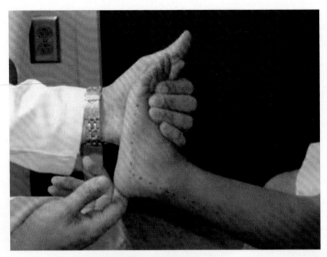

FIGURE 1.69 Clinical photograph of the left foot in a patient with an equinus (ankle plantar flexion) contracture. This is most commonly due to a tight heelcord/Achilles tendon.

2. **Extensor lag.** This term describes the difference between active knee extension and passive knee extension. A difference between the two is expressed as an extensor lag of XX degrees and usually indicates weakness or insufficiency of the quadriceps muscle or extensor mechanism (quadriceps-patella-patellar tendon complex).
3. **Recurvatum, procurvatum.** These terms describe deformity of the lower limb (femur, tibia, or knee) in the sagittal plane. Procurvatum describes anteriorly angulated deformity and recurvatum describes posterior angulated deformity. An example of recurvatum is hyperextension of the knee. An example of procurvatum is anterior bowing of the tibia.
4. **Contracture, laxity.** Contracture describes loss of range of motion of a joint. For example, if an ankle joint, when maximally stretched, is 10° short of a right angle, this is expressed as a 10° equinus contracture (**Figure 1.69**). Laxity describes excessive range of motion of a joint such as hyperextension of a knee (**Figure 1.70**) or elbow or instability of a joint such as in a shoulder dislocation or ACL injury in a knee.

Joints

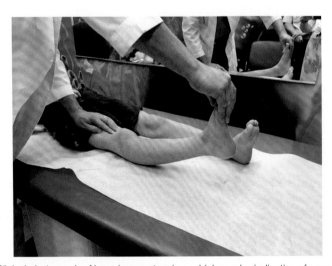

FIGURE 1.70 Clinical photograph of knee hyperextension, which can be indicative of generalized joint laxity.

Effusion and Synovial Thickening

An effusion is a finding of noticeable increased fluid within a joint. It can be detected on physical examination for joints close to the skin (fingers, knee, ankle, and wrist) but requires ultrasound or MRI to detect for deeper joints (ie, hips). Synovial thickening is a finding of joint inflammation where the lining of the joint is noticeably thicker than normal. This is seen in superficial joints in patients with chronic inflammation (juvenile rheumatoid arthritis).

Muscles

1. **Grades of strength**. There are several strength grading systems, but the most commonly used is a scale of 0 to 5.
   0 = no flicker of muscle activity
   1 = flicker only with no movement
   2 = movement only in the horizontal plane (no resistance to gravity)
   3 = movement against gravity but not against resistance
   4 = movement against resistance but not normal strength
   5 = normal strength
2. **Spasticity, dystonia, and athetoid.** Spasticity is the most common muscle problem in cerebral palsy. It is defined as velocity-dependent resistance to motion. The joint can move through a larger range of motion when it is moved slowly but much less so when moved quickly. Dystonia is subtler and can be concealed by concurrent spasticity. With dystonia, the movements are involuntary, often twisting and sometimes repeating. Athetoid movements are rhythmic, repeating movement and less common than the others.

● *Surgical Nomenclature*

Reduction—Definition

Fracture "reduction" is the act of manipulating the limb/bone to correct the amount of displacement or angulation.

Closed Versus Open Reduction

Reduction can be performed by either "closed" or "open" means. Closed reduction means manipulating the fracture without making a surgical incision, while open reduction refers to manipulating the bone directly via a surgical incision over the fracture site.

Fixation Options

While obtaining an adequate fracture reduction is the overall goal of fracture treatment, maintaining the reduction can be achieved in a multitude of ways.

1. *Percutaneous pinning:* No formal incision is made, and hardware is punctured through the skin into the bone (**Figure 1.71**).
2. *Internal fixation:* Fixation hardware remains deep to the skin.
3. *External fixation:* Hardware is visible and fixated outside the skin (**Figure 1.64**).
4. *Plate:* Hardware is typically placed on top of the bone's cortex and held with screws (**Figure 1.72**).
5. *Intramedullary nail:* Hardware is inserted within the intramedullary canal of a long bone.
   a. *Rigid nail versus flexible nail* (**Figure 1.73**).

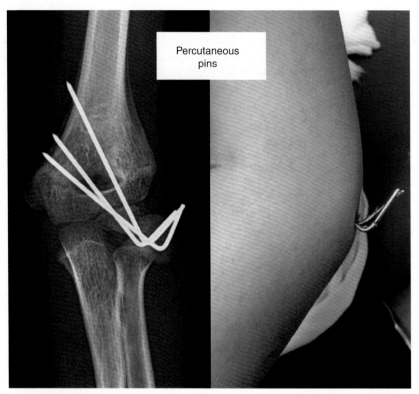

FIGURE 1.71 Anteroposterior (AP) radiograph (left panel) and clinical image (right panel) of a patient with percutaneous pin fixation of an elbow fracture.

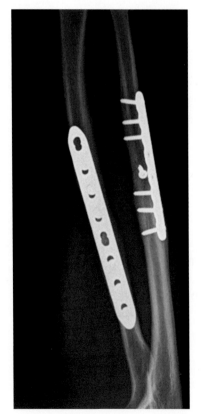

FIGURE 1.72 Anteroposterior (AP) forearm radiograph showing plate and screw fixation of the radius and ulna.

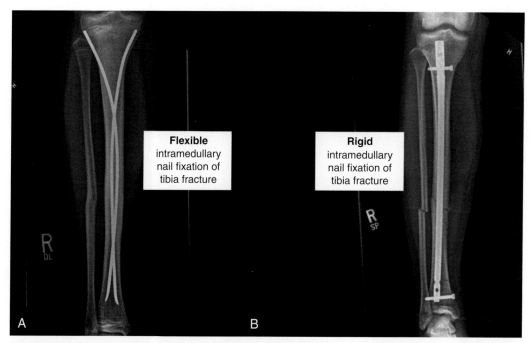

FIGURE 1.73 Anteroposterior (AP) tibia radiographs displaying two different types of intramedullary (IM) nail fixation: A, flexible; B, rigid IM nail fixation.

Procedures

Pediatric orthopedic surgeons often perform surgery to correct deformities in the limbs or spine, and correction can be achieved in a variety of ways.

1. *Growth plate:* Growth plate modulation (guided growth) can be used to affect the growth of skeletally immature bone.
   a. *Epiphysiodesis:* Surgical fusion of the physis to halt growth.
   b. Hemiepiphysiodesis: Decreasing the growth of a portion of the physis to influence angular growth (**Figure 1.74**). With this method, the implant spans the growth plate on the convexity of the deformity one wishes to correct.
2. *Bone:* In addition to surgical manipulation of the growth plate, orthopedic surgeons can more directly correct bony deformity by performing an *osteotomy* (cutting of the bone) or *osteoclasis* (cutting or physical destruction of the bone in multiple locations typically followed by fixation) to achieve the desired correction.
3. *Soft tissue:* The soft tissues surrounding the bone can also be an important contributor to deformity, and surgeons can address the soft tissues by performing:
   a. *Tenotomy:* Cutting of tendons.
4. Tendon Z-lengthening: Stepwise cutting of tendon to make it longer. This can be done open or percutaneously.
   a. *Recession:* Lengthening of the muscle fascia.

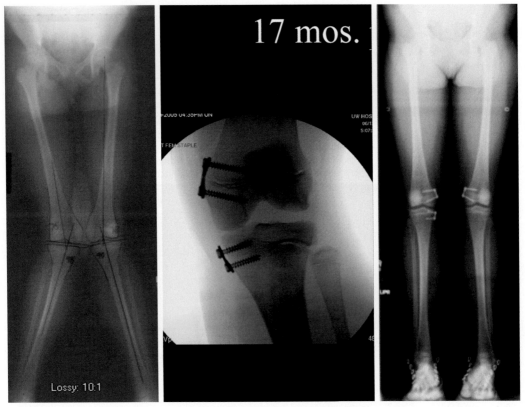

FIGURE 1.74 Preop teleroentgenogram (left panel), intraop fluoroscopic imaging (middle panel), and postoperative teleroentgenogram (right panel) of genu valgum correction via hemiepiphysiodesis.

    b. *Fasciotomy*: Incising the muscle fascia.
    c. *Tendon/ligament advancement*: Shortening of an abnormally lengthened tendon/ligament.
    d. *Neurolysis:* Surgical release of a constricted peripheral nerve.
    e. *Nerve transfer*: Surgically moving a peripheral nerve to a new anatomic location/position.

● Nomenclature Related to Casts, Splints, and Braces

Materials

Plaster Versus Fiberglass

Contemporary casting/splinting materials are typically made of either *plaster of Paris* or synthetic *fiberglass*. Both materials rely on a chemical reaction (after dipping into water) to convert the underlying material from one that is easily pliable (ie, to wrap around limbs/joints) into one that is rigid and can provide structural support and immobilization to a limb or joint. When plaster casts cure, they can generate a lot of heat and can burn patients.

Cast Definition

Casts provide circumferential immobilization to an affected limb and are described based on their anatomic location and the joints spanned on the affected limb. Common examples include:

Upper Extremity

1. Long arm, short arm (**Figure 1.75**), Muenster, thumb spica.

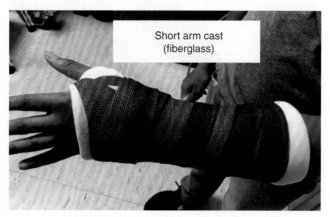

FIGURE 1.75 Clinical photograph of a short-arm fiberglass cast.

Lower Extremity

1. *Long-leg* (**Figure 1.76**), *short-leg* (**Figure 1.77**), and *cylinder cast (a long-leg cast that does not include foot).*

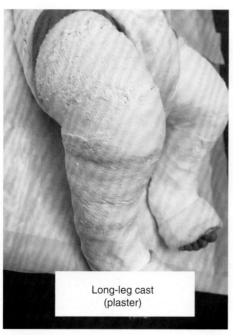

FIGURE 1.76 Clinical photograph of a long-leg plaster cast. In this example, the long-leg cast is used as a treatment for clubfoot.

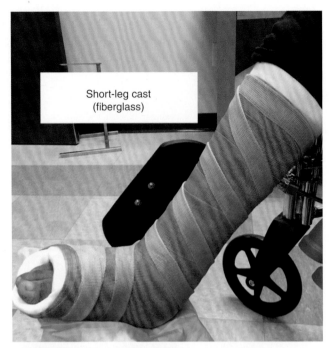

FIGURE 1.77 Clinical photograph of a short-leg fiberglass cast.

2. Hip spica cast (**Figure 1.78**).

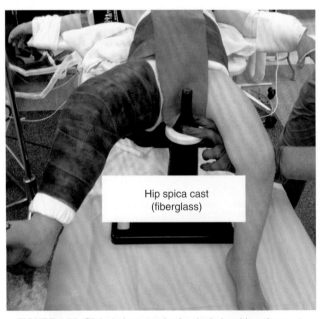

FIGURE 1.78 Clinical photograph of a single-leg, hip spica cast.

Spine

1. *Mehta cast* (**Figure 1.79**).

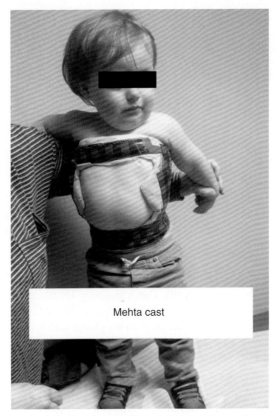

Mehta cast

FIGURE 1.79 Clinical photograph of a patient in a Mehta cast. This cast is used in young children with early-onset (<5 years old) scoliosis. It allows for scoliosis curve control without surgery.

Splints

Splints are noncircumferential and can be made in the clinic or obtained from commercial vendors. They are also described based on anatomic location and can be additionally described based on which side of the affected limb the splint is applied to (ie, *volar wrist splint, long-leg posterior splint, short-leg posterior splint*, etc.).

Brace Types

Braces refer to prefabricated or custom-made durable medical equipment used to address specific anatomic and/or biomechanical abnormalities.

Foot/Ankle

1. *UCBL* orthosis. "University of California Biomechanics Laboratory" orthosis provides contoured support to the plantar foot surface as well as the medial and lateral sides of the foot for maximum foot control without extending above the ankle. Typically used for flatfoot deformities.

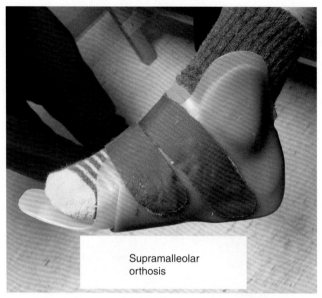

FIGURE 1.80 Supramalleolar orthosis (SMO) used to treat a variety of foot conditions.

2. *SMO.* Supramalleolar orthosis (**Figure 1.80**). This is similar to UCBL, except that it extends above the ankle (eg, supramalleolar). Used to help control varus/valgus of the ankle joint.

3. *AFO.* Ankle foot orthosis. Orthosis that extends from the plantar surface of the foot proximally above the ankle and below the knee (eg, stops at the calf level). Used for a variety of conditions to provide external support for the foot and ankle with the goal of providing a stable, plantigrade foot and to facilitate shoe wear.

Hip/Leg

1. *KAFO.* Knee-ankle-foot orthosis. Orthosis that extends from the plantar surface of the foot to the ankle and proximally above the knee joint and stops at thigh level. Provides support for the foot, ankle, and knee. Those that extend above the hip are HKAFO's.

2. *Pavlik harness.* Used for developmental dysplasia of the hip (DDH) in infants and femur fractures in children less than 6 months. Maintains the hip in a flexed and abducted position to facilitate acetabular development in DDH and provides splinting for femur fractures in young children.

Spine

1. *TLSO.* Thoracolumbosacral orthosis. Used in scoliosis to help control curvature of the spine. The Boston TLSO is designed to be worn full-time, whereas the Providence TLSO is designed to be worn at nighttime only. The Boston brace is fitted to conform to the patient's current curvature while the Providence brace is fitted to provide some curve correction. The Providence brace is worn at nighttime only because in order to provide correction, the brace "pushes" on the patient's curve and is therefore uncomfortable to wear during activities of daily living.

2. *Halo.* This is a form of external fixation of the skull with the goal of controlling the patient's spine through traction. In children with spine deformities, it can be used to provide spinal traction to provide provisional, gradual deformity correction in preparation for definitive surgery (**Figure 1.81**).

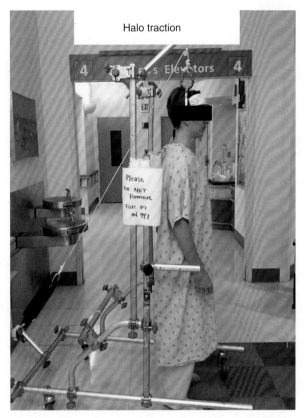

FIGURE 1.81 Clinical photograph of a patient in a halo traction setup to provide preoperative scoliosis curve correction.

Differences Between Pediatric and Adult Musculoskeletal Systems

James G. Jarvis and Megan E. Johnson

Introduction

There are anatomical and physiological differences between the pediatric and adult musculoskeletal systems. Certain anatomical differences of the bones and joints in children combine to produce unique and variable responses to injuries and healing that are not seen in the mature skeletons of adults. Furthermore, due to the presence of growth plates, there are also different physiological factors at play. Neurological development and milestones, remodeling accelerated by growth, and the effects of increased body mass index (BMI) on the growing skeleton are just some of the special features and unique aspects that must be considered when examining and treating pediatric patients.

Anatomical Differences and Their Potential Clinical Importance

Bone

At birth, bone is relatively less dense, less lamellar, and has increased porosity relative to a mature bone[1-3]. With increasing age, adaptive changes occur that result in progressive formation of lamellar and osteon bone within the diaphysis compared to the spongy, trabecular bone of the metaphysis and epiphysis. Immature bone has a lower elastic modulus than mature bone. It bends to a greater extent when stressed and absorbs more energy before it breaks. These differences in architecture result in different healing patterns with buckle fractures in the softer spongy bone of the metaphysis and greenstick fractures and plastic deformation in the diaphysis of the long bones (**Figure 2.1A-C**).

One of the most distinguishing differences between the bones of a child and an adult is the presence of a thick and robust periosteum. This layer is strong but is easily lifted by hematoma or purulence and is less likely to rupture than in adults. This thick bridge adds stability to fractures, is instrumental in the remodeling and correction of longitudinal deformities (**Figure 2.2A-C**), and also accounts for the rapidity with which infant and toddler fractures heal relative to their adult counterparts (**Figure 2.3**). While periosteum is an important aid in fracture remodeling, it can also be a block to reduction. For instance, it can often be found in the fracture site on the tension side of a displaced epiphysis (eg, distal tibia) or through an apophyseal injury (tibial tubercle avulsion).

Growing bone is constantly changing due to the endochondral ossification process (**Figure 2.4**). The chondro-osseous epiphyses are variably radiolucent, especially in the very young, and can be difficult to interpret on plain radiographs. Similarly, the physis (growth plate) is constantly changing in appearance making interpretation of radiographs more challenging. Physeal injuries often need to be inferred on the basis of sound clinical judgment coupled with an accurate physical examination, rather than on the radiographic appearance. In cases where fractures are suspected, a contralateral radiograph can allow one to distinguish between subtle injury and normal developing bone. Of course, once periosteal new bone has appeared 10 days after the injury, the diagnosis can be confirmed in retrospect (**Figure 2.5**).

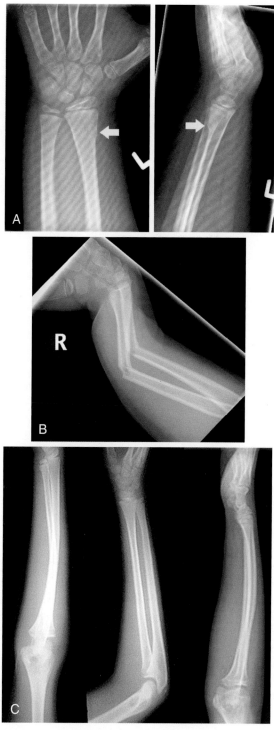

FIGURE 2.1 A, Buckle fracture (arrows) in a seven-year-old girl. The soft spongy bone of the metaphysis is more susceptible to bending or "buckling" than a more brittle mature bone, which tends to break. B, Greenstick fracture (seven-year-old girl). This greenstick fracture shows how the child's softer bone can break on only one side and bend on the other. The fracture does not extend all the way through the bone. C, Plastic bowing of the forearm. Due to the thinner cortex and higher elasticity of the bone in children, bending or plastic bowing of the entire bone is not unusual (when subjected to angulated longitudinal forces). (C, From Andrew F. Kuntz MD, Wei-Shin Lai MD, et al. University of Virginia Health Sciences Center, Department of Radiology.)

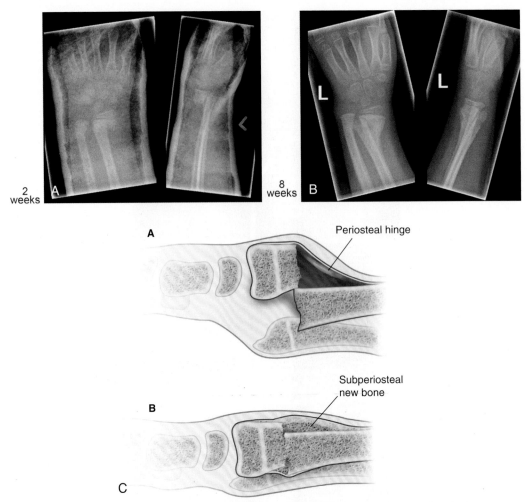

FIGURE 2.2 Periosteal healing—distal radius fracture in a six-year-old girl. A, 2 weeks post injury. B, 8 weeks post injury. Notice the rapid remodeling of this distal radius fracture due to the robust periosteal healing. C, Periosteal healing.

Joints

Normal infants can have joint contractures as a result of intrauterine positioning that will eventually stretch out. For instance, infants have 70° to 80° of passive and active hip external rotation, and this progressively resolves as they become ambulatory. It is well known that toddlers and young children are very flexible and with time, the joints become stiffer. Increased ligamentous laxity can be associated with hereditary diseases of connective tissue such as Ehlers-Danlos, Marfan, and Down syndromes. Nonsyndromic ligamentous laxity is often familial and is seen in 10% to 15% (this likely factors into many common conditions such as hip dysplasia, recurrent patellar subluxation, and flexible flat feet). Generalized ligamentous laxity can be established clinically based on the thumb-to-forearm distance, hyper extensibility of the long fingers, and hyper extensibility of the elbow and knee joints[4] (**Table 2.1**; **Figure 2.6**).

Growth Plates

The most distinct structural difference between young and mature bone is the presence of the physis or growth plate. The anatomy and function of the various layers and components of this structure are well defined (**Figure 2.7**). The zone of hypertrophy is where chondrocytes are undergoing enlargement

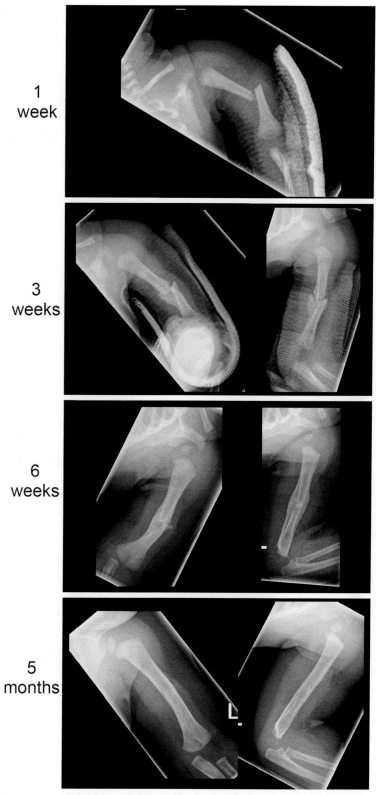

1 week

3 weeks

6 weeks

5 months

FIGURE 2.3 Robust periosteal healing. Birth fracture humeral shaft. Nearly complete regeneration of the humeral shaft is due to the powerful periosteal remodeling potential in a newborn.

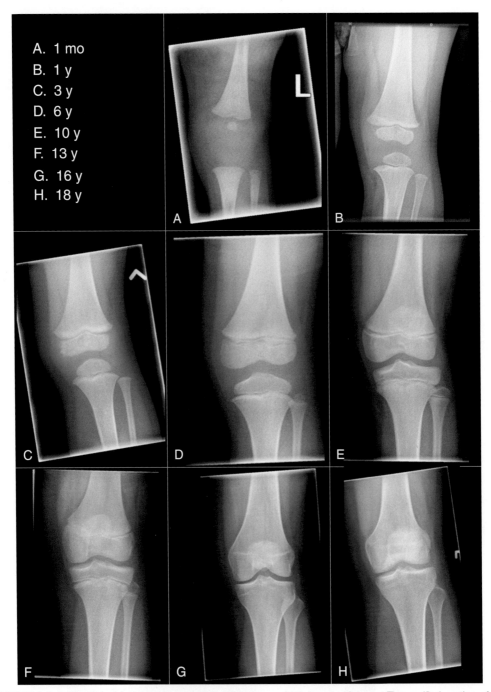

A. 1 mo
B. 1 y
C. 3 y
D. 6 y
E. 10 y
F. 13 y
G. 16 y
H. 18 y

FIGURE 2.4 Sequential endochondral ossification of the knee—birth to age 18 years. The ossified portion of the distal femoral epiphysis is very small at birth. Notice how it progressively enlarges with growth to ultimately "cap" the end of the bone at maturity.

and programmed cell death (apoptosis). This region is very susceptible to shear forces and represents the weakest and most vulnerable area of the growth plate. Although deriving some mechanical protection from the perichondrial ring of Lacroix, the weakness of the hypertrophic zone is associated with, or affected by, many common childhood conditions as noted below.

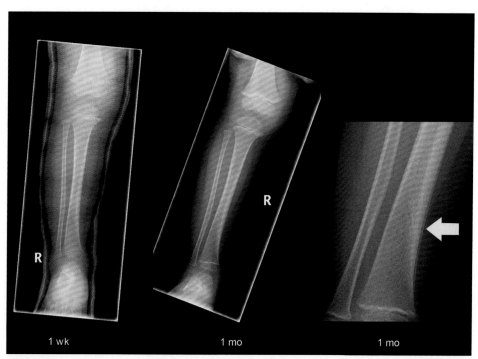

1 wk   1 mo   1 mo

FIGURE 2.5 Toddler fracture of the tibia in a two-year-old boy. Barely perceptible "toddler fracture" of the tibia, confirmed one month post injury by evidence of healing periosteal new bone (yellow arrow) along the distal tibial shaft (arrow).

Slipped capital epiphysis of the proximal femur likely represents an admixture of pubertal hormonal imbalance which may widen the growth plate and, coupled with increased shear forces, can overload the hypertrophic zone leading to gradual or abrupt slipping of the femoral head (**Figure 2.8**). In rickets, due to defective mineralization, the hypertrophic zone becomes disorganized and expanded (**Figure 2.9**). Skeletal dysplasias also affect this zone, leading to progressive deformity (**Figure 2.10**).

Another major difference in the growing skeleton is the presence of the apophysis, which is basically a growth plate under tension from the insertion of large tendons. These growth plates do not lengthen the bone much, yet can be a location of acute injury or chronic irritation. In adults, a rapid increase in tension at a tendon can lead to rupture while overuse can lead to painful mid-substance tendonitis. In children, similar acute stress on the strong tendon will lead to failure through the apophysis as opposed to adult tendon rupture. Chronic overuse can lead to clinical inflammation and pain at the insertion of the tendon and not along the tendon itself as seen in adults. With chronic apophysitis, radiographs will show fragmentation and irregular bone at the insertion site. Osgood-Schlatter disease of the tibial tubercle is an example of abnormal bone development due to repetitive traction through strong ligaments (**Figure 2.11**).

Table 2.1	Criteria for Generalized Ligamentous Laxity

1. Passive dorsiflexion and hyperextension of the fifth MCP joint beyond 90°.
2. Passive apposition of the thumb to the flexor aspect of the forearm.
3. Passive hyperextension of the elbow beyond 10°.
4. Passive hyperextension of the knee beyond 10°.
5. Active forward flexion of the trunk with the knees fully extended so that the palms of the hands rest flat on the floor.

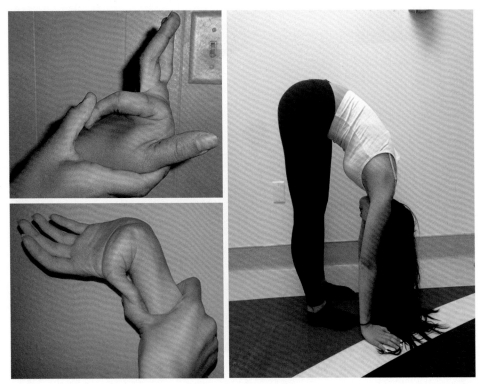

FIGURE 2.6 Criteria for generalized ligamentous laxity. Metacarpophalangeal hyperextension, passive apposition of the thumb, and excessive trunk forward flexion (also see **Table 2.1**). (A, From https://en.wikipedia.org/wiki/Ligamentous_laxity. B, From The Pediatric Upper Extremity. 1811-1821.)

In acute trauma, it is important to remember that the tendon and ligaments are stronger than the bone and the growth plate. Suspicion of these growing conditions should direct the examination to bone rather than the ligaments. Many "ankle sprains," "medial collateral ligament strains," and other injuries in growing children are actually Salter-Harris type 1 fractures and not sprains at all. This can easily be differentiated on examination by accurately localizing the area of maximal tenderness to the bone and not the ligament.

● *Physiological Differences and Their Potential Clinical Importance*

Growth and Milestones

During infancy, the child is completely dependent on its parents. Various developmental steps and abilities are typically reached at the following times[5] (**Table 2.2**; **Figure 2.12**). An understanding of these milestones will help guide the examiner in interpreting possible aberrations. For example, the immature gait of the early walker is typically unsteady and wide-based with irregular cadence. This results from several factors including a relatively high center of gravity and low muscle-to-body weight ratio, in addition to immaturity of the nervous system and postural control mechanisms. However, it is completely normal (▶ **Video 2.1**). The timing of some events such as the development of hand dominance is controversial, but a consistent hand preference begins to emerge between ages 2 and 4, and most children entering kindergarten (age 5-6) have established a definite hand preference for using a pencil and scissors. Hand dominance prior to age 2 may imply a neurological deficit on the nondominant side.

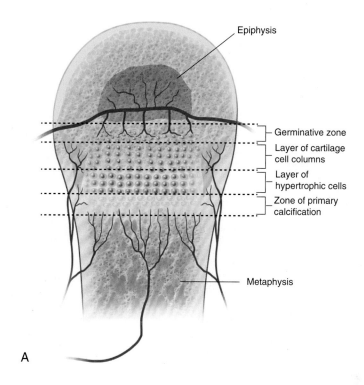

Epiphysis

Germinative zone

Layer of cartilage cell columns

Layer of hypertrophic cells

Zone of primary calcification

Metaphysis

A

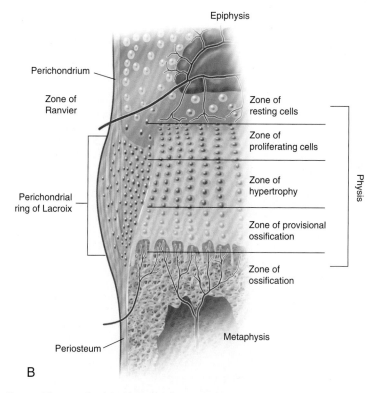

Epiphysis

Perichondrium

Zone of Ranvier

Zone of resting cells

Zone of proliferating cells

Zone of hypertrophy

Perichondrial ring of Lacroix

Zone of provisional ossification

Physis

Zone of ossification

Periosteum

Metaphysis

B

FIGURE 2.7 A, Zones of the growth plate. Note that the zone of hypertrophy is the weak link and most growth plate fractures fall through this zone. B, Histology of the growth plate.

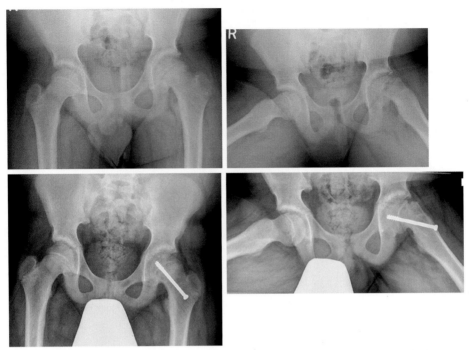

FIGURE 2.8 Slipped capital femoral epiphysis in an 11-year-old boy (before and after pinning). Slippage of the femoral epiphysis through the zone of hypertrophy in a preteen who is going through a growth spurt. Stabilized with internal fixation/cannulated screw.

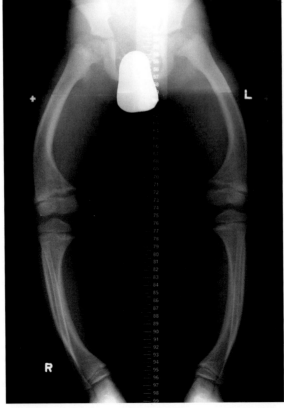

FIGURE 2.9 Lower extremity bowing deformity in rickets. Note the widened, distal femoral growth plate with associated bowing in this child with rickets.

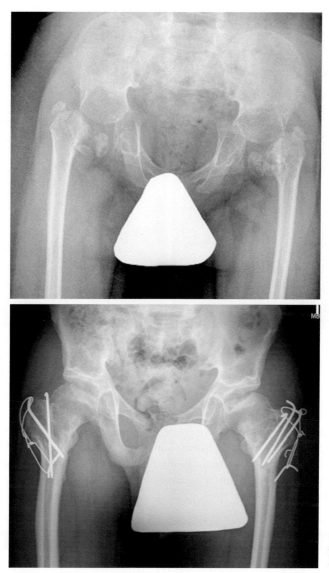

FIGURE 2.10 Progressive coxa vara in a 10-year-old boy with spondyloepiphyseal dysplasia (before and after correction). Note the bilateral failure and wide displacement of the proximal femoral epiphysis leading to severe coxa vara. Corrected by bilateral proximal femoral valgus osteotomies.

Normal Growth Patterns for Children and Adolescents

Growth after age 3 proceeds at a relatively linear and constant rate (**Figures 2.13** and **2.14**) while adolescence is characterized by accelerated growth with the physical changes associated with sexual maturation and the pubertal growth spurt[6] (**Figures 2.15** and **2.16**).

Body proportions change dramatically in the first few years of life. The relatively large head size of the infant and toddler is quickly eclipsed by the growth of the lower extremities, which contributes a far greater percentage of growth in height than does trunk growth (**Figure 2.17**). Total body length is doubled by the 4th year and tripled by the 13th year. The height of an adult is about twice the height of a two-year-old child.

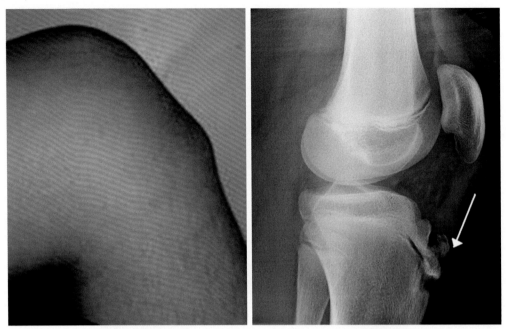

FIGURE 2.11 Osgood-Schlatter disease. Chronic traction/"overuse" by the patellar ligament on the relatively weaker proximal tibial growth cartilage in this teenager leads to chronic swelling and inflammation. (https://en.wikipedia.org/wiki/Osgood%E2%80%93Schlatter_disease.)

Predication of skeletal maturity and the end of growth is important in determining the impact of different disorders which effect the growth plate. For instance, a growth plate injury in a two-year-old could lead to a profound length discrepancy but a similar injury in an older child/adolescent may not. In order to judge the potential impact, we often have to predict the end of growth and this can typically be determined by several means. On history, menarchal status is an important landmark and most girls stop growth within two years post menarche. Physical examination is directed toward Tanner

Table 2.2	**Typical Developmental Milestones**
AGE IN MONTHS	**ABILITY**
2-5	Smiles spontaneously
2-4	Head control
2-6	Turns from prone to supine and vice versa
5-8	Sits independently
6-9	Pulls up using furniture and starts to stand
9-13	Says mommy/daddy
10-16	Drinks from a cup
11-16	Walks independently
14-22	Climbs stairs
14-30	Combines two different words
20-30	Puts on clothing
22-30	Hops on the spot

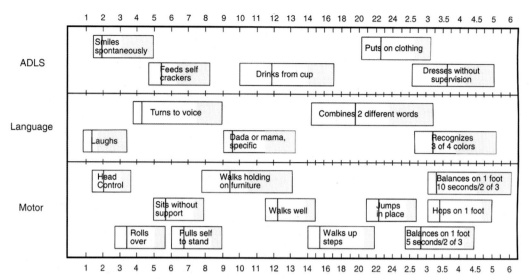

FIGURE 2.12 Denver developmental screening. The average child can cruise around furniture at 9 months and walk independently at about 12 months of age. ADLS, activities of daily living. (From Weinstein SL. *Practice of Pediatric Orthopedics*. Philadelphia, PA: Lipincott Williams & Wilkins; 2001.)

staging (**Figure 2.18**). Radiographic assessment of growth includes bone age determination from hand and wrist radiographs (**Figure 2.19**). Pelvis radiographs can help judge maturation when managing scoliosis and closure of the triradiate cartilage usually precedes peak height velocity (PHV). After the PHV, Risser sign will become evident and will progress to full fusion of the iliac apophysis (Risser 5) (**Figure 2.20**). Other indicators of increased maturation include closure of the olecranon apophyses (**Figure 2.21**).

Growth and Remodeling

Multiple different disorders can lead to systemic differences in growth in children. Increased limb size can be seen with Proteus syndrome, Klippel-Trenaunay-Weber syndrome, Beckwith-Wiedemann syndrome, and neurofibromatosis to name a few. A common idiopathic overgrowth of one side of the body is called hemihypertrophy (**Figure 2.22**) and should be distinguished from the previously mentioned syndromic causes with the aid of a genetic evaluation (**Figure 2.23**).

The immature skeleton of the child has the unique ability to adapt and remodel in response to local stress or injury—a phenomenon not seen in adults. This is due to the growth potential of the physeal plate and the remodeling potential of the thick and strong periosteum. Although this is typically seen in the long bones, it can also occur in the vertebrae and smaller bones. Increased localized growth can be seen in patients with regional inflammatory response such as in juvenile arthritis, periphyseal neoplasia, and trauma. Increased growth can be asymmetric after certain fractures adjacent to the growth plate or decreased growth can be asymmetric as a result of injury to the physis, which leads to partial growth plate closure (**Figures 2.24** and **2.25**).

Growth and the Effects of Increased BMI

The growth plate is the weak link in the developing skeleton and can be susceptible to increased BMI; compressive forces perpendicular to a growth plate can retard growth and lead to skeletal deformity. Tibia vara or Blount disease is a progressive bowlegged deformity due to altered growth at the knee and it appears in two forms. The infantile form is typically seen in heavyset children who walk at an early

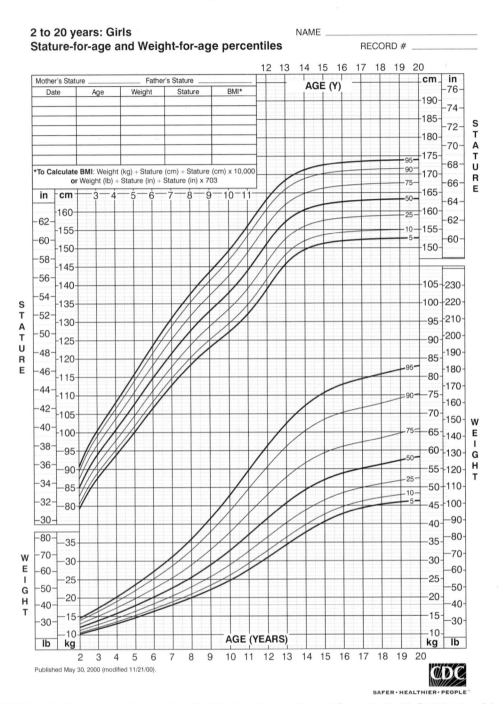

FIGURE 2.13 Standard growth charts for girls. (Developed by the National Center for Health Statistics in collaboration with the National Center for Chronic Disease Prevention and Health Promotion. Available at http://www.cdc.gov/growthcharts.)

age, putting excessive forces on the medial tibial growth plate causing growth retardation (**Figure 2.26**). The adolescent variety is usually seen in overweight individuals and is felt to be secondary to markedly increased mechanical stress on the medial tibial growth plate (**Figure 2.27**) and occasionally the distal femoral growth plate.

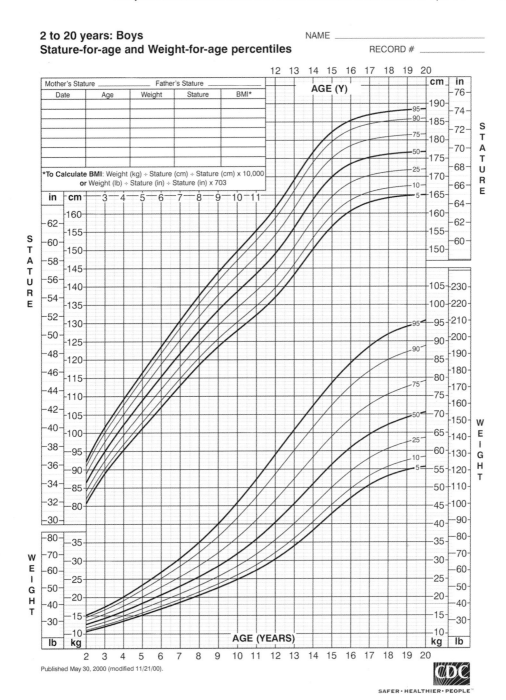

FIGURE 2.14 Standard growth charts for boys. (Developed by the National Center for Health Statistics in collaboration with the National Center for Chronic Disease Prevention and Health Promotion. Available at http://www.cdc.gov/growthcharts.)

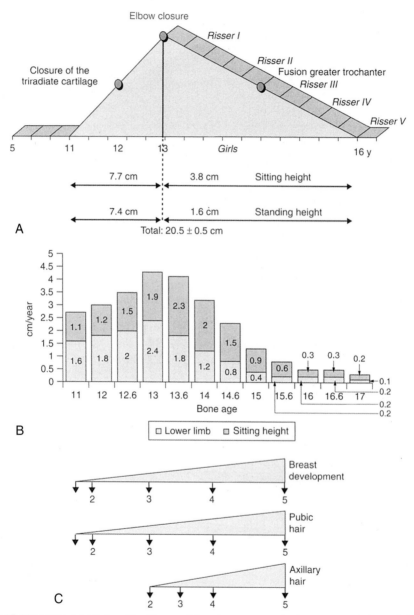

FIGURE 2.15 Maturation graphs for girls. Closure of the olecranon apophysis corresponds to peak height veloc-ity in both boys and girls. Growth tends to slow down thereafter. Growth milestones in girls are generally 2 years advanced compared to boys. (From Dimeglio A. *Growth in Pediatric Orthopaedics*. In: *Lovell and Winter's Pediatric Orthopaedics*. 6th ed. Philadelphia, PA: Lippincott Williams & Wilkins; 2005.)

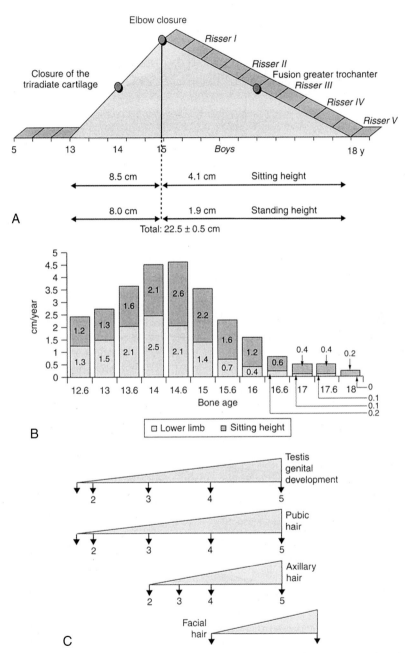

FIGURE 2.16 Maturation graphs for boys. (From Dimeglio A. *Growth in Pediatric Orthopaedics*. In: *Lovell and Winter's Pediatric Orthopaedics*. 6th ed. Philadelphia, PA: Lippincott Williams & Wilkins; 2005.)

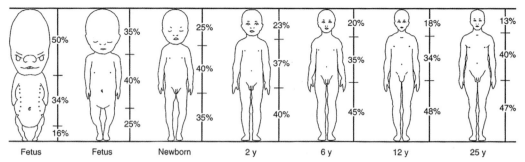

FIGURE 2.17 The proportions of the body as they change with growth. In contrast to infants and toddlers, most growth occurs in the lower extremities in older children. The adult is about twice the height of the two-year-old child. (From Dimeglio A. *Growth in Pediatric Orthopaedics*. In: *Lovell and Winter's Pediatric Orthopaedics*. 6th ed. Philadelphia, PA: Lippincott Williams & Wilkins; 2005.)

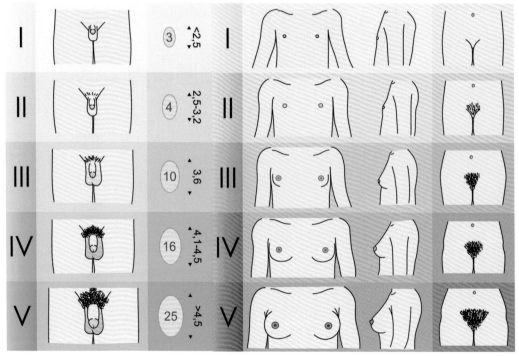

FIGURE 2.18 Tanner staging. (From https://openi.nlm.nih.gov/detailedresult.php?img=PMC4478390_fnhum-09-00344-g001&req=4.)

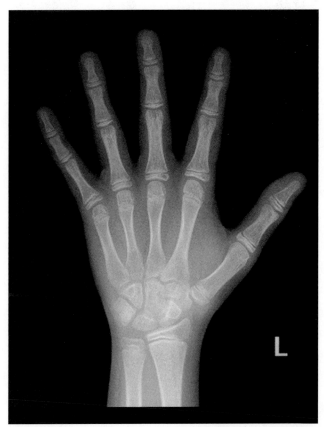

FIGURE 2.19 Bone age wrist radiograph. Growth plate closure occurs sequentially, beginning in the distal phalanges and progressing proximally toward the wrist.

Excessive BMI can also increase shear forces applied obliquely to a growth plate and can result in mechanical failure. For instance, slipped capital femoral epiphysis results from an interplay of pubertal hormonal changes coupled with mechanical overload and increased shear forces on the vulnerable growth plate.

Growing Pains

Growing pains can occur at night in children from 5 to 10 years of age and are usually bilateral lower extremity pains and achiness that resolve with local supportive measures. These pains tend to be focused at the knee and lower legs and can come and go over months to years. The diagnosis should be considered a diagnosis of exclusion (**Table 2.3**). Patients with concurrent systemic symptoms or activity-related pain during the day should be studied carefully for other causes of pain. Growing pains do not affect the upper extremities or the spine and a careful review of systems is needed to rule out pathologic processes that are more likely to be unilateral, not restricted to nighttime and in those who may have systemic symptomology. The clinician who ascribes back pain to "growing pains" is at risk of missing a more sinister diagnosis.

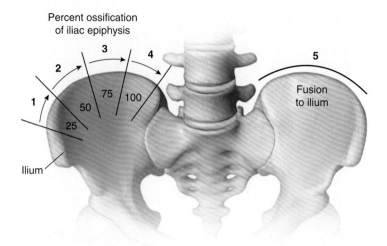

FIGURE 2.20 Risser sign. Ossification of the ischial apophysis progresses from lateral to medial during the last year of growth.

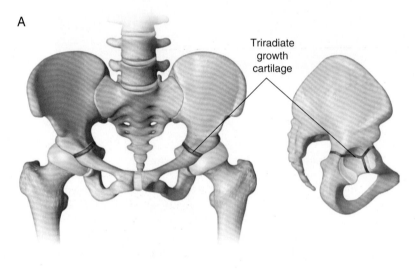

FIGURE 2.21 A, Triradiate cartilage. An open triradiate cartilage indicates that the child is still rapidly growing. B, Olecranon apophysis closure pattern. Closure of the olecranon apophysis is coincident with the end of the maximal growth velocity. This occurs 2 years earlier in girls than in boys.

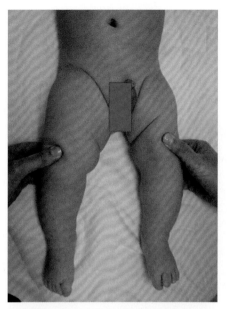

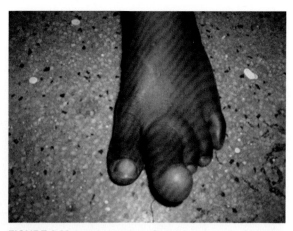

FIGURE 2.23 Local gigantism. Severe overgrowth of the second toe is seen in this girl with localized gigantism.

FIGURE 2.22 Hemihypertrophy, marked overgrowth of the left lower extremity in a child with idiopathic hemihypertrophy.

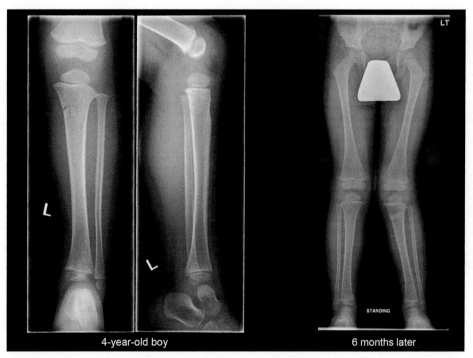

4-year-old boy

6 months later

FIGURE 2.24 Cozen phenomenon. Valgus angular growth due to asymmetric growth plate stimulation following fracture of the proximal left tibia in a four-year-old boy. This asymmetric growth may be due to enhanced vascularity in the vicinity of the incomplete fracture (on the medial side).

6-year-old girl

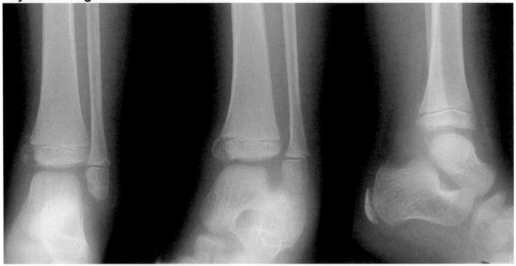

6 mo

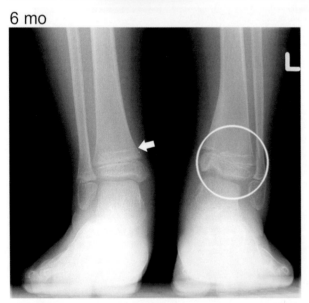

FIGURE 2.25 Salter-Harris type 4 fracture with growth arrest showing convergent Park-Harris growth arrest lines (inside circle) and subsequent varus ankle deformity. Note symmetric growth of the opposite normal tibia (arrow).

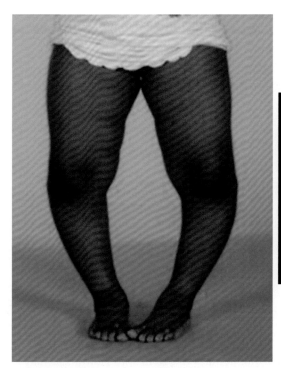

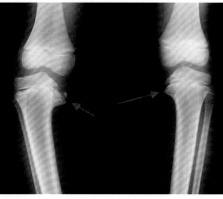

FIGURE 2.26 Infantile Blount disease. Note irregularity and fragmentation of the medial growth plate in this early-walking toddler with infantile Blount disease.

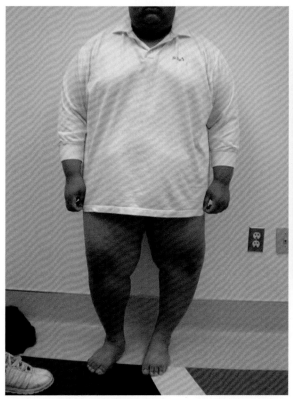

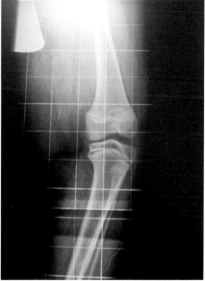

FIGURE 2.27 Adolescent Blount disease. Excessive mechanical stress on the medial growth plate of the proximal tibia can cause disrupted growth and subsequent varus deformity—seen here in a heavy-set teenager with adolescent Blount disease.

Table 2.3	Definition of 'Growing Pains'—Inclusion and Exclusion Criteria	
PAIN FACTORS	**INCLUSION CRITERIA**	**EXCLUSION CRITERIA**
Nature of pain	Intermittent Some pain-free days and nights	Persistent increasing intensity
Unilateral or bilateral	Bilateral	Unilateral
Location of pain	Anterior thigh, calf, posterior knee—in muscles	Upper extremity joint pain Back Pain
Onset of pain	Evening or at night	Pain still present next morning
Physical examination	Normal	Swelling, erythema, tenderness Local trauma or infection Reduced joint range of motion Limping
Laboratory tests	Normal	Objective findings, eg, ESR, X-ray, bone scan abnormalities
Limitation of activity	Nil	Reduced physical activity

Conclusion

In summary, there are many fundamental differences between the pediatric and adult musculoskeletal systems. In children, differing physical examination features will occur with growth and thus it is important for the clinician to appreciate how growth and development will change the examination over time. A working knowledge of the various anatomic and physiologic differences is paramount to conducting an accurate and successful physical examination in the pediatric setting.

References

1. Hefti F. *Basic Principles*. In: *Pediatric Orthopedics in Practice*. Berlin Heidelberg: Springer-Verlag; 2007.
2. Ogden J. *Injury to the immature skeleton*. In: *Skeletal Injury in the Child*. New York, NY: Springer-Verlag; 2000.
3. Weiner D. *Basic considerations in growing bones and joints*. In: *Pediatric Orthopedics for Primary Care Physicians*. 2nd ed. New York, NY: Cambridge University Press; 2004.
4. Beighton P, Solomon L, Soskolne CL. Articular mobility in an African population. *Ann Rheum Dis*. 1973;32:413-418.
5. Staheli L. *Growth in: Practice of Pediatric Orthopedics*. Philadelphia, PA: Lippincott Williams & Wilkins; 2001.
6. Dimeglio A. *Growth in pediatric Orthopaedics*. In: *Lovell and Winter's Pediatric Orthopaedics* 6th ed. Philadelphia, PA: Lippincott Williams & Wilkins; 2005.

Pearls and Pitfalls of the Pediatric Musculoskeletal Examination

Andrew Howard, Martin Herman, and Michael Wolf

● Introduction

The clinical history and physical examination are the basis for diagnosis. The clinic visit is also used to establish rapport and trust, to convey information, to assess understanding, to advise about treatment options, and to assist in making a treatment decision.

Pediatric musculoskeletal conditions range from trivial to significant, can involve any part of the body, and can present before birth or in fully grown young adults. In addition, a full spectrum of pathophysiology includes congenital abnormalities, developmental conditions, infections, benign and malignant tumors, neurodevelopmental conditions, syndromes, genetic and metabolic diseases, inflammatory problems, and of course traumatic conditions. The children with these conditions may have developmental differences or medical comorbidities. Children are seen with parents or caregivers representing the entire spectrum of adults and the entire spectrum of family and social circumstances.

Pearl: In pediatrics, the family and caregivers are an inseparable part of evaluation of a patient.

Pitfall: Do not address the parents and ignore the patient. This is important at all ages, not just teens!

● What You Know Before Entering the Room

Most orthopedic consultations start with information in hand—sometimes considerable information. This comes from the referring physician, the medical charts, and existing imaging studies. In many cases, the definitive diagnosis may be made by reviewing radiographs or other studies before seeing the patient. *This is no way reduces the importance of taking a history and performing a clinical examination*, although it may guide the process considerably. Even if you think you know what is wrong with the patient, you need to confirm that the diagnosis you are considering matches the patient's concerns and that it is correct. Some diagnoses need to be made on the first encounter and acted on immediately to prevent the patient from further harm. These include child abuse, septic arthritis, slipped epiphysis, and malignant tumors. A table outlining key features on history and physical examination is provided (**Table 3.1**).

Pearl: Every diagnosis is a "working" diagnosis—question, confirm, and verify!

Pitfall: What is the easiest diagnosis to miss? The second one…

  Do not miss an asymptomatic contralateral slipped epiphysis.

  Do not miss a second spinal/cervical spine fracture in a trauma patient.

Table 3.1	Do Not Miss Diagnoses in Children's Orthopedics, With Key Findings on History and Physical Examination		
	HISTORY	**PHYSICAL EXAMINATION**	**OTHER**
Slipped capital femoral epiphysis	• Insidious onset of painful limp in adolescent	• Shorter stance phase • Trendelenburg lurch toward the affected side • Externally rotated foot progression • Obligatory external rotation of thigh with passive hip flexion • Pain with hip IR	• Usually more evident on lateral than anteroposterior view • Contralateral hip involved in 20% at presentation • MRI may be required for "preslip"
Child abuse	• May be inconsistent with injury seen, vague, or changing • May have multiple health care or injury visits • Developmentally disabled child • Psychosocial stressors • Unrelated adult caregiver, stepparent	• Skin injuries • Patterned injuries • Burns • Bruising • Oral injury • Genital injury • Apprehensive or hypervigilant child	• Multiple fractures • "Corner" metaphyseal fractures • Rib fractures • Skull fractures • Any pattern of long bone injury that does not fit the reported mechanism
Malignancy	• Limb pain not associated with activity • Night pain • Enlarging mass • Weight loss • Fever, unwellness, constitutional symptoms	• Deep, firm, fixed mass • Warm • Hypervascular • May be tender	• Bony destruction • Reactive bone formation
Septic arthritis (hip)	• Limb pain or disuse in an unwell child or infant	• Limb held flexed and externally rotated • Febrile • Will not weight bear • Toxic appearing • Pain with ranging hip, especially extension, IR	• High white cell count, ESR, CRP • Not all findings present in early cases

● *Who Is Who?*

Children rarely come alone and sometimes come with a considerable entourage. Introduce yourself to the child first, and tell them briefly what will happen in the visit. Then ask who is accompanying the child to introduce themselves, and establish their relationship to the child. This can be done in a confirmatory manner if the chart is open, for example say "and are you Wendy, Peter's mother?," or you may simply ask. If there are a lot of people in the room and/or relationships are unclear, just ask.

Pearl: Doctors may also come with an entourage! Introduce yourself, state your role in the team, and introduce the rest of the team who are or will be there.

Pitfall: Family structures are varied, complex, fluid, and may be unstable or dysfunctional. Know who is who!

Language

Having an interpreter present, or using a phone link to an interpreter service, is very helpful for understanding medical concepts for many people who have English as a second language. Ideally, this is arranged beforehand but now is a good time to ask if an interpreter is desired.

Pearl: In the interest of clinic efficiency, consider having a another team member articulate the assessment and plan with the aid of a translator. Let the family know you will be back at the end to confirm all questions are answered.

Pitfall: Even if a relative has come as an interpreter, it is often better to use a neutral, professional interpreter instead. Some hospitals require a certified medical translator for all of these clinics.

Developmental Delay

Developmentally delayed children *always* communicate, even if it is limited to parents interpreting gestures or expressions. Some have considerable scope for detailed expression and/or have tremendous receptive language. Address the child first, as you would a child with evidently normal development. If appropriate, then ask the caregiver how does the child communicate best. Everybody has heard of people with disabilities creating sophisticated art and literature—remember that you may be meeting such a child.

Pearl: Developmentally delayed children may have substantial ability to communicate, even if not readily apparent.

Pitfall: In families with high medical need children, the siblings can often be ignored and may spend their childhood living in the shadow of their sister or brother. Say hi to them, and engage them if only for just a short bit.

The Uncooperative/Crying/Anxious Toddler

Toddlers and behaviorally challenged children can be difficult to evaluate and anxiety (stranger danger) will demand that the clinician have a stealthy approach to examining the uncooperative or crying child. Observational examination begins as the child walks through the hall to the clinic room and may be most useful, especially with props and toys (▶ **Video 3.1**). In children with obvious fear, it may be beneficial to keep the clinic door open in order to reduce anxiety. It may be best to stand in the doorway, avoid eye contact, and completely ignore the child and talk with the parents. Many components of the examination can be passively observed and elicited by playing with child, which may also settle him or her down. When it becomes time to examine the child, engage a parent or sibling and perform a basic examination (eg, internally and externally rotating a hip) on one of these family members. Once the examination begins, always start at unaffected areas away from the site of the chief complaint. A forceful examination or examination with patient restrained by parents is not effective and potentially leads to missed diagnosis. However, be careful not to obtain insufficient information by evaluating a patient on a parent's lap (▶ **Video 3.2**).

Pearl: Remember you can have the family return at a later date in those instances where the child is completely uncooperative and the examination is critical in the decision-making process.

Pitfall: Hip internal and external rotation is best documented in the prone position, which makes toddlers nervous. You can get the same information by having the child lay supine (where they can watch you) with their knees flexed over the edge of the bed.

Chief Complaint

In older less anxious children, first ask why they have come to clinic, even if it is obvious that the parent will have to answer for them to get the real information. An engaged, interested child who feels involved often warms up and interacts more readily and without fear or apprehension. Asking a few questions like how old are you or who are your brothers and sisters will engage a younger child in a nonthreatening and familiar manner. With a teenager, we explore the chief complaint more fully *before* turning to the parent for their own perspective. After speaking with the child, ask their permission, or tell them, that you are going to ask the parent(s) some questions as well. Include both parents. Different people have different concerns. Try to find out what concern, expectation, or meaning is attached to the condition.

Pearl: Always start with the child. This is especially important with adolescents. Ask an open-ended question, and listen.

Pitfall: Some doctors cut in, take over, and direct the conversation too quickly. Do not ignore the parent's perspective.

● Clinical Strategies in the Age of Electronic Medical Records

You now have a computer in your room with your patient. It may contain substantial useful information about your patient, which may be easy or difficult to access on the fly. It is also quite likely that you need to put substantial amounts of information into the computer at some stage in the clinical encounter, whether by typing, clicking boxes, or dictating.

If there is a substantial amount of information about the current complaint from a referring provider or from relevant past history, it can be efficiently summarized for the patient/parent to confirm or ask for differences. If it is irrelevant to the current encounter, it can be ignored.

The patient or parent has also likely spent some internet time researching their condition. There is no need to be covert about this. They may be well informed, misinformed, or overinformed. Everybody knows that there is unreliable information on the internet, and most people are glad to be directed to reliable sources such as those from professional organizations, government agencies, and patient groups.

Sometimes the most difficult parents are those with a technical or scientific bent who get into the primary medical literature far enough to recognize broad gaps and inconsistencies. Accept and acknowledge when people come in with reams of information. Rather than getting into arguments or reconciliation sessions with Dr Google, we prefer to take control of the conversation, gather the clinical information we want, and be detailed and specific in giving our own interpretation—including options or controversies. A detailed letter copied to the parents allows them to go home and digest or compare information on their own.

Pearl: The computer is there to work for you and your patient. If your institution allows the use of a scribe…it is well worth it.

Pitfall: The EMR is not the center of the encounter and try to look at the patient when using it. Asking tickbox questions from EMR prevents you from hearing the patient's perspective, which is what they have come to address.

● Physical Examination

Setting the stage for a successful orthopedic examination must be considered and implemented before the visit begins and requires continued effort throughout the patient's examination.

Patient Privacy

Clinicians and support staff must be mindful of patient privacy. Health Insurance Portability and Accountability Act regulations require that sensitive patient information be appropriately protected. Regardless of the setting (waiting room, emergency department, clinic, pre/post op, fracture bay, patient room), active measures must be taken to respect patient privacy. Proper privacy improves thoroughness of the history, especially for sensitive questions, and relaxes the patient for the examination. A private examination area also allows for the parent to leave so that the clinician may speak to the patient alone if needed.

Examination Space

Preparing an adequate examination space is crucial. The table must be long enough for a supine examination. The examiner should ideally have access to both sides of the table; if the examination table is against a wall, then the patient should be asked to change head/foot position during the examination. A stool should be in the room for the physician to sit down on for parts of the examination. All necessary examination tools should be readily available including computers and light boards to review nondigital imaging with the patient. A long hallway or large examination space allows for an extended distance for observation of gait, a critical part of the musculoskeletal examination (see ▶ **Video 3.3**).

First Impressions

The clinicians and staff should focus on making a good first impression. Instruct all staff to dress modestly and appropriately for an interaction with children and families. All who interact with patients should introduce themselves and describe their role, including physicians and physician extenders, residents and other trainees, and students. An attempt should be to acknowledge and understand the relationship to the patient of all people in the room. Sit at eye level or squat down when first addressing children and speak directly to them when age-appropriate. We prefer to take a history from verbal patients directly first, and then ask follow-up questions to the parents.

Patient Modesty

The clinicians and support staff must be sensitive to patient modesty. Always knock and ask permission to enter the patient's room and then wait for a response before entering. Consider taking a history before the patient changes into a gown. When gowning, consider a gown for the front and a gown for the back. During the examination, keep the patient covered when possible. Consider an additional gown or other drape to cover the patient when the supine examination exposes private areas. Trainees and other observers should be positioned in the room to allow for proper observation but no unnecessary exposure of the patient. ALWAYS include a nurse or medical assistant of the same gender for older teens and young adults if the parent or guardian is not able to be present for the examination. Before discussing the assessment and plan, have patients redress so that they are more comfortable and able to focus better on your comments.

● *Diagnostic Tests*

Diagnostic testing in children needs special consideration. Tests that are relatively safe and easy for adults can be challenging in children given the need to stay still, fear of testing and needles, and the exponential risks of radiation exposure contributing to potential malignancy. Evaluation of musculoskeletal complaints often requires plain radiographs, utilizing advanced imaging only to identify specific diagnoses. When possible, we utilize MRI over CT or bone scan to minimize the radiation exposure, abiding by the principle of ALARA, an acronym for "as low as (is) reasonably achievable." This concept states that every reasonable effort should be made to maintain exposures to ionizing radiation as far below the dose limits as is practical to obtain diagnostic information.

The clinician must be thorough in the explanation of any recommended diagnostic tests. To begin, explain the rationale for diagnostic testing, including the purpose, benefits, and risks. Describe the physical act of the test in as simple terms as possible (eg, MRI will require you to lay in small tube for about an hour, but nothing will touch you) and inform of the patient and family about any invasive components of testing (eg, IV needed for contrast) that may be uncomfortable. For each test, the need for sedation must be considered. Additionally, explain any necessary preauthorization or referral steps the family must take before obtaining and consider having staff available to assist with scheduling and authorization.

Always discuss with the patient and the family what the possible diagnostic outcomes of the test may be, including potential serious disease processes such as malignancy if this is in the differential diagnosis. While it is easy to vague about the diagnostic possibilities, it is our practice to at least prepare the families for the most likely outcomes. The possibility of needing further testing depending on the outcome of testing should also be discussed (eg, another imaging study or a biopsy). It is preferable, when possible, to deliver the results yourself, as opposed to having a secretary or assistant read a report over the phone; serious findings should always be discussed face-to-face when possible.

Discussion of Diagnosis/Prognosis

Stating a diagnosis is the most efficient way to begin a discussion with a trained medical professional. For patients, stating the working or established diagnosis is also an excellent starting point for most discussions. However, it is important to define the diagnosis in lay terms and provide some additional information to help to frame it. People like to know how common their diagnosis is, how important it is, how it affects daily life, and whether it will worsen with time or resolve. Discussion of the meaning of the diagnosis, as well as the prognosis, is the first step to having an informed patient. If health care is to be patient-centered and patients/families are to take control of their own health, then at a minimum, they need to know what they have and what it means.

Some diagnostic terms are emotionally laden. Cerebral palsy, osteogenesis imperfecta, bone tumors, and other conditions come with many mild variants, but not every parent recognizes this. Parents may assume that a condition is progressive or severe when the diagnostic label includes a large spectrum of pathology. We prefer to use the correct diagnostic term, but immediately place the child's condition in the appropriate place along the spectrum of disease and reassure the parent that the child will be monitored closely.

Pearl: A teenager or parent should be able to tell you their diagnosis and what it means to them.

Pitfall: Some diagnostic terms are emotionally laden and patients can use these terms without knowing what they mean.

Discussion of Treatment Plan

Discussion of plans for investigation and treatment is helped by clarifying how long the patient is likely to be under care in the orthopedic clinic. We find the concept of the "clinical home" useful in framing such discussions. Some conditions will require ongoing follow-up, perhaps until maturity, while many conditions allow discharge after a treatment episode. Some conditions are primarily orthopedic, other patients have orthopedic manifestations of primary conditions which may be neurodevelopmental, metabolic, or related to other chronic conditions. Considering the orthopedic diagnosis in the context of the child's other diagnoses, and the local situation of ongoing care, allows one to determine whether the child's ongoing clinical "home" will be the orthopedic clinic and also to think about how care will be divided between different primary care providers and specialists. For example, screening ultrasounds for cardiac/renal abnormalities associated with some orthopedic conditions may be better ordered by a primary care provider or pediatrician, if that person is going to follow up on abnormal findings.

Shared Decision-Making is the cornerstone of considering, discussing, and effectuating a treatment plan. One way to frame this is to consider three separate discussions:

Team talk: "Let us work as a team to make a decision that suits your child/family."
Option talk: "Let us compare the possible options."
Decision talk: "Tell me what matters most to you for this decision."

Once an orthopedic treatment plan is made, a decision about operative treatment is often needed. This requires discussion and documentation of

- the diagnosis
- the treatment or operation proposed

- the nature of the operation—what actually happens
- the expected results of the operation—how it affects prognosis, chances of success
- material risks of the treatment proposed, including common or important complications
- alternatives to the treatment proposed, and their consequences (including no treatment)
- a discussion demonstrating that the child and parent understand the treatment decision

Parents and families usually like to discuss decisions among themselves, and then rediscuss with a surgeon—often with more specific and relevant questions. A copy of a detailed clinic letter, and a recommendation for credible online information resources, can help families have more informed discussions at home. For emergency conditions, they can be given time to discuss alone and the clinician can come back.

Many parents will bring lists of questions in first or especially subsequent clinic visits when planning treatment. You should ask for the list rather than having them read questions one at a time—that way you can scan it and make sure to discuss what is important to them first. For questions that relate to mechanics of perioperative care, make sure the right person (nurse, physio, etc) is answering these questions with sufficient detail.

Pearl: Be clear with parents which aspects of investigation and treatment belong in the orthopedic clinic and which belong elsewhere.

Pitfall: For simple conditions or decisions, the entire process may take place in a single initial clinic visit. A single visit suffices for time-dependent conditions requiring urgent operative management. However, for many conditions, the treatment decisions may take two or more clinic visits to fully discuss and clarify.

Special Circumstances

Certain diagnosis and conditions listed below will require focused consideration.

Malignancy

It is important to remember that leukemias present with musculoskeletal manifestations in about 1/3 of cases, and orthopedic surgeons may be the first to encounter the fatigued patient with bone pain. History, physical findings, plain film findings, and peripheral blood counts all provide clues to the diagnosis, which is likely to be confirmed by a bone marrow biopsy done by a hematologist.

Malignant tumors are rare in children's orthopedics and benign bone tumors are very common and a large majority of these (eg, osteochondromas) can be definitively diagnosed with imaging studies alone and most do not require biopsy. Other processes require biopsy to be certain, but are still more likely benign.

Patients with a lower probability of malignancy should wait until the biopsy is back before having extensive discussions about prognosis, treatment, and implications. Many conditions in the differential diagnosis may require simple or no treatment. If the "worst-case" scenario occurs, making a diagnosis in a timely fashion and arranging appropriate treatment are likely to yield excellent results for the vast majority of patients in high income countries in this day and age.

Having a workup for a potential malignancy is a frightening experience for parents and for children. Patients with an obvious sarcoma are often referred to a multidisciplinary clinic early in the course of the workup and have access to pediatric oncologists and support services. Focusing on treatment allows an always positive view of the future even in the case of a devastating diagnosis.

Pearl: With potential malignancies, reassure them that there is an excellent system for dealing with the "worst-case" scenario, but do not have extensive and detailed discussions when not needed.

Pitfall: Remember that parents may confuse "tumor" with "malignancy" and may be inappropriately worried about benign lesions.

Children With Chronic Conditions

Some chronic conditions that children have make a greater impact on health and even on life expectancy than do malignancies. Muscular dystrophies, neurodevelopmental conditions, and severe skeletal dysplasias may all have significant impact on the child and family's life and future.

Children with these conditions often come to the orthopedic clinic with the diagnosis already made. Confirm that the patient has appropriate pediatric care and rehabilitation access for the primary condition.

If the diagnosis is newly made in the orthopedic clinic, set up the medical and rehabilitation referrals. Discuss the overall prognosis, as well as specific orthopedic concerns. These discussions may span many visits. Allow parents' permission to ask questions at every visit, and direct them to the best place to get answers for the nonorthopaedic ones.

Multidisciplinary clinics are useful for many children with chronic or long-term conditions, especially those that require extensive rehabilitation care. Goal setting for orthopedic interventions is improved by input from rehabilitation services, and operative aftercare often involves heavy involvement of rehabilitation services. It can be tremendously useful to have the child's therapist present during clinic visits.

Pearl: In children who will likely require multiple procedures (eg, congenital short femur), it may be best to spend the first few appointments answering questions and getting to know the family and the patient. Let the treatment plan crystalize as families adjust to the challenge.

Pitfall: Avoid laying out a lifetime of treatment requirements and likely outcomes for a child with significant disability as this can overwhelm the families.

Complications

Your patients **will** have complications. Most of the time, they will be complications that you have already discussed with them in your surgical planning. This helps. Most of the time, they will be common complications without long-term significance. This also helps.

When a complication occurs, treat it as any other diagnosis. State the diagnosis, and interpret it. Provide additional information—severe or not severe, common or not, lasting or resolving—as well as discuss how you suggest treating it and what the options are. As with any other diagnosis, you want to know that the parents and patient understand, so you want to hear some of this back in their own words.

Most patients prefer the complication to be treated by the original surgeon. After all, you know the most about what went on during the initial operation, and you have a vested interest in the recovery—as does your patient! Communicate as if you are both on the same side. Yet it is advantageous to involve other surgeons or physicians in the treatment of a complication. Oftentimes it is hard to critically evaluate and appropriately intervene when you are emotionally affected. In addition, families appreciate that you are utilizing every resource to help the child. In any of these cases, it is best to remain actively involved in the care and present to the family and patient.

Pearl: When (not if) complications happen, be open, be honest, and be there with the family. They need your help and support more than ever.

Pitfall: Complications are painful and the natural response is to avoid contact with the patient and family. See them more frequently and give them 24-hour access to your phone, they need to see that you are sharing their pain.

Second Opinions

You will see patients for second opinions; some parents like to shop around for information, others are not happy with what they have heard or what has happened. There are important things to consider as the families are asking you to *judge* what has happened or been recommended and they may ask you to *treat* the child.

1. Ask the parents why they wanted a second opinion specifically.
2. Outline aspects of your opinion that are similar to the first one, and then discuss explicitly where the opinion differs and why.
3. There is no role in the consultation room for criticizing the care or the decisions made by a colleague. Avoid being judgmental, it helps to disclose that not all of your patients have fared perfectly.

It is possible to express a difference of opinion without criticizing someone else's judgment. Getting into long discussions about past decisions and "what-ifs" is rarely helpful in planning how to get a patient better. On the other hand, parents may need some degree of closure over what they perceive as an adverse event or may themselves feel guilty for. Find out what they really care about, address it objectively, and try to move the discussion to the future.

At this stage, there is an option for the parents to continue care where they started, to transfer care to you, or for shared care. Always suggest continued care with the original surgeon and that you are happy to help. Again, it is important to be open about this discussion, explicit, and objective.

Pearl: Send a letter back to the original provider. It would be very rare for the parents to object to this.

Pitfall: Do not assume that giving a second opinion means taking over care.

Difficult Parents

Few things are as distressing as watching your children lose their health—especially where there is uncertainty over the severity, duration, and consequences. Compared with the amount of stress parents go through in the clinical setting, we see surprisingly little bad behavior. Acknowledge the emotion that you see. Ask why they are upset. You may be surprised at the answer and it may have little to do with you. You may be able to help them. It is useful to document when people are angry and what they say is upsetting them. They may have a legitimate issue to be solved.

You will encounter parents who are pushy, selfish, obnoxious, unpleasant, disrespectful, demeaning of yourself or your staff, or otherwise display significantly bad behavior. If they are angry or emotionally overwrought, this may be a temporary manifestation. You cannot blame the child for the parent's behavior, and for the sake of the child, the best response to bad behavior is to ignore it. Do not move people ahead, nor punish them by making them wait longer. Do not spend more time, or less. Occasionally, you may have to "call" people on their behavior and refocus them on the task at hand which involves the care of their child.

Some parents are litigious and may sue you; if there is an open lawsuit against you, then the doctor-patient relationship no longer exists and you should not be seeing the family in the clinical setting. Sometimes a family is consulting you to gain perspective for a lawsuit against another doctor, it is better to sign a medicolegal consent and to proceed in an open manner at an appropriate time and place outside of the clinic.

Pearl: Try to remember that caring for their child is one of the most stressful things for a parent and most would gladly trade places with their child.

Pitfall: When feeling alienated by obnoxious parents, have empathy for the child who lives with it every day and who needs your help.

Conclusion

Mastering the pediatric musculoskeletal office visit takes attention, thought, and practice. Given the wide range of diagnoses, patient characteristics, and family dynamics, it is crucial to have a framework for an orthopedic visit. The clinical history and physical examination are the basis for diagnosis. However, during the visit, it is also essential to establish rapport, to convey information, to assess understanding, to advise about treatment options, and to assist in making a treatment decision.

When you enter a room, be sure to introduce yourself, state your role in the team, and introduce the rest of the team. Then ask who is accompanying the child to introduce themselves and establish their relationship to the child. The family and caregivers are an inseparable part of evaluation of a patient.

It is common in orthopedic consultation to have information before entering the examination room. This does not reduce the importance of the history and physical examination. Every diagnosis is a "working" diagnosis and needs to be continually reevaluated. Direct, thorough, and thoughtful communication is essential when discussing diagnostic tests, diagnosis, prognosis, and treatment plans.

Strategies need to be in place to optimize the use of EMR, ensure patient privacy, and provide adequate examination space. An approach with a focus on patience and planning is needed with challenging and potentially time-consuming visits, including those requiring language interpretation; patients with developmental delay, chronic conditions, malignancy, or complications; difficult and uncooperative patients and/or parents; and second opinions.

The pediatric musculoskeletal office is filled with challenges and potential pitfalls. However, using clinical pearls to develop an effective communication-based approach is as crucial to the success of an orthopedic surgeon as development of his or her surgical skills.

Observational Gait Analysis and Correlation With Static Examination

Robert M. Kay, Susan A. Rethlefsen, and Tom F. Novacheck

Introduction

Locomotion is how one moves from place to place. For most people, walking is the primary mode used for the majority of the day, and "gait" describes the pattern with which one walks. The assessment of gait is something we all do in our daily lives, both in our jobs as healthcare professionals and in the community.

Human gait is a complex movement with many components, but there are many characteristic walking patterns encountered in children and young adults. In this chapter, we will explore some of the basics of gait, how to look at gait, and how to identify some of the most common walking abnormalities seen in children.

Basics of Gait

Despite individual variations in walking pattern, there are certain underlying features of normal gait. Gage[1] described the five prerequisites of normal gait: (1) stability in stance, (2) foot clearance in swing, (3) prepositioning of the foot for initial contact, (4) adequate step length, and (5) energy conservation.

In typical gait, 80% of the gait cycle is spent in single-limb stance (one foot on the ground) and the other 20% in double-limb stance (both feet on the ground) (**Figure 4.1**). Problems which compromise

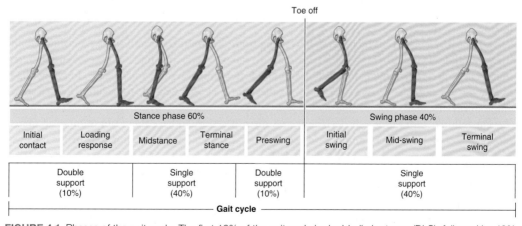

FIGURE 4.1 Phases of the gait cycle. The first 10% of the gait cycle is double-limb stance (DLS), followed by 40% single-limb stance (SLS), another 10% DLS, and the final 40% being SLS. The first 60% of the gait cycle is stance phase and the final 40%, swing phase. (From Louis ED, Mayer SA, Rowland LP. *Merritts Neurology*. Philadelphia, PA: Wolters Kluwer; 2016:Figure 14.1.)

one's stability when walking typically decrease the amount of single-limb stance on the affected side, resulting in a corresponding increase in double-limb stance.

For typical gait, the gait cycle breaks down as follows: the first 10% of the gait cycle is double-limb stance (both feet on the ground), then 40% of single-limb stance, an additional 10% of double-limb (DL) stance, and the last 40% are again single-limb (SL) stance.[1,2] Because of symmetry of the two legs in typical gait, one can think of this simply as 10-40-10-40 timing of the gait cycle (10% DL, 40% SL, 10% DL, and 40% SL). This results in each limb contacting the ground for 60% of the gait cycle (the so-called stance phase) and being in the air for the remaining 40% (so-called swing phase) (**Figure 4.1**).

Looking more closely at stance phase, based on the 10-40-10-40 timing cited above, the first 10% of the gait cycle is double-limb stance. This starts with the foot contacting the ground after being in swing. It therefore starts with initial contact. At initial contact, the hip is maximally flexed, the knee is fully extended, and the ankle is in neutral dorsiflexion. The first 10% of the gait cycle (initial contact and loading response) mainly entails the transfer of all the body weight onto this limb as the other limb is getting ready for swing phase.

The next 40% of the gait cycle is single-limb stance (called midstance and terminal stance) and basically entails progressing one's weight forward while the stance phase foot remains in contact with the ground. During midstance and terminal stance, the body is advancing over a fixed foot, resulting in progressive ankle dorsiflexion (usually to a maximum of approximately 10°) in terminal stance. By the end of terminal stance, the hip and knee are fully extended, facilitating a long step length.

The next 10% of the gait cycle (the final 10% of stance phase for this limb) is double-limb stance. This 10% is called preswing and involves the processes of readying this stance-phase limb for swing phase, which requires transferring of all the weight off this limb to the other limb. Preswing is marked by rapid hip and knee flexion so that facilitating foot clearance.

The final 40% of the gait cycle is swing phase and involves the progression of the swing phase limb. In mid- and terminal swing, there is progressive hip flexion and knee extension, also allowing limb advancement and a long step length. Swing phase ends with initial contact and the process repeats.

● Principles of Observational Gait Analysis

The most reliable observation of a child's gait is when the child does not think he/she is being watched. As healthcare providers, this puts us at a significant disadvantage.

In general, it is best to observe the child walking in a long hallway (at least 15 m long, if possible), while barefoot and wearing shorts and sometimes even taping up long shorts (to expose as much of the legs as possible). This is very important since pathology at one level in the extremity(ies) often affects other levels.

Optimally, the child is observed when walking from the front, back, and sides. Assessing stability in stance and foot clearance in swing is important. In stance, observe for hip and knee extension in terminal stance, progressive ankle dorsiflexion from mid- to terminal stance, and balance. In swing phase, observe for hip and knee flexion and ankle dorsiflexion (to at least neutral) to facilitate foot clearance and limb advancement.

For children with subtle gait deviations, it is often necessary to have them run to more accurately assess gait pathology. For very mildly involved children with hemiplegia, running may be the only way to elicit significant gait pathology (▶ **Video 4.1**).

Make sure to look at the child in his/her entirety. Asymmetry of the trunk and upper extremities may be the most evident sign of a neurologic disorder.

For children with braces, they should also be observed walking in their braces. Children who sometimes use walking aids (eg, crutches, walkers, gait trainers, etc) should be observed with and without the devices, whenever possible.

In many cases, the best data regarding someone's gait are obtained by watching the child walk toward the examining room before seeing the healthcare provider or when leaving the clinic after seeing the healthcare provider. In such circumstances, the child will walk with a more typical gait pattern for that child (since he/she is not consciously trying to perform a "clinic walk" for the medical personnel).

If there is even a remote concern for neuromuscular involvement, a few quick tests can provide useful additional information. Having the child get up from the middle of the floor and looking for a Gowers sign is often useful in young children with toe walking (▶ **Video 4.2**). Also, having a child toe walk and heel walk can be useful in assessing strength and muscle control.

For young and/or anxious children, getting them to walk may be challenging in the office environment. Having them walk toward their parents, mobile phones, tablets and/or having a ready supply of toys and/or treats may provide sufficient enticement to get even the most hesitant child to walk for you.

When assessing intoeing, it can be useful to put a sticker over the anterior patella and watch the child walk. This will help in the assessment of potential internal hip rotation during gait.

Until one has gained significant experience with observing gait, it is often best to first systematically evaluate one joint/body part at a time. For instance, one may initially focus attention at the ankle and evaluate that joint throughout the gait cycle, before turning attention to the knee, then the hip. This sequential pattern of analysis done in both the frontal and side view.

With the advances in mobile phone technology, we all typically carry a video recording device with us throughout the day. Using one's mobile phone can facilitate the evaluation of a child's gait. Numerous apps are available for mobile devices which allow for stop frame, slow motion, marking joint angles, etc (such as Coach's Eye, Dartfish, Hudl and Kinovea, among others). Health Insurance Portability and Accountability Act (HIPAA) concerns exist, however, in the use of images on unencrypted devices.

● *Observing Gait From the Side*

When observing from the side, focus on the sagittal (flexion/extension) plane of movement. There are just a few main points in the gait cycle to focus on to get a good handle on the child's gait pattern.

Looking at the pelvis can be difficult. A very helpful tip-off for anterior pelvic tilt is if there is evident lumbar lordosis (swayback) seen from the side during gait.

At the hip, there should be maximal flexion in terminal swing and initial contact. There is then progressive hip extension throughout stance until maximum hip extension occurs at terminal stance. There is then rapid hip flexion in preswing as the leg readies for swing phase.

At the knee, the main times to focus on are terminal stance and terminal swing (which are both characterized by maximal knee extension) and preswing until initial swing (rapid knee flexion) to facilitate foot clearance in swing.

The ankle has mild plantar flexion in loading response, progressive dorsiflexion in mid- to terminal stance, and then plantar flexion in preswing as the limb gets ready for swing phase. In swing phase, the ankle is basically in neutral dorsiflexion.

● *Observing From the Front and Back*

When observing from the front and back, the main planes assessed are the coronal plane (looking for abduction and adduction) and the transverse plane (rotational problems such as intoeing and outtoeing). It is important to assess the foot position as well.

Typical gait does not have much excursion in the coronal plane. The pelvis, hips, and knees only vary about 10° total throughout the gait cycle. The legs should be essentially vertical throughout the vast majority of the gait cycle.

In the transverse plane, one can assess rotation, intoeing, and outtoeing. There is mild rotation of the pelvis (slight internal rotation of the pelvis in terminal swing through loading response and mild external rotation in terminal stance). The hips rotate in the opposite direction from the pelvis—mild external rotation in terminal swing and mild internal rotation in terminal stance.

When looking at the transverse plane, one should assess the foot progression angle (FPA), ie, is the foot pointed inward or outward during gait? The average FPA is 10° to 15° external. Similarly, when evaluating gait, one should look at the knee progression angle (KPA). The KPA should be approximately neutral throughout the gait cycle. If there is a significant difference between the KPA and FPA, then there is deformity below the knee, usually tibial torsion and/or a foot deformity.

When looking at the foot from the front and back, look for abnormal positioning and weight-bearing. The foot should be in a relatively neutral position throughout the gait cycle. In valgus feet, there is excessive medial weight-bearing. For varus feet, the weight-bearing is lateral, and it is useful to assess whether this varus is continuous or in only stance or swing phase.

● Specific Gait Deviations

Some common gait deviations are seen in **Table 4.1**.

Table 4.1	Common Gait Deviations and Causes
DEVIATION	**COMMON CAUSES**
Intoeing	Excessive femoral anteversion
	Internal tibial torsion
	Metatarsus adductus
Outtoeing	External hip muscle contracture (seen in toddlers)
	External tibial torsion
	Valgus foot
	Compensation for ankle pain which decreases ankle dorsiflexion
	Compensation for foot drop
Unilateral toe walking	Hemiplegia (eg, due to cerebral palsy)
	Compensation for heel pain
	Compensation for short leg gait
Bilateral toe walking	Idiopathic toe walking
	Toe walking due to sensory processing dysfunction
	Cerebral palsy
	Duchenne muscular dystrophy
Trendelenburg gait	Childhood hip disorders (slipped capital femoral epiphysis [SCFE], developmental dysplasia of the hip [DDH], Legg-Calvé-Perthes)
	Weak hip abductors (eg, spina bifida)
Lumbar lordosis	Compensation for anterior pelvic tilt
	Weak hip extensors as in spina bifida
	Tight hip flexors
	Spine deformity
Crouch gait	Compensation for leg length discrepancy (on long leg)
	Neuromuscular diseases (eg, cerebral palsy ([CP]) or spina bifida)
Varus foot	Neuromuscular disease (eg, CP, spina bifida, Charcot-Marie-Tooth disease)
Valgus foot	Idiopathic
	Tarsal coalition
	Neuromuscular disease

● *Antalgic Gait (*▶ *Video 4.3)*

Often, when a layperson says someone is "limping," this is a reference to an antalgic gait pattern. Pain causes the individual to try to avoid putting weight on the affected limb, thus resulting in decreased time spent in stance phase on the affected limb. The child will be noted to "favor" the affected leg. Since less time is spent on the affected side, the step length on the nonpainful limb will be shortened (since there is little time on the painful limb and the attempt to avoid force in the painful limb).

An antalgic gait may be accompanied by other gait deviations. For instance, if someone has heel pain, they may walk on their tiptoes to avoid exacerbating the heel pain, while someone with pain in the forefoot may walk on their heels. Toddlers with pain below their knee may choose to crawl around the house rather than walk.

Physical examination should be correlated with the gait examination. For infants and toddlers, refusal to walk in a child who appears to crawl fine typically indicates a problem below the knee. In children who have difficulty or inability to convey the site of pain, a thorough examination of the spine, pelvis, and lower extremities is necessary to evaluate the site of pathology. The hips, knees, and ankles should be ranged and the osseous structures palpated. Decreased and painful internal hip rotation suggests the hip as the site of pathology. A positive figure-4 or FABER (hip **FL**exion, **Ab**duction, and **E**xternal **R**otation) suggest sacroiliac (SI) joint pathology. Refusal to allow spine flexion, especially in the absence of normal lumbar lordosis, suggests discitis. Referred pain to distant sites, such as to the hips and lower extremities from the spine or to the thigh and knee from the hip, should be considered as well.

● *Trendelenburg Gait (*▶ *Video 4.4)*

A Trendelenburg gait refers to a person who leans his or her body over the affected hip in stance phase. It can occur due to weakness (such as those with altered hip mechanics like abductor muscle weakness, trochanteric overgrowth, or hip displacement). Trendelenburg gait will also occur as one will shift their center of gravity to the affected side to decrease hip pain. The trunk lean to the affected hip minimizes the joint reaction force at the hip and can decrease hip pain if present. Patients with pain will not only shift the center of gravity to the affected side but will also have decreased time in stance phase (antalgic gait). Among the numerous causes of hip pain include acute infection, toxic synovitis, and the sequelae of typical childhood hip disorders (including Legg-Calvé-Perthes disease [LCPD], developmental dysplasia of the hip [DDH], and slipped capital femoral epiphysis [SCFE]).

● *Short Limb Gait (*▶ *Video 4.5)*

Common causes of short limb gait include true limb length discrepancy (LLD) or functional LLD. It is easy to understand how an anatomically shortened femur or tibia could affect gait. On physical examination, an LLD is best appreciated by having the child stand with the feet together and the knees extended. In the case of LLD, the pelvis will be tilted when the child stands in this way. The examiner can place the index finger at the top of the iliac crest on each side to easily demonstrate the discrepancy. Placement of blocks of different heights under the short leg can be done until the pelvis is level. Most patients with a significant LLD will feel that the amount of lift which is required to actually level the pelvis makes the short leg actually feel overcorrected.

Less intuitive are patients who walk with an apparently shortened limb as a result of joint pathology. A patient with a fixed knee flexion contracture or a dislocated hip will make that side seem short. Conversely, a fused knee or fixed equinus contracture will make that side seem long.

For children with a short limb gait, there are some common compensations made to functionally equalize the limb lengths during gait, thus keeping the pelvis level and decreasing the vertical excursion of the center of gravity during the gait cycle. Previous authors have reported that LLD exceeding 3.7% of limb length resulted in significant gait asymmetry.[3] The most common deviations with LLD include the following, in isolation or combination: (1) toe walking on the short side, (2) walking with a bent knee on the long side, (3) tilting the pelvis, and (4) abducting or adducting the hip.

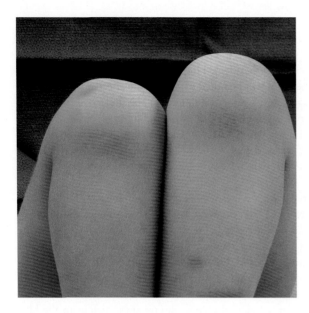

FIGURE 4.2 With the child supine and the hips flexed to 90°, a Galeazzi sign is checked. Knee height inequality, as in this case, is indicative of unilateral hip dislocation. (Image with permission of the Children's Orthopaedic Center, Los Angeles.)

Gait Deviations Associated With Hip Pathology

DDH: In a patient with a unilateral dislocated hip; the child may walk on their toe on the affected side as well as a Trendelenburg lurch as well as LLD gait. The contralateral knee may be more flexed in stance phase. In patients with unilateral DDH, they will typically have a positive Galeazzi sign (unequal knee heights when the hip and knee are flexed, **Figure 4.2**). The walking-age child with DDH will also have decreased hip abduction of the dislocated hip. For those patients with bilateral DDH, the legs will appear equal in length, and there will not be any short limb gait compensation; both hips will have limited hip abduction. They will have waddling Trendelenburg gait as a result of functional hip weakness, and they will have hyperlordosis to accommodate the hip flexion posture.

SCFE: A child with unstable SCFE has severe pain (think pain from a hip fracture) and will not bear weight on the affected side even with crutches. Gait associated with a stable slipped capital femoral epiphysis can have a combination of different gait abnormalities. These older children and adolescent patients can be in pain (and have an antalgic gait = decreased stance phase), and there is routinely a trunk lean to the affected side in stance (Trendelenburg gait). Since the hip is externally rotated throughout the gait cycle, there is an external foot progression (as well as external knee progression). Children with SCFE typically can't get the hip into a trailing position in terminal stance. Since approximately 10% to 20% of children with SCFE present with bilateral SCFE, this gait pattern may be evidenced bilaterally. For a child with SCFE, physical examination is most notable for obligate external hip rotation when the affected hip is flexed (**Figure 4.3**). Hip flexion and hip abduction are typically decreased in patients with SCFE.

LCPD: Children with LCPD will also have a Trendelenburg gait due to associated hip pain and, typically, hip abductor weakness. Their rotation is more neutral, but they often have trouble getting the hip into a trailing position. These children are typically younger than those with SCFE (often 5-8 years), with a preponderance of males. In LCPD, hip internal rotation and abduction are routinely decreased and cause discomfort.

Duchenne Muscular Dystrophy (▶ Video 4.6)

Duchenne muscular dystrophy (DMD) is the most common muscular dystrophy seen in children. As an x-linked recessive gene, it occurs almost exclusively in males and affects approximately 1 in every 3000 male births.

Initially, the first clues of the disease may be a delay in walking and new-onset toe walking. The calves are enlarged (pseudohypertrophy) in the vast majority of these children but not all.

The gait deviations in DMD have been well described.[4] Early on, there may be few changes in gait, other than decreased ankle dorsiflexion and mildly increased hip flexion during gait. As the disease

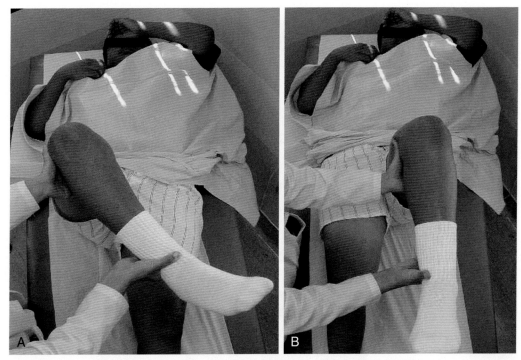

FIGURE 4.3 A, Obligate external rotation typical in slipped capital femoral epiphysis (SCFE) as the right hip is flexed. The examiner flexes the hip, while attempting to maintain neutral rotation, but the hip falls involuntarily into external rotation. B, In contrast, the left hip flexes and remains in neutral rotation since this child did not have an SCFE on the left. (Images A and B with permission of the Children's Orthopaedic Center, Los Angeles.)

progresses, the children have hip abductor weakness and walk with a broad base with increased shoulder movement and waddling-bilateral Trendelenburg gait. As a result of decreased hip extensor power, they will also develop progressive anterior pelvic tilt with significant lumbar lordosis as well. These children will often have significant difficulty getting up from the floor or from a chair and often find climbing onto the examination table difficult. Physical examination shows diffuse weakness of the upper and lower extremities. Weakness is greater proximally than distally. More than 80% of these children have pseudohypertrophy of the calves, with large, firm calves, despite calf weakness. Early loss of dorsiflexion range on physical examination of the ankles is typical. A Gowers sign is classic as these children "walk up" their legs as they rise from the floor (**Figure 4.4**).

Ataxic Gait (▶ Video 4.7)

Children with a variety of neuromuscular disorders may walk with an ataxic gait. An ataxic gait is characterized by lack of balance and coordination of movements. These children are often "shaky" and typically walk with a broad base (feet far apart). Because of their instability during walking, most of the gait cycle is spent with both feet on the ground, resulting in very slow and labored gait. Physical examination shows difficulty with multiple tests. The Romberg test will show instability. The child will also have difficulty with finger-to-nose testing and rapid alternating movements. Nystagmus is often evident as well.

Intoeing/Outtoeing

Many children are brought to healthcare professionals due to family concerns of their feet turning in or out during gait. In most instances, there is no associated pain or functional deficit. The main things to assess and to compare are both the FPA and the KPA. Think about the FPA as the sum total of rotational

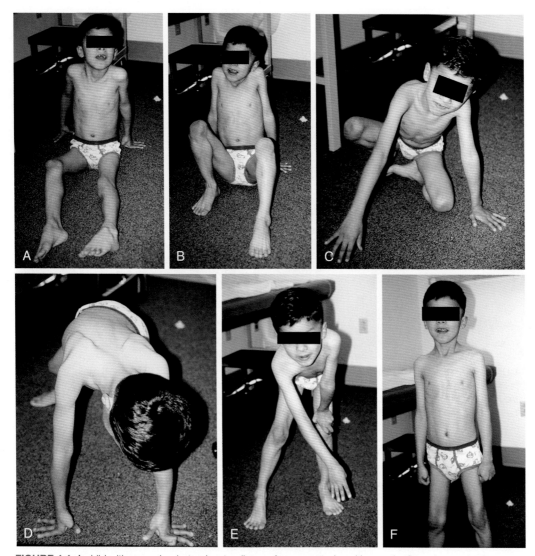

FIGURE 4.4 A child with muscular dystrophy standing up from a seated position on the floor, demonstrating a positive Gowers sign as he has to "climb up" his legs to a standing position due to proximal muscle weakness. (Images A-F with permission of the Children's Orthopaedic Center, Los Angeles.)

profile of the lower limb. For instance, let us assume the child's foot is normal; if the patient has a positive or negative FPA and KPA is neutral (which is normal), then the rotation is coming from below the knee with likely tibial torsion. If the FPA and the KPA are internal, then at least some of the internal rotation is coming from above the knee with likely excessive femoral anteversion. On occasion, a child will walk with a neutral FPA despite having significant internal KPA; in this case, the child must have compensatory external tibial torsion that compensates for femoral torsion. In patients with concordant knee pain, this alignment has been termed miserable malalignment.

Physical examination can quickly differentiate the various common causes of intoeing. In children who like to "W sit" (**Figure 4.5**), excessive femoral anteversion is typical. With the child in the prone position, the hips are internally and externally rotated. A significant difference in hip rotation (eg, much more internal than external rotation) is consistent with excessive femoral torsion (**Figure 4.6**). With the child still in the prone position, the thigh foot angle is checked and transmalleolar angle may also be

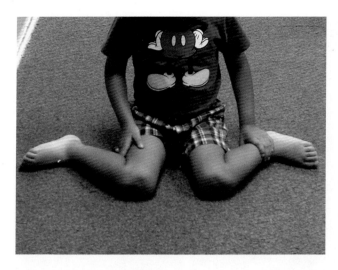

FIGURE 4.5 A child with femoral anteversion sitting in the "W position." (Image with permission of the Children's Orthopaedic Center, Los Angeles.)

checked prone or sitting (**Figure 4.7**). If this is significantly internal or external (normal is ~10° external), then there is tibial torsion. The borders of the feet are checked and should be straight. If the medial border of the foot is curved inward, then the intoeing is likely due, at least in part, to metatarsus adductus or a varus foot.

Cerebral Palsy

Cerebral palsy (CP) is the most common motor disease of childhood and affects 1 in every 300 to 400 children. Most children with CP walk (either with or without assistive devices), and there are many well-described gait deviations associated with CP, depending on the child's function and degree of involvement.[5-9] In these patients, it is important to look at all levels of the lower extremities when assessing gait. Some common gait deviations are discussed below.

Crouch (▶ Video 4.8)

In general terms, when someone walks with bent knees, they are referred to as having "crouch gait." There are three main types of "crouch gait," which vary based on the status and the position of ankle, knee, and hip during gait.[10] In calcaneal crouch (or "true" crouch), the ankles are bent excessively up

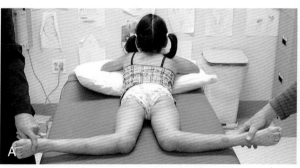
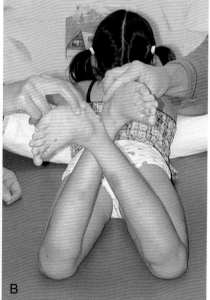

FIGURE 4.6 Marked asymmetry of hip internal rotation (A) and external rotation (B) in the prone position in this child with marked femoral anteversion. (Images A and B with permission of the Children's Orthopaedic Center, Los Angeles.)

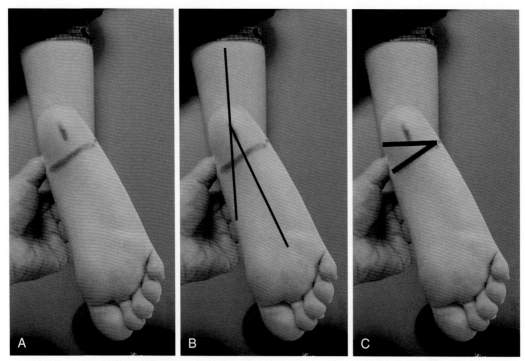

FIGURE 4.7 A, Short longitudinal mark and a longer transverse mark on the foot of a child whose torsional profile is being checked. B, The image shows how the thigh foot angle (TFA) is measured between a longitudinal axis down the femur and the longitudinal axis of the foot. C, Measurement of the transmalleolar angle as the angle subtended by a line along the axis between the malleoli and a second through the transverse axis of the knee. (Images A-C with permission of the Children's Orthopaedic Center, Los Angeles.)

(usually due to triceps surae weakness) and the hip and knee must compensate to a flexed position to keep the child upright. In these children, with the ankles bent excessively upward, the potential of functional long-term walking is very limited without stabilizing the excessive dorsiflexion of the foot. In apparent equinus crouch, the knee is primarily flexed due to muscle or joint contracture. The ankle does not dorsiflex excessively, but is in a neutral position. If this child were able to get the knee extended "normally" in stance phase, then he/she would not be toe walking. The third type of crouch is called jump gait. In this form of crouch, the child walks on his toes due to a combination of ankle equinus (plantar flexion), and the child's knee being excessively flexed for some, if not all of the gait cycle. In those in whom the knee extends essentially fully in terminal stance, it is excessively flexed from at least the end of swing phase through a portion of stance phase. On physical examination, the lower extremities are checked for spasticity and range of motion. Specifically, the ankles are checked for range of motion (amount of dorsiflexion) with the knee flexed and extended. Tightness with the knee flexed indicates a greater degree of tightness (with involvement of both the gastrocnemius and the soleus muscles). Hamstring range of motion and knee flexion contractures are checked as well. If the hamstrings and knee are not tight, but the patient has crouch gait, then the source of the knee flexion during gait is at a level other than the knee.

● "Scissor" Gait (▶ Video 4.9)

Though there is mild "tilt" of the pelvis during walking, the thighs remain in a relatively vertical position during walking. The tight groin muscles (adductors) are often overactive in cerebral palsy. This results in the leg(s) crossing the midline while walking and the child "scissors." Seen from the front or back, the child is noted to have his legs cross the midline of his/her body, which often interferes with the ability of the other leg to progress without catching on the first leg. Physical examination entails checking for hip abduction with the hips in flexion and in extension. The hips are typically significantly tighter in this patient population with the hips extended, the position in which we typically walk.

Toddler With Hemiplegia

Most children with spastic diplegia of variable severity have significant delays in motor milestones which alert the family and the providers to a diagnosis of developmental delay. Children with mild hemiplegia often walk independently before 18 to 24 months of age, and a diagnosis of cerebral palsy is often delayed. When walking, they may walk on their toes, or their gait may appear near normal. Having them run often accentuates the abnormalities of gait (▶ **Video 4.1**). In particular, running often results in the child "posturing" with the affected arm. In such situations, the child typically holds the elbow (and often the wrist) in a flexed position.

Physical examination may not demonstrate any fixed contractures. It is important to assess the tone of the muscles. The pronators are often spastic, and they can be tested by grasping the child's hand and rapidly pronating and supinating the forearm; this will often reveal even subtle spasticity. Fine motor control is often quite limited, and trying to get the child to use the nondominant hand to grasp for objects is helpful. Remember to ask the parents about when the child demonstrated hand dominance or hand preference; this should NOT be evident before 2 to 3 years of age.

Stiff Knee Gait (▶ Videos 4.4 and 4.10)

One of the prerequisites of normal gait is foot clearance in swing. Normally, the hip and knee rapidly flex in preswing and initial swing to allow the foot to clear the floor in swing phase. Unfortunately, many ambulatory children with cerebral palsy have a stiff knee in swing phase which interferes with foot clearance in swing. The stiff knee makes the leg seem longer functionally in swing phase. This typically results in dragging the toes and tripping. This tripping is exacerbated in children who also have equinus in swing phase. The prone rectus (or Duncan-Ely) test can help demonstrate rectus femoris spasticity. The child is placed in the prone position and the knee flexed rapidly by the examiner. An ipsilateral hip rise indicates rectus spasticity and may implicate this muscle in knee stiffness in swing.

Equinus Gait

Equinus gait refers to the ankle being in a plantarflexed (downward) position during gait and may be a component in crouch gait described above. There are various patterns of equinus, and physical examination of the ankle is important to be certain whether the ankle is in a position of fixed equinus or spastic equinus and thus in plantar flexion in both swing and stance phase. In some children, the ankle equinus is not fixed or has a spastic component and only drops into equinus during swing phase (when the foot is in the air). This is the so-called "drop foot" in swing and can be a result of weakened ankle dorsiflexors. Some children have severe drop foot and have to rapidly hyperflex the knee and hip during swing phase to clear the foot; another term for this is called a "steppage gait" (▶ **Video 4.11**). If a child with a steppage gait is provided with an appropriate brace which controls the drop foot, the compensatory hip and knee flexion will typically resolve.

In other children, the equinus occurs throughout the gait cycle, so they walk on their toes throughout stance phase, and the ankle is also in equinus in swing (when the foot is in the air). On visual gait assessment, observers tend to overestimate equinus.[11] The child has to accommodate the equinus and can do so in two ways. Primarily, this is accommodated in stance phase by flexing the knee as seen in crouch gait described above; this is common in cerebral palsy as patients may have concurrent hamstring contracture which also promotes knee flexion. Alternatively, the ground reaction force moves anteriorly and the equinus may be associated with an ipsilateral knee extensor thrust and/or knee hyperextension during gait (▶ **Video 4.10**). This is called a "back-knee gait," and the knee will often be seen to "snap back" in stance phase, typically at a time when the ankle is in a significant amount of equinus.

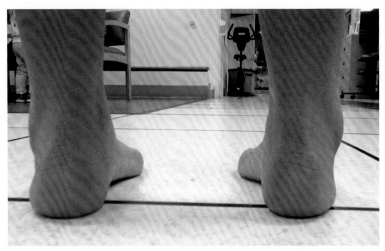

FIGURE 4.8 Picture from behind showing a varus hindfoot on the right but not the left, with the heel being medial to the weight-bearing axis of the tibia on the right but not the left. (Image with permission of the Children's Orthopaedic Center, Los Angeles.)

Equinovarus Foot Gait

Equinovarus gait is the combination of equinus (as described above) and varus of the hindfoot. Varus refers to the position when walks on the lateral border of the foot and can be due to contracture or spasticity of the tibialis posterior or tibialis anterior. By walking on the lateral border of the foot, less of the foot surface area contacts the ground and the child is less stable when he/she walks. In addition to the findings regarding equinus gait, the instability which results from the child walking on the lateral border of the foot causes the child to spend relatively little time in single-limb stance phase (less time with only the equinovarus foot) compared to usual and more time with both feet on the ground than other children. The heel (calcaneus) is medial to the weight-bearing axis of the tibia when there is a varus foot (**Figure 4.8**). In some children, the varus positioning will be present throughout the entire walking (gait) cycle, while in others, it occurs in stance or swing phase. On physical examination, calf contracture and/or spasticity is assessed as noted above. It is important to assess the rigidity of the varus deformity. The foot can be grasped and manipulated toward a valgus position. If the varus of the foot can be fully corrected, and overcorrected into valgus, then the deformity is flexible. The confusion test can also be performed in order to determine if the anterior tibialis is contributing to the varus positioning. The child is instructed to flex his hip actively; the tibialis anterior usually fires (due to a mass action pattern) and if the foot supinates, then the anterior tibialis is deemed to be a contributing factor to the varus foot (▶ Video 4.12).

Valgus Foot Gait

Flatfeet or planovalgus feet can lead to outtoeing and can be a result of connective tissue disorders such as Marfan syndrome or Ehlers-Danlos syndrome. Children with fixed equinus contractures can get midfoot collapse which leads to valgus hindfoot. Valgus foot position/outtoeing may also be seen in patients with tarsal coalition.

Conclusion

The underpinnings of understanding pathologic gait are based on the understanding of typical gait. The 10-40-10-40 framework of the gait cycle provides a scaffold upon which to build an understanding of gait. The ability to assess a child's walking is a critical portion of the assessment of children with many disorders of childhood. Abnormal gait may be the first sign leading to an accurate diagnosis of an underlying disorder (such as toe walking in a young child with DMD) or may be the manifestation of a much simpler disorder (eg, unilateral toe walking following a calcaneal stress injury in a toddler). Observational gait analysis often provides many useful clues to the underlying pathology and will greatly assist in the diagnostic matrix.

References

1. Gage JR. *Gait Analysis in Cerebral Palsy*. Oxford, UK: MacKeith Press; 1991.
2. Perry J, Burnfield JM. *Gait Analysis: Normal and Pathological Function*. 2nd ed. Thorofare, NJ: SLACK Incorporated; 2010.
3. Kaufman KR, Miller LS, Sutherland DH. Gait asymmetry in patients with limb-length inequality. *J Pediatr Orthop*. 1996;16(2):144-150.
4. Sutherland DH, Olshen R, Cooper L, et al. The pathomechanics of gait in Duchenne muscular dystrophy. *Dev Med Child Neurol*. 1981;23(1):3-22.
5. Davids JR, Bagley AM. Identification of common gait disruption patterns in children with cerebral palsy. *J Am Acad Orthop Surg*. 2014;22(12):782-790.
6. Gage JR, Schwartz MH, Koop SE, Novacheck TF. *The Identification and Treatment of Gait Problems in Cerebral Palsy*. 2nd ed. London: MacKeith Press; 2009.
7. Kay RM. Lower-extremity surgery in children with cerebral palsy. In: Skaggs DL, Kocher MS, eds. *Master Techniques in Orthopaedic Surgery*. 2nd ed. Philadelphia: Wolters Kluwer; 2016:149-192.
8. Novacheck TF, Trost JP, Sohrweide S. Examination of the child with cerebral palsy. *Orthop Clin North Am*. 2010;41(4):469-488.
9. Rethlefsen SA, Blumstein G, Kay RM, Dorey F, Wren TA. Prevalence of specific gait abnormalities in children with cerebral palsy revisited: influence of age, prior surgery, and Gross Motor Function Classification System level. *Dev Med Child Neurol*. 2017;59(1):79-88.
10. Rodda J, Graham HK. Classification of gait patterns in spastic hemiplegia and spastic diplegia: a basis for a management algorithm. *Eur J Neurol*. 2001;8(suppl 5):98-108.
11. Wren TA, Rethlefsen SA, Healy BS, Do KP, Dennis SW, Kay RM. Reliability and validity of visual assessments of gait using a modified physician rating scale for crouch and foot contact. *J Pediatr Orthop*. 2005;25(5):646-650.

Diagnostically Directed Examination for Neurological Disorders

M. Wade Shrader and A. Noelle Larson

Introduction

Patients with neurological conditions present with discrete physical examination findings. Pattern recognition is important for diagnosis and treatment. Although in many instances, the condition is evident at birth, other presentations may be subtle and are identified by the orthopedic surgeon in infancy, childhood, or even adolescence. Thus, a basic neurologic examination should be routinely performed for all patients, especially those presenting with gait disturbance or spinal complaints. Further, pattern recognition and familiarity with common presentations is needed to promptly diagnose specific disease entities and conditions.

Cerebral Palsy

With an incidence of 2 to 4 per 1000 live births, cerebral palsy (CP) is the most common motor disability of childhood. CP is a static encephalopathy characterized by an upper motor neuron disease that causes abnormality in muscle tone, selective motor control, strength, balance, and coordination. Typically caused by an ischemic event, the most common etiology today is periventricular leukomalacia (PVL) from prematurity. Hypoxic birth events and intrauterine strokes are less common but constitute a small percentage of patients with CP. Although the neurological injury is static and does not change over time, the effects of time, growth, and developmental delay along with the abnormal muscle tone make the clinical picture of CP quite variable over a child's growth. One common way to characterize severity is with the Gross Motor Functional Classification System (GMFCS) (**Figure 5.1**), which is reliable and repeatable over time and correlates closely with other measures of function. In this system a patient is classified as follows: **Level I:** walks and runs without difficulty; **Level II:** walks; no aids; needs support for stairs or uneven ground; **Level III:** walks with aids (canes, walker); **Level IV:** stands or weight bears for transfers with assistance; predominately uses wheelchair for mobility; and **Level V:** no functional weight bearing; wheelchair for mobility.

Other neurological conditions mimicking a CP-like condition include perinatal infections with subsequent encephalopathy, congenital brain malformations (such as Dandy-Walker syndrome or agenesis of the corpus callosum), postnatal hypoxic events (like nonaccidental trauma or near drowning), or certain chromosomal disorders. Hereditary spastic paraplegia may have a similar presentation as CP, but patients experience progressive spasticity in the legs only.[1] These "CP-like" conditions are subtly different than the typical ex-preemie with PVL or a child with perinatal hypoxic event, but the majority of the clinical features of these disorders can be grouped together with CP, and significant efforts should not be expended to parse those patients away from a typical CP-clinic environment.

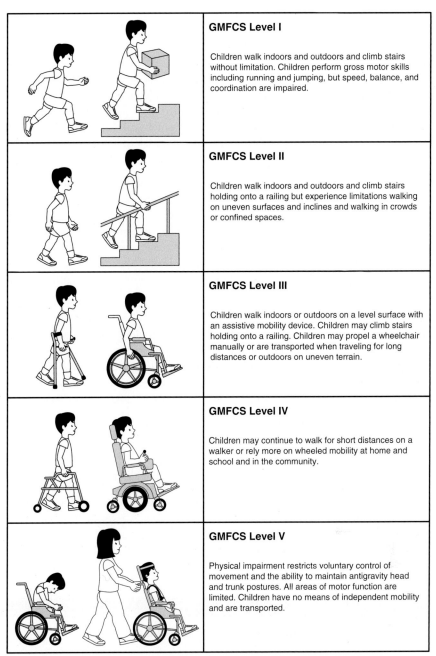

GMFCS Level I

Children walk indoors and outdoors and climb stairs without limitation. Children perform gross motor skills including running and jumping, but speed, balance, and coordination are impaired.

GMFCS Level II

Children walk indoors and outdoors and climb stairs holding onto a railing but experience limitations walking on uneven surfaces and inclines and walking in crowds or confined spaces.

GMFCS Level III

Children walk indoors or outdoors on a level surface with an assistive mobility device. Children may climb stairs holding onto a railing. Children may propel a wheelchair manually or are transported when traveling for long distances or outdoors on uneven terrain.

GMFCS Level IV

Children may continue to walk for short distances on a walker or rely more on wheeled mobility at home and school and in the community.

GMFCS Level V

Physical impairment restricts voluntary control of movement and the ability to maintain antigravity head and trunk postures. All areas of motor function are limited. Children have no means of independent mobility and are transported.

FIGURE 5.1 The Gross Motor Function Classification System (GMFCS) allows caregivers to quantitate the functional ambulatory ability of children with cerebral palsy. (Used with permission from Palisano RJ, Rosenbaum P, Walter S, Russell D, Wood E, Galuppi B: Development and reliability of a system to classify gross motor function in children with cerebral palsy. *Dev Med Child Neurol.* 1997;39(4):214-223. Illustrated by Kerr Graham and Bill Reid, The Royal Children's Hospital, Melbourne.)

Specific Physical Examination Findings

Neurological Examination

Spasticity—Ashworth Scale

The Ashworth scale is the most common method to quantify increased motor tone. This scale is a manual scale that evaluates resistance of motion of a specific joint (**Table 5.1**). The original scale was only designed to measure hypertonicity or spasticity. The modified scale allows the examiner to document hypotonia, which can be found in children with CP. This common scale is unfortunately very subjective and at times difficult for the examiner to differentiate overall muscle stiffness from spasticity.[3]

Deep Tendon Reflexes

The Babinski sign is a test to determine an upper motor brain lesion, which is common in CP. The lateral side of the foot is rubbed with a relatively sharp, but blunt instrument, and it is run from the heel along a curve to the toes. A normal flexor response, the toes flex in response. An extensor, or abnormal response, the big toe extends, and the other toes fan out. This is a positive sign that indicates an upper motor neuron deficit (brain or spinal cord). Deep tendon reflexes (DTRs) in the child with CP may be markedly abnormal. For those patients with significant hypertonicity, the DTRs will likely be brisk and abnormal. Along with the increased DTRs, the patient may have significant ankle clonus with sustained beats.

Dystonia

Dystonia is a movement disorder that has a torsional component along with muscle contractions with recurrent major movement patterns. Dystonia may occur in a single limb, in a single joint, or as a whole-body generalized movement pattern. Dystonia is a movement disorder that is very common in CP. Although patients may have a primary spastic pattern of CP, there are some common elements of underlying dystonia. Dystonia can be measured using the Hypertonia Assessment Tool.[4]

● Hip

Children with CP are at risk for progressive hip displacement, and this can lead to stiffness; limited motion; difficulty with sitting and perianal cares; and possibly pain from late arthrosis. The rate of hip displacement increases with the clinical severity; for instance, patients who have spastic quadriplegia who are nonambulatory (GMFCS V) may have hip subluxation/dislocation in 75% of cases. The hip examination in children with CP is a crucial part of the physical assessment. Attention to detail and reproducible measurements is vital to help determine changes in the pathophysiology and can help predict which patients are prone to hip displacement even before hip radiographs are obtained.

Table 5.1	Ashworth Scale
SCORE	**DESCRIPTION OF THE MUSCLE TONE**
00	Hypotonia
0	Normal tone
1	Slight increase (slight catch and release or minimal resistance to joint ROM)
1+	Slight increase (slight catch and minimal increased resistance to joint ROM for more than half the joint range)
2	More marked increase through most of the whole joint range, but affected joint is easily moved
3	Considerable increase (passive movement difficult but possible)
4	Joint cannot be moved

General Examination

Range of motion is assessed in all planes: flexion-extension, internal-external rotation, and abduction-adduction. Sagittal plane motion (flexion and extension) is best measured in the supine position, with the limb of interest slightly off the edge of the table so you can determine true extension. Many children with CP will have hip flexion contractures, which is masked by compensatory lumbar lordosis. In these cases, the Thomas test is performed as described below.

Rotation is best measured prone, where the examiner can truly determine the rotational profile of the entire lower extremity including the tibia. With care taken to keep the pelvis neutral and level, the knee is flexed to 90°, rotated outwardly to the maximal excursion to measure hip internal rotation, and rotated inwardly to measure hip external rotation (**Figure 5.2**).

15 Degrees Internal Rotation   85 Degrees Internal Rotation

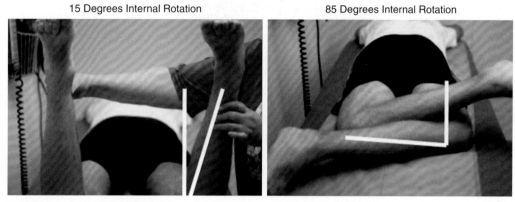

FIGURE 5.2 Hip internal and external rotation is best assessed in the prone position. This child has 15° of right hip internal rotation with 85° of external rotation.

Hip Abduction

The measurement of hip abduction is especially important in CP; patients with severe limited hip abduction are considered at risk for hip displacement and radiographs are indicated (**Figure 5.3**).

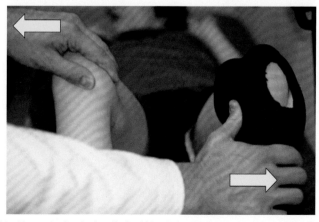

FIGURE 5.3 This child with cerebral palsy has limited hip abduction in the supine position. These hips are at risk for displacement and a radiograph should be obtained to assess hip status.

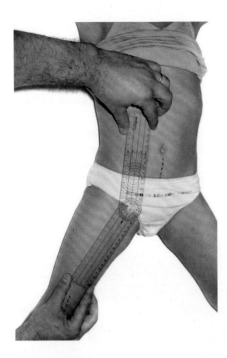

FIGURE 5.4 A goniometer can be used to quantitate the amount of hip abduction, usually with the hip extended. (Figure provided by Dr. Ismat Ghanem.)

Hip abduction can be measured with a goniometer with the hips and knees extended in order to isolate the effects of hamstring tightness on abduction (**Figure 5.4**). While abduction in extension, the examiner should have his/her hand on the pelvis to make sure there is no coronal plane pelvic rotation. Asymmetric hip abduction should be a warning sign to the examiner of the higher risk of hip dysplasia and should trigger an anteroposterior (AP) pelvis radiograph.

The spasticity of the hip adductors can be an important factor when measuring hip abduction. For this reason, two measurements of hip abduction with knee/hip flexion is important to measure: the modified Tardieu joint angles, R1 and R2. R1 is the measurement of hip abduction in a fast, initial movement of maximum attempted hip abduction; the maximum hip abduction will be halted by the catch or clonus that is the hallmark of spasticity. R2 is the second measurement with a slower, more gradual hip abduction maneuver. This allows the examiner to account some of the effect of true spasticity on this important angular measurement.

Galeazzi Sign

The difference in apparent limb length with the hips and knees flexed to 90° is a positive Galeazzi sign (**Figure 5.5**). Usually, this indicates significant hip dysplasia and possible hip dislocation, and the examiner should ensure that an AP pelvis radiograph is obtained.

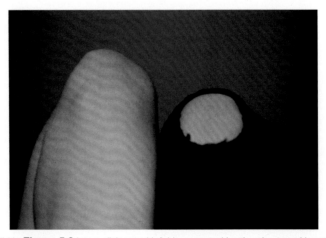

FIGURE 5.5 The child in **Figure 5.3** has a dislocated left hip as noted by the shortened length of the femur, otherwise known as a positive Galeazzi sign.

Thomas Test and Modified Thomas Test

Hip flexion contracture is a common pathology in ambulatory CP; yet it can be hard to detect as pelvic and lumbar lordosis can mask a true hip flexion contracture. The Thomas test can be performed to detect and measure a hip flexion contracture. With the patient supine on the examination table, the contralateral limb is flexed to the chest, and the examiner attempts to fully extend the opposite limb. When the examiner is holding the opposite knee to the chest, it flattens out the lumbar lordosis and keeps the pelvis relatively stable. If a hip flexor contracture (usually iliopsoas) is present on the other side, the affected limb will not be able to lay flat on the examination table (**Figure 5.6**). Examination tip: The examiner must remember that many patients who are being tested for hip flexion contractures can have concurrent knee flexion contractures which can prevent the leg from lying flat during the Thomas test and thus imply that there is a flexion contracture. In these patients, the hip to be tested for hip flexion contracture should have the leg and foot hanging over the edge of the bed.

On occasion, the rectus femoris muscle can contribute to hip flexion contracture (**Figure 5.7A**) and can be suspected when the rectus tendon is well defined and easily palpated from the rest of the quadriceps tendon above the patella (**Figure 5.7B**). Rectus tightness becomes highly suspected when the affected limb is taken off of the table and the knee does not fully flex with gravity (**Figure 5.7C**); rectus tightness is confirmed when further knee flexion (modified Thomas test) causes the hip to flex (**Figure 5.7D**).

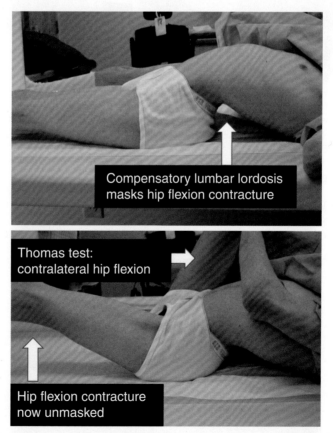

FIGURE 5.6 In the top panel, the child's legs lay flat on the bed and a hip flexion contracture is accommodated by the compensatory lumbar lordosis. The Thomas test is used in the lower panel to assess for hip flexion contracture: by flexing the hip, the opposite hip flexion contracture is now unmasked.

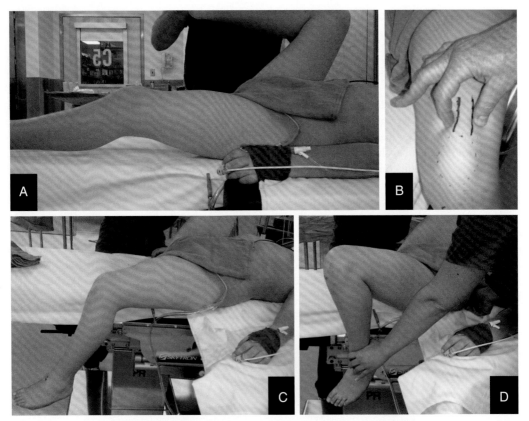

FIGURE 5.7 A hip flexion contracture can be due to psoas and/or the rectus femoris tightness. In Panel A, this patient has a positive Thomas test. In Panel B, the clinician is palpating a very tight rectus femoris tendon which could be the cause of the contracture. In Panel C, the clinician allows the leg to hang over the side of the bed. The fact that the thigh can lay flat implies the psoas is not the cause of the hip flexion contracture. When the knee is flexed in Panel D, tightening the quadriceps, there is further hip flexion, confirming the rectus femoris is tight.

Craig Test to Assess Femoral Anteversion

Although most normal adults have some amount of femoral anteversion (around 15°-20°), many patients with CP have excessive femoral anteversion (>45°) and are noted with significantly more internal rotation than external rotation in the prone position (**Figure 5.8**). The test to measure femoral anteversion

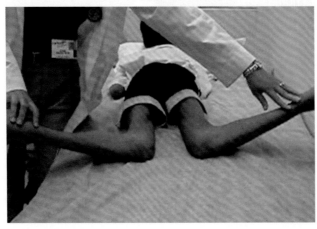

FIGURE 5.8 This child with spastic diplegia has excessive femoral anteversion, as noted by internal rotation of the hip to 80°.

Craig test:
quantitate anteversion

Rotate limb until trochanter is most prominent

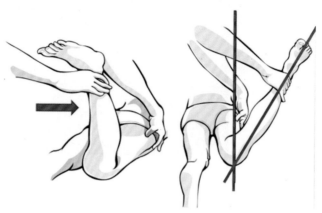

FIGURE 5.9 The Craig test allows one to estimate anteversion: The hip is internally rotated until the greater trochanter is most prominent. The angle of the femur to a perpendicular line suggests the amount of anatomic anteversion of the femoral neck in relation to the shaft of the femur.

is also known as the Craig test. The patient's hip and knee are flexed to 90° of flexion. The examiner rotates the hip medially and laterally, while palpating the greater trochanter area, until the outward most point is found in the lateral aspect of the hip (the greater trochanter is parallel to the table at this point) (**Figure 5.9**). In individuals with severely limited hip motion, this examination may be difficult. The examiner then measures the angle of the hip to determine the amount of anteversion, using the long axis of the tibia.

Unique Hip Positions

In most patients with CP, there is a predominance of increased tone and contractures of the psoas and adductor tendons and the leg is flexed and adducted. With this pattern the hip can become dislocated, and in these instances the hip is usually dislocated in a posterior-superior direction (**Figure 5.10**). In

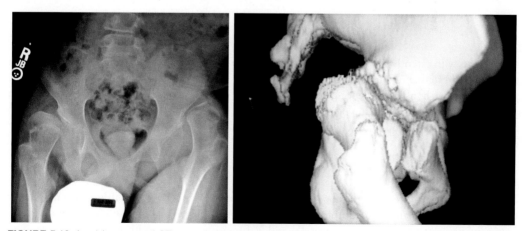

FIGURE 5.10 A pelvis x-ray and CT scan demonstrate superior and posterior displacement of the proximal femur in this child with spastic quadriplegia who is a GMFCS Level V. Most hip displacements in these patients are in this direction as a result of hip flexion and adduction contractures.

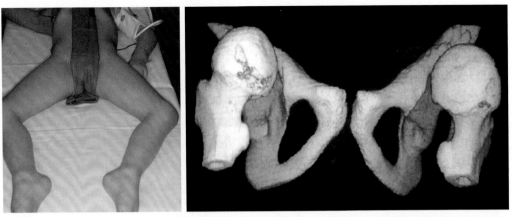

FIGURE 5.11 This child has rare anterior dislocations of the femoral heads. On the clinical picture to the left, one can note the prominences of the femoral head in the groin. In contrast to the prior patient in **Figure 5.10**, this child has hip abduction and extension contractures. The CT scan demonstrates the femoral head to be dislocated anteriorly.

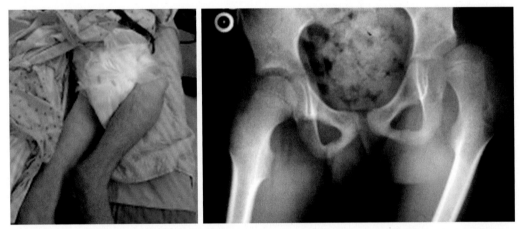

FIGURE 5.12 A windswept hip deformity is noted clinically by having one hip abducted and the contralateral hip is adducted. The adducted hip is prone to hip displacement as noted in the pelvis x-ray.

rare patients with extensive tone in the hamstrings and hip extensor muscles, the hips are abducted with extension and external rotation. In some of these patients, the hip can be displaced anteriorly and these patients will have bony prominence palpable in the groin (**Figure 5.11**). Finally, in some patients with asymmetric tone, a windswept hip positioning (sometimes this is an iatrogenic problem from treatment) can occur with one hip abducted while the other hip is adducted (and at this latter hip) and is at risk for dislocation (**Figure 5.12**).

● *Knee*

The knee examination is typically focused on ambulatory patients with CP, although nonambulators may have important knee pathology, as well, such as patellar instability and fixed contractures. Typically, patients with GMFCS Levels IV and V function tolerate mild to moderate knee flexion contractures, and treatment for these contractures that do not interfere with quality of life is unnecessary.

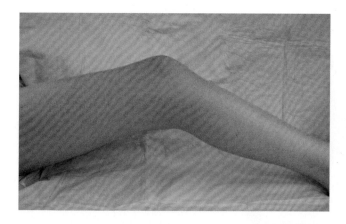

FIGURE 5.13 This child has a knee flexion contracture approaching 30°. The knee flexion contracture is assessed with the hip extended to remove any effect from hamstring tightness.

General Examination

The knee examination in CP usually is focused on range of motion. There is rarely ligamentous instability in CP, but a general stability examination of the knee joint should be performed. It is important to determine active and passive ROM and further to understand the difference between tight hamstrings and knee flexion contractures. CP patients with tight hamstrings may have knees that can fully extend (no knee flexion contracture); but all CP patients with knee flexion contractures (**Figure 5.13**) have tightened hamstrings. Rarely patients can have severe quadriceps spasticity and muscle tightness that lead to extension contractures (inability to flex the knee) (**Figure 5.14**). These are rare patterns and can be seen in patients with total brain injury that occur postnatally (near drowning patients).

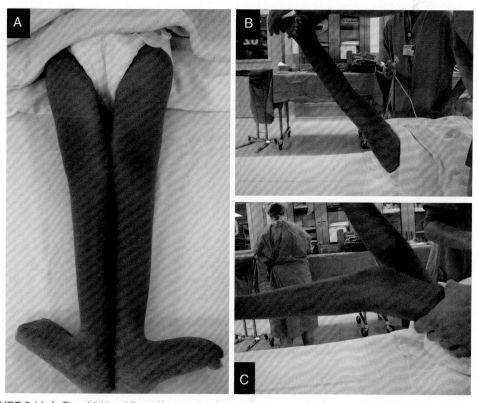

FIGURE 5.14 A, The child has bilateral knee extension contractures and calcaneus foot deformity. B, Knee hyperextension is noted on exam. C, There is also restricted knee flexion.

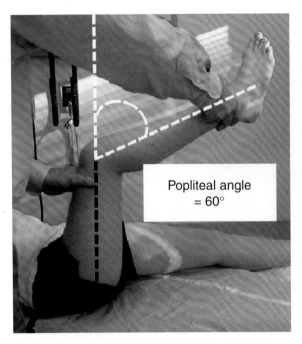

Popliteal angle = 60°

FIGURE 5.15 The popliteal angle allows one to quantitate the amount of hamstring tightness. With the patient supine, the hip is flexed at 90° (which tensions the hamstrings) and the knee is extended until resistance is met.

Popliteal Angle

The classic knee physical examination finding in CP is an increased popliteal angle due to hamstring tightness or spasticity. This is characterized by decreased knee extension when the hip is flexed to 90° by the examiner and is a result of the fact that the spastic and tight hamstrings (which originate from the pelvis) must lead to knee flexion as the hip is flexed. The popliteal angle is measured with the contralateral limb fully extended and flat on the table. When the knee extension becomes harder to obtain and pelvis starts to move, that is the angle of the knee that gives the popliteal angle, measured from the horizontal (**Figure 5.15**). As the hamstrings get tighter, and especially with increasing flexion contracture, the popliteal angle increases. As aforementioned, severe and long-standing hamstring tightness can occasionally lead to knee flexion contractures, which is characterized by the inability to straighten the knee when the hip is extended. This should be carefully evaluated and followed over time as the child grows as this is an important functional implication of increased muscle tone, hamstring tightness, and progressive contracture that has functional implications for the child and adolescent.

Extensor Lag

Some children with CP do not have a true knee flexion contracture but have significant quadriceps weakness, which can contribute to crouched gait. Many of these children will have true extensor lag of the knee, measured by full passive extension of the knee in the seated position, but decreased active knee extension. The extensor lag is the discrepancy between passive extension that can be obtained by the examiner and the amount of extension that the patient can produce.

Ely Test

Some patients with CP walk with minimal knee flexion in swing phase, which has been coined a "stiff knee gait" (▶ **Video 5.1**). In addition to diminished knee flexion, they have to lurch to the other side and swing the limb wide in order to clear the toe. For some patients this is due to persistent rectus femoris activity during swing phase. The Ely test is used to measure the degree of rectus femoris spasticity. The patient is placed prone and the knee is flexed rapidly. The examiner carefully observes if and when the pelvis may raise off the examination table, indicating significant rectus femoris spasticity, which may indicate the need for rectus transfer or resection (▶ **Video 5.2**). The Ely test can be determined in a binary fashion (positive or negative) or the angle of knee flexion that caused the first rise of the pelvis can be recorded.

Patella Alta and Patellar Stability

The patellar height should also be evaluated, especially in ambulatory children with CP. Patella alta is often a physical examination finding that can easily be palpated, although the exact value of patella

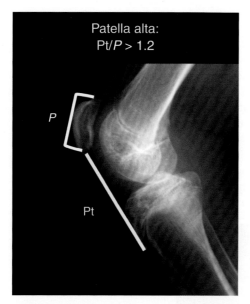

Patella alta:
Pt/*P* > 1.2

P

Pt

FIGURE 5.16 Many ambulatory children with crouched gait will have patella alta as a result of elongation of the patella tendon. Radiographically this is noted by a ratio of the patellar tendon to patella lengths greater than 1.2.

alta is measured on the lateral knee radiograph (**Figure 5.16**). The normal ratio of the patella tendon to patella is 0.8 to 1.2; ratios greater than 1.2 imply a diagnosis of patella alta.

Some children with CP will occasionally have some element of patellar instability. A careful patellar stability examination in both the supine and the flexed knee position may give the examiner some idea if there is patellar laxity that could be causing anterior knee pain.

● *Foot and Ankle*

The foot and ankle examination in CP is especially important. Spasticity can lead to predictable and progressive deformities that are initially flexible and later, with more bone and joint abnormality, can become rigid and fixed. Treatment priorities are different based upon different levels of GMFCS function. Children at GMFCS Levels I-III have the potential for ambulation, and thus the foot examination is geared to determine which anatomic pathologies can lead to impairments in walking. A reliable, plantigrade foot (or one that can be braced in a functional position) is essential for efficient human ambulation. Sometimes a child has contractures that affect foot position and may require surgery (▶ **Video 5.3**). Other patients can have weakness such as in the hemiplegic patient with a drop foot in swing phase that can be helped with a brace (▶ **Video 5.4**). Conversely, children at GMFCS Levels IV and V are marginal or nonambulators; the examination and subsequent treatment is geared toward producing a braceable foot to help with transfers and for shoe wear to protect the foot from the environment.

General Examination

As with the hip and knee, a thorough range of motion evaluation is important. Specific ankle dorsiflexion and planar flexion measurements should be documented and serially recorded to determine if a change has occurred. A general, qualitative assessment of the flexibility of the subtalar joint is also important. Any pain that occurs with palpation or with range-of-motion assessment should be thoroughly evaluated, typically with radiographs. Careful examination of the plantar aspect of the foot can reveal where abnormal pressures are being applied (**Figure 5.17**).

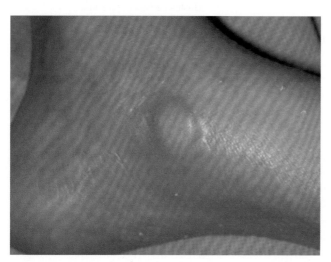

FIGURE 5.17 Many children with cerebral palsy will have tight tendoachilles, which leads to midfoot collapse and a prominent talar head which can develop calluses (as seen here).

Silfverskiold Test

The classic examination of the equinus ankle in neuromuscular disease is the Silfverskiold test, which differentiates isolated contracture of the gastrocnemius from the combined contracture of the gastrocnemius and soleus complex (**Figure 5.18**). This examination is predicated on the anatomical differences between these plantar and flexor muscles, since the gastrocnemius crosses two joints (the ankle and the knee), while the soleus only crosses the ankle. Passive dorsiflexion is tested with the knee bent to 90° (when the gastrocnemius is relaxed) and again with the knee in full extension (when the gastrocnemius would be fully engaged). Any limitation in dorsiflexion with the knee flexed is a true measurement of soleus contracture, where the lack of dorsiflexion with the knee fully extended is a measurement of gastrocnemius contracture. This differentiation allows for the targeted treatment of the location of pathology, especially when performing a selected fascial lengthening using the concept of "Surgical Dose" where only the shortened muscle complex is lengthened.

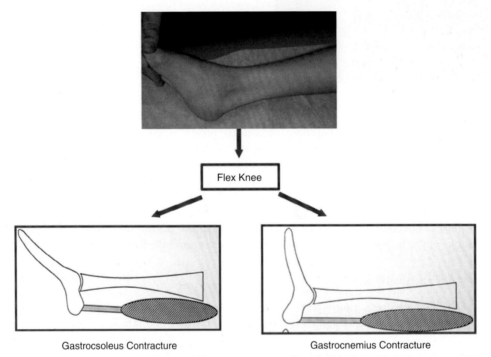

Flex Knee

Gastrocsoleus Contracture   Gastrocnemius Contracture

FIGURE 5.18 The Silfverskiold test allows one to determine whether limited ankle dorsiflexion is due to gastrocnemius contracture or both gastrocnemius and soleus tightness. When the knee is flexed 90°, the clinician is testing the soleus muscle alone. When the knee is extended, the clinician is testing for tightness in both muscles. Therefore, if the ankle has limits in dorsiflexion in both knee positions, both muscles are affected. If dorsiflexion is just limited in extension but not with knee flexion, the gastrocnemius alone is tight.

Planovalgus

Planovalgus foot deformities are extremely common in children with CP, across all GMFCS functional levels (**Figure 5.19**). It is felt that the tight tendoachilles contracture leads to excessive midfoot stress that leads to a flatfoot appearance. Many times, CP children will have flexible flat feet when they are young; as adolescents, the deformity may progress and become more fixed. The calcaneus will assume more of a valgus position which can be inspected with a weight bearing examination. Also viewing medially will reveal a significant loss of the midfoot arch with a prominence plantarly that is both the subluxated talonavicular joint with a prominent talar head. The midfoot collapse leads to forefoot abduction and makes the limb appear outtoed (**Figure 5.20**). With a planovalgus foot, the peroneal tendons may be

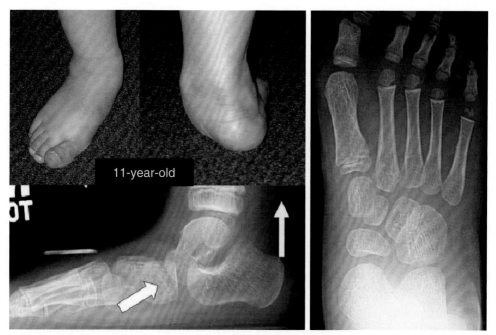

FIGURE 5.19 Most children with spastic cerebral palsy have tight tendoachilles. The inability to dorsiflex the ankle due to the Achilles contracture leads to midfoot breach as seen in this 11-year-old with a vertically positioned talus.

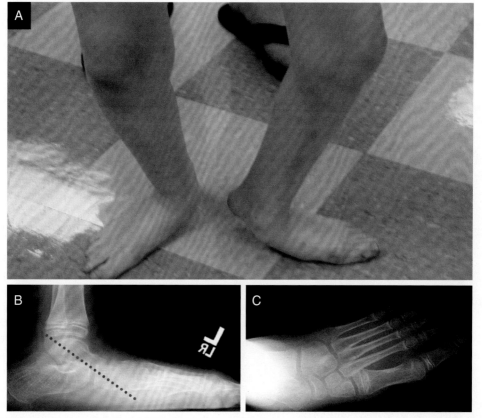

FIGURE 5.20 A, This adolescent has severe midfoot break and an external foot progression angle secondary to Achilles contractures. B and C, This results in uncoverage of the talar head which can frequently be a pressure point and area of skin breakdown.

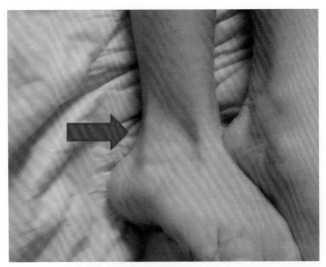

FIGURE 5.21 In addition to tight Achilles tendons, spasticity and contracture can be found in multiple tendons which can cross the ankle, such as in this child with very tight peroneal tendons (red arrow).

tight and contracted, especially in nonambulators (**Figure 5.21**). Both peroneal longus and brevis may be palpable laterally. With the progressive foot deformity and loss of functional subtalar motion, these contracted tendons become fixed and nonfunctional in the nonambulatory patient.

As the deformity progresses, this hindfoot position will become more fixed and rigid. The patient may complain tenderness over the prominent talar head, and callosities may be present medially (**Figure 5.17**). The patients will frequently have a loss of subtalar motion as the calcaneus is fixed into valgus with subluxation of the subtalar joint. A foot that can be passively corrected is usually braceable with orthotics. Once the deformity becomes fixed, however, surgical treatment may be required to bring the foot into a more neutral position.

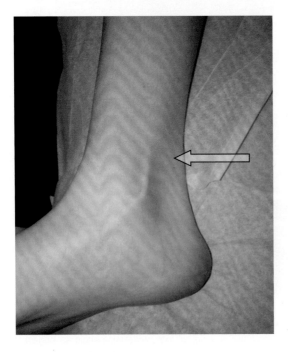

Equinovarus

While planovalgus deformities are present in all of the different GMFCS levels, equinovarus foot deformities tend to occur in more ambulatory patients. The equinus ankle position typically leads to a varus hindfoot when the foot is supple (▶ **Video 5.5**). Unilateral or bilateral toe walking is a common presentation for patients with CP. Either the posterior tibialis (**Figure 5.22**) or the anterior tibialis (and occasionally both) can be the primary forces for driving the foot into a varus position. Patients with diplegia distribution will many times have equinovarus feet when they are younger, but the natural history often changes as they grow into adolescence, when their larger body

FIGURE 5.22 This child has a very prominent posterior tibialis tendon, as noted by the yellow arrow behind the medial malleolus.

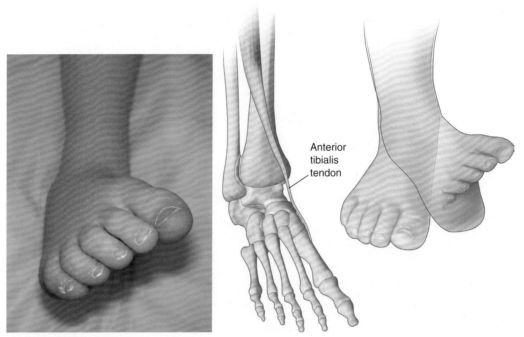

FIGURE 5.23 This child has dynamic spasticity of his anterior tibialis tendon which leads to forefoot supination, especially in the swing phase of gait.

weights help push the feet into a more planovalgus position. However, patients with hemiplegia will typically remain with the equinovarus deformities throughout their growth and development.

A detailed observational gait examination with special detail during swing phase is the most important determination of which tibialis tendon is the most important contributor to the varus foot position. If the foot is supinated during the swing phase (**Figure 5.23**), then it is likely the anterior tibialis that is driving the varus; if, however, significant supination is not seen during swing phase, then it is more likely the posterior tibialis is the culprit (▶ **Video 5.6**). A hindfoot varus position in stance also points toward tibialis posterior pathology.

The confusion test has classically been used to help differentiate the causative factor for equinovarus foot positioning, especially during the swing phase of the gait cycle. The test is performed by having the patient sit on an examination table with the knee flexed to 90°. The examiner asks the patient to flex their hip against resistance; a positive confusion test is when the patient co-contracts and dorsiflexes his ankle with foot supination while flexing their hip (▶ **Video 5.7**). This positive result implies that the anterior tibialis is a major factor in the equinovarus foot position, especially in swing phase, and that a split anterior tibialis transfer may improve foot positioning.[2]

Dorsal Bunion

Dorsal bunions are common in the setting of CP, especially in spastic quadriplegia.

This deformity is caused primarily due to an overpull of the tibialis anterior raising the first metatarsal with powerful toe flexors causing flexion of the distal phalanx of the great toe (**Figure 5.24**). The flexibility and passive ROM of the great toe metatarsophalangeal (MTP) joint is determined with special determination of fixed contractures. Also, the examiner should determine if the anterior tibialis is extremely tight and palpable.

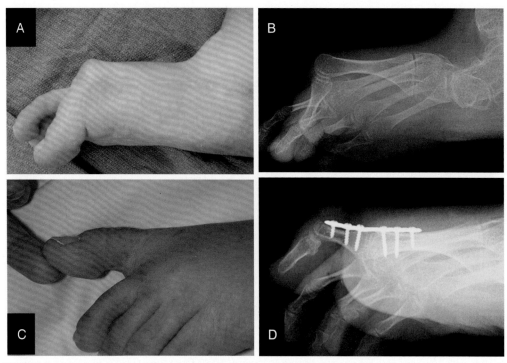

FIGURE 5.24 Great toe deformities can also exist in children with cerebral palsy such as this child with a dorsal bunion noted (Panels A and B). Subsequent fusion of the first metatarsal phalangeal joint corrects this deformity (Panels C and D).

Hallux Valgus

Hallux valgus deformities also occur in the CP population. Careful examination of the great toe and any overlapping of the second toe should be noted (the great toe may come over the top or under the second toe) (**Figure 5.25**). Patients may have difficulty with hygiene or with pressure injuries between the two toes.

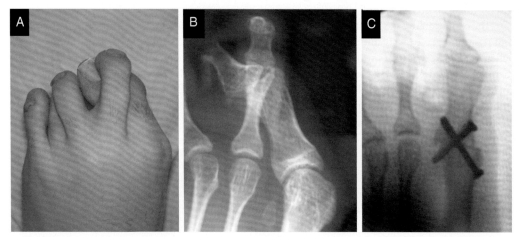

FIGURE 5.25 A, Hallux valgus deformity seen clinically. B, Hallux valgus deformity on radiograph. C, Due to underlying spasticity, hallux valgus in cerebral palsy patients is best treated with a first metatarsal phalangeal joint fusion.

The MTP joint should be carefully examined to determine if it is subluxated. The MTP should be axially loaded to perform a "grind test" to see if there is any crepitus or pain, which may be indicated by early degenerative changes of the MTP joint.

● Spine

Examination of the spine should be done with the child undressed and the back observed in a sitting position (**Figure 5.26**). Many children with CP do not have the motor control to sit independently. However, these children still spend a majority of their day seating in their wheelchair; their spine deformity is much different even in a supported seating environment, compared to a supine position. That is why an assisted sitting position is of significant importance in the spine examination, as a supine examination may hide significant spinal deformity.

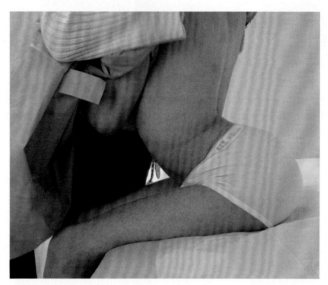

FIGURE 5.26 Excessive lumbar lordosis is commonly seen in children with cerebral palsy.

Manual Flexibility

Also known as the "Miller test," this is an examination to manually determine spine curve flexibility. Patients with CP and scoliosis are typically small for their age, and many times, they are still small enough to be held like a small child. The examiner holds the child in a lateral position. If the scoliosis is flexible, then the child will be able to bent over the knee and reverse the curve. More stiff, rigid curves will not bend out in this fashion, and that may indicate the need for more significant surgical intervention.

Pelvic Obliquity

Oftentimes, the pelvic obliquity is the most clinically significant part of their spine deformity. Along with examining the spine in a seated or assisted sitting position, the examiner should pay close attention to the pelvic obliquity in that seating position. Any pelvic-rib abutment should be noticed, and a careful skin examination should be done on the downside of the pelvic obliquity, as that is a frequent place for pressure injuries (**Figure 5.27**).

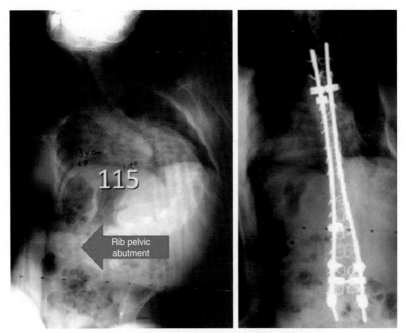

FIGURE 5.27 Children with cerebral palsy have long sweeping scoliosis curves, which are different than that seen in idiopathic scoliosis. This child has pelvic obliquity, and the ribs are abutting the pelvis.

Upper Extremity

The upper extremity examination of children with CP can be complex and difficult. Oftentimes, upper extremity issues in these children are referred to pediatric hand specialists, and those detailed examinations are beyond the scope of this chapter. This section will focus on the overall examination of what the general pediatric orthopedist or what the pediatric specialist in CP may need to focus on.

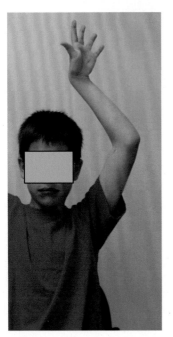

A general range of motion examination should be performed to determine overall functional range and if any contractures are present. The classic upper extremity examination in hemiplegia includes a propensity for elbow flexion, decreased supination, wrist flexion, and ulnar deviation and difficulty with grasp and release (▶ **Video 5.8**). Shoulder internal rotation and limited abduction are commonly found in nonambulatory CP (**Figure 5.28**). Elbow flexion contractures are also common, and a careful examination should be performed to determine if hygiene or skin issues are occurring due to severe contractures (**Figure 5.29**). A palpable, dislocated radial head is also common in patients with GMFCS Level IV or V function; this is usually an incidental finding and is not commonly painful.

Wrist deformities are also common in patients and are usually in flexion with ulnar deviation (**Figure 5.30**). Over time these

FIGURE 5.28 Upper extremity involvement is commonly seen in cerebral palsy. This boy with spastic hemiplegia with limited elbow extension has a flexed and ulnarly deviated hand which is in a pronated position.

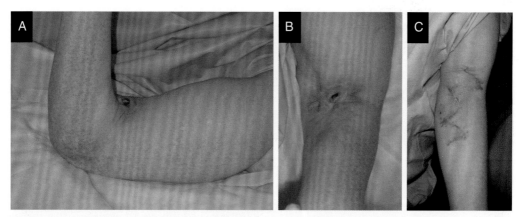

FIGURE 5.29 A, Severe biceps contractures can lead to skin break down and difficulty with daily cares. B, Anterior view of resulting skin breakdown due to poor access for hygiene in the antecubital fossa. C, Resolution of skin breakdown after surgical release.

can become fixed wrist flexion contractures that can make hygiene and dressing difficult (**Figure 5.31**). The volar wrist crease must be inspected for hygiene and skin issues. The dorsal surface may have palpable subluxated carpus bones that may be painful.

A sensory examination is important if the wrist flexion position is found to be flexible, and a tendon transfer is being considered. At least a rudimentary proprioceptive sense is important for successful tendon surgery, such as the FCU to ECRB transfer in patients with hemiplegia.

Finger deformities are also common, and these may include thumb-in-palm deformity (**Figure 5.32**) and either boutonniere deformities or swan neck deformities of the fingers (**Figure 5.33**). Subluxation and frank dislocation of the MTP and PIP joints may occur, and these should be differentiated with a careful examination of the stability of these joints.

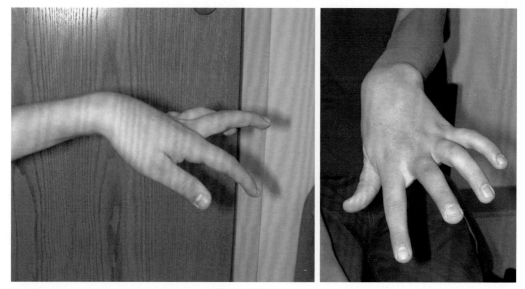

FIGURE 5.30 This child with hemiplegia has difficulty with wrist extension and hyperextension of his third, fourth, and fifth digits, while some lag of his index finger is noted.

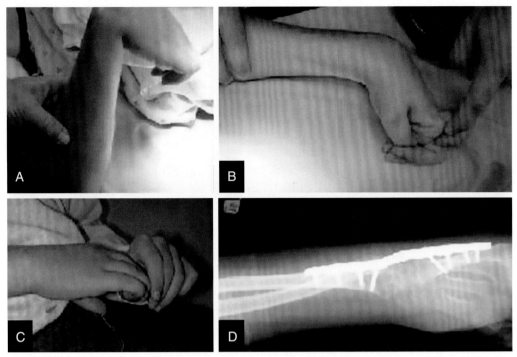

FIGURE 5.31 Similar to severe biceps contractures, wrist flexion contractures can lead to difficulty with daily cares. This child with severe wrist contractures (Panels A and B) undergoes wrist fusion with a good clinical and radiographic result (Panels C and D).

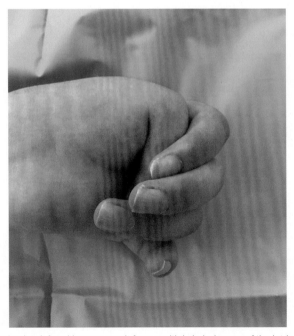

FIGURE 5.32 Thumb and palm deformities can result from multiple imbalances of the intrinsic and extrinsic muscles of the thumb.

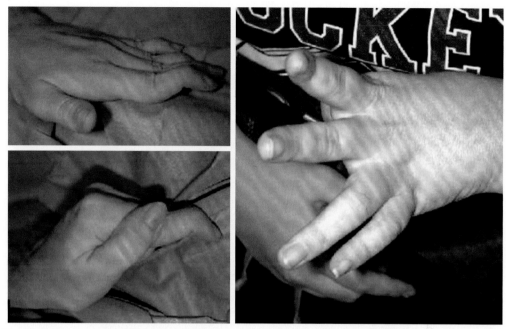

FIGURE 5.33 Swan neck deformities and boutonniere deformities can also exist in the fingers of children with cerebral palsy. This child has the typical swan neck appearances of the fingers.

Myelomeningocele

Spina bifida or myelomeningocele is a neural tube defect, leading to in utero exposure of the neural elements and malformation of the spinal cord. Widespread neurologic involvement is frequent and may include developmental delay, syrinx, Chiari II malformation (**Figure 5.34**), hydrocephalus, myelodysplasia, and tethered cord, as well as downstream effects such as spinal deformity (scoliosis and kyphosis),

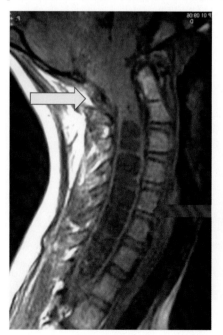

paralysis, sensory loss, joint contractures such as hip dysplasia, and neurogenic bowel and bladder. Interestingly, upper extremity function may also be impaired in patients with myelomeningocele. Infants born with spina bifida can have significant skeletal deformities that include kyphosis (**Figure 5.35**), fixed hip dislocation, congenital dislocation of the knee (**Figure 5.36**), severe stiff clubfoot (**Figure 5.37**), and calcaneal foot positions (**Figure 5.38**).

As affected children age, the physical examination vary by age and by level of involvement, but should always include an assessment of functioning muscle groups and their nerve function. Neurologic function may change over time as the child develops and thus detailed serial examinations are recommended. Patients with *thoracic level*

FIGURE 5.34 An MRI scan demonstrates a very large herniation of the cerebellar tonsils into the foramen magnum, otherwise known as a Chiari malformation. Subsequent dilatation of the cervical spine cord is present with the very large cervical syrinx.

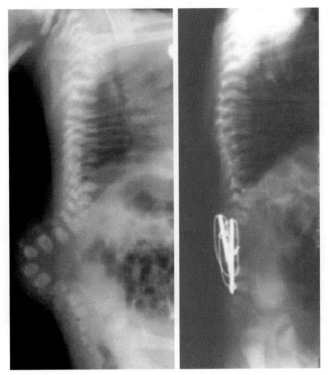

FIGURE 5.35 This child with myelodysplasia, or spina bifida, has severe congenital kyphosis associated with the spinal cord dysplasia.

myelomeningocele will be nonambulatory and have no voluntary motor control below the waist, although spastic involuntary movement may be noted. Patients with *upper lumbar level* function (L1 or L2) will have voluntary hip flexor and some hip adductor function. Some of these patients can stand for short periods with extensive orthotic apparatus. Yet most of these patients spend the bulk of their time being wheelchair-dependent and thus prone to sacral decubitus ulcers in their insensate skin. These patients will rarely have

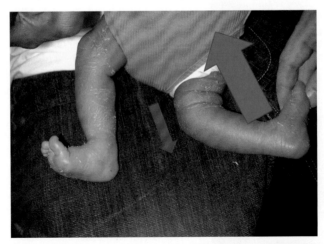

FIGURE 5.36 Knee extension contractures can be present in children with muscle imbalance as a result of strong quadriceps tendon (strong L3 motor level) in the face of weak hamstring power (absent L4 motor functioning).

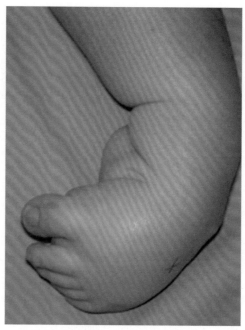

FIGURE 5.37 Many children with spina bifida will have very severe teratologic clubfoot deformities, as noted here. These clubfoot deformities are much stiffer than idiopathic clubfeet.

any meaningful community ambulatory ability and many will have hip dislocations (located hips are not necessary in this group and surgical treatment is not recommended) (**Figure 5.39**). *Lower lumbar level* function assumes strong L1 and L2 function in addition to L3 (active quadricep function) or L4 level of function (active quadriceps and medial hamstring function). These patients may have community ambulatory potential with crutches and KAFO (knee ankle foot orthosis) or AFO (ankle foot orthosis). Patients with L5 *level of function* can be good ambulators as they have much stronger hamstring functioning and weak

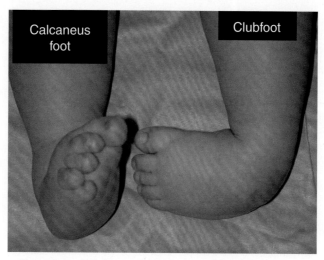

FIGURE 5.38 This boy with myelodysplasia has two opposite foot deformities. On the right side he has a calcaneus foot as a result of weak gastrocsoleus muscle in the face of very strong foot dorsiflexor power. The other side is a classic teratologic clubfoot.

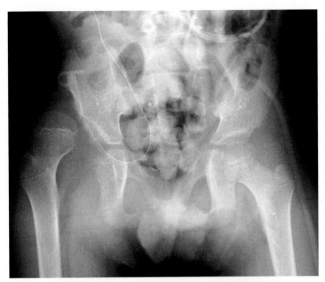

FIGURE 5.39 Children with spina bifida will often have dysplasia or dislocation of their hips. This is due to weak hip abductors and extensors. The pathology is considered different than that seen in cerebral palsy. In cerebral palsy, the hips dislocate due to extremely spastic hip flexors and hip adductors. Conversely, in spina bifida, there is weakness in the hip abductors and extensors which leads to migration of the hips.

hip abduction; unfortunately, they can have a severe calcaneus deformity as a result of good anterior tibialis function in the face of a paralyzed gastrocsoleus complex. Sacral level patients will have good ambulatory ability yet can develop cavovarus foot positioning and clawing of the toes as a result of poor foot intrinsic muscle function and the fact that the strong posterior tibialis tends to invert the foot and is not balanced by equal power in the peroneal muscles which evert the foot (**Figure 5.40**).

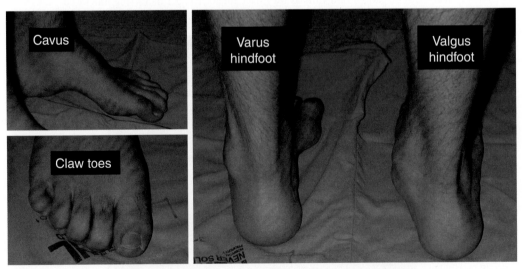

FIGURE 5.40 Cavovarus foot deformities are almost always associated with some form of a neurologic disorder. This child has a unilateral cavovarus foot with clawing of the toes and is likely due to some abnormality in the spinal cord. Patients with bilateral cavovarus feet may have a hereditary sensory motor neuropathy that requires referral to pediatric neurology.

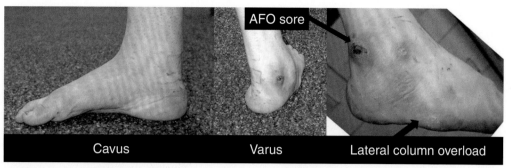

FIGURE 5.41 Children with a cavovarus foot can develop lateral column overload and pressure sores from ill-fitting prostheses.

At each clinic examination, the child is examined and the level of motor control is assessed and compared to prior exams. Any decreases in motor level or gait pattern should prompt evaluation for worsening hydrocephalus, shunt malfunction, tethered cord, or other central nervous system process. It is critical to remember that these patients are insensate and thus are unable to detect sacral decubitus ulcers in thoracic level patients and foot sores in the lower lumbar level and sacral level patients (**Figure 5.41**). A lumbar level myelomeningocele patient may develop a painless red, hot swollen limb, which may suggest infection. Yet in fact the most likely diagnosis is fracture, healing is robust and prompt, so radiographs are indicated.

Children with myelomeningocele walk with certain gait patterns and can have rotational deformities of the femur and tibia. Patients with myelomeningocele may have weak quadriceps and calf muscles, resulting in a crouch gait pattern. Although young patients can be supported in KAFOs and HKAFOs, good quadriceps strength is essential for long-term ambulation. Weak hip abductors result in a significant Trendelenburg gait, which is almost ubiquitous in the myelomeningocele population. Ground reaction AFOs may help provide stability.

Muscular Dystrophy

There are several types of muscular dystrophy seen in children, and Duchenne is the most common type of muscular dystrophy, present in 1 in 20,000 live births. Patients present with progressive weakness around 3 to 6 years of age with new onset toe walking and clumsiness. On physical examination, they have trouble getting up off of the floor and classically with a positive Gowers sign (**Figure 5.42**), pseudohypertrophy of the calf muscles (**Figure 5.43**), and gait disturbances. The patient may accommodate for hip extensor weakness resulting in lumbar lordosis (**Figure 5.44**). A Trendelenburg gait may be present due to hip abductor weakness. The Meryon sign reflects shoulder girdle weakness, where in attempting to pick up the child by the chest, the arms slide the grasp due to weakness. Prompt referral to neurology for diagnosis is appropriate for a patient with suspected muscular dystrophy. As the disease progresses, many patients become nonambulatory and may develop severe equinovarus foot deformities and knee and hip flexion contractures. Treatment with corticosteroids has delayed the presentation and severity of scoliosis and may prolong ambulation. Becker muscular dystrophy is a variant of Duchenne and with a variable natural history; some patients can develop spine deformity, and this should be treated as these children can survive into their late adulthood. Many children with muscular dystrophy are affected in the hips with weak hip extensor power, which leads to compensatory lordosis and knee flexion (**Figure 5.45**).

Facioscapulohumeral muscular dystrophy is another common muscular dystrophy in which the muscles of the face, shoulder blades, and upper arms are among the most affected. Facial weakness may

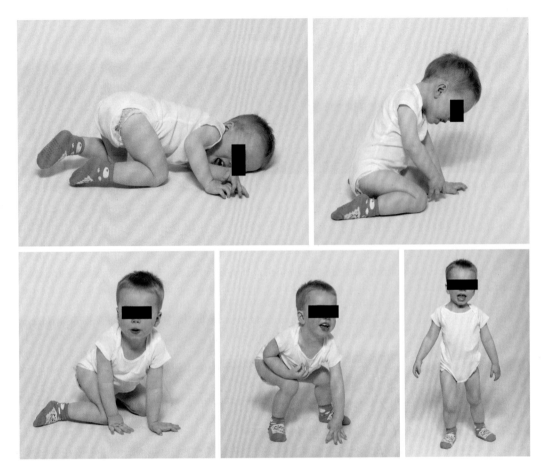

FIGURE 5.42 Stepwise progression as an attempt to stand in a child with positive Gowers sign, secondary to Duchenne muscular dystrophy. He has proximal weakness, which requires using his upper extremity to rise from a supine position.

result in limited movements of the lips, causing difficulties whistling or pursing the lips (**Figure 5.46**). Affected individuals may develop a "mask-like" facial appearance. The atrophy around the shoulders can be picked up on physical examination by noticing wasting of the periscapular region (**Figure 5.47**). Functionally shoulder weakness presents with limited shoulder abduction and winging of the scapula (▶ **Video 5.9**). With limited function and pain, some patients may opt for surgical stabilization of the shoulder blade via fusion to the ribcage.

● Spinal Muscular Atrophy

Spinal muscular atrophy (SMA) is the most common lethal inherited disease of infancy, with an incidence of 1 in 20,000 live births. It is caused by deterioration of the anterior horn cells, due to a mutation in the survival motor neuron 1 gene. In 2016, nusinersen was approved by the FDA, which is an antisense oligonucleotide, which upregulates survival motor neuron 2 gene expression. Other treatments, including gene therapy, are in development. These treatments, particularly with early initiation, are changing the disease phenotype. Some patients with SMA Type 1 and 2 are able to ambulate, which previously was not the case.

On examination, legs are typically flexed, abducted, and externally rotated. Development of hip dysplasia is common, as is scoliosis. Muscle weakness is more pronounced proximally rather than distally

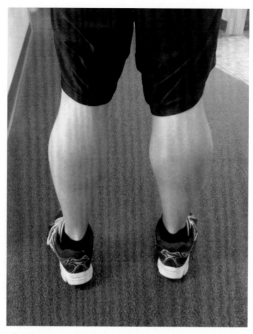

FIGURE 5.43 Calf hypertrophy seen in a boy with limb-girdle muscular dystrophy.

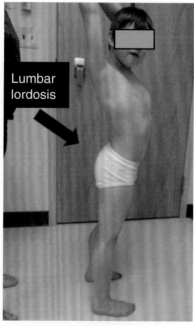

FIGURE 5.44 This boy with Duchenne muscular dystrophy has excessive lordosis, secondary to weak hip extensor power.

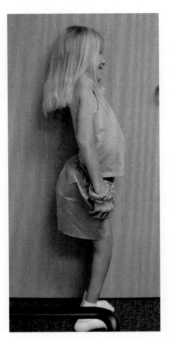

FIGURE 5.45 Another child with hyperlordosis, secondary to muscular dystrophy.

and lower extremities greater than upper extremities. Tongue fasciculations may be present as well as tremors in the hand. Reflexes may be preserved early on but become absent as the disease progresses. Hip, knee, and ankle and equinovarus foot deformities develop in nonambulatory patients. Hyperlordosis and sometimes thoracic kyphosis are features of the condition.

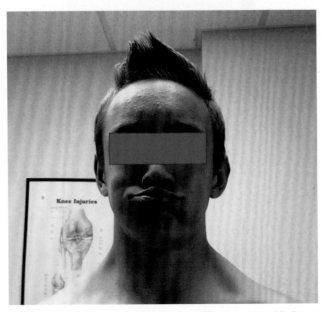

FIGURE 5.46 This boy with facioscapulohumeral dystrophy has difficulty pursing his lips, secondary to weakness of his facial muscles.

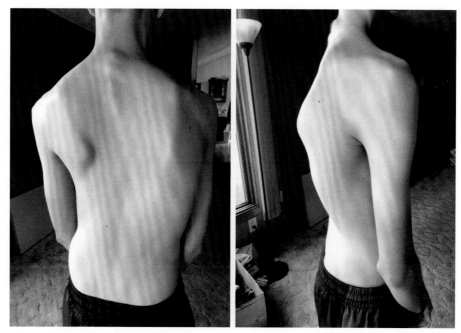

FIGURE 5.47 This boy with facioscapulohumeral dystrophy and scoliosis has severe atrophy and wasting around his scapula.

● *Other Conditions*

New neurologic conditions are frequently detected in the pediatric orthopedic clinic. For instance, children with structural spinal cord problems can first present to the orthopedist for lost function or deformity such as differences in foot size (**Figure 5.48**). It can be difficult to diagnose spinal cord pathology in pediatric patients as there can be significant compressive lesions or instability prior to the development of symptoms. Classic upper motor neuron findings will precede symptoms and include hyperreflexia, Hoffman sign, Babinski sign, and clonus. Upper cervical spine myelopathy may present with torticollis,

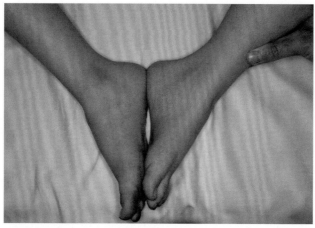

FIGURE 5.48 This child with asymmetric foot size is likely secondary to abnormal neurologic involvement, and detailed neurological examination is warranted.

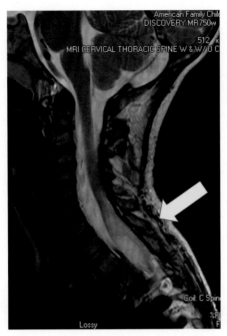

FIGURE 5.49 This child with an asymmetric gait and torticollis presents with a cervical spine tumor.

cranial nerve involvement, or ataxia. Torticollis may be the first sign of a cervical spinal cord tumor (**Figure 5.49**). Symptoms when they occur include early fatigue, loss of fine motor coordination, bowel or bladder dysfunction, and gait changes (▶ **Video 5.10**). Children with some skeletal dysplasia (especially Morquio syndrome and diastrophic dysplasia) and specific syndromes (Down, Larson, etc.) should be screened for myelopathic signs as a result of upper cervical spine instability. Children with Down syndrome tend to be low tone and may have unusual gait patterns at baseline; thus, myelopathy can be difficult to detect.

Patients with tethered cord may also present with gait disturbance, tight hamstrings, and hyperreflexia. Patients with Chiari malformation, syrinx, and tethered cord may present with atypical scoliosis, including left-sided thoracic curve, kyphosis in the thoracic spine, asymmetric abdominal reflexes (▶ **Video 5.11**), and unilateral cavovarus foot (**Figure 5.40**). In general, unilateral cavus feet indicate the need for an MRI scan to rule out the above deformities.

Presence of a bilateral cavovarus foot deformity should prompt referral to a pediatric neurologist. A family history should be taken to see if there is a hereditary propensity for these foot deformities which can result from undiagnosed hereditary motor and sensory neuropathy (Charcot-Marie-Tooth syndrome). Patients with HMSN usually have detectable weakness of tibialis anterior or peroneal musculature. They may or may not have clawing of the toes. They may present with a history of frequent ankle sprains. Hands should be examined for atrophy of the intrinsic muscles and clawing of the fingers (**Figure 5.50**). The Coleman block test can be useful to evaluate for the rigidity of the hindfoot varus. The examiner places a 1-cm-thick block under the lateral foot allowing the first and second rays to drop off the edge of the block. If the hindfoot deformity corrects, then the varus deformity is flexible, and much of the varus position of the foot is compensating for the cavus component.

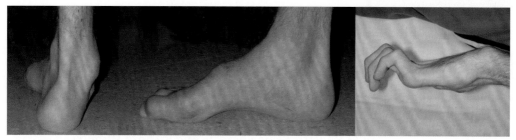

FIGURE 5.50 This adult male with Charcot-Marie-Tooth disease has cavovarus deformity of the feet which is secondary to intrinsic and extrinsic muscle imbalance. In addition, he has severe clawing of his hands, secondary to similar muscle imbalances about the hand and wrist.

Summary

Many pediatric neurologic conditions have an effect on the growing skeleton, and pediatric orthopedists are often the first to suspect and assist in making these diagnoses. It is critical to suspect that what you are evaluating in the face of pain, loss of function, and deformity may not be a primary orthopedic condition but a manifestation of a neurologic condition. Always remember that although you may not have seen a number of these disorders, they may have seen you.

References

1. Cooley WC, Melkonian G, Moses C, Moeschler JB: Autosomal dominant familial spastic paraplegia: description of a large New England family and a study of management. *Dev Med Child Neurol.* 1990;32:1098-1104.
2. Davids JR, Holland WC, Sutherland DH. Significance of the confusion test in cerebral palsy. *J Pediatr Orthop.* 1993;13(6):717-721.
3. Mutlu A, Livanelioglu A, Gunel MK. Reliability of Ashworth and Modified Ashworth scales in children with spastic cerebral palsy. *BMC Musculoskelet Disord.* 2008;9:44. doi:10.1186/1471-2474-9-44.
4. Marsico P, Frontzek-Weps V, Balzer J, van Hedel HJ. Hypertonia Assessment Tool. *J Child Neurol.* 2017;32(1):132-138. doi:10.1177/0883073816671681.

Physical Examination for Unusual and Syndromic Conditions

Pooya Hosseinzadeh, Ron El-Hawary, Craig Eberson, and Kishore Mulpuri

Unusual Conditions

Patients present to orthopedic surgeons for management of their musculoskeletal problems. It is imperative for the clinician to realize that these issues may exist in the setting of a genetic/syndromic condition. It is important to realize this for two reasons: first, a known diagnosis may point toward potential areas of concern, facilitating early diagnosis of an associated orthopedic issue; second, by recognizing potential associations, the child presenting with an orthopedic concern (ie, scoliosis) can be examined with the intention to seek other underlying conditions (ie, Marfan syndrome [MFS]). It is often the other associated abnormalities of the specific underlying condition that represent the largest health risk (ie, aortic aneurism).

In other chapters of this book, we focus on how examination of different areas can aid in making a diagnosis of a limb or spine deformity. Many different disorders such as skeletal dysplasia can have effects on the pediatric skeleton in multiple locations. Children with neurofibromatosis may have severe scoliosis and tibial pseudarthrosis in addition to neurofibromas. Children with marfanoid characteristics can have limb deformity, scoliosis, foot deformities, and other conditions. In this chapter, we discuss some of these unusual syndromes and disorders. Instead of looking at a presenting deformity in search of a diagnosis, we consider the whole child with a known diagnosis and look for orthopedic deformities. In addition, we will discuss the evaluation of children with chronic regional pain syndrome.

Neurofibromatosis

Type 1 neurofibromatosis (NF-1), also known as von Recklinghausen disease, is a condition involving overgrowth of neural tissue leading to multisystem involvement. Orthopedic manifestations and concerns are many.

Pathophysiology

NF-1 is inherited in an autosomal dominant pattern with roughly half of cases arising from spontaneous mutation. The orthopedic management of NF-1 can be challenging and often requires a multidisciplinary approach.

Diagnosis and Physical Examination Findings

The diagnosis of NF-1 is made by establishing the presence of several physical features (**Table 6.1**).

Café au lait spots are hyperpigmented lesions that are present in the majority of patients with NF-1 (**Figure 6.1**).

Cutaneous neurofibromas are mixed cell tumors, consisting predominantly of Schwann cells, and present in late childhood. They are seen on the surface of the skin as well-circumscribed grayish tumors. Plexiform neurofibromas are diffuse tumors that are present under the skin. Lesions that cross the

Table 6.1	Diagnostic Criteria for Neurofibromatosis

More than six café au lait spots (15 mm in adults, 5 mm in children)
Two or more neurofibromas or one plexiform neurofibroma
Axillary or inguinal freckling
Optic glioma
Two or more Lisch nodules (iris hamartomas)
Bone lesions (sphenoid dysplasia, long bone thinning with or without pseudarthrosis)
A first-degree relative with NF-1
Can be remembered with the mnemonic "CAN FOOL" (café au lait, axillary freckling, neurofibromas, first-degree relative, optic glioma, osseous lesion, Lisch nodule)

National Institutes of Health Consensus Development Conference Statement: neurofibromatosis. Bethesda, Md., USA, July 13-15, 1987. *Neurofibromatosis*. 1988:1(3):172-178.

midline on both sides of the spine often arise from the spinal canal. They have a "bag of worms" appearance and have the potential to undergo transformation to malignant peripheral nerve sheath tumors. This transformation, which often occurs 10 to 20 years after the original tumors present, is usually heralded by sudden onset of pain, enlargement, and new neurological deficits. Axillary Freckling (**Figure 6.2**) is the second most common feature seen in NF-1.

Other skin findings include macrodactyly, elephantiasis (large soft-tissue masses), and overgrowth of the skin with a velvety, soft, papillary quality, known as verrucous hyperplasia. Children with NF-1 are also known to have an increased risk of developmental delay, stroke, psychiatric disorders, and heart disease.

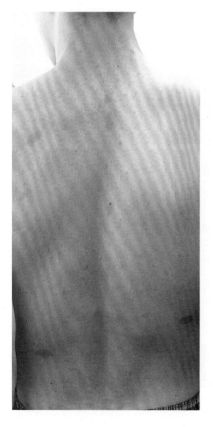

FIGURE 6.1 Multiple café au lait spots in a patient with neurofibromatosis.

Orthopedic Manifestations

Roughly half of patients with NF-1 will have a spinal deformity. While many present with curves which resemble idiopathic scoliosis, these curves may undergo transformation to the dystrophic curves characteristic of NF-1 (**Figure 6.3**).

Nondystrophic curves progress in a manner similar to adolescent idiopathic scoliosis, but dystrophic curves can progress rapidly and relentlessly. The later curves are usually short, sharply angular, and may have significant kyphosis (**Table 6.2**).

Bony abnormalities include vertebral wedging, narrowing of the pedicles, and dural ectasia, which erode into the vertebral body. This leads to vertebral scalloping and thinning of the pedicles, factors that may make fixation during surgery difficult. Magnetic resonance imaging should be considered for patients with NF-1 presenting with scoliosis to screen for intraspinal tumors.

Other orthopedic manifestations include congenital pseudarthrosis of the tibia, as well as other bony dysplasias. While the tibia is the most commonly affected, other bones can be involved as well (**Figure 6.4**).

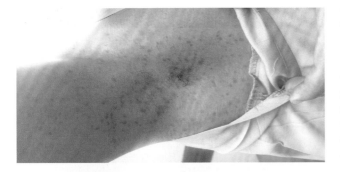

FIGURE 6.2 Axillary freckling in a patient with neurofibromatosis.

The term "congenital pseudar-throsis of the tibia" is confusing to many and would imply that children are born with a nonunion of their tibia. The confusion rests in the fact that most children with this condition are born without an established

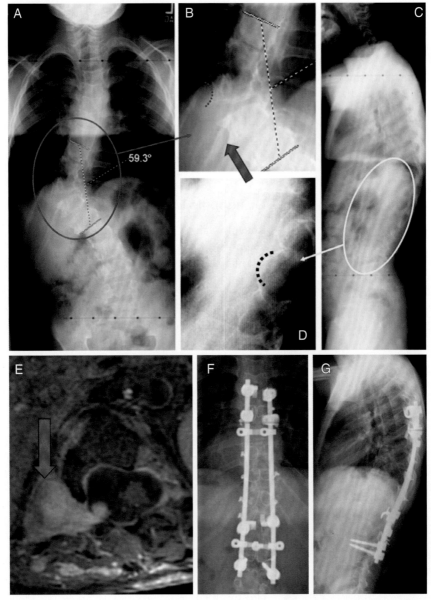

FIGURE 6.3 A, This 10-year-old boy with NF-1 has a 60° scoliosis. B, A close-up view of the curve demonstrates dystrophic changes with vertebral scalloping (dashed red line) and rib penciling (red arrow). C, Lateral X-ray. D, A close-up of the lateral X-ray demonstrates further vertebral scalloping which is likely due to dural ectasia. E, MRI demonstrates a large neurofibroma is the concavity of the curve. F and G, This child underwent anterior and posterior spine fusion.

Table 6.2	Dystrophic Spinal Changes in NF-1

Dural ectasia leading to vertebral scalloping
Foraminal enlargement from dumbbell neurofibromas
Rib penciling
Short, sharply angular curves
Dysplastic pedicles
Kyphoscoliosis

fracture with just anterolateral bowing of the tibia (and often the fibula) and with time, the tibia will fracture and not heal. Adding further confusion is the reality that not all children with NF-1 and antero-lateral bowing will ever fracture. Treatment is complex and fraught with difficulties.

Limb overgrowth is an additional finding on examination. Limb hyperplasia and overgrowth are common. Subperiosteal bone growth has also been noted and may be responsible for irregular bone elongation.

Differential Diagnosis

The diagnosis of NF-1 is usually easy to make based upon the presence of nonorthopedic lesions such as café au lait spots and axillary freckling. When faced with a child with hemihypertrophy, NF-1 should stay on the list of possible causes until definitive diagnosis is made. Other causes include Proteus syndrome, Klippel-Trenaunay-Weber (KTW) syndrome, and Beckwith-Wiedemann syndrome.

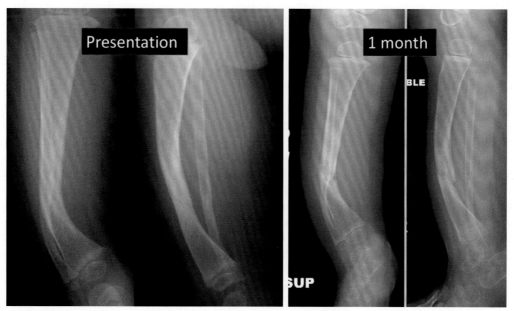

FIGURE 6.4 This girl with NF-1 was born with anterolateral bow of the tibia that one month later developed fracture and worsening deformity.

● *Hemihypertrophy*

Hemihypertrophy is a rare condition where one side of the body is enlarged compared to the other side of the body. Based on the degree of enlargement, patients may present during infancy or not until they are school-aged.

Pathophysiology

The mechanism of enlargement in patients with hemihypertrophy is unknown and may affect an entire side of the body or often it may affect just one of the lower extremities. In classic hemihypertrophy, the femur and the tibia on the affected side are longer than the femur and tibia on the normal side and the affected foot is usually larger (**Figure 6.5**).

In evaluated children with apparent hemihypertrophy, one should recognize that it may not be enlargement of one limb but actually atrophy of the other limb secondary to other causes.

Differential Diagnosis and Physical Examination Findings

In mild cases of hemihypertrophy, it may be difficult to differentiate one from having a hypoplastic limb on the other side. Recent work has provided normative data for the developing child's upper limb length, girth, and circumference to aid the practitioner. In other cases, the upper and lower limbs are markedly enlarged and the diagnosis is obvious (**Figure 6.6**).

The practitioner should look for signs and symptoms of associated conditions such as NF-1 (see above), Proteus syndrome (asymmetric enlargement) (**Figure 6.7**), Beckwith-Wiedemann (enlarged tongue), and KTW syndrome (port-wine stains and vascular abnormalities under the skin) (**Figures 6.8** and **6.9**).

Orthopedic Manifestations

An enlarged limb can lead to limb length discrepancy that may require treatment. As outlined in the chapter on limb length discrepancy, treatment may include a shoe lift for minor discrepancies in symptomatic patients, growth arrest timed to effectuate correction, or limb lengthening of the short limb. Parents and patients often relate difficulty with shoe wear for the differences in foot size and can be bothered by cosmetic differences in limb girth. Unfortunately, little corrective treatment can be done for these issues and accommodative measures with different shoe sizes are usually all that is available.

Differential Diagnosis

The list of conditions that can cause atrophy can include hemiplegia or other neurologic disorders as well as congenital limb deficiency syndromes. Toddlers with mild congenital short femur can be misdiagnosed with hemihypertrophy of the normal limb. As the child ages, it becomes clear that only the femur is affected and other signs such as genu valgum and anterior knee laxity (absent cruciate ligament) confirm that the short limb is the abnormal limb. True limb enlargement (hemihypertrophy) is discussed above and includes Proteus syndrome, NF-1, KTW, and Beckwith-Wiedemann syndrome. Advanced imaging studies such as angiography and magnetic resonance imaging are often sufficient for a diagnosis of the associated conditions, but biopsy of suspected neurofibroma may be required to diagnose NF-1. In KTW, "benign" vascular tumors and arteriovenous malformations can lead to high-output cardiac failure if sufficiently large. Even when small, these lesions can be infiltrative, disfiguring, and painful. In children with apparent idiopathic hemihypertrophy, it is critical to consider that this may actually represent Beckwith-Wiedemann syndrome with a risk for development of intraabdominal tumors. Routine abdominal ultrasounds should be obtained every 3 to 4 months in patients with hemihypertrophy until the age of seven.

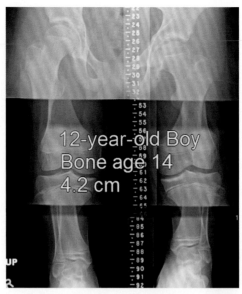

FIGURE 6.5 This 12-year-old boy with hemihypertrophy has a 4.2 cm discrepancy, 2.4 cm in the femur, and 1.8 cm in the tibia.

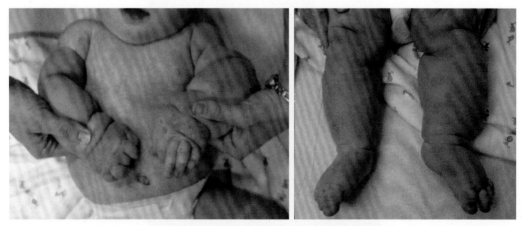

FIGURE 6.6 This 4-month-old baby has enlargement of his upper and lower extremity consistent with a diagnosis of hemihypertrophy. Abdominal ultrasound examinations must be obtained every 3 to 6 months to rule out tumor such as hepatoblastoma or Wilms tumor that are seen in Beckwith-Wiedemann syndrome.

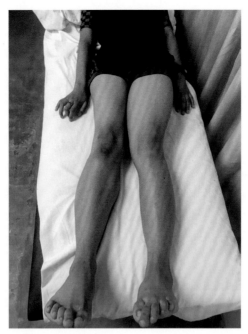

FIGURE 6.7 This Honduran boy with Proteus syndrome has hypertrophy of the left thigh and foot with hypertrophy of the right calf.

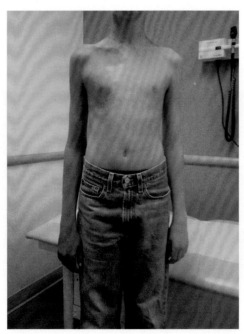

FIGURE 6.8 This boy with Klippel-Trenaunay-Weber syndrome has port-wine stain of the right upper extremity. His arm is longer and his hand is larger.

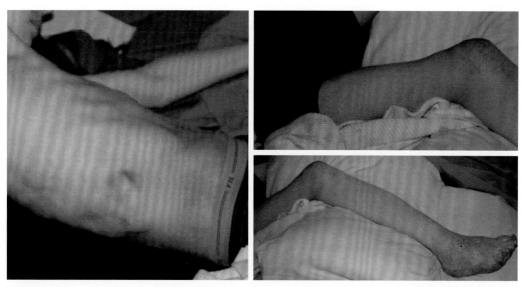

FIGURE 6.9 This boy with severe Klippel-Trenaunay-Weber syndrome has vascular malformations on the right side of his body from his trunk, to his thigh, and down to his foot.

● Marfan Syndrome

MFS is a disorder of connective tissue that results in many different orthopedic deformities and can have varying effects on the patient's appearance and function. The systemic scoring system for the diagnosis of MFS is a helpful guide to the features of MFS (**Table 6.3**).

It is important to diagnose the condition as some may have life-threatening cardiovascular pathology. The phenotype may range from classic MFS with ocular and cardiovascular pathology to patients who have "marfanoid characteristics" with a few features such as increased height, arachnodactyly, and pectus excavatum or carinatum.

Pathophysiology

MFS is an autosomal dominant disorder resulting from an abnormality in the fibrillin 1 gene on chromosome 15. Careful evaluation may reveal the clinical findings that lead to the diagnosis, potentially avoiding long-term sequelae of the disease.

Diagnosis and Physical Examination Findings

Cardiovascular findings include aortic root dilatation and dissection, mitral valve prolapse, pulmonary artery enlargement, and left ventricular disease. Ocular manifestations include lens dislocation, glaucoma, cataracts, and retinal detachment. Patients often have high arched palates. Frequently, the orthopedic manifestations of the disease are the first symptoms that warrant medical attention. In these cases where the patient presents with a constellation of orthopedic features of MFS, the provider is well justified in referral to genetics and cardiology.

Orthopedic Manifestations

The physical examination findings of MFS are paramount in raising suspicion of the disease and prompting further workup. Chest wall deformities are common such as pectus excavatum or carinatum (**Figure 6.10**).

Table 6.3	Systemic Scoring System for the Diagnosis of Marfan Syndrome
FEATURE (POINTS)	**MAXIMUM POSSIBLE SCORE**
Chest deformity	2
Pectus carinatum deformity (2)	
Pectus excavatum (1)	
Chest asymmetry (1)	
Dural ectasia (2)	2
Facial features[a] (1)	1
Foot deformity	2
Hindfoot deformity (2)	
Pes planus (1)	
Mitral valve prolapse, all types (1)	1
Myopia >3 diopters (1)	1
Pneumothorax (2)	2
Protrusio acetabuli (2)[b]	2
Reduced elbow extension (1)	1
Reduced US/LS ratio[b], increased arm/height, and no severe scoliosis (1)	1
Skin striae (1)	1
Spine deformity	1
Scoliosis (1)	
Thoracolumbar kyphosis (1)	
Wrist and thumb deformities	3
Wrist sign (1)	
[a]Thumb sign (1)	
Wrist and thumb signs (3)	
Maximum total score	20

[a]Presence of three of the following features: dolichocephaly enophthalmos, downslanting palpebral fissures, malar hypoplasia, retrognathia.
[b]LS, lower segment; US, upper segment. US length is the total arm span from each finger. LS is measured from the top of the symphysis pubis to the floor.
Adapted with permission from Loeys B, Dietz H, Braverman A, et al. The revised Ghent nosology for the Marfan syndrome. *J Med Genet*. 2010;47(7):476-485.

Arachnodactyly is a prominent feature of MFS. The wrist (Walter Murdoch sign) and thumb (Steinberg sign) features should be sought (**Figure 6.11**).

Musculoskeletal findings include asymmetric genu valgum (▶ **Video 6.1**), spinal deformity, pes planus (**Figure 6.12**), and protrusio acetabuli.

Protrusio acetabuli refers to an abnormally deep hip socket, which leads to the femoral head migrating medially and protruding into the pelvic cavity (**Figure 6.13**).

Spinal deformity in MFS is typically rapidly progressive. Curve patterns vary from idiopathic type to kyphoscoliosis. Dural ectasia often results in changes in vertebral morphology, scalloping of vertebral bodies, and small pedicles. Fusion for these patients should encompass all curves and often requires fairly long constructs (**Figure 6.14**).

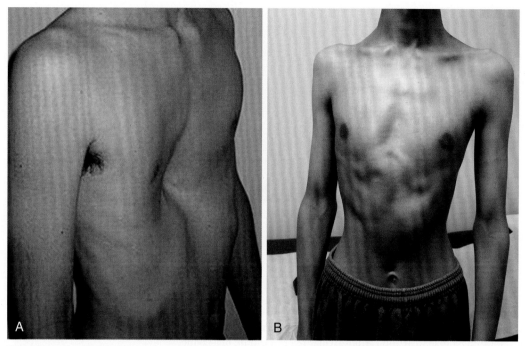

FIGURE 6.10 Chest wall deformity commonly seen in Marfan syndrome. A, Pectus excavatum. B, Pectus carinatum.

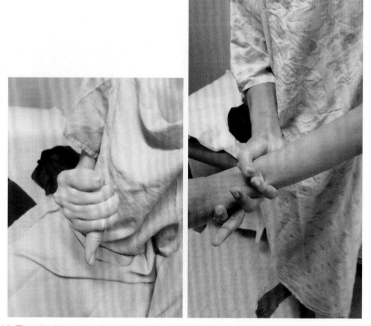

FIGURE 6.11 Thumb sign and wrist encirclement are common findings in patients with Marfan syndrome.

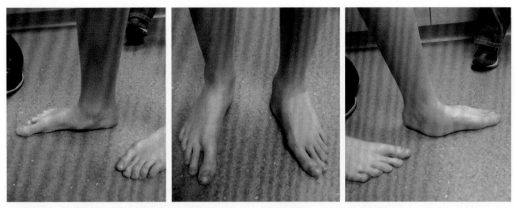

FIGURE 6.12 This child with marfanoid characteristics has arachnodactyly and severe pes planus (flatfeet). She does not have cardiac or ocular pathology.

Differential Diagnosis

The differential diagnosis includes other connective tissue disorders such as Ehlers-Danlos syndrome, Loeys-Dietz syndrome, homocystinuria, and Beals syndrome. A referral for genetic analysis is crucial in establishing a diagnosis and cardiovascular referral can be life-saving.

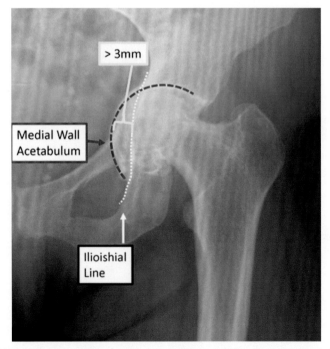

FIGURE 6.13 A right hip X-ray demonstrates acetabulum protrusio as defined by the method of Armbruster wherein the acetabular wall is shown to protrude ≥3 mm medial to the ilioischial (Kohler) line.

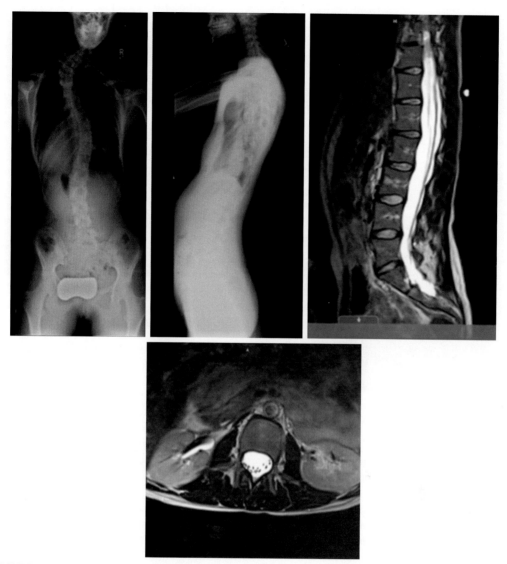

FIGURE 6.14 A 15-year-old child with Marfan syndrome (MFS). Radiographs show typical MFS curves, atypical in nature when compared to idiopathic, including a thoracolumbar kyphosis. MRI shows expansion of the spinal canal from dural ectasia, a common finding in these patients.

Down Syndrome

While the pathology of Down syndrome (DS) resulting from trisomy 21 is well known, there are comorbidities in this population that affect the diagnosis and management of their disease. The primary care provider has to be cognizant of orthopedic concerns that may be present as 20% of children will have musculoskeletal involvement. The orthopedist has to be aware of medical morbidities that can affect their treatment.

Diagnosis and Physical Examination Findings

The general physical examination features of children with DS are usually easily recognized by their characteristic facial appearance and constellation of developmental abnormalities. The physical examination of children with DS will reveal certain characteristic features. Their hands reveal a single palmar ("Simian") crease and small finger hypoplasia or clinodactyly (**Figure 6.15**).

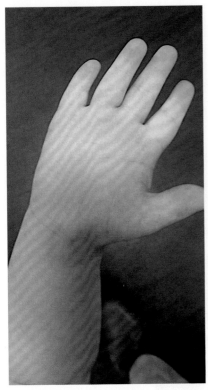

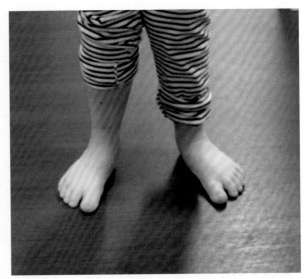

FIGURE 6.16 Pes planovalgus in a Down syndrome patient.

Orthopedic Manifestations

The majority of these patients will have notable ligamentous laxity. This is often manifested through widespread joint involvement.

FIGURE 6.15 Simian crease and clinodactyly (bent finger) of the fifth finger seen in a Down syndrome patient.

Foot Deformities: Flat feet (pes planovalgus) (**Figure 6.16**) are common, and often, medial column collapse results in hallux valgus as well. Children with DS have varying levels of hypotonia, which often results in delayed walking. This, combined with joint laxity, often makes orthotic support a helpful adjunct to physical therapy. A referral to an orthopedic specialist can often facilitate proper brace management of foot deformity. Surgical management for flat feet or hallux valgus is usually not required.

Knee Problems: DS patients can have increased genu valgum and patella femoral instability may be present in patients with or without limb deformity. Some of these patients will be asymptomatic and some may have symptoms that require treatment. Yet, surgical treatment for patella instability has high recurrence rate as a result of ligaments and soft tissues restretching out (**Figure 6.17**).

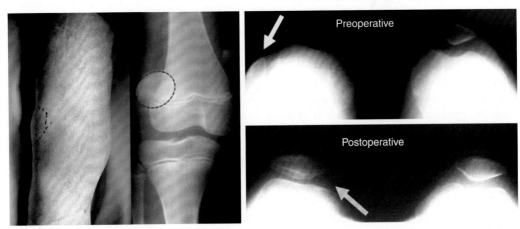

FIGURE 6.17 This 12-year-old girl has lateral patella subluxation (red circle) that completely dislocates with knee flexion (yellow arrow). Following reconstruction, her patella is centered over a dysplastic lateral femoral condyle (orange arrow).

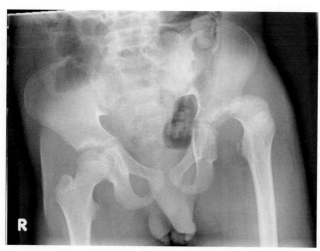

FIGURE 6.18 This child with Down syndrome presented to the emergency department after rolling over in bed and complaining of hip pain. He was diagnosed with a hip dislocation and reduced. He subsequently required periacetabular osteotomy to restore stability to the joint.

Hip Problems: Limping or hip pain should prompt AP pelvis and frog-leg lateral radiographs to rule out hip instability or slipped capital femoral epiphysis. Children with DS can have hip instability as a result of their hip capsule being highly pliable and the propensity to stretch out (**Figure 6.18**). These children will have a history of popping hips during diaper changes or certain positions and this condition can be present in all ages. Most of the time, the hips are not painful until later in life as a result of osteoarthritis. Surgical treatment is often extensive and is fraught with high recurrence rates.

Slipped capital femoral epiphysis can also occur in children with DS (**Figure 6.19**). These patients need to have blood testing for thyroid dysfunction. Treatment includes pinning of both hips as the rate of contralateral slip is high in patients with endocrinopathy and children. DS children are not reliable historians for onset of symptoms.

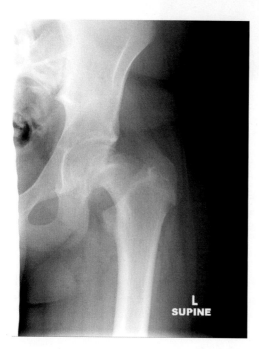

Spine Issues: Spinal hypermobility, in addition to bony deformity of the occipital condyles, can result in occipitocervical and atlantoaxial instability. A history of increased falling, balance difficulties, worsening gait, or neck pain should be thoroughly investigated. Abnormal deep tendon reflexes, weakness, ataxia, or decreased cervical spine range of motion should prompt cervical spine radiographs. Any concern of instability should be investigated with computed tomography or magnetic resonance imaging (**Figure 6.20**).

Scoliosis is also seen in children with DS. Long-cassette posteroanterior and lateral views of the entire spine should be ordered if there is a concern of scoliosis on examination.

FIGURE 6.19 Slipped capital femoral epiphysis on a patient with Down syndrome. In addition to urgent surgical fixation, the child will require screening for hypothyroidism.

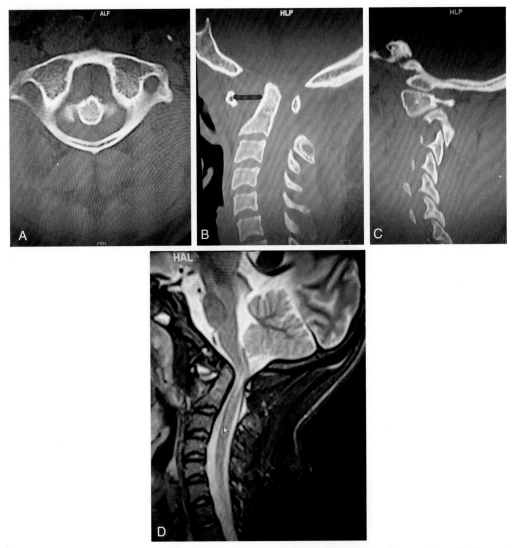

FIGURE 6.20 Patient with Down syndrome presenting with lower extremity weakness after wrestling with his cousin. A and B, CT scan demonstrates increased atlantodental interval (red line). C, Flattening of the C1 articulation with the occipital condyles is also seen on the lateral side (*); this often leads to C1-occipital instability as well. D, MRI shows significant spinal cord compression. This patient had his deformity reduced in traction and then underwent occiput to C3 fusion.

Musculoskeletal Pain: Children with DS can present with complaints of pain and difficulty with ambulation. It is critical to rule out cervical spine instability, yet vague musculoskeletal complaints can be a result of arthropathy of DS (multiple joint arthritis), thyroid dysfunction, or leukemia.

● *Achondroplasia*

Achondroplasia is the most common and well-known form of disproportionate dwarfism recognizable at birth. Like many skeletal dysplasias, many orthopedic manifestations can be present at multiple levels. Most children function very well into adulthood and without the need for surgical intervention.

Pathophysiology

Achondroplasia is a result of a mutation in the fibroblast growth factor receptor-3 (*FGFR-3*) gene, with an incidence of 1 in 30,000 and is autosomal dominant, yet the bulk of patients result from sporadic mutations. Altered FGF-3 receptor activity results in growth retardation in the proliferative zone of the growth plate.

Differential Diagnosis and Physical Examination Findings

The clinical features include short stature with normal trunk length, frontal bossing, and the bridge of the nose is depressed. There is characteristic rhizomelic shortening of the arms and legs, mild flexion deformity of the elbows, genu varum, and a trident hand. A gibbus may be present in the thoracolumbar region.

● *Nonorthopedic Manifestations*

Stenosis of the foramen magnum and the upper cervical spine may result in symptoms within the first two years of life. These include hypotonia, delayed development, weakness, and apnea. The diagnosis is confirmed through a sleep study and MRI. Some patients may require surgical decompression to avert serious neurological compromise. Other problems include recurrent otitis media, obstructive sleep apnea, and decreased respiratory function.

Orthopedic Manifestations

Spinal Abnormalities: In addition to foramen magnum stenosis, infants may have thoracolumbar kyphosis that is noticed when the child begins to sit. It usually starts to resolve when the child begins to start walking. Progressive kyphosis with vertebral wedging may be managed with bracing when out of bed and surgical stabilization may be needed in severe kyphosis (**Figure 6.21**).

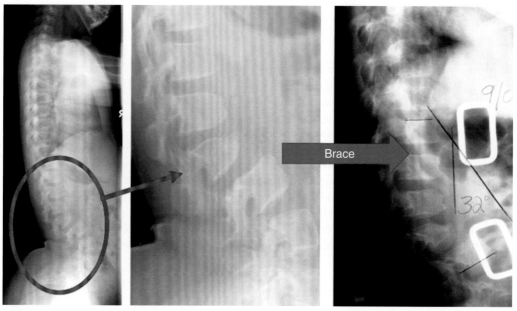

FIGURE 6.21 This toddler with achondroplasia with lumbar kyphosis and vertebral wedging is treated with a brace to improve her kyphosis.

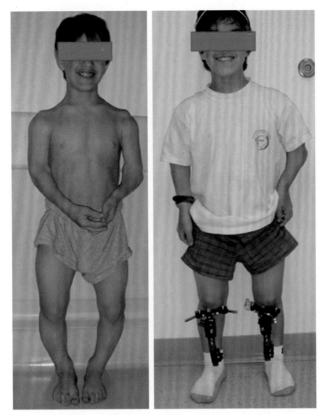

FIGURE 6.22 This 15-year-old boy with achondroplasia has bilateral genu varum that underwent proximal tibial osteotomy with application of external fixation.

The stenosis is common due to progressive reduction of interpedicular distances from L1 to L5 and shortening of the pedicles. Symptomatic stenosis usually occurs in the adults but may occur earlier; severe stenosis requires decompression concurrent spinal stabilization.

Lower Extremity: Children with achondroplasia will have genu varum as a result of deformity in the tibia, femur, knee, or as a combination of deformity from all of three locations (▶ **Video 6.2**).

Even though genu varum is common, the natural history suggests that it is relatively well tolerated and does not lead to total knee replacement in most adults with genu varum. Surgical treatment for varus is indicated for the rare patient with pain, and osteotomies are performed at the site of the deformity (**Figure 6.22**).

Proximal tibia oblique osteotomies can correct both varus and internal rotation. Limb lengthening for stature has been performed for children with achondroplasia. It is more commonly performed in Europe and South America for a variety of reasons.

Upper Extremity: Patients will occasionally have elbow flexion contractures and radial head subluxation/dislocation has been detected. These deformities are usually asymptomatic and rarely require treatment.

● Diastrophic Dysplasia

Children with diastrophic dysplasia (DD) have very severe rhizomelic dwarfism with marked short stature and disproportionately short limbs with classic orthopedic deformities that are often resistant to treatment. The skull is of normal size and left palate is present in nearly half of these children. Children are recognized with their classic cauliflower-shaped ears (**Figure 6.23**).

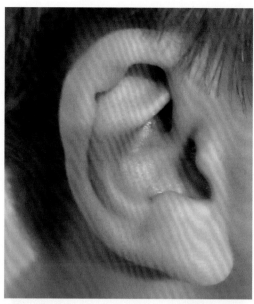

FIGURE 6.23 Cauliflower ears are a classic sign seen in patients with diastrophic dysplasia.

Pathophysiology

DD is an autosomal dominant inheritance and is caused by abnormalities in the sulfate transporter gene. The disease primarily affects proteoglycan molecules in cartilage and results in abnormalities in growth cartilage (shortening) as well as in articular cartilage (joint dysplasia).

Orthopedic Manifestations

Upper Extremity: The thumbs are widely abducted (hitchhiker thumbs). (**Figure 6.24**).

Spine: Scoliosis is common, and the deformity may become very severe. Cervical kyphosis is occasionally seen in patients and can resolve with time and growth, but surgery is required if progression is noted.

Lower Extremity: In addition to skeletal shortening, children with DD have severely dysplastic and contracted joints, which have a propensity for developing osteoarthritis with time (**Figure 6.25**).

Joint releases have limited value and corrective osteotomies are needed (▶ **Videos 6.3 and 6.4**).

Rigid foot deformities (clubfoot and skew foot) are characteristic and are often resistant to standard joint releases which are performed in severe idiopathic clubfeet (**Figure 6.26**).

In DD, the articular surfaces of joints are markedly incongruous; thus, release of the capsule (which is the problem in idiopathic clubfeet) is doomed to fail.

● *Osteogenesis Imperfecta*

Osteogenesis imperfecta (OI) is a hereditary disorder that affects bone strength and has a wide spectrum of involvement that can range from severe infantile osteopenia that can be fatal, to a child with frequent fractures, progressive deformity, and chronic bone pain, to a normal statured adolescent who breaks a few bones. Depending on the severity of disease, treatment can vary from counseling and avoiding high-risk behavior in mild cases to medical treatment and possible surgical reconstruction in more severe cases.

Pathophysiology

Most patients with a clinical diagnosis of OI are positive for a mutation in one of the two genes that encode α chains of type I collagen (*COLIA* and *COL2A*). These defects can affect both the amount and the quality of the collagen, which makes up the tensile strength component of bone.

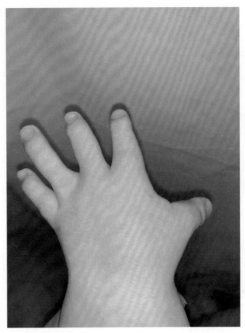

FIGURE 6.24 This boy with diastrophic dysplasia has classic hitchhiker thumbs.

Diagnosis

The diagnosis is typically made clinically in a child with multiple low energy long bone fractures. Genetic studies are typically performed to confirm the diagnosis.

Differential Diagnosis

Since these patients present at a young age with a low energy fracture, the first differential diagnosis list often includes nonaccidental trauma.[9] Metabolic bone disorders and skeletal dysplasia can also be in the differential diagnosis in some patients.

Classification System

The Sillence classification system can broadly classify patients. Type I is a mild disorder with blue sclerae and multiple bone fractures during childhood, but is less common in adolescence. Type II is the lethal manifestation noted in infants with fractured femurs; mortality results from respiratory insufficiency due to rib involvement. Type III is the most severe type. Children have large skulls with triangular facial appearance and initially blue sclerae. Over time, the multiple fractures can lead to long bone deformity and vertebral fractures can lead to spinal deformity. Many patients use wheelchairs for mobility. Type IV is not as severe as Type III as these patients are ambulatory with short stature, bowed bones, and vertebral fractures. Most of the time, their sclera is white.

Treatment

The treatment of OI focuses on the prevention of joint contractures, improving bone fragility, and fracture fixation and deformity correction. Physical therapy is used to help with mobility and prevention of joint contractures. Medical treatment in the form of bisphosphonates (BPs) has been helpful in improving bone density and fracture prevention. Surgical treatment is considered for acute fracture fixation and correction of deformed extremities.[8]

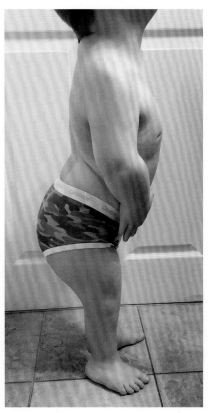

FIGURE 6.25 This boy with diastrophic dysplasia has rhizomelic shortening with severe hip and knee flexion contractures.

Nonorthopedic Manifestations

Teeth: Some forms of OI affect teeth causing opalescent teeth called dentinogenesis imperfecta.

   Face: Some patients with OI have triangular faces (**Figure 6.27**).

   Chest: Barrel chest deformity is seen in some forms of OI.

   Eye: Sclera in some patients with OI has a blue-gray color. This is typically caused by thinning of the sclera showing through the choroidal veins (**Figure 6.28**).

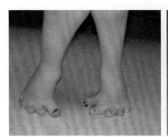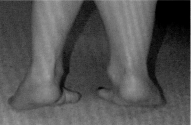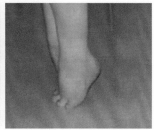

FIGURE 6.26 This seven-year-old girl with diastrophic dysplasia has severe foot deformities. Severe metatarsus adductus and equinus are noted.

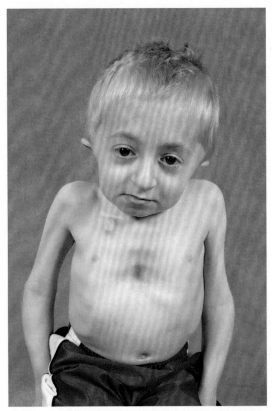

FIGURE 6.27 Triangular face and barrel chest in a child with osteogenesis imperfecta. (Courtesy of Michael P Whyte, MD, Center for Metabolic Bone Disease and Molecular Research at Shriners Hospital for Children, St. Louis.)

Orthopedic Manifestations

Long Bones: Depending on the severity of the disease, the quality of the bones can vary and children can have multiple fractures or gradual deformation, which can result in deformity, and as the deformity increases, the number of fractures can increase (**Figure 6.29**).

The radiographic quality of bone can be improved with the use of oral IV BPs which prevent osteoclastic resorption. Many consider BPs to be the standard of care in moderate and severe OI forms. BPs have reliably shown to increase BMD in OI, and there have been multiple promising reports of reduced fracture risk.

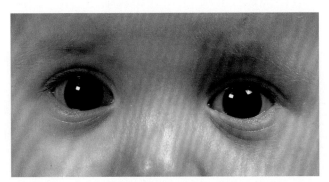

FIGURE 6.28 Blue sclera in a young child with osteogenesis imperfecta. (Courtesy of Michael P Whyte, MD, Center for Metabolic Bone Disease and Molecular Research at Shriners Hospital for Children, St. Louis.)

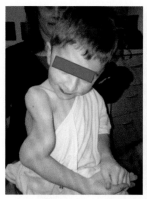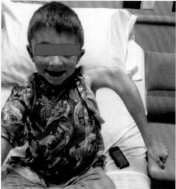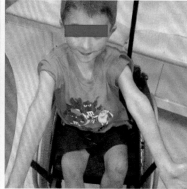

FIGURE 6.29 This boy with Type III osteogenesis imperfecta has severe humerus deformity that required corrective osteotomies and intramedullary fixation.

Surgical methods can be used to correct deformity through osteotomy, which is stabilized by intramedullary devices, which can elongate as the child grows (**Figure 6.30**).

The frequency of fractures can be reduced by these devices and in severe cases, the rods can be inserted before the child begins to walk.

Spine: Patients with Type III and Type IV can develop scoliosis as a result of gradual bone wedging and may require spinal fusion to prevent progression. Bracing is not effective for OI. Surgery typically is indicated at 35° for severe forms of OI and at 45° for mild forms (**Figure 6.31**).

Hypophosphatemic Rickets

Hypophosphatemic rickets is a genetic disorder affecting phosphate reabsorption in the proximal tubule leading to excess phosphate excretion impairing bone mineralization.[10] The most common form is X-linked inherited but autosomal forms also exist.

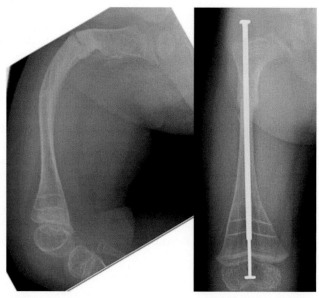

FIGURE 6.30 This 20-month old with severe osteogenesis imperfecta has deformity in the right femur, which was corrected with osteotomy and placement of a lengthening nail. The parallel lines in the femur are growth lines from bisphosphonate treatment.

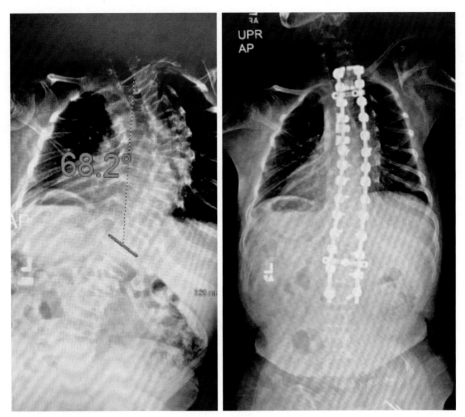

FIGURE 6.31 This 13-year-old with progressive scoliosis and osteogenesis imperfecta underwent posterior spine fusion.

Pathophysiology

PHEX is the most commonly affected gene in hypophosphatemic rickets. PHEX gene mutation results in increased levels of serum fibroblast growth factor 23 (FGF-23) leading to decreased phosphate reabsorption in the proximal tubule.[11] Hypophosphatemia impairs bone mineralization resulting in the clinical features of rickets.

Physical Findings

Children with hypophosphatemic rickets typically have short stature with small lower extremities (**Figure 6.32**).

Hypophosphatemia may cause muscle weakness that can delay walking in the affected children. Dolichocephaly (elongation of the skull from front to back) and craniosynostosis (premature closure of the skull sutures in an infant) are seen in some children (**Figure 6.33**).

Abnormal bone mineralization in the lower extremities can result in lower extremity deformities typically in the form of genu varum or genu valgum (**Figure 6.34**).

Bone pain and tenderness at the tendon insertion sites (enthesopathy) are also commonly seen in the affected children and adults.[11,12]

Diagnosis

Diagnosis is typically confirmed with low serum phosphorus level in a patient with the clinical symptoms described especially when a strong family history is present. Genetic studies can be done to confirm the diagnosis.[11]

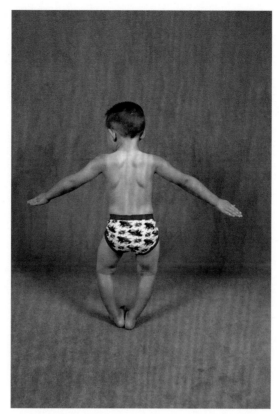

FIGURE 6.32 A child with X-linked hypophosphatemic rickets. Short stature, genu varum, and short lower extremities are shown. (Courtesy of Michael P Whyte, MD, Center for Metabolic Bone Disease and Molecular Research at Shriners Hospital for Children, St. Louis.)

Differential Diagnosis

Other forms of rickets (nutritional, vitamin D resistant, etc.) and some forms of skeletal dysplasia may have similar clinical features. Although rare in children, tumor-induced osteomalacia can result in low energy fractures, bone pain, and low serum phosphorus level.[13]

Treatment

Medical treatment with phosphorus and active form of vitamin D is the mainstay of treatment.[14] Surgical treatment may be required for the correction of limb deformities.[10]

● *Complex Regional Pain Syndrome*

Introduction

Terminology

Complex regional pain syndrome (CRPS) was first described over 150 years ago and is characterized as a chronic pain condition affecting a single extremity.[1] There are dozens of different names for this condition, including reflex sympathetic dystrophy (RSD), causalgia, Sudeck atrophy, shoulder hand syndrome, transient osteoporosis, algodystrophy, post-traumatic osteoporosis, and regional migratory osteoporosis.[1] CRPS is the "officially endorsed" term by a working group for the International Association for the Study of Pain. It is subdivided into CRPS 1 if it is not associated with a nerve injury (formerly known as reflex sympathetic dystrophy) and CRPS 2 if it is associated with a nerve injury (formerly known as causalgia).[1]

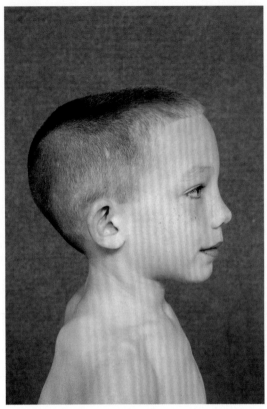

FIGURE 6.33 Plagiocephaly in a child with hypophosphatemic rickets. (Courtesy of Michael P Whyte, MD, Center for Metabolic Bone Disease and Molecular Research at Shriners Hospital for Children, St. Louis.)

Pathophysiology

There are numerous theories on the pathophysiology of CRPS, which includes an inflammatory process, a sympathetically mediated process, central sensitization, ischemia-reperfusion injury, neuropathy, and autoimmune process.

Pediatric Versus Adult CRPS

Pediatric CRPS is not as common as adult CRPS and rarely occurs under the age of 6 years. Most typically, it occurs in the adolescent years, is more common in females, and more common in the lower extremities.[2]

Clinical Significance

For children with CRPS, most of the inciting injuries are relatively minor and are often not related to fractures. As a result, it may take several months before CRPS is diagnosed and ultimately treated.[3] An understanding of the history and physical examination findings is key in order to avoid delays in diagnosis and treatment of this condition.

Physical Examination

Diagnostic Criteria

For adults with CRPS, the Budapest clinical diagnostic criteria have been found to be 85% sensitive and 69% specific.[4] There is no consensus-based diagnostic criteria for CRPS in children; however, the Budapest criteria is currently being evaluated for its reliability in the pediatric population:

1. Patients must report continuing pain that is disproportionate in time or degree to the usual course of pain after any trauma or other inciting event.

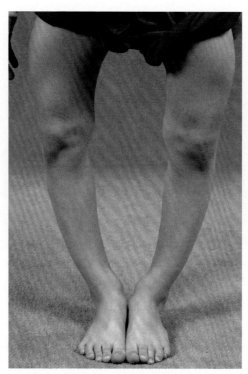

FIGURE 6.34 Bilateral genu varum in hypophosphatemic rickets. (Courtesy of Michael P Whyte, MD, Center for Metabolic Bone Disease and Molecular Research at Shriners Hospital for Children, St. Louis.)

2. Patients must report at least one symptom in three of the four following categories:
   a. Sensory: hyperalgesia (that is, exaggerated pain to a painful stimulus, such as pinprick) and/or allodynia (that is, pain elicited by a normally nonpainful stimulus, such as light touch).
   b. Vasomotor: skin color changes and/or skin color asymmetry and/or temperature asymmetry.
   c. Sudomotor/edema: edema and/or sweating changes and/sweating asymmetry.
   d. Motor/trophic: decreased range of motion and/or motor dysfunction (weakness, tremor, dystonia) and/or trophic changes/asymmetry involving nails, skin, and/or hair.

Pediatric Physical Examination

The physical examination for children sometimes differs as compared to the examination findings for adults (**Figure 6.35**).

In the pediatric population, the extremity may be cold and blue at the onset of symptoms and may not be very swollen or edematous. This is opposed to a warm, red, and swollen extremity in the adult population.[5]

● Diagnostic Tests/Advanced Imaging

It is common that children undergo imaging as part of their investigation into the etiology of their symptoms. In one study on 20 children with CRPS, the most common imaging modalities used were plain radiography (95%), three-phase technetium bone scan (70%), and MRI (45%). Initially radiographs were used to rule out fracture, while later on, radiographs were found to demonstrate generalized osteopenia. Bone scans were often obtained within 3 months from the onset of symptoms and showed inconsistent patterns of uptake: diffuse hypoperfusion, normal perfusion, and, less commonly, diffuse hyperperfusion (**Figure 6.36**).[3]

Treatment

Once diagnosed, effective treatment of CRPS requires a dedicated multidisciplinary approach. This approach often requires a combination of psychology, physiotherapy, and medication.[3]

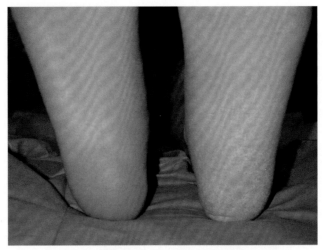

FIGURE 6.35 Clinical pictures of a child with right foot reflex sympathetic dystrophy. She has different color and sweat pattern on the plantar aspect of the right foot in comparison to the left.

Psychology

As anxiety and pain-related fear have been identified as being associated with a poor outcome with CRPS, psychological treatment is extremely valuable.[3] The goals of treatment are to improve pain management skill and promote normal activity levels through behavioral and cognitive-behavioral interventions. Psychological interventions are key if the patient is missing school, as normalizing life activities (school, sports, sleep, and social) is key element to improving CRPS.

Physiotherapy

Daily home exercises and mirror therapy are the cornerstones of effective physical treatment of CRPS.[6] To ensure return to physical function, physiotherapy is an integral part of the management of patients

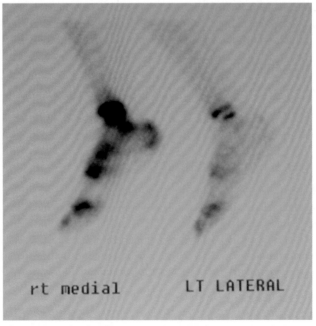

FIGURE 6.36 Bone scan of the same child with right foot reflex sympathetic dystrophy. This demonstrates increased uptake in right foot.

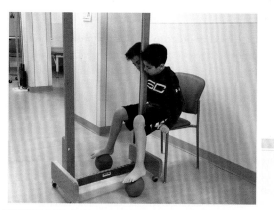
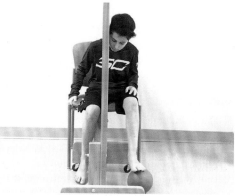

FIGURE 6.37 A 10-year-old male basketball player with a right ankle injury and subsequent reflex sympathetic dystrophy (RSD). His RSD is being treated by mirror therapy utilizing his unaffected left lower.

who are experiencing CRPS.[3] However, the primary challenge for the physiotherapist in this regard is the pain that is often experienced by the patient with CRPS. Options for therapeutic and functional movement are often limited by the patient's symptom presentation. Facilitating movement without increasing pain is much more pleasant to patients. Mirror therapy is a technique that "moves without moving" the affected extremity thereby not increasing the patient's overall pain (**Figure 6.37**; ▶ **Video 6.5**).

The mirror visual feedback is perceived as movement of the painful extremity without the experience of pain associated with actual movement. In essence, through mirror visual feedback, the patient is engaging the cortical regions of his brain responsible for movement of his affected extremity. Mirror therapy can provide significant analgesic benefit, which will then enable the patient to participate in more conventional movement-based therapeutic exercise. Mobile applications are available to assist with patients performing these exercises at home (**Figure 6.38**).

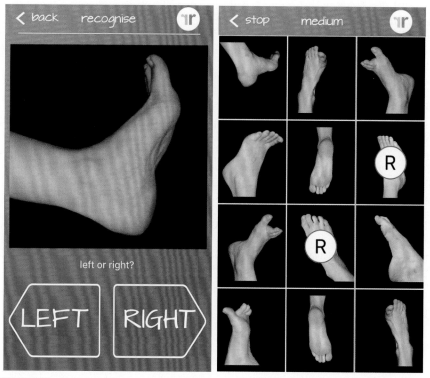

FIGURE 6.38 The Recognise™ app can be used to treat CRPS through a graded motor imagery program.

Medication

Medications such as amitriptyline and gabapentin can be used in order to improve symptoms enough to allow for physiotherapy of their affected extremity.[3] For more refractory cases, inpatient treatment with continuous regional anesthesia (epidural or peripheral nerve) and inpatient physiotherapy may be required.[7]

References

1. Dutton K, Littlejohn G. Terminology, criteria, and definitions in complex regional pain syndrome: challenges and solutions. *J Pain Res*. 2015;8:871-877.
2. Logan DE, Carpino EA, Chiang G, et al. A day-hospital approach to treatment of pediatric complex regional pain syndrome: initial functional outcomes. *Clin J Pain*. 2012;28(9):766-774.
3. Low AK, Ward K, Wines AP. Pediatric complex regional pain syndrome. *J Pediatr Orthop*. 2007;27(5):567-572.
4. Harden RN, Bruehl S, Perez RS, et al. Validation of proposed diagnostic criteria (the "budapest criteria") for complex regional pain syndrome. *Pain*. 2010;150(2):268-274.
5. Borchers AT, Gershwin ME. Complex regional pain syndrome: a comprehensive and critical review. *Autoimmun Rev*. 2014;13(3):242-265.
6. Moseley GL. Graded motor imagery is effective for long-standing complex regional pain syndrome: a randomised controlled trial. *Pain*. 2004;108(1-2):192-198.
7. Donado C, Lobo K, Velarde-Álvarez MF, et al. Continuous regional anesthesia and inpatient rehabilitation for pediatric complex regional pain syndrome. *Reg Anesth Pain Med*. 2017;42(4):527-534.
8. Burnei G, Vlad C, Georgescu I, Gavriliu TS, Dan D. Osteogenesis imperfecta: diagnosis and treatment. *J Am Acad Orthop Surg*. 2008;16(6):356-366.
9. Kocher MS, Kasser JR. Orthopaedic aspects of child abuse. *J Am Acad Orthop Surg*. 2000;8(1):10-20.
10. Sharkey MS, Grunseich K, Carpenter TO. Contemporary medical and surgical management of X-linked hypophosphatemic rickets. *J Am Acad Orthop Surg*. 2015;23(7):433-442.
11. Pavone V, Testa G, Gioitta Iachino S, Evola FR, Avondo S, Sessa G. Hypophosphatemic rickets: etiology, clinical features and treatment. *Eur J Orthop Surg Traumatol*. 2015;25(2):221-226.
12. Reid IR, Hardy DC, Murphy WA, Teitelbaum SL, Bergfeld MA, Whyte MP. X-linked hypophosphatemia: a clinical, biochemical, and histopathologic assessment of morbidity in adults. *Medicine (Baltimore)*. 1989;68(6):336-352.
13. Sahoo J, Balachandran K, Kamalanathan S, et al. Tumor(s) induced osteomalacia – a curious case of double trouble. *J Clin Endocrinol Metab*. 2014;99(2):395-398.
14. Petersen DJ, Boniface AM, Schranck FW, Rupich RC, Whyte MP. X-linked hypophosphatemic rickets: a study (with literature review) of linear growth response to calcitriol and phosphate therapy. *J Bone Miner Res*. 1992;7(6):583-597.

Suggested readings

Bitterman A, Sponseller P. Marfan syndrome: a clinical update. *J Am Acad Orthop Surg*. 2017;25(9):603-609.

Caird MS, Wills BP, Dormans JP. Down Syndrome in children: the role of the orthopaedic surgeon. *J Am Acad Orthop Surg*. 2006;14(11):610-619.

Crawford AH, Schorry EK. Neurofibromatosis in children: the role of the orthopedist. *J Am Acad Orthop Surg*. 1999;7(4):217-203.

DE MAio F, Fichera A, Deluna V, Mancini F, Caterini R. Orhtopedic aspects of marfan syndrome: the experience of a referral center for diagnosis of rare diseases. *Adv Orthop*. 2016;2016:8275391.

Feldman DS, Jordn C, Fonseca L. Orthopedic manifestations of neurofibromatosis type 1. *J Am Acad Orthop Surg*. 2010;18(6):346-357.

Hankinson TC, Anderson RC. Craniovertebral junction abnormalities in down syndrome. *Neurosurgery*. 2010;66(3 suppl):32-38. doi:10.1227/01.NEU.0000365803.22786.F0.

7

Diagnostically Directed Examination for Infectious, Inflammatory, and Neoplastic Conditions

Jonathan G. Schoenecker, Stephanie N. Moore-Lotridge, Samuel Johnson, and Alexandre Arkader

● Introduction

Pediatric musculoskeletal infections are challenging. Given the potential for devastating complications, such as avascular necrosis, growth compromise, joint destruction, thrombosis, and even death, few consults in pediatric orthopedics provoke more apprehension and concern than a child with a potential infection. Bacteria express virulence factors that promote tropism for damaged and regenerating tissue,[1] and given that the developing musculoskeletal system in children and regenerative tissues share many common features (ie, growth factors, angiogenesis, newly forming matrices), there is an increased prevalence of infection in children as compared to adults, even independent of injury.[2] The principal cause of morbidity and mortality in patients with pediatric musculoskeletal infections is a prolonged or exuberant host response to the injury, referred to as the acute phase response (APR). Prior to antibiotics, the mortality rate of acute hematogenous osteomyelitis in children was nearly 50%.[3,4] Fortunately, through the advent of antibiotics and the ability to perform surgical debridement of infected tissues, the mortality rate from pediatric infections has dropped tremendously.[2,5,6]

In the modern era, while cases of isolated infections do occur, infections that lead to death or disability typically involve infection of multiple tissues of the same anatomic location (eg, bone, muscle, and joint), or systemic infections involving multiple body parts (eg, bone and lung)[6-8] (**Figure 7.1**). Opposed to single isolated infections, the APR to combinatory infections is more exuberant, correlating with the amount of tissue infected and the duration of the infection. Furthermore, pathogens have developed the capacity to "hijack" acute phase reactants, thus pathologically driving inflammation and coagulation, driving thrombotic complications, such as septic pulmonary emboli, deep vein thrombosis, and potentially death.[9] Given the essential role for vascularity in developing bone, thrombosis following an exuberant APR can also lead to avascular necrosis of the epiphysis, metaphysis, or diaphysis, potentially leading to loss of joint function and abnormal limb development. For these reasons, rapid diagnosis and application of the appropriate antibiotics and/or surgical intervention are essential to mitigate an exuberant or prolonged APR.

In this chapter, we will examine the epidemiology and clinical presentation of common musculoskeletal infections afflicting the pediatric population, discuss the diagnostic tools available (imaging and laboratory assessments) for evaluation of infection location and progression, and highlight evidence-based treatment practices aimed at reducing the time patients spend in an exuberant survival APR to improve patient outcomes and mitigate complications. In addition, we will highlight some findings that are common to pediatric musculoskeletal neoplasia and noninfectious inflammatory conditions.

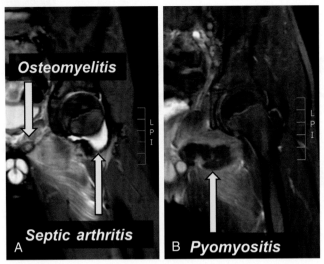

FIGURE 7.1 Infection involving multiple tissues surrounding the hip. Most severe cases of musculoskeletal infections of the hip or the knee do not involve an isolated tissue type. In these MRI cuts, there is evidence of both (A) osteomyelitis in addition to possible septic arthritis (vs reactive joint effusion) and (B) pyomyositis in the same patient within a localized environment. This is typical of cases of hip infections where pathogens rarely stay isolated to the joint. (Images reproduced with permission from Monroe Carell Jr. Children's Hospital at Vanderbilt, Nashville, TN.)

● *Musculoskeletal Infection Epidemiology*

In the pediatric population, infections of the hip and knee predominate as anatomical characteristics of the bone, joint, and muscles surrounding the hip and knee predispose them to be the most common sites of infection in children.[10] Pyogenic organisms are the most common causative pathogens of pediatric musculoskeletal infections with *Staphylococcus aureus* being responsible for 40% to 90% of cases.[4,11] However, the patterns of epidemiology related to pediatric musculoskeletal infections are regularly changing, attributable to dynamic mutations in the bacterial genome, use of antibiotics, and vaccinations. For example, with the advent of routine infant vaccination against *Haemophilus influenzae*, incidence of musculoskeletal infection caused by *H. influenzae* has decreased substantially.[12] In another example, a 2008 study found that zero children were treated for a methicillin-resistant *Staphylococcus aureus* (MRSA) infection in 1982; yet from 2002 to 2004, MRSA was isolated as the causative organism in 30% of children.[2] Thus, the epidemiology for musculoskeletal infections is ever-changing and an up-to-date understanding of disease incidence and common pathogens must be considered when diagnosing and directing treatment for patients with musculoskeletal infections.

Osteomyelitis

Acute hematogenous osteomyelitis (AHO) is defined as an inflammatory infection of the bone that will often extend to the subperiosteal space, surrounding muscle or joint. The physical examination will vary with location and severity of disease. Osteomyelitis in the extremity can lead to global limb swelling, warmth, and redness. Painful palpation and limited joint motion can be present in all infections of the limb, and differential diagnosis can be difficult to differentiate among cellulitis, pyomyositis, septic arthritis, and osteomyelitis (**Figure 7.2**).

Most AHO in children involves the appendicular skeleton at the metaphyseal region of long bones such as the femur, tibia, and humerus[13] (**Figure 7.3**). In the United States, AHO has an estimated annual incidence rate of 1 in 5000 in children younger than 13 years of age.[14] Prior studies have demonstrated that the rate of osteomyelitis is higher in males than in females.[15] Several studies conducted in the United States demonstrate an increase in AHO: a research team at the University of Texas Southwestern

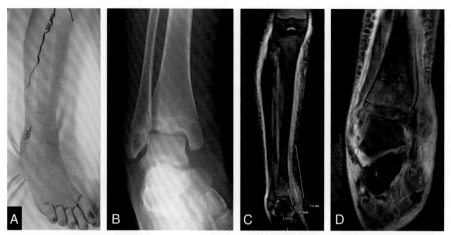

FIGURE 7.2 Osteomyelitis of the distal tibia. A, This girl has an inflamed leg with swelling, redness, pain, and warmth. The extent of inflammation has been marked in order to follow disease progression. B, With early presentation of osteomyelitis, the radiographs are negative. C, MRI of the entire leg demonstrates diffuse inflammation that correlates with the clinical examination. D, More limited MRI demonstrates that the infection is based in the distal tibia metaphysis. (Images reproduced with permission from CHOP Orthopedics, Philadelphia, PA.)

reported a 2.8-fold increase in the incidence of osteomyelitis from 1988 to 2008[2]; researchers at the Mayo Clinic found an increase in osteomyelitis between 1969 and 2009, citing changes in diagnosing patterns or increases in risk factors (eg, diabetes) among patients.[15]

While *S. aureus* remains the most common causative organism in patients with osteomyelitis,[4,11,16-19] other organisms, such as coagulase-negative *Staphylococcus*, group A β-hemolytic *Streptococcus*, *Streptococcus pneumoniae*, and group B *Streptococcus*, are also common.[10] As highlighted above, due to antibiotic administration and subsequent pathogen evolution, physicians are now observing an increased rate of patients with MRSA-associated osteomyelitis. Importantly, compared to non-MRSA osteomyelitis, patients with MRSA have been shown to endure a more robust APR, have a longer hospital stay, and experience a higher rate of complications.[20]

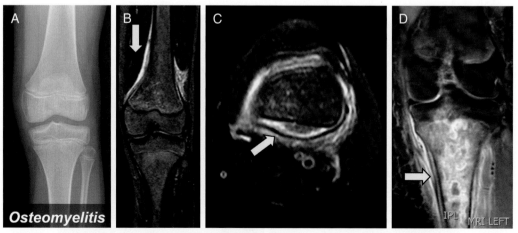

FIGURE 7.3 Osteomyelitis at the metaphysis. Osteomyelitis in the metaphysis can spread to the subperiosteal or extraperiosteal space. Radiographic (A) and MRI identification (B) of a distal femoral osteomyelitis with subperiosteal abscess of the distal femur that has spread into muscle. Radiographic (C) and MRI identification (D) of proximal tibial osteomyelitis of the proximal tibia with subperiosteal abcess. Yellow arrows indicate infection site. (Images reproduced with permission from Monroe Carell Jr. Children's Hospital at Vanderbilt, Nashville, TN.)

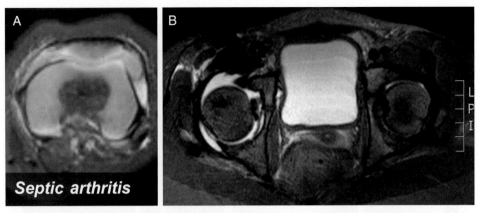

FIGURE 7.4 Septic arthritis. A, MRI of septic arthritis of the knee. B, MRI of septic arthritis of the hip. (Images reproduced with permission from Monroe Carell Jr. Children's Hospital at Vanderbilt, Nashville, TN.)

Septic Arthritis

Septic arthritis is an infection in a joint space, with no extension to the surrounding musculature or bone[21] (**Figure 7.4**). It occurs almost twice as often as AHO and most frequently affects children under the age of 10, with 50% of cases occurring in children younger than 2 years of age. Unlike AHO, septic arthritis presents as a near equal distribution among males and females.[5] However, upon presentation, septic arthritis can be difficult to differentiate from conditions like transient synovitis (discussed in more detail below), which poses no long-term sequela. Importantly, septic arthritis is associated with marked complications, such as early osteoarthritis of the joints, developmental deformities of the infected joint, or spreading to a systemic infection.

Hematogenous-derived septic arthritis can develop in the shoulder, elbow, and ankle, but is most prominently observed in the hip and knee joints.[6,22,23] Septic arthritis can also result from either direct inoculation following a traumatic injury or contamination from an adjacent infection, such as epiphyseal osteomyelitis (**Figure 7.5**). Importantly, there are a few metaphyses that are intra-articular and if affected with AHO, they could lead to a higher chance of a secondary septic arthritis. These include the proximal humerus, proximal radius, proximal femur, and distal fibula.

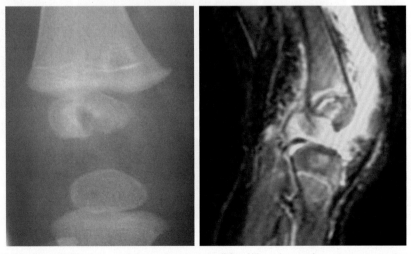

FIGURE 7.5 Septic arthritis from epiphyseal osteomyelitis. Although rare, hematogenous osteomyelitis can begin in the epiphysis and spread to the joint presenting with septic arthritis. (Images reproduced with permission from CHOP Orthopedics, Philadelphia, PA.)

While *S. aureus* is the most common pathogen overall, there is a significant increase in the incidence of *Kingella kingae*, especially in children younger than 2 years old.[24] Importantly, unlike *Staphylococcus* species, *K. kingae* is a less virulent gram-negative bacillus that is associated with a lower rate of complications and joint damage compared to *Staphylococcus* species. Furthermore, if *K. kingae* is suspected, cultures should be held for 10 days to increase the recovery rate for *K. kingae*. In addition, yield is considerably higher when a specimen is inoculated into enriched blood culture media. PCR testing for *K. kingae* is now used routinely in areas of high prevalence.

Pyomyositis

Pyomyositis is defined as an infection isolated to the musculature with no extension into the bone or nearby joint. On physical examination, this usually presents with swollen and painful limb. Sometimes the child can present with compartment syndrome–like signs such as pain with passive stretch (**Figure 7.6**).

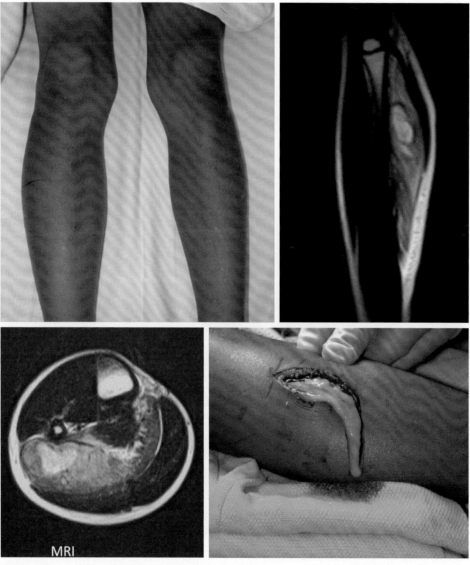

FIGURE 7.6 Pyomyositis of the leg. Clinical examination demonstrates a swollen calf that is tender. The child resists dorsiflexion of the foot and has pain with passive stretch. MRI exam demonstrates an abscess in the posterior compartment that requires surgical drainage. (Images reproduced with permission from CHOP Orthopedics, Philadelphia, PA.)

Pyomyositis can affect multiple muscle groups, varies in severity (associated with the amount of tissue infected), and frequently affects the musculature of the hip. It can be difficult to clinically differentiate between proximal femoral osteomyelitis, septic arthritis of the hip, or pyomyositis. In recent years, pyomyositis has been reported with greater frequency in large part due to the increased use of MRI in cases of pediatric musculoskeletal infections[25-28] (**Figure 7.7**). A prospective study conducted at Vanderbilt Children's Hospital from 2010 to 2012 found that in children consulted for an acutely irritable hip, cases of pyomyositis outnumbered cases of septic arthritis at a rate of 2:1.[29] As such, proper identification of pyomyositis (rather than septic arthritis) allows patients to be treated without the need for joint debridement. *S. aureus* has been reported as the most common pathogen in up to 90% of cases.

Necrotizing Fasciitis

Necrotizing fasciitis is a rare infectious process that primarily involves the deep dermis and underlying fascia of musculoskeletal tissue. Necrotizing fasciitis can occur idiopathically or be brought on by a number of identifiable causes, such as minor trauma, major trauma, or postoperatively.[30-32] Although it has been estimated that 70% of cases are of the lower extremity, upper extremity involvement has been described.[33,34]

While Group A *Streptococcus* remains the primary cause of monomicrobial infections, most cases of necrotizing fasciitis are caused by two or more bacterial species that work synergistically to seize control of the host APR. The mortality rate of necrotizing fasciitis in children has been reported in the range of 5% to 20%, making it one of the most feared and life-threatening orthopedic infections.[35-38]

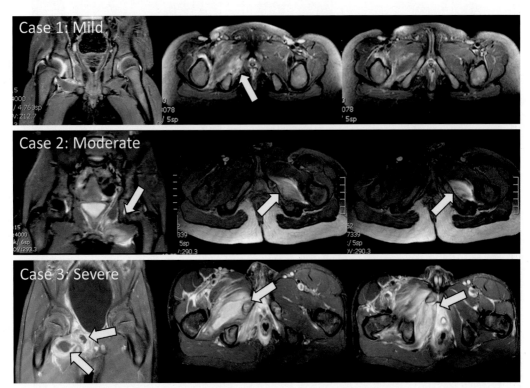

FIGURE 7.7 Varying severity of pyomyositis in musculature around the hip. Three pediatric cases with MRI imaging demonstrating mild, moderate, and severe cases of pyomyositis surrounding the hip. (Images reproduced with permission from Monroe Carell Jr. Children's Hospital at Vanderbilt, Nashville, TN.)

● *Pathophysiology of Disease: Acute Phase Response—The Double Edge Sword in Infection*

Musculoskeletal tissue injury evokes a cascade of carefully regulated pathways that are collectively known as the APR. The two principle roles of the APR are (1) survival and (2) tissue repair. These objectives are tackled in a temporal order, such that during the "survival" phase, damage control is initiated by a coordinated effort between coagulation and the survival inflammatory response to temporarily seal off compartments with a fibrin/platelet seal. Additionally, this sealant promotes egress of survival inflammatory cells, which help reduce the susceptibility to infection. For example, neutrophils, in cooperation with the host's coagulation response, work to trap bacteria in DNA nets and fibrin webs and release chemotoxins to kill pathogens while macrophages clear the trapped bacteria. Once survival is ensured, the APR transitions to a reparative inflammatory response that paves the way for revascularization and regeneration of the damaged tissues.

In the context of an isolated injury, the APR is a regulated and coordinated series of events occurring over 6 weeks, allowing for a timely recovery[9,54] (**Figure 7.8A**). When the APR is insufficient, as commonly observed in patients with liver damage or cirrhosis (the liver is the principal effector organ of the APR), patients can experience hemorrhage, greater susceptibility to infection, and subsequently impaired tissue regeneration. Alternatively, an over exuberant or prolonged "survival" APR can drive excessive inflammation and a coagulopathic state, enough to increase the risk for complications, such as thrombosis, systemic inflammatory response syndrome, multiorgan dysfunction, and death (**Figure 7.8B**).[55] If the patient survives and enters into the repair phase, a prolonged survival phase can promote delays in healing or potential failure of the reparative phase, resulting in chronic nonhealing wounds, tissue fibrosis, and impaired tissue function.[56,57]

In the context of infection, the regulated and coordinated nature of the APR can be lost.[1,9] After invading the body, bacterial proliferation and the expression of virulence factors allow pathogens to evade the host containment mechanisms (fibrin/DNA webs) and migrate through tissue planes, causing damage to neighboring tissue. As the infection progresses, injury to the surrounding tissues is continuous, which, along with the bacteria's capacity to hijack many of the acute phase reactants, leads to an exuberant "survival" APR (**Figure 7.9A**).

Antibiotics and surgical debridement are paramount for cessation of the continuous injury[1,9] (**Figure 7.9B**). As noted above, regulation of the APR is critical, such that continuous exuberant activation can lead to devastating complications, accounting for the majority of morbidity and mortality in pediatric patients with musculoskeletal infections. Therefore, the APR may be viewed as a "double-edged sword." While a well-coordinated APR is essential for combating and eliminating an infection, a prolonged, excessive APR can drive devastating complications.[9] Together, these concepts present a paradox for surgeons and health care providers caring for these patients.

To assist in overcoming this paradox, timely identification and diagnosis of musculoskeletal infections, serial monitoring of the APR, and application of the appropriate antibiotics and/or surgical intervention are essential to mitigate an exuberant or prolonged APR, thus reducing the risk of complications, patient morbidity, and mortality.

Bacterial Hijacking of the APR

To combat the body's host response to infection, pathogenic bacteria have developed virulence factors that provide them the ability to invade, persist, and disseminate within the human body.[1] While bacteria travel through the circulation and the musculoskeletal systems every day, they rarely take hold to cause clinical infection. Though chance will play a role in determining when and where musculoskeletal infections occur, it has been established that "trauma" to musculoskeletal tissue is a major predisposing factor as to where infections establish.[58,59] For example, when a traumatic injury occurs in the skeletal muscle, a hematoma can form and serve as a focal nidus for infection.[60] Furthermore, in the developing musculoskeletal system of pediatric patients, unique characteristics of the physis, such

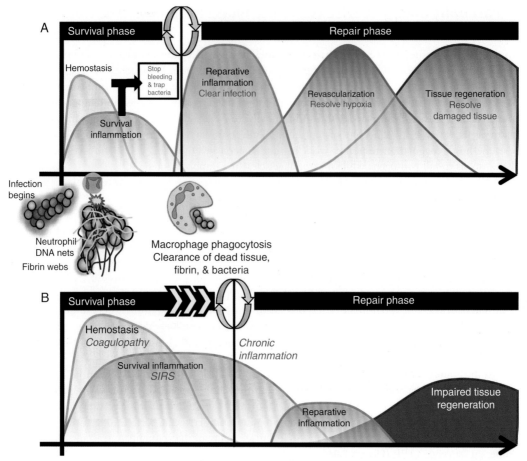

FIGURE 7.8 The acute phase response—the body's response to injury. A, Following the establishment of an infection and the associated tissue destruction, the body must first resolve bleeding and contain the bacteria via neutrophil-derived DNA nets and fibrin webs. Together, hemostasis and the survival inflammatory response comprise the "survival phase" of the APR, which is essential to preserve life. Once bleeding has been stopped and the bacteria are contained, the body can transition to the "reparative phase" where inflammatory components, such as macrophages, can enter the tissue and begin to clear dead cellular debris, bacteria, and the previously established fibrin matrices. Once cleared, revascularization and tissue regeneration of the damaged tissues can occur to reestablish the preinfection physiologic state. B, In cases of severe injury, the APR can be overexuberantly activated, provoking complications in both the "survival phase" and "repair phase." APR, acute phase response.

as robust vascularity and its relative immune privilege nature, may predispose this site to initiation of infections. For example, the tortuous anatomy of the vasculature of the zone of ossification in the metaphysis has been demonstrated to cause turbulent blood flow, thereby permitting bacterial accumulations.[61] Additionally, developing bone produces factors that inhibit innate immune cell activity in the metaphysis, but not the diaphysis.[62] Therefore, taken together, these anatomical characteristics make the metaphysis a more permissive and nutrient-rich region in which pathologic bacteria can take hold.

Because of coevolution over millions of years, bacteria have developed mechanisms to "hijack" and utilize the APR to their advantage to support dissemination and evade the host immune response. As discussed above, coagulation during the survival phase of the APR serves as one of the initial defense mechanisms against bacterial invasion by immobilizing bacteria with fibrin clots and recruiting leukocytes to the site of infection through integrin expression on fibrin.[1] However, bacteria like *S. aureus*

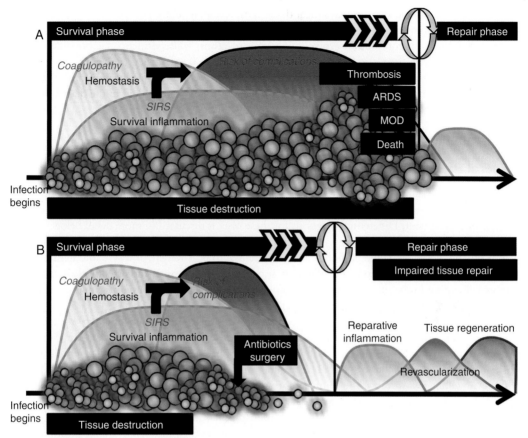

FIGURE 7.9 The acute phase response following infection. A, As infection progresses, the survival phase of the APR will become exuberantly activated, as it attempts to respond to the progressing infection and tissue destruction. Time spent under these two systemic states increases the patient's risk for complications. B, Through intervention with surgical debridement and antibiotic administration, the pathogen onslaught can be reduced, allowing the survival phase of the APR to be sufficient to stop bleeding and trapping the remaining bacteria, though patients may still experience impaired tissue healing in response to a dysregulated APR. ARDS, acute respiratory distress syndrome; MOD, multiple organ dysfunction.

utilize the coagulation system to their benefit by producing virulence factors, such as coagulase (Coa) and von Willebrand factor binding protein (vWBP), which activate prothrombin to thrombin, thereby catalyzing the cleavage for fibrinogen to fibrin. Fibrin then surrounds the bacteria and forms a protective abscess from incoming neutrophils and macrophages, thus allowing the bacteria to proliferate.[1] As the abscess grows, *S. aureus* produces SpA (staphylococcal protein A) and Emp, an envelope associate protein, to impede phagocytosis and promote abscess stabilization/adherence in tissues, respectively.[63] Once quorum is reached and the abscess can no longer support further bacterial growth, *S. aureus* utilizes plasmin, a critical fibrinolytic enzyme, to break apart the fibrin abscess allowing the bacteria to disseminate.[1]

Unsurprisingly, many bacteria have developed virulence factors that manipulate the fibrinolytic system to avoid being trapped by procoagulant factors like fibrin. As plasmin is the critical protease for the fibrinolytic system, *Streptococcus pyogenes*, *S. aureus*, *Escherichia coli*, *Borrelia burgdorferi*, *Neisseria meningitidis*, and *Pseudomonas aeruginosa* all hijack plasmin activity as a means to cleave fibrin clots, laminin basement membranes, and DNA nets to escape containment to disseminate.[1] Together, these virulence factors help to explain why bacteria commonly associated with musculoskeletal infections often disseminate among various anatomical tissue compartments (bone, muscle, joint space, and circulation). This ongoing evolutionary battle between the host APR and the pathogen's capacity to hijack these mechanisms will continue to evolve going forward. Thus, while virulence factors differ significantly between bacterial species (eg, *S. aureus* compared to *K. kingae*), they evolve toward the same goal: to better serve bacterial survival. Therefore, awareness and continual reeducation of the interplay between the APR and bacterial infections of the musculoskeletal system will aid in the diagnosis, prognostication, and treatment of infections going forward.[1,9,11]

● Clinical Presentation of Musculoskeletal Infections

General Presentation

Unfortunately, the signs and symptoms of musculoskeletal infections, focal trauma, and cancer around the hip and knee present in a similar manner. Thus, the ability to discern these pathologies is critical to direct proper treatment. Differential diagnosis for these cases is discussed in more detail below.

Independent of the musculoskeletal infection type, pediatric patients commonly present with complaints of pain, decreased range of motion, inability/refusal to bear weight, and systemic signs of infection, such as a fever. While deep tissue infections, such as deep pyomyositis and osteomyelitis, may show minimal alteration to the skin, soft tissue infections, such as superficial pyomyositis, may present with erythema and a swollen appearance (**Figure 7.6**).

Because of significant swelling associated with musculoskeletal infections, pediatric patients can experience pain, effusion that hinders motion, and subsequent anxiety associated with pain.[39] As such, when the hip is involved, patients most often hold their hips in a flexed, abducted, and externally rotated position (**Figure 7.10; ▶ Video 7.1**). When the knee or elbow is involved, patients will likewise present with an unwillingness to move the joint, adopting a semi-flexed position of the joint, which can be released following joint aspiration (**Figure 7.11**). As an infection progresses, further tissue damage and swelling can cause increased pressure within the joint capsule, ultimately depriving the joint from its necessary blood supply. For this reason, patients should be left in their most comfortable position rather than immobilized in an extended position.[40,41]

Special consideration must be made for the neonate or premature infant in the ICU. These children have minimal immunological capabilities. As such, temperature may not be elevated and blood work may be normal with little rise in the acute phase reactants. In these cases, the key findings are redness, swelling, and decreased use of the extremity (**Figure 7.12**). Many of these neonates will have multiple sites of infection and those joints that cannot be assessed well (hip and shoulder) should have screening ultrasound and aspiration if positive.

Presentation of Osteomyelitis Versus Septic Arthritis Versus Pyomyositis

It can be difficult to discern septic arthritis, periarticular osteomyelitis, and pyomyositis. Patients with metaphyseal periarticular osteomyelitis may develop a reactive effusion that limits motion, causes pain, and mimics the clinical presentation of septic arthritis (**Figure 7.13**). If the osteomyelitis is more meta-diaphyseal in location, patients commonly lack the joint irritability found in pediatric patients with septic arthritis and will instead exhibit tenderness to palpitation of the affected bone. Likewise, pyomyositis is most commonly found in pediatric patients around the hip joint (pericapsular pyomyositis) and can present similarly to septic arthritis, including joint irritability, pain, and reduced range of motion.

Furthermore, clinical examination and laboratory markers often fail to distinguish pyomyositis from septic arthritis and osteomyelitis. In a two-year prospective study for septic hip consults, only 15% were found to have a confirmed septic hip, while the remaining patients were alternatively found to have transient synovitis (38%), pericapsular pyomyositis (32%), proximal femur osteomyelitis (6%), or a differential diagnosis such as leukemia or neuroblastoma (ie, other) (9%).[29]

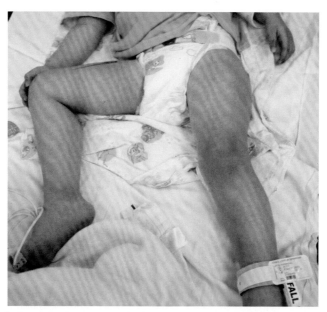

FIGURE 7.10 Exam findings of a flexed externally rotated and abducted hip are the most concerning for infection around the hip in children. (Images reproduced with permission from Monroe Carell Jr. Children's Hospital at Vanderbilt, Nashville, TN.)

Septic elbow prior to aspiration

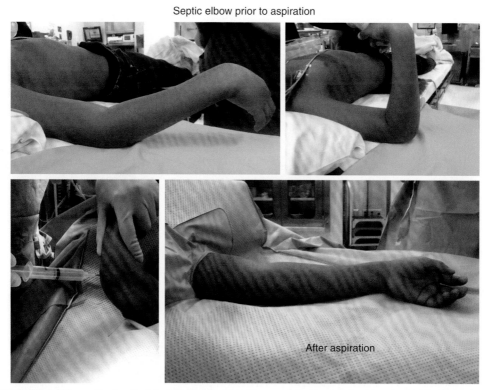

After aspiration

FIGURE 7.11 Elbow effusion that limits motion. This 10-year-old boy presents with severe elbow pain with laboratory studies that point toward septic elbow. Even asleep, the child's elbow did not flex more than 95° and lacked 30° of extension with gravity. Immediately after elbow aspiration, the arm would passively extend with gravity. (Images reproduced with permission from CHOP Orthopedics, Philadelphia, PA.)

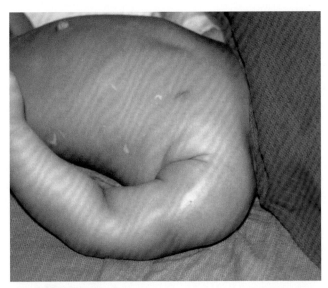

FIGURE 7.12 Swollen shoulder in neonate. Progressive swelling and decreased use of the extremity by the infant should be considered infectious until proven otherwise. (Images reproduced with permission from CHOP Orthopedics, Philadelphia, PA.)

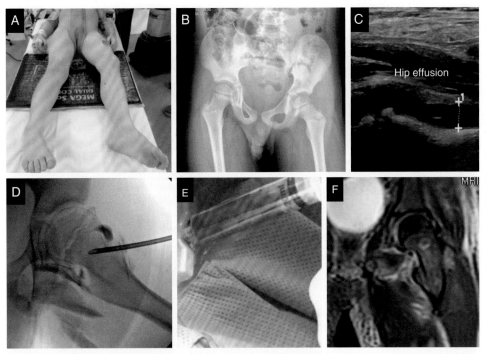

FIGURE 7.13 Physical examination for proximal femoral osteomyelitis. A, This child presents with signs and symptoms consistent with septic arthritis of the left hip (flexion and external rotation of the hip). B, Radiographs of the left hip are negative for bony lesions. C, Ultrasound demonstrated an effusion that when aspirated was negative for pus. D and E, A large needle was placed in the femoral metaphysis, which yielded purulence confirming osteomyelitis. F, Later MRI was positive for osteomyelitis.

MRI is the best imaging modality to diagnose infection around the hip or knee, given its ability to delineate the source of infection. If the child is young enough to necessitate sedation for a full MRI to be performed, alternatively, a FAST-sequence MRI can be employed to effectively delineate the source of infection. Furthermore, as many infections around the hip and knee are not isolated to one specific anatomic location, MRI evaluation is helpful in identifying all sources of an infection prior to surgical intervention that may be occurring in the contiguous areas around the joint (**Figure 7.1**). Through use of MRI, it has been demonstrated that the incidence of pyomyositis is greater than previously believed. In patients with admission for septic hip, it has been demonstrated that the obturator musculature situated deep within the pelvis is infected in more than 60% of cases.[29]

● *Differential Diagnosis*

As highlighted above, unfortunately, the signs and symptoms of musculoskeletal infection, focal trauma, and malignancy may present in a similar manner—pain, tenderness, swelling, and radiographic abnormalities. Additionally, soft tissue infections, such as necrotizing fasciitis, erysipelas, and cellulitis can appear similar at presentation but vary drastically in severity (**Figure 7.14**). To help differentiate these conditions, there are several distinguishing features that an astute physician can use to delineate these conditions and direct appropriate and timely treatment.

When assessing soft tissue infections, the rate of spread can be very useful in discerning if a patient is suffering from a mild infection, such as cellulitis and/or erysipelas, versus necrotizing fasciitis, which is rapidly progressive and necessitates emergent attention. While each of these conditions can present with focal redness, warmth, and tenderness, patients with necrotizing fasciitis may also describe pain that does not align with the presenting erythema, followed by numbness to the same area because of superficial nerve damage. Upon presentation, the margins of the erythema should be noted (**Figure 7.2**). In cases of necrotizing fasciitis, the infection will rapidly progress, resulting in significantly different margins in just a few hours. Alternatively, cellulitis and erysipelas will not spread rapidly (**Figure 7.15**). Early and emergent surgical intervention in cases of necrotizing fasciitis is critical to avoid devastating consequences.

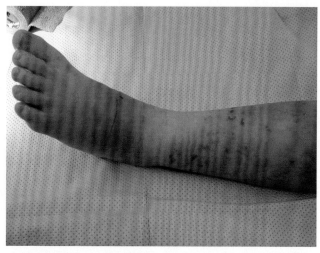

FIGURE 7.14 Physical examination for cellulitis. This patient presents with just cellulitis that was managed with antibiotics. The clinical appearance is not too dissimilar to a child with distal tibial osteomyelitis shown in **Figure 7.2**. (Images reproduced with permission from CHOP Orthopedics, Philadelphia, PA.)

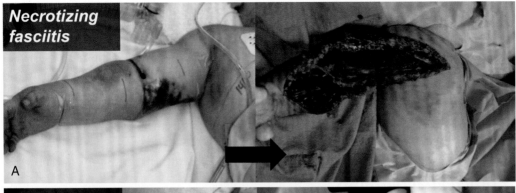

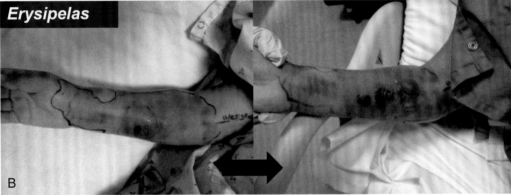

FIGURE 7.15 Differentiating necrotizing fasciitis from erysipelas. Upon presentation, both necrotizing fasciitis and erysipelas can appear as swollen tissues, accompanied by redness and tenderness to the infected site. A, Necrotizing fasciitis progresses rapidly causing massive tissue destruction, dissemination of bacteria, and liquefactive necrosis beneath fascial planes, dissecting the muscular compartments independent of surgeon's knife. B, Erysipelas does not progress, yet appearance of the infection can change to appear like a burn, including blisters. (Images reproduced with permission from Monroe Carell Jr. Children's Hospital at Vanderbilt, Nashville, TN.)

● Tools for Evaluation

Accurate and timely initial evaluation by physicians is crucial to determine (1) if a child has an infection, (2) where the infection is located, (3) what tissues are affected, and (4) the severity of the infection to direct optimal treatment and combat the potential of an over exuberant APR. Imaging can be useful for determining each of these factors, though each imaging modality possesses strengths and limitations for evaluation of musculoskeletal infections.

Laboratory Tests

Blood and tissue cultures, antibody titers (such as Lyme), or genetic analysis (PCR) can each be utilized to confirm the presence of an infection and potentially identify the causative pathogen. Culture tests may require several days until results are available, and it is important to note that culture negative results do not specifically indicate that the patient is not infected. Rather, negative results may occur for several reasons: the causative organism may be difficult or unable to culture, joint aspiration can be challenging (especially outside of the operating room), and if the infection is diffuse with no local abscess, isolating a concentrated source of bacteria can be difficult.

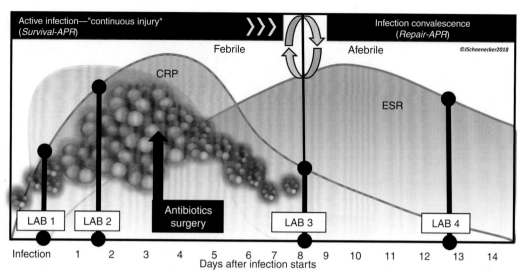

FIGURE 7.16 APR—laboratory utility. Acute phase response markers and infection. Levels of acute phase reactants following tissue injury change dramatically and rapidly. IL-6 (yellow curve) is the first acute phase reactant to increase, followed closely by procalcitonin (not depicted) and then CRP (pink curve). In cases of severe tissue injury, CRP reaches levels more than 100 times preinjury values. Fibrinogen (also measured as ESR, green curve) increases to a lesser degree and takes weeks to return to its preinjury levels. The extent and duration of an acute phase response are dependent upon the severity of a tissue injury and resulting production of inflammatory cytokines such as IL-6. The magnitude of the acute phase reaction can be quantified by both the peak concentration of an acute phase reactant as well as the total amount of that reactant over time (area under the curve).

In addition to identifying the pathogens responsible for infection through culture, laboratory tests aimed at monitoring the dramatic changes of the APR can be effective in assessing the severity of disease and the patient's prognosis (**Figure 7.16**). Though commonly measured, white blood cell count is the least sensitive assessment in the context of pediatric musculoskeletal infections. Prior studies have demonstrated a wide range in incidence of elevated WBC (25%-73%) of patients with osteomyelitis, and similar results have been reported in patients with septic arthritis.

Measures of inflammation such as C-reactive protein (CRP) are effective in the early diagnosis of infection (within 4-6 hours), such that higher CRP levels are associated with increasing disease severity and more severe outcomes, including a longer length of stay in the hospital (**Figure 7.17**).[8] If a treatment is effective, the CRP and other acute phase reactants should begin to return to normal levels, with an expected spike associated with any surgical intervention.[9] If values are not returning to normal, this indicates that further intervention is likely necessary. Another commonly measured value, the erythrocyte sedimentation rate (ESR) is a less sensitive marker for the APR and can also produce misleading data for assessing infections, given that confounding conditions, such as pregnancy, obesity, and anemia, all result in an elevated ESR.[42,43] On the other hand, monitoring ESR may be useful to assess long-term recovery of patients.[44]

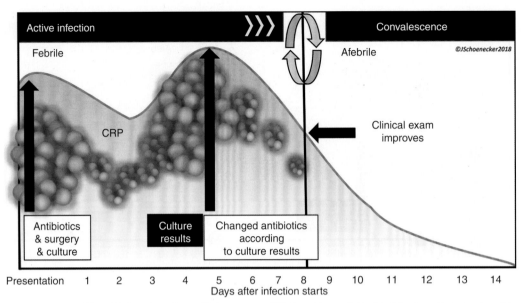

FIGURE 7.17 APR and labs changing within a case. CRP trend in pediatric hip infection. Early treatment is essential in treating hip infection, with antibiotics and surgery leading to a decrease in CRP over the first 2 days. However, it began increasing again over days 3 and 4. At that time, culture results showed inadequate antibiotic therapy. The antibiotics were adjusted on day 5 and the CRP once again began trending in the correct direction and the clinical examination improved. The body had entered the convalescent stage as tissue repair began. This case highlights the importance of culture directed therapy. It is essential to obtain culture material during debridement to guide antibiotic therapy.

Radiographs

Traditionally, radiographs of the affected location, can assist physicians in delineating pathologies that mimic symptoms of infection, including trauma or malignancy. Subtle edema resulting in enlargement of the adjacent muscle layers is detectable as early as 3 days following the onset of infection. Yet, bony changes caused by infection will not be visible on plain radiographs until approximately 7 days following the onset of infection.[18,45] In general, bone that is infected tends to develop areas of bone lysis. As such, use of radiographs of the affected and the unaffected contralateral limb can be beneficial for identifying subtle differences such as swelling or effusion of the joint.

Ultrasound

Ultrasound is frequently utilized to identify joint effusions and periosteal abscesses (**Figure 7.18**). While the cost-effectiveness, lack of ionizing radiation, and relative accessibility may make ultrasound an attractive tool to physicians, ultrasound is limited by its inadequate specificity, inability to image marrow, and critical dependence on operator skill. There has been considerable investigation into the utility of ultrasound in the context of musculoskeletal infections, but results, to this point, have been disappointing and highlight the insufficiency and lack of reliable diagnosis by present-day ultrasound technology. Importantly, reliable differentiation between septic arthritis and benign conditions, including toxic synovitis, cannot be done with ultrasonography alone.

Magnetic Resonance Imaging

MRI has become the gold standard for accurately determining the anatomical location(s) and tissue types infected. Thus, many physicians strongly advocate for MRI when there is concern for

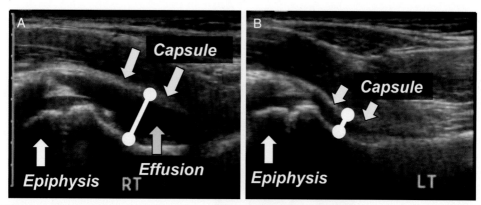

FIGURE 7.18 Ultrasound for hip effusion. A, Ultrasound is an effective imaging method for identifying hip effusion. You can see the capsule elevated from the right proximal femur with increased fluid in the joint. However, it is not specific for infection and does not show additional sites of infection. B. Comparison ultrasound of the unaffected left hip. (Images reproduced with permission from Monroe Carell Jr. Children's Hospital at Vanderbilt, Nashville, TN.)

musculoskeletal infections as MRI provides superior soft-tissue resolution and can be utilized to accurately detect abscesses and differentiate pyomyositis, osteomyelitis, and septic arthritis.[46,48] Furthermore, as many infections around the hip and knee are not isolated to one specific anatomic location, MRI evaluation is helpful in identifying individual sources of infection (**Figure 7.1**). Furthermore, the high resolution of soft tissue offered by MRI can be helpful in directing the approach for joint aspiration. Extraosseous infection and other associated complications can also be discovered using MRI. *S. aureus* musculoskeletal infections, in particular, have been linked to high rates of extraosseous infection and thrombotic complications, including deep vein thrombosis. Finally, postoperative MRI can be helpful to identify persistent infection if the patient is not demonstrating the expected clinical improvement. Infection, like tumors, can be viewed as a form of continuous injury, which will drive the APR until the aggravating factor is resolved. Thus, MRI is a helpful tool to manage an over exuberant APR, reducing the risk of associated complications.

Aspiration

In cases of suspected septic arthritis, aspiration of the affected joint should be performed as soon as possible to finalize the diagnosis and decrease the intracapsular pressure. Aspiration of a joint with an 18- or 20-gauge spinal needle is generally performed under ultrasound guidance to ensure safe entry into the joint and/or effusion (**Figure 7.19**). The fluid obtained is subsequently transferred into the appropriate culture media and/or tubes for laboratory analysis, culture, PCR (in the case of suspected cases of *Kingella* or Lyme arthritis), gram stain, leukocyte count, and polymorphonuclear cell percentage.

Aspiration is also a valuable technique when evaluating suspected osteomyelitis. When performing this, it is a good idea to aspirate as the needle hits the bone, as there may be a subperiosteal abscess. Then the needle can be driven into the bone and a specimen from the metaphysis can be obtained and the appropriate cultures can be sent (**Figures 7.13 and 7.20**). Importantly, as illustrated in **Figure 7.1**, many times patients can experience multiple foci of infected tissues. Thus, when performing an aspiration, prior MRI imaging can be useful to ensure that you are not passing through a soft tissue abscess on the way to collect from the bone or joint. This knowledge helps ensure that the specimen collected is from the desired tissue of interest and also reduce the potential of inoculating a potentially noninfected area such as the joint space.

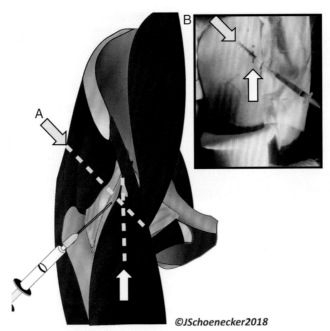

©JSchoenecker2018

FIGURE 7.19 Hip aspiration technique. A, The aspiration technique centers on the hip flexion crease (yellow arrow) and the rectus tendon (white arrow). The approach is from the lateral inferior quadrant of the two lines aiming where they intersect. B, The yellow and white arrows once again show the hip flexion crease and rectus tendon with the approach demonstrated with needle and syringe.

● Treatment and Pathology Management

Antibiotic

Antibiotics are the first line of therapy for musculoskeletal infections. Appropriate timing of administration and selection of antibiotics, guided by clinical evaluation and culture results, is essential to provide optimal treatment. When an infection is suspected, recent clinical studies have suggested that antibiotic therapy *should not* be held prior to obtaining cultures since administration of antibiotics did not reduce culture yields from the site of infection.[49,50] Selection of antibiotic is dependent on both the suspected pathogen and patient factors. For example, neonates are at an increased risk of exposure to hospital acquired pathogens, such as MRSA, Candida, Enterobacteriaceae, or group B streptococcus,[51-53] and therefore should be treated with ampicillin, cefotaxime over gentamycin, acyclovir, and vancomycin is used in regions where MRSA is prevalent.[52,54] Alternatively, if the child is less than 4 years of age, *K. kingae* should be considered and if suspected, ceftriaxone should be administered.

The duration of antibiotics administered is dependent on the institutional experience, the patient's response, as well as the tissue type affected. For example, 2 to 4 weeks of IV antibiotics is often recommended for osteomyelitis, followed by oral antibiotics for a total of 6 to 8 weeks. Some institutions have promoted shorter durations of IV antibiotics until CRP has decreased by 50%, followed by 2 to 4 weeks of oral antibiotics.[54] In cases of septic arthritis and pyomyositis, treatment regimens are typically shorter and can be limited to 2 to 3 weeks of large dose oral antibiotic after the initial infection has been managed with intravenous antibiotics and surgical drainage. Finally, when considering treatment strategies for patients with combinatory infections (osteomyelitis and pyomyositis), antibiotics should be administered according to the longest course necessary to cover all tissue types.

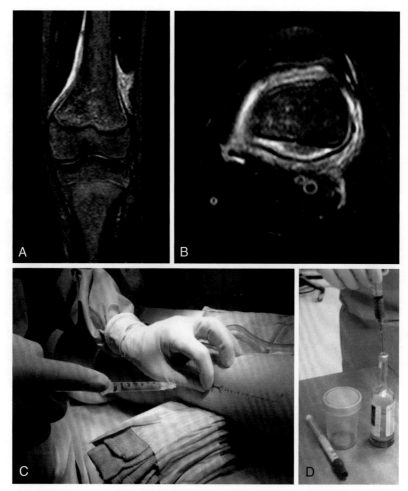

FIGURE 7.20 Aspiration and surgical treatment of subperiosteal osteomyelitis. A and B, MRI imaging of a subperiosteal abscess. C and D, A sample has been isolated for culturing. In addition to aspiration of the abscess prior to the initial incision, collection of intraoperative bone cultures and swabs should be taken to identify the responsible pathogen. By collecting various culture sources, physicians can increase their likelihood of obtaining a positive culture. (Images reproduced with permission from Monroe Carell Jr. Children's Hospital at Vanderbilt, Nashville, TN.)

Operative Management

Septic Arthritis

Septic arthritis should be treated with irrigation and debridement in an urgent manner, through the most direct access to the joint. As an example, the hip is most commonly drained through the anterior approach[55] (**Figure 7.21**). However, if the infection involves multiple tissues, the choice of approach should consider not only access to the joint space, but also access to the affected musculature or bone. In addition to an open approach, septic arthritis of larger joints can be debrided arthroscopically with excellent results.[56-58] In most cases of septic arthritis, a drain is left in place and removed 2 to 3 days after surgery once inflammatory markers have decreased and the patient has improved clinically. Persistent clinical symptoms and elevated inflammatory markers after 48 hours suggest recurrence, inadequate debridement, adjacent infection, or need for alternate antibiotic therapy.

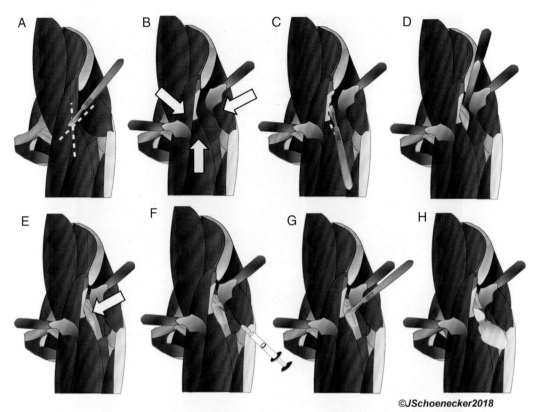

©JSchoenecker2018

FIGURE 7.21 Anterior debridement of the hip. A, Identify the intersection of the hip flexion crease (yellow dotted line) and the interval between the sartorius and tensor fascia lata (white dotted line). Make an incision along the hip flexion crease through skin and subcutaneous tissue centered mostly lateral to this intersection. B, Develop the plane between the sartorius and tensor fascia lata (white arrows). Identify the conjoint rectus tendon (yellow arrow). C, Make an incision along the lateral border of the rectus tendon at which the gluteus minimus attaches to the tendon. D, Use a Cobb to peel gluteus minimus off the hip capsule. E, Exposing the hip capsule. F, With the capsule exposed aspirate synovial fluid for culture. G, Take a 1 cm cube of hip capsule for culture, and H, irrigate copiously. A drain is placed after debridement is complete.

Osteomyelitis

If abscess forms either in the intraosseous, subperiosteal, or extraperiosteal space, surgical debridement is often performed. The goal of debridement is to obtain a culture and debulk the infection and necrotic bone (▶ **Video 7.2**). If the infection is present within the subperiosteal or extraperiosteal space, prior to the incision, aspiration of the abscess should be obtained and sent for culture (**Figure 7.20**).

Pyomyositis

The first line of treatment is antibiotic administration, and surgical intervention is based upon severity and response to treatment. Upon identification of abscess formation and location by MRI, surgical debridement and irrigation are warranted (**Figure 7.6**).[59] When the obturator musculature situated deep within the pelvis is infected, as estimated to be infected in more than 60% of cases,[34] a medial approach can be utilized to safely assess the obturator musculature through either the adductor brevis or the obturator foramen (**Figure 7.22**).

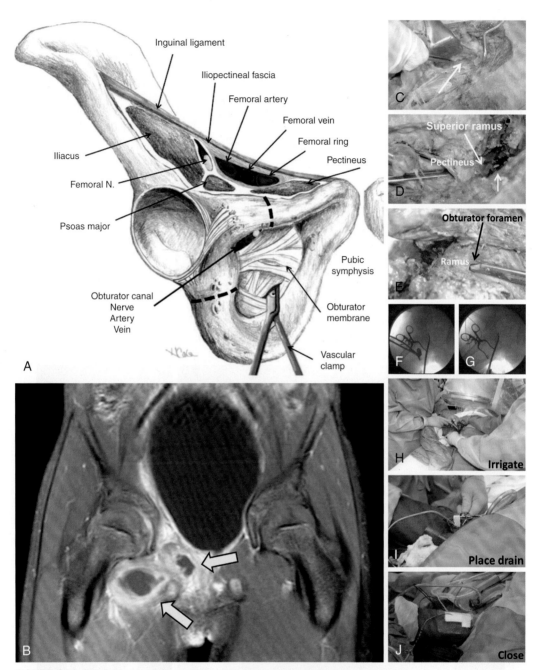

FIGURE 7.22 Surgical approach to drain obturator internus infection. A, The obturator canal allows passage of the obturator nerve, artery, and vein and is located in the superior-lateral portion of the obturator membrane. To avoid these structures, a clamp is bluntly passed medial and inferior to the obturator canal to gain access to the obturator internus. B, MRI demonstrating location of pyomyositis infection within the obturator internus. C-J, Detailed surgical approach demonstrating access to the obturator internus (in a cadaveric study), interoperative images visualizing placement of clamp prior to (H) irrigation, (I) drain placement, and (J) closure with drain placement. (Images reproduced with permission from Monroe Carell Jr. Children's Hospital at Vanderbilt, Nashville, TN.)

● Beyond Infection: Discerning Malignancy and Inflammatory Conditions

Malignancy Mimicry

Like infection, pediatric patients suffering from a neoplasia can present with similar, nonspecific systemic symptoms, such as pallor, malaise, fever, weight loss, lymphadenopathy, hemorrhagic events, hepatosplenomegaly, and others. Adding to the difficult task of distinguishing neoplasia from musculoskeletal infections, patients in both cohorts may complain of body pain, neurologic symptoms, palpable masses, and "bone pain" that awakens the child from sound sleep (**Figure 7.23**).

While differentiating tumors from infection may be challenging, there are a few key points that can assist in making this differentiation. Leukemia is the most common malignancy in children and often presents with diffuse bone pain, anemia, and bleeding. Acute lymphoblastic leukemia, the most common type of leukemia, will be diagnosed with an abnormal manual differential on peripheral blood smear; however, in ~10% of cases, these tests will be inconclusive and clinicians will need to exercise their suspicion to obtain further imaging and invasive testing (bone marrow aspirate) as needed. Radiographic analysis can be helpful to detect lucent metaphyseal bands helping to distinguish these symptoms from infection.[60,61] Furthermore, while some patients may experience pathologic fractures and significant demineralization of the bone, others will only experience marrows change detectable by MRI (**Figure 7.24**).

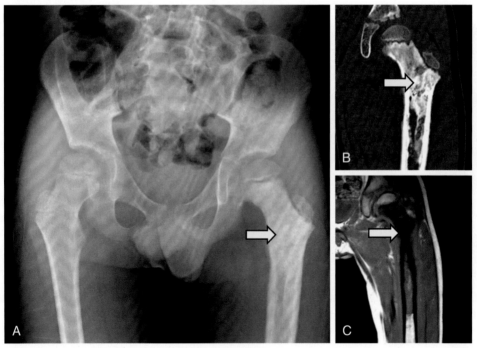

FIGURE 7.23 Use of radiographs to rule out differential diagnoses. The main role of radiographs in hip infection is ruling out other pathology, such as fracture, or in this case malignancy, as children often present with hip pain and refusal to bear weight in cases of cancer of the hip as well. This 6-year old presented with hip pain and was found to have osteosarcoma of the proximal femur. A, Radiograph demonstrated radiodensity of the proximal femur which was confirmed on CT scan (B). C, MRI documents marrow changes well beyond that noted in on plain radiographs and the CT scan. (Images reproduced with permission from Monroe Carell Jr. Children's Hospital at Vanderbilt, Nashville, TN.)

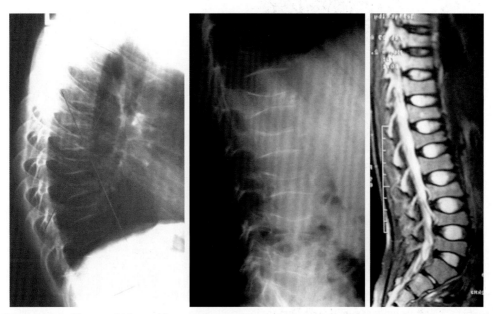

FIGURE 7.24 A 10-year-old boy with acute lymphoblastic leukemia who presents with fatigue and back pain. Radiographs demonstrate multiple compression fractures in his spine, and MRI reveals uniform marrow changes from the leukemia. (Images reproduced with permission from CHOP Orthopedics, Philadelphia, PA.)

In young children, metastatic neuroblastoma or eosinophilic granuloma (EG) should be considered while in older children, Ewing or osteogenic sarcoma (**Figure 7.25**) is more common.[62-64] While Ewing sarcoma classically presents as a bone lesion associated with a large soft tissue mass, the initial presentation can be subtler and limited to "just a limp." Furthermore, radiographically, Ewing sarcoma can be very similar to acute osteomyelitis with minimal periosteal reaction and no soft tissue mass (**Figure 7.26**). While infection is more common than a primary sarcoma, when considering surgical intervention, it is important to consider tissue sampling for both bacterial cultures as well as for histology. No matter how convinced the team is that the problem is an infection or a tumor…it is important to remember to "Always culture a tumor and always biopsy an infection."

Furthermore, several benign bone tumors, most notably chondroblastoma (**Figure 7.27**), Langerhans cell histiocytosis (LCH), and osteoid osteoma can likewise mimic infection. Clinically, chondroblastoma can present in a manner similar to subacute osteomyelitis with patients complaining of joint-related pain with movement. On imaging, chondroblastoma can appear just like subacute epiphyseal osteomyelitis and present as a well-defined lytic lesion within the epiphysis with significant surrounding edema on MRI.[65] EG has been referred to as the "great imitator" and can present with localized pain, mild swelling, and other nonspecific signs. When one considers infection as a likely cause, they would be wise to consider EG as a possible confounding diagnosis. LCH can also present as a disseminated, systemic disease with hepatosplenomegaly, lymphadenopathy, skin involvement, and constitutional symptoms among others[66] (**Figure 7.28**). Finally, patients with osteoid osteoma classically present with pain that wakes them from sound sleep, but is readily relieved by NSAIDS. Overall, the diagnosis of osteoid osteoma can be particularly deceptive, especially in young children, as MRI imaging can demonstrate significant edema and soft tissue inflammation, mimicking an infectious process[67] (**Figure 7.29**). Thin-cut CT scan may be needed to document the small nidus of tissue with surrounding sclerosis that is missed on MRI scans.

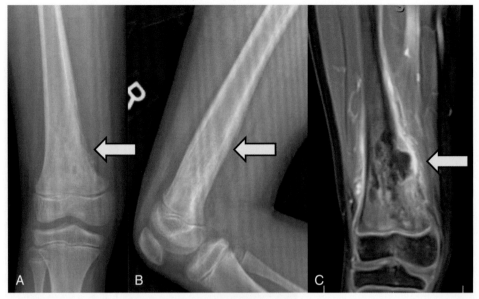

FIGURE 7.25 Soft tissue mass with Ewing sarcoma. An 11-year-old boy who presented with few months history of knee/thigh pain and a mass, associated with difficulty in walking and running. AP and lateral radiographs of the distal femur (A and B) demonstrate an ill-defined, permeative, aggressive looking lytic lesion with disorganized periosteal reaction. C, T1 contrasted coronal MRI shows the extent of marrow involvement and a soft tissue mass associated to the lesion. Biopsy was consistent with Ewing sarcoma. (Images reproduced with permission from CHOP Orthopedics, Philadelphia, PA.)

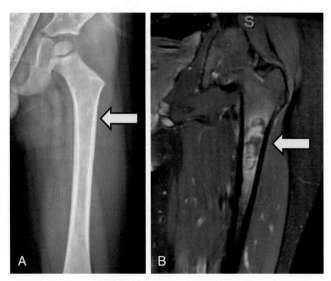

FIGURE 7.26 Ewing sarcoma without soft tissue mass. A 5-year-old boy, otherwise healthy, presented with a few days history of a limp and mild fever. Blood work indicated mildly elevated inflammatory markers. AP radiograph (A) of the proximal femur demonstrates a lucent area in the proximal femur (arrow) without any periosteal reaction, bone destruction, or other signs. T1-contrasted coronal MRI demonstrates a well-defined area of marrow abnormality with no soft tissue extension. Open biopsy and intraoperative frozen sections were done at the time of planned debridement for a presumed osteomyelitis and was indicative of Ewing sarcoma. (Images reproduced with permission from CHOP Orthopedics, Philadelphia, PA.)

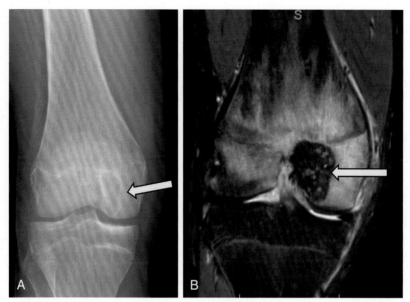

FIGURE 7.27 Chondroblastoma. Chondroblastoma in a 4-year-old male who presented complaining of several month history of pain with activities and inability to run. A, AP radiograph of the distal femur demonstrates a well-defined lytic lesion within the epiphysis (arrow). B, T1 STIR MRI shows significant amount of surrounding edema associated to this chondroblastoma. (Images reproduced with permission from CHOP Orthopedics, Philadelphia, PA.)

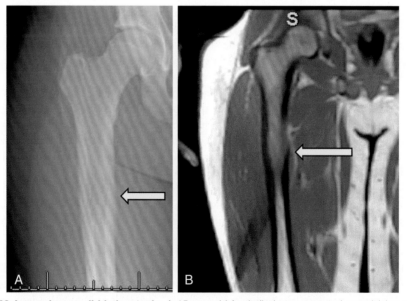

FIGURE 7.28 Langerhans cell histiocytosis. A 15-year-old football player presented complaining of thigh pain since the season was over 3 months prior. He denied any other symptoms and only had mildly elevated inflammatory markers. The AP femur radiograph (A) demonstrates a well-defined lytic lesion in the proximal femoral diaphysis, associated to mild cortical scalloping, and periosteal reaction; T1 coronal MRI shows no soft-tissue mass (B). Biopsy confirmed Langerhans cell histiocytosis. (Images reproduced with permission from CHOP Orthopedics, Philadelphia, PA.)

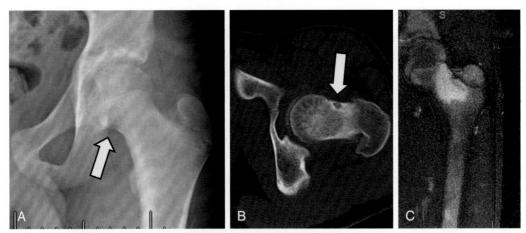

FIGURE 7.29 Osteoid osteoma. A 14-year-old male presented with several month history of left hip pain with activities and also awakening him at night. The pain was responsive to NSAIDS. AP radiograph of the hip (A) does not show any definitive obvious lesions, and just very mild cortical thickening (arrow) is observed; T2 coronal MR image shows significant area of marrow edema concerning for an infectious or chronic trauma etiology (B); axial CT (C) successfully demonstrates the small osteoid osteoma nidus (arrow). (Images reproduced with permission from CHOP Orthopedics, Philadelphia, PA.)

Differentiating Inflammatory Disorders

In addition to malignancy, one of the most difficult differentials with infection is discerning these from inflammatory, or reactive, conditions. The physical signs of these pathologies are similar, including joint pain and limp with prolonged ambulation, progressing to difficulty to bear weight. As highlighted previously, untreated septic arthritis can cause permanent articular cartilage damage within 8 hours; this highlights the importance of urgent diagnosis and distinction from toxic or transient synovitis, a reactive effusion of the joint. Traditionally, the "Kocher criteria"[68] have been used to help distinguish between septic arthritis and transient synovitis in the hip. These criteria provide a valuable framework to consider when evaluating a child with an inflamed hip. Problems are encountered when these criteria are applied to joints other than the hip, or when it is used to distinguish septic arthritis from other infections like osteomyelitis or pyomyositis. Subsequent studies and application of these algorithms at different institutions have produced conflicting results in their efficacy to discern septic arthritis from other pathologies.[69] While the Kocher criteria are a valuable way to consider the different diagnosis and likely probabilities, differentiation between septic arthritis and toxic synovitis in an acutely ill child must depend upon the experience and acumen of the providers.

While being less common than toxic synovitis, juvenile idopathic arthritis (JIA) and rheumatic fever can likewise present with pain and swelling of the afflicted joint and an associated fever. JIA is an autoimmune-mediated version of chronic arthritis commonly seen in children 7 to 12 years of age (6 per 100,000).[70] Though commonly mistaken for infection, JIA can be distinguished by its gradual onset, polyarticular nature (akin to leukemia), and radiographic presentation in which the joint typically appears worse than it functions. In cases of rheumatic fever, joint pain is typically greater than cases of JIA, yet the joint will appear seemingly normal. Rheumatic fever, a sequela of group A streptococcal infection, predominantly affects the knees, ankles, elbows, and wrists.[71] Pain secondary to rheumatic fever is typically evanescent and migratory in nature. While the Jones criteria can be utilized to help diagnose rheumatic fever, the diagnosis of poststreptococcal reactive arthritis can likewise be applied to patients with a documented history of group A strep, but fail to meet all components of the Jones criteria.[72] While the incidence of complications from poststreptococcal reactive arthritis remains unclear, the implementation of long-term antibiotics remains controversial.

● Conclusion

Given the challenging nature of pediatric musculoskeletal infections and the potential for devastating complication, a thorough understanding of the epidemiology and optimal clinical evaluation practices are essential for residents in training and attending physicians alike. Imaging, specifically MRI, can provide critical information about the location of the infection and tissues involved, the severity of the infection, and aid in identifying persistent infections if the patient is not demonstrating the expected clinical improvement. Thus, when available, MRI should be considered the gold standard in diagnostic imaging for pediatric musculoskeletal infections. As highlighted throughout, the APR elevates in response to the severity of the infection and, if too exuberant, can lead to complications such as thrombosis and avascular necrosis potentially leading to loss of joint function and abnormal limb development. For these reasons, rapid diagnosis (utilizing imaging, joint aspiration, and laboratory tests) and application of the appropriate antibiotics and/or surgical intervention are essential to mitigate an exuberant or prolonged APR, ultimately providing better care to patients.

References

1. An TJ, Benvenuti MA, Mignemi ME, Thomsen IP, Schoenecker JG. Pediatric musculoskeletal infection: hijacking the acute-phase response. *JBJS Rev.* 2016;4(9). doi:10.2106/JBJS.RVW.15.00099.
2. Gafur OA, Copley LA, Hollmig ST, Browne RH, Thornton LA, Crawford SE. The impact of the current epidemiology of pediatric musculoskeletal infection on evaluation and treatment guidelines. *J Pediatr Orthop.* 2008;28(7):777-785.
3. Ciampolini J, Harding KG. Pathophysiology of chronic bacterial osteomyelitis. Why do antibiotics fail so often? *Postgrad Med J.* 2000;76(898):479-483.
4. Song KM, Sloboda JF. Acute hematogenous osteomyelitis in children. *J Am Acad Orthop Surg.* 2001;9(3):166-175.
5. Dodwell ER. Osteomyelitis and septic arthritis in children: current concepts. *Curr Opin Pediatr.* 2013;25(1):58-63.
6. Mignemi ME, Benvenuti MA, An TJ, et al. A novel classification system based on dissemination of musculoskeletal infection is predictive of hospital outcomes. *J Pediatr Orthop.* 2018;38(5):279-286.
7. Amaro E, Marvi TK, Posey SL, et al. C-reactive protein predicts risk of venous thromboembolism in pediatric musculoskeletal infection. *J Pediatr Orthop.* 2019;39(1):e62-e7.
8. Copley LA, Barton T, Garcia C, et al. A proposed scoring system for assessment of severity of illness in pediatric acute hematogenous osteomyelitis using objective clinical and laboratory findings. *Pediatr Infect Dis J.* 2014;33(1):35-41.
9. Benvenuti M, An T, Amaro E, et al. Double-edged sword: musculoskeletal infection provoked acute phase response in children. *Orthop Clin North Am.* 2017;48(2):181-197.
10. Wang CL, Wang SM, Yang YJ, Tsai CH, Liu CC. Septic arthritis in children: relationship of causative pathogens, complications, and outcome. *J Microbiol Immunol Infect.* 2003;36(1):41-46.
11. Blyth MJ, Kincaid R, Craigen MA, Bennet GC. The changing epidemiology of acute and subacute haematogenous osteomyelitis in children. *J Bone Joint Surg Br.* 2001;83(1):99-102.
12. Peltola H, Kallio MJ, Unkila-Kallio L. Reduced incidence of septic arthritis in children by Haemophilus influenzae type-b vaccination. Implications for treatment. *J Bone Joint Surg Br.* 1998;80(3):471-473.
13. Conrad DA. Acute hematogenous osteomyelitis. *Pediatr Rev.* 2010;31(11):464-471.
14. Sonnen GM, Henry NK. Pediatric bone and joint infections. Diagnosis and antimicrobial management. *Pediatr Clin North Am.* 1996;43(4):933-947.
15. Kremers HM, Nwojo ME, Ransom JE, Wood-Wentz CM, Melton LJ III, Huddleston PM III. Trends in the epidemiology of osteomyelitis: a population-based study, 1969 to 2009. *J Bone Joint Surg Am.* 2015;97(10):837-845.
16. Karwowska A, Davies HD, Jadavji T. Epidemiology and outcome of osteomyelitis in the era of sequential intravenous-oral therapy. *Pediatr Infect Dis J.* 1998;17(11):1021-1026.
17. Khachatourians AG, Patzakis MJ, Roidis N, Holtom PD. Laboratory monitoring in pediatric acute osteomyelitis and septic arthritis. *Clin Orthop Relat Res.* 2003(409):186-194.
18. Jackson MA, Nelson JD. Etiology and medical management of acute suppurative bone and joint infections in pediatric patients. *J Pediatr Orthop.* 1982;2(3):313-323.

19. Green NE, Edwards K. Bone and joint infections in children. *Orthop Clin North Am*. 1987;18(4):555-576.

20. Saavedra-Lozano J, Mejias A, Ahmad N, et al. Changing trends in acute osteomyelitis in children: impact of methicillin-resistant Staphylococcus aureus infections. *J Pediatr Orthop*. 2008;28(5):569-575.

21. Alshryda S, Huntley JS, Banaszkiewicz PA. *Paediatric Orthopaedics: An Evidence-Based Approach to Clinical Questions*. 1st ed. New York: Springer International Publishing; 2017:543.

22. Frank G, Mahoney HM, Eppes SC. Musculoskeletal infections in children. *Pediatr Clin North Am*. 2005;52(4):1083-1106, ix.

23. Street M, Puna R, Huang M, Crawford H. Pediatric acute hematogenous osteomyelitis. *J Pediatr Orthop*. 2015;35(6):634-639.

24. Yagupsky P, Erlich Y, Ariela S, Trefler R, Porat N. Outbreak of Kingella kingae skeletal system infections in children in daycare. *Pediatr Infect Dis J*. 2006;25(6):526-532.

25. Browne LP, Mason EO, Kaplan SL, Cassady CI, Krishnamurthy R, Guillerman RP. Optimal imaging strategy for community-acquired *Staphylococcus aureus* musculoskeletal infections in children. *Pediatr Radiol*. 2008;38(8):841-847.

26. Karmazyn B, Kleiman MB, Buckwalter K, Loder RT, Siddiqui A, Applegate KE. Acute pyomyositis of the pelvis: the spectrum of clinical presentations and MR findings. *Pediatr Radiol*. 2006;36(4):338-343.

27. Marin C, Sanchez-Alegre ML, Gallego C, et al. Magnetic resonance imaging of osteoarticular infections in children. *Curr Probl Diagn Radiol*. 2004;33(2):43-59.

28. Theodorou SJ, Theodorou DJ, Resnick D. MR imaging findings of pyogenic bacterial myositis (pyomyositis) in patients with local muscle trauma: illustrative cases. *Emerg Radiol*. 2007;14(2):89-96.

29. Mignemi ME, Menge TJ, Cole HA, et al. Epidemiology, diagnosis, and treatment of pericapsular pyomyositis of the hip in children. *J Pediatr Orthop*. 2014;34(3):316-325.

30. McHenry CR, Brandt CP, Piotrowski JJ, Jacobs DG, Malangoni MA. Idiopathic necrotizing fasciitis: recognition, incidence, and outcome of therapy. *Am Surg*. 1994;60(7):490-494.

31. Lee A, May A, Obremskey WT. Necrotizing soft-tissue infections: an orthopaedic emergency. *J Am Acad Orthop Surg*. 2019;27(5):e199-e206.

32. Wong CH, Chang HC, Pasupathy S, Khin LW, Tan JL, Low CO. Necrotizing fasciitis: clinical presentation, microbiology, and determinants of mortality. *J Bone Joint Surg Am*. 2003;85(8):1454-1460.

33. McCarthy JJ, Dormans JP, Kozin SH, Pizzutillo PD. Musculoskeletal infections in children: basic treatment principles and recent advancements. *Instr Course Lect*. 2005;54:515-528.

34. Hankins CL, Southern S. Factors that affect the clinical course of group A beta-haemolytic streptococcal infections of the hand and upper extremity: a retrospective study. *Scand J Plast Reconstr Surg Hand Surg*. 2008;42(3):153-157.

35. Bingol-Kologlu M, Yildiz RV, Alper B, et al. Necrotizing fasciitis in children: diagnostic and therapeutic aspects. *J Pediatr Surg*. 2007;42(11):1892-1897.

36. Brook I. Aerobic and anaerobic microbiology of necrotizing fasciitis in children. *Pediatr Dermatol*. 1996;13(4):281-284.

37. Eneli I, Davies HD. Epidemiology and outcome of necrotizing fasciitis in children: an active surveillance study of the Canadian Paediatric Surveillance Program. *J Pediatr*. 2007;151(1):79-84.

38. Tang JS, Gold RH, Bassett LW, Seeger LL. Musculoskeletal infection of the extremities: evaluation with MR imaging. *Radiology*. 1988;166(1 pt 1):205-209.

39. Peltola H, Vahvanen V. A comparative study of osteomyelitis and purulent arthritis with special reference to aetiology and recovery. *Infection*. 1984;12(2):75-79.

40. Nade S. Acute septic arthritis in infancy and childhood. *J Bone Joint Surg Br*. 1983;65(3):234-241.

41. Soto-Hall R, Johnson LH, Johnson RA. Variations in the intra-articular pressure of the hip joint in injury and disease. A probable factor in avascular necrosis. *J Bone Joint Surg Am*. 1964;46:509-516.

42. Bottiger LE, Svedberg CA. Normal erythrocyte sedimentation rate and age. *Br Med J*. 1967;2(5544):85-87.

43. Sox HC Jr, Liang MH. The erythrocyte sedimentation rate. Guidelines for rational use. *Ann Intern Med*. 1986;104(4):515-523.

44. Michail M, Jude E, Liaskos C, et al. The performance of serum inflammatory markers for the diagnosis and follow-up of patients with osteomyelitis. *Int J Low Extrem Wounds*. 2013;12(2):94-99.

45. Capitanio MA, Kirkpatrick JA. Early roentgen observations in acute osteomyelitis. *Am J Roentgenol Radium Ther Nucl Med*. 1970;108(3):488-496.

46. Jaramillo D, Treves ST, Kasser JR, Harper M, Sundel R, Laor T. Osteomyelitis and septic arthritis in children: appropriate use of imaging to guide treatment. *AJR Am J Roentgenol*. 1995;165(2):399-403.

47. Mazur JM, Ross G, Cummings J, Hahn GA Jr, McCluskey W. Usefulness of magnetic resonance imaging for the diagnosis of acute musculoskeletal infections in children. *J Pediatr Orthop*. 1995;15(2):144-147.

48. Modic MT, Feiglin DH, Piraino DW, et al. Vertebral osteomyelitis: assessment using MR. *Radiology*. 1985;157(1):157-166.

49. Benvenuti MA, An TJ, Mignemi ME, Martus JE, Thomsen IP, Schoenecker JG. Effects of antibiotic timing on culture results and clinical outcomes in pediatric musculoskeletal infection. *J Pediatr Orthop*. 2016;39(3):158-162.

50. Zhorne DJ, Altobelli ME, Cruz AT. Impact of antibiotic pretreatment on bone biopsy yield for children with acute hematogenous osteomyelitis. *Hosp Pediatr*. 2015;5(6):337-341.

51. Frederiksen B, Christiansen P, Knudsen FU. Acute osteomyelitis and septic arthritis in the neonate, risk factors and outcome. *Eur J Pediatr*. 1993;152(7):577-580.

52. Ish-Horowicz MR, McIntyre P, Nade S. Bone and joint infections caused by multiply resistant *Staphylococcus aureus* in a neonatal intensive care unit. *Pediatr Infect Dis J*. 1992;11(2):82-87.

53. Wong M, Isaacs D, Howman-Giles R, Uren R. Clinical and diagnostic features of osteomyelitis occurring in the first three months of life. *Pediatr Infect Dis J*. 1995;14(12):1047-1053.

54. Castellazzi L, Mantero M, Esposito S. Update on the management of pediatric acute osteomyelitis and septic arthritis. *Int J Mol Sci*. 2016;17(6):855.

55. Souza Miyahara H, Helito CP, Oliva GB, Aita PC, Croci AT, Vicente JR. Clinical and epidemiological characteristics of septic arthritis of the hip, 2006 to 2012, a seven-year review. *Clinics (Sao Paulo)*.. 2014;69(7):464-468.

56. Edmonds EW, Lin C, Farnsworth CL, Bomar JD, Upasani VV. A medial portal for hip arthroscopy in children with septic arthritis: a safety study. *J Pediatr Orthop*. 2018;38(10):527-531.

57. Nusem I, McAlister A. Arthroscopic lavage for the treatment of septic arthritis of the hip in children. *Acta Orthop Belg*. 2012;78(6):730-734.

58. Sanpera I, Raluy-Collado D, Sanpera-Iglesias J. Arthroscopy for hip septic arthritis in children. *Orthop Traumatol Surg Res*. 2016;102(1):87-89.

59. Spiegel DA, Meyer JS, Dormans JP, Flynn JM, Drummond DS. Pyomyositis in children and adolescents: report of 12 cases and review of the literature. *J Pediatr Orthop*. 1999;19(2):143-150.

60. Rogalsky RJ, Black GB, Reed MH. Orthopaedic manifestations of leukemia in children. *J Bone Joint Surg Am*. 1986;68(4):494-501.

61. Hann IM, Gupta S, Palmer MK, Morris-Jones PH. The prognostic significance of radiological and symptomatic bone involvement in childhood acute lymphoblastic leukaemia. *Med Pediatr Oncol*. 1979;6(1):51-55.

62. Cabanela ME, Sim FH, Beabout JW, Dahlin DC. Osteomyelitis appearing as neoplasms. A diagnostic problem. *Arch Surg*. 1974;109(1):68-72.

63. Lindenbaum S, Alexander H. Infections simulating bone tumors. A review of subacute osteomyelitis. *Clin Orthop Relat Res*. 1984(184):193-203.

64. Willis RB, Rozencwaig R. Pediatric osteomyelitis masquerading as skeletal neoplasia. *Orthop Clin North Am*. 1996;27(3):625-634.

65. Roberts JM, Drummond DS, Breed AL, Chesney J. Subacute hematogenous osteomyelitis in children: a retrospective study. *J Pediatr Orthop*. 1982;2(3):249-254.

66. Arkader A, Glotzbecker M, Hosalkar HS, Dormans JP. Primary musculoskeletal Langerhans cell histiocytosis in children: an analysis for a 3-decade period. *J Pediatr Orthop*. 2009;29(2):201-207.

67. Chai JW, Hong SH, Choi JY, et al. Radiologic diagnosis of osteoid osteoma: from simple to challenging findings. *Radiographics*. 2010;30(3):737-749.

68. Kocher MS, Zurakowski D, Kasser JR. Differentiating between septic arthritis and transient synovitis of the hip in children: an evidence-based clinical prediction algorithm. *J Bone Joint Surg Am*. 1999;81(12):1662-1670.

69. Luhmann SJ, Jones A, Schootman M, Gordon JE, Schoenecker PL, Luhmann JD. Differentiation between septic arthritis and transient synovitis of the hip in children with clinical prediction algorithms. *J Bone Joint Surg Am*. 2004;86(5):956-962.

70. Behrens EM, Beukelman T, Gallo L, et al. Evaluation of the presentation of systemic onset juvenile rheumatoid arthritis: data from the Pennsylvania Systemic Onset Juvenile Arthritis Registry (PASOJAR). *J Rheumatol*. 2008;35(2):343-348.

71. Working Group on Pediatric Acute Rheumatic Fever and Cardiology Chapter of Indian Academy of Pediatrics; Saxena A, Kumar RK, Gera RP, et al. Consensus guidelines on pediatric acute rheumatic fever and rheumatic heart disease. *Indian Pediatr*. 2008;45(7):565-573.

72. Mignemi ME, Martus JE, Bracikowski AC, Lovejoy SA, Mencio GA, Schoenecker JG. The spectrum of group A streptococcal joint pathology in the acute care setting. *Pediatr Emerg Care*. 2012;28(11):1185-1189.

8

Evaluation for Nonaccidental Trauma

Karen L. Lakin

Introduction

Orthopedic injuries are common in childhood. Fractures accounted for 788,925 visits to the emergency department in the United States in 2010.[1] Although most fractures are accidental, the clinician must be alert to injuries that are the result of child abuse. The orthopaedist must also be alert to other nonorthopedic injuries that may be red flags for abuse. Failure to recognize these injuries could result in a child at risk for continued abuse, or worse, death. Over diagnosing abuse may result in separation of a child from caregivers resulting in further emotional and psychological trauma to the child. Failing to diagnose a medical condition that can lead to bone fragility can also delay possible treatment.

Epidemiology

In the United States, approximately 4.1 million referrals were made to Child Protective Services for allegations of child maltreatment in 2017, of which 9.6% were made by medical personnel. Reports were substantiated for 674,000 child victims of abuse or neglect, with 1720 child fatalities reported in 2017 directly attributed to abuse or neglect, or as a contributing factor for the death.

There are four major categories of child maltreatment. Neglect refers to failure to provide for a child's basic needs resulting in physical, emotional, psychological, or education harm. This is the largest category of abuse, approximately 74.9% of all cases reported. Physical abuse, which comprises 18.3% of reported cases, is the second most common type of child maltreatment. Physical abuse is defined as infliction of injury as the result of punching, beating, kicking, biting, burning, shaking, or otherwise harming a child. Sexual abuse makes up 8.6 % of reported cases. Psychological or emotional abuse is reported in 5.7% of cases. The remaining cases involve types of maltreatment that do not fit into the major categories such as drug exposed infants and medical child abuse.[2]

Multiple studies have identified factors associated with an increased risk for abuse. These include child-specific factors including age of the victim, history of prematurity, chronic illness, and developmental delay.[3,4] Children under the age of one have the highest incidence of abuse, 25.2 per 1000 children. Females are at a slightly increased risk for abuse than males; however, males are more likely to die from abuse with a rate of 2.68/100,000 compared to females at 2.02/100,000.[2]

Perpetrator risk factors include alcohol and drug abuse by the caregiver, young parenthood, low educational status, mental health issues, and lower socioeconomic status. Lack of understanding by the caregiver of normal childhood behavior and development often leads to frustration of the caregiver with the victim. Parents are implicated as perpetrators in 77.6% of the reported cases. Environmental factors in the home include a history of domestic violence/abuse, a nonbiological caregiver present in the home, and social isolation. Community factors include neighborhood violence and poverty.[5]

Fractures are the second most common injury identified in inflicted injury, behind soft tissue injuries. Children under the age of three have the highest incidence of nonaccidental fractures, with 69% under the age of one.[6] Understanding the mechanisms required to result in specific types of fractures in conjunction with the developmental stage of the child is critical in considering whether an injury is the result of abuse.

The Medical Evaluation

History of Present Illness

As with all medical conditions, evaluating the pediatric patient with an orthopedic injury begins with a comprehensive history of the present illness. The caregiver needs to provide a detailed history with information about the circumstances of the injury: mechanism of injury, positioning of the child, specifics regarding the distances, objects, etc, who was present, when the patient showed symptoms, intervening treatment, and when medical care was obtained. Although we accept the history as reported by the caregivers initially, the plausibility of the history should be compared with the objective diagnosis of the patient. Considerations that may increase the level of suspicion that the history is unreliable include mechanism of injury reported inconsistent with the fracture pattern, severity of injury inconsistent with the mechanism, and an injury inconsistent with the developmental stage of the child. An unwitnessed injury is particularly concerning in young children due to concerns for lack of supervision.

Changing histories are also concerning, but consider small variations in history may be reported by a distressed caregiver. For example, in a crisis, the caregiver may report the patient seized for 10 minutes when it was less than 3 minutes. Discrepancies in location of individuals present at the time of the incident are significant and a red flag for a changing history that may indicate possible abuse.

The developmental stage of the child as well as the plausibility of the reported mechanism in relation to the degree of injury must be assessed. Careful attention should be made to the reported history by the caregiver, however, because semantics matter. For example, one would not expect a three-week-old infant to be able to "roll over"; however, a caregiver may report that the patient "fell" off a couch. Even an inanimate object may fall if placed in an unstable position. It is important to clarify descriptions of the circumstances when taking a history from the caregiver.

Past Medical History

Past medical history provides additional information that is important in your assessment. This includes history of birth, nutrition, medications, and development. Birth history is important as birth trauma may result in fractures at the time of delivery, particularly for a large infant or difficult presentation. Common fractures reported include clavicle, humerus, and femur fractures. Although the birth records may not specifically note "trauma," information may be obtained from the caregivers and other family members regarding bruising noted at birth, observed lack of movement of a limb, prolonged labor, and a history of use of instrumentation at delivery.

Nutritional information is important since breast-fed infants may require vitamin D supplementation, especially in darker pigmented infants and infants born in the winter months. As the child gets older, toddler diets lacking in vitamin D or nutritional problems may contribute to osteopenia. Medications such as diuretics, antiepileptic medications, and steroids may also affect bone loss. Nonweight bearing children, such as children with cerebral palsy, may have diffuse osteopenia, as well as children with medical conditions affecting absorption of calcium and vitamin D such as cystic fibrosis.

Because the developmental stage of the child is essential in assessing the plausibility of the reported cause of the injury, a careful history of the developmental milestones of the patient should be taken and documented. In addition, information regarding possibility of developmental delay could identify a known risk factor for abuse.[7]

Family History

Family history may provide clues to genetic conditions that may predispose a patient to orthopedic injuries. These include a history of Ehlers-Danlos syndrome, osteogenesis imperfecta, X-linked hypophosphatemia, and neuromuscular diseases. Family may often not know the actual diagnosis, so questions related to frequent fractures, early hearing loss, and dental issues may provide clues to guide your evaluation.

Social History

It is important to know the context of the child's social environment and how it affects the patient's risk for abuse. The primary caregivers and their relationship to the child should be documented as well as other caregivers that may have access to the child, including babysitters and extended family members. Information regarding other children in the home should be obtained to have children formally interviewed as potential witnesses and more importantly, also examined for signs of abuse. The home environment is also helpful to note including what type of bed the child sleeps in, the type of flooring, stairs present, etc. Prior history with child protective services and/or law enforcement should be noted as well as any history of domestic violence or illicit drug use.

Physical Examination

The general appearance of the child should be documented including height, weight, head circumference in infants, overall nutritional status, and hygiene of the patient. The neurological status of the patient should be evaluated as well as documentation of development.

The physical examination should be thorough and begin with examination of the skin. Cutaneous injuries are the most common injuries in abused children. Bruises, abrasions, ecchymosis, and burns should be documented. Photographs can be helpful, and should be taken for medical purposes, ie, to follow progression of a lesion. If abuse is suspected, it is important that caregivers or legal authorities photograph injuries for evidence purposes.

The lack of bruising does not mean the child has not been exposed to nonaccidental orthopedic injuries.[8,9] However, 90% of physical abuse victims present with cutaneous injuries, including bruising, abrasions, alopecia, scars, burns, and bite marks.[10] The location and pattern of a cutaneous injury gives clues as to whether the injury is accidental or nonaccidental. Bruising in nonambulating children is almost always concerning for abuse. Young children who are mobile tend to fall forward, resulting in bruising to foreheads, elbows, knees, and shins. Injuries around the ear, abdomen, genitals, back, and buttocks are less likely to be injured from falls. Common patterns of bruising include implement-shaped lesions such as belts, cords, and paddles (**Figures 8.1** and **8.2**).

Oval-shaped bruising in clusters may be indicative of knuckles or fingerprints (**Figure 8.3**). Multiple fine lines, evenly spaced, may signify a handprint (**Figure 8.4**). Although hematomas often have certain patterns of coloration, bruising cannot be dated.[11]

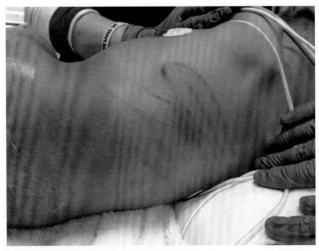

FIGURE 8.1 Three-year-old with cord marks from beating with an extension cord. The patient also suffered partial thickness burns to the buttocks, genital area, and bilateral feet.

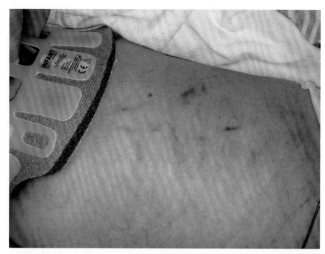

FIGURE 8.2 Rectangular patterned bruising in a toddler struck with a belt.

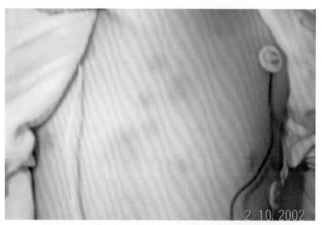

FIGURE 8.3 Two-year-old critically ill toddler with internal injuries and head trauma. Multiple oval-shaped bruises are noted from knuckles.

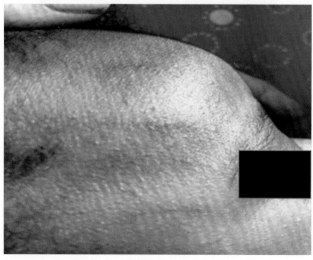

FIGURE 8.4 Seven-month-old with patterned facial bruising. Linear marks are a result of the leakage of blood into the tissue from the capillaries forming a negative imprint of the offending hand.

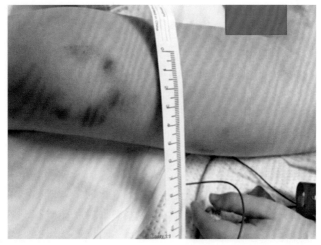

FIGURE 8.5 Bite mark on a three-year-old who was sexually and physically abused.

Other external injuries that may be present on physical examination that are suspicious for non-accidental trauma (NAT) in young children include bite marks, torn frenulum from forced feeds, and auricle hematomas (**Figures 8.5** and **8.6**). Petechiae may be present because of blunt trauma, friction, choking, or vomiting (**Figure 8.7A** and **B**).

Bruising in nonambulatory infants is especially concerning and may be a red flag for more serious injury, particularly if there is bruising to the face.[12] Suspicion for abusive head trauma warrants a comprehensive evaluation for intracranial trauma, possible presence of retinal hemorrhages, and skeletal trauma (**Figure 8.8**).

Always pay attention to the sclera and teeth as blue sclera or altered dental development may indicate osteogenesis imperfecta (**Figure 8.9**).

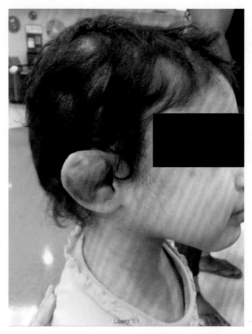

FIGURE 8.6 Auricle hematoma and alopecia in a five-year-old with malnutrition, healing fractures, and old subdural hemorrhage. No history of trauma was given.

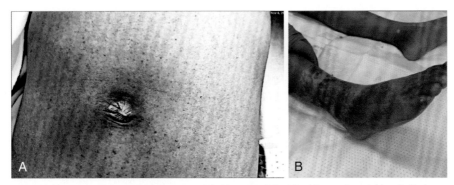

FIGURE 8.7 A, Developmentally delayed five-year-old with periumbilical bruising and petechiae. B, Patient sustained circumferential partial thickness burns to right foot and splash burn to left foot while in the care of mother's boyfriend.

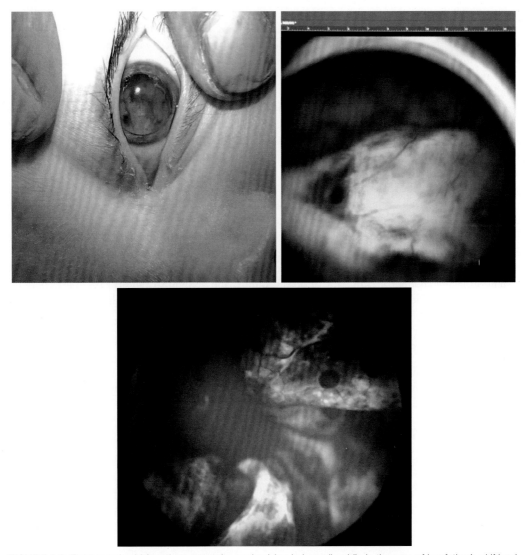

FIGURE 8.8 Eight-month-old found unresponsive and seizing in her crib while in the care of her father's girlfriend. On physical examination, the patient had right scalp soft tissue swelling and bruising to the right ear. The patient was diagnosed with bilateral retinal hemorrhages, vitreous hemorrhage, acute bilateral subdural hemorrhages, and a posterior rib fracture of the left ninth rib.

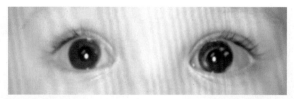

FIGURE 8.9 Blue sclera seen in patients with osteogenesis imperfecta.

Abusive head trauma is the most lethal form of child abuse and is a leading cause of death in children less than 2 years of age.[13] The term abusive head trauma is used to describe all forms of intracranial injury from nonaccidental or inflicted trauma. The most common intracranial injury seen in NAT is a subdural hemorrhage; however, subarachnoid hemorrhages, parenchymal contusions, and epidural hemorrhages may occur in NAT. The traumatic intracranial injury is often found in association with retinal hemorrhages, usually complex, and fractures, especially rib fractures inconsistent with the history of trauma. Injury to the spine including vertebral fractures, spinal cord contusions, and ligamentous injuries may also be found in cases of abusive head trauma. The mechanism may involve blunt force trauma to the head as well as violent shaking alone or with direct impact.[14] Clinically, infants may present with a wide spectrum of non-specific symptoms including irritability, vomiting, altered mental status, seizures, coma, and death. Infants that have an evolving subdural hemorrhage over time may present with an enlarging head circumference, irritability, and a history of vomiting that may have previously been diagnosed as gastroesophageal reflux.[15]

Burns are often seen in NAT in children under the age of 5 years.[16] The typical pattern of burn is an immersion burn involving the lower extremities, buttocks, and perineum. The pattern of injury gives a clue as to the mechanism of injury. Typically, both feet and ankles are burned circumferentially, with a similar depth and there is well-demarcated line of burn to noninjured skin present. This pattern is often described as a "stocking" distribution. There are rarely splash marks, and flexion creases, as well as the soles of the feet, may be spared. There is often a "doughnut" distribution of burn to the buttocks area, which describes sparing of the central area of the buttocks. This spared area represents the part of the buttocks that is held against the bottom of the tub, which limits exposure of the hot water to that area. Intentional burns of the upper extremities may also be seen (**Figure 8.10**). Immersion burns of the upper extremities are circumferential and appear in a "glove distribution" (**Figure 8.11**).

Visceral injuries may present on physical examination with bruising over the abdomen, abdominal distension, acute abdominal pain, lack of bowel sounds, and abdominal rigidity. The most common visceral injuries include liver and spleen lacerations, retroperitoneal hematomas, duodenal hematomas, and pancreatic injury[17] (**Figure 8.12**).

Orthopedic Examination

The physical examination of the musculoskeletal system may reveal obvious abnormalities, such as swelling, erythema, or deformity of the bone. Pain on movement or palpation, crepitus, or palpable callus under the skin may be found in the injured area.

● Laboratory Testing

Basic trauma laboratory tests are recommended when there is a concern for NAT. The laboratory tests include those of complete metabolic profile, complete blood count, coagulation profile, amylase, lipase, and urinalysis. Testing for metabolic bone disease and genetic syndromes that may predispose the patient to fractures should be guided by the physical examination, medical history, and family history.

● Imaging

The physical examination will guide you on the plain radiographs to order. In children <2 years of age, the American Academy of Pediatrics (AAP) recommends a skeletal survey to evaluate for occult fractures.[18] A skeletal survey includes anteroposterior and lateral views of the skull, chest, oblique views of the ribs,

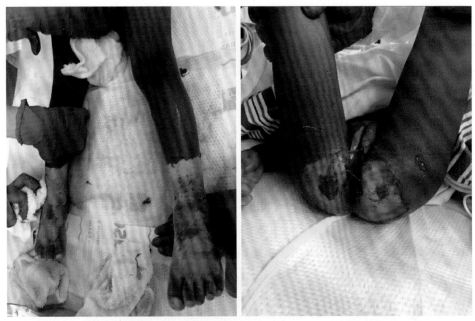

FIGURE 8.10 Two-year-old with partial thickness burns to bilateral lower extremities and burns to the buttocks and perineum. No splash burns are present and patient has a "doughnut" pattern of burn to the buttocks area indicating forced immersion.

lateral views of the spine, anteroposterior views of the pelvis, long bones of the extremities, and feet and posteroanterior oblique views of the hands. Whole body X-rays, also known as baby grams, should not be performed because they are not sensitive enough to detect occult fractures. Fractures that are highly suspicious for abuse, that is rib fractures and metaphyseal fractures, are most often detected only after a skeletal survey has been performed. Acute fractures, particularly rib fractures, may not be seen on the initial films and a repeat skeletal survey is recommended 2 weeks after the initial evaluation. It is at this time point that periosteal reaction and exuberant bone formation will herald the presence of a rib fracture.

Computed tomography, CT, of the head is performed on any patient with neurological status changes, history of head trauma, and all children under the age of 6 months with any concerns for physical abuse. Three-dimensional reconstruction of the skull on CT can help differentiate between true skull fractures and accessory sutures (**Figure 8.13**).[19] Imaging of the spine is also recommended to evaluate for

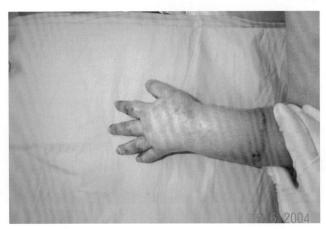

FIGURE 8.11 Fourteen-month-old with partial thickness immersion burn to left hand and forearm.

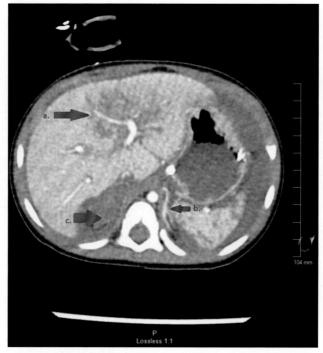

FIGURE 8.12 One-year-old found unresponsive and in hypovolemic shock. No history of trauma. Patient reportedly had decreased activity, anorexia, vomiting, and diarrhea beginning 5 hours prior to presentation. Multiple areas of bruising and abrasions are seen on physical examination. CT of abdomen is significant for a. liver laceration, b. adrenal hematoma, and c. adrenal hemorrhage. Patient was also found to have buckle fractures of the left anterolateral seventh and eighth ribs.

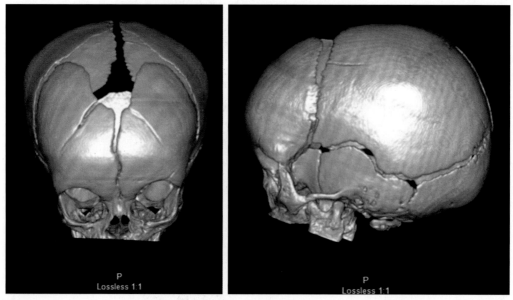

FIGURE 8.13 Complex skull fracture in a 6-month-old with no history of trauma and associated chronic and acute subdural hematomas.

spinal trauma. Magnetic resonance imaging, MRI, of the head and spine may detect injuries not seen on CT scan. These include shearing injuries, ischemia, and parenchymal hemorrhages. Spinal subdural hemorrhages as well as ligamentous injury may also be appreciated on MRI.[20]

● Fracture Types

All fractures can occur from accidents as well as from inflicted, or nonaccidental, trauma and no fracture is pathognomonic for abuse if witnessed accidental trauma occurs. Certain fractures are more commonly described in association with NAT especially if the purported circumstances and mechanism of injury are not concordant.

The age and developmental stage of the patient must also be considered as well. Eighty percent of abusive fractures were found in children less than 18 months of age[21] (**Figure 8.14**).

For example, a "toddler's fracture" or distal tibial fracture for an ambulatory child of 18 months is generally considered accidental. The same fracture pattern in 4-month-old, obviously

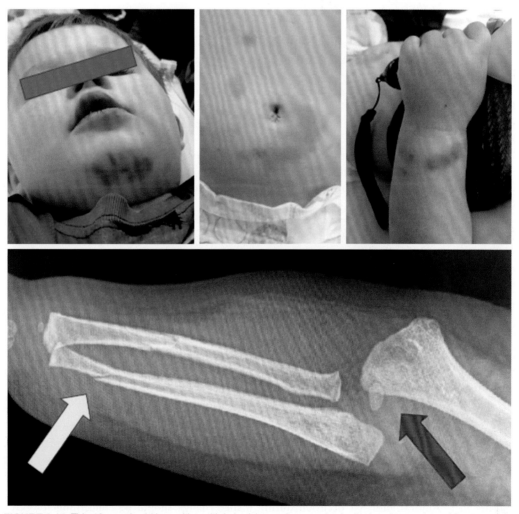

FIGURE 8.14 This 18-month-old boy with multiple bruising and a completely displaced transphyseal fracture of the humerus (red arrow) with same sided forearm fracture (yellow arrow).

nonambulatory, would be considered suspicious for inflicted trauma. Any fractures with no history of trauma, significant fractures sustained, and delay of care noted are concerning for abuse. In addition, it is important to understand the mechanisms of injury that cause the morphology of the fracture.

Biomechanical characteristics of the bones of children result in patterns of fractures that are commonly seen in pediatrics, but not in adults. Children's bones are more porous, covered in a thicker periosteum, and have growth plates at the ends of long bones.[22] These properties result in children's bones that may bend before they break, which in fact dispels the myth that is often suggested by investigators that a child's fracture was the result of an accident since the child has "weaker" bones.

● Common Fracture Patterns Seen in Accidental Trauma and NAT

Torus or buckle fractures are incomplete fractures, usually of the distal radius or tibia, as the result of a compressive force.

Greenstick fractures are also incomplete fractures that occur when there is a force that causes bending of the bone resulting in disruption on the tension side. The force is usually not sufficient enough to lead to transverse fracture.

Transverse fractures at the midshaft of bones usually occur as a result of direct trauma or as a result of indirect trauma such as a fall on the outstretched hand.

Ping pong fractures are depressed skull fractures that occur when the inner calvarium of young infants buckles as a result of blunt force trauma. These may also occur in association with difficult extraction during birth.

Simple linear skull fractures may be seen after falls in infants. It is always important to consider, however, the distance and velocity of the fall, and the surface material where the child landed. A complex skull fracture, including comminuted, depressed, or open fractures, is associated with a greater impact.

Spiral fractures of long bones are a result of twisting and torsional mechanisms. The common mechanism includes a toddler who is running and whose foot gets caught and the twisting of his leg with forward momentum of his body leads to a toddler's fracture (spiral tibial fracture) (**Figure 8.15**).

Compression fractures of the vertebral bodies may result from axial force such as a fall from a great height or motor vehicle accident. Children with osteoporosis may be at greater risk of these patterns. These can also occur from NAT.

● Common Fracture Locations

Fractures that are considered highly suspicious for abuse in infants and children include rib fractures, classic metaphyseal corner fractures, sternal fractures, spinous process fractures, and scapular fractures. The mechanisms required to result in these unusual fractures are not seen in normal handling of infants or childhood accidents.[23] Other fracture patterns that may be more concerning for abuse include multiple fractures, especially multiple fractures at different stages of healing. Vertebral body fractures and digital fractures are unusual in infants and toddlers and may be suspicious for abuse.

Femur Fractures

Femur fractures are often seen in abused children; however, they are also seen in accidental injury. Despite a long-held belief that "a femur fracture in a child is abuse until proven otherwise," most femur fractures in ambulatory children are not abuse.[24]

It is important to correlate the fracture pattern with the reported mechanism. A spiral femur fracture in a 9-month-old that occurred during diaper change should be concerning for NAT (**Figure 8.16**).

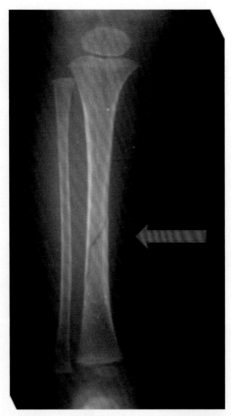

FIGURE 8.15 This spiral tibial fracture is otherwise known as a toddler fracture. It can happen with NAT too.

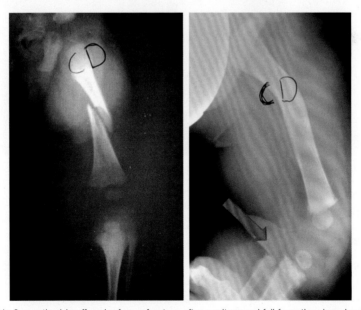

FIGURE 8.16 This 6-month old suffered a femur fracture after a witnessed fall from the changing table. The mechanism of injury seemed consistent. Routine follow-up radiographs 6 months later demonstrate good healing but also a recent fracture of the proximal tibia was serendipitously noted (red arrow). The child was referred to child protective services where NAT was confirmed.

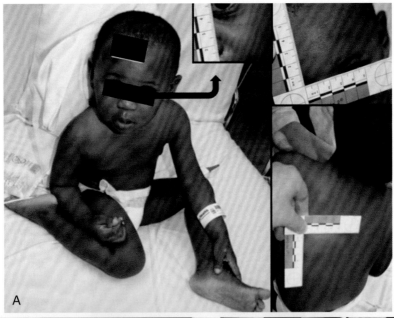

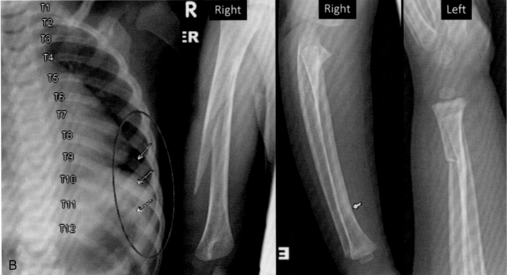

FIGURE 8.17 A, This two-year-old toddler has pain and decreased use of both arms as well as bruising on his face and back. B, Skeletal survey documented rib fractures (red circle), acute right humerus fracture, healed right forearm fracture (yellow arrow), and acute left forearm fracture. The combination of bruising, rib fractures, and multiple fractures in various stages of healing is diagnostic for nonaccidental trauma.

Rib Fractures in Infants

Posterior rib fractures are often seen in association with abusive head trauma. The mechanism of injury involves anterior posterior compression of the rib cage resulting in fractures occurring particularly along the posterior aspect over the spinous processes (**Figure 8.17A** and **B**).

Classic Metaphyseal Fractures

The classic metaphyseal fracture, also known as "corner" or "bucket-handle" fracture, occurs in association with shearing forces or torsion of the long bone (**Figure 8.18**).

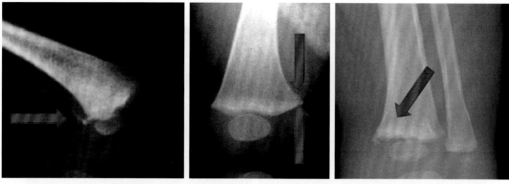

FIGURE 8.18 Metaphyseal corner fractures at varying locations and which are highly suggestive for NAT.

Transphyseal Fractures of the Distal Humerus

This variant of the supracondylar fracture is usually encountered in infants and young toddlers. The affected child will have a swollen elbow that is painful (**Figure 8.19**).

There may be muffled crepitance on examination. Radiographs are difficult to confirm the diagnosis and advanced imaging such as ultrasound or MRI may be helpful (**Figures 8.20** and **8.21**).

Sternal Fractures

Sternal fractures occur as the result of blunt force trauma to the chest. Significant force is required, and this type of fracture occurs in association with motor vehicle accidents.

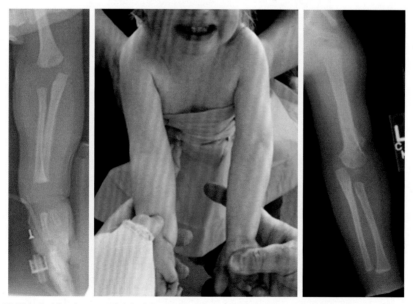

FIGURE 8.19 This toddler has a painful, deformed, and swollen left elbow and has a radiographic evidence of a distal humerus transphyseal fracture.

Normal   Fracture

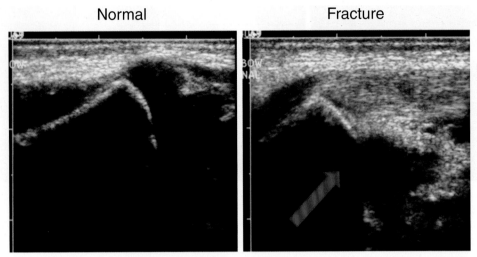

FIGURE 8.20 Ultrasound images of a child with displaced transphyseal fracture of the distal humerus, which was difficult to see radiographically. Ultrasound is a preferable examination to MRI as it does not require general anesthesia.

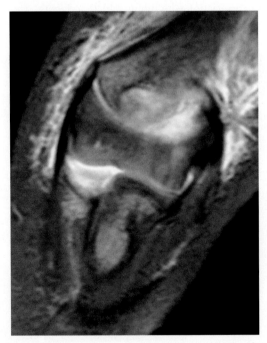

FIGURE 8.21 MRI examination of the distal humerus of a child who was initially referred for septic elbow but was found to have a transphyseal supracondylar humerus fracture. MRI can clearly demonstrate the cartilage that is not seen on radiographs. MRI is not normally used for evaluation of this injury.

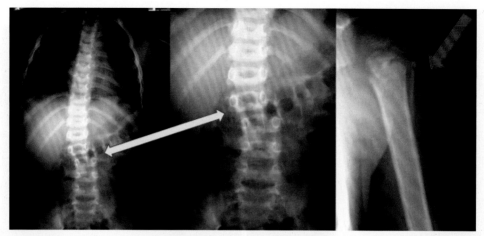

FIGURE 8.22 This child was suspected of NAT based upon a displaced spinal fracture from falling down the stairs (yellow arrow). Skeletal survey documented a healing proximal humerus fracture (red arrow) and NAT was confirmed.

Spine Fractures

Spinous process fractures can result from hyperflexion and hyperextension as well as from direct trauma. More severe trauma is required to disrupt the spinal column (**Figure 8.22**).

Scapular Fractures

High energy, blunt trauma is required to cause a scapular fracture, and this fracture is usually accompanied by traumatic soft tissue injuries to the chest. A developmental variant of the scapula, OS acromiale, occurs when the distal acromion fails to fuse. A healing fracture of the scapula may be incorrectly diagnosed. The absence of additional traumatic injuries of the chest as well as follow-up imaging can be used to distinguish this normal variant from a healing fracture.[25]

● *Differential Diagnosis and Confounding Medical Circumstances*

Accidental trauma, preexisting medical conditions, as well as metabolic diseases that may be related to a predisposition to fracture should be considered in the evaluation of pediatric fractures.

Children that are born prematurely may have decreased mineralization of the bones that should normalize with appropriate nutrition by 1 year. Children who are of low birth weight, require total parenteral nutrition for prolonged periods, or have medical conditions requiring long-term treatment with medications that affect bone mineralization such as steroids or diuretics may also be at risk. Nutritional compromise can be either due to medical conditions associated with the prematurity or by choice. For instance, exclusive breastfeeding of infants without vitamin D supplementation may result in nutritional rickets, placing the child at risk for fractures. Laboratory studies should include serum calcium, phosphorus, alkaline phosphatase, parathyroid hormone, 25-hydroxy vitamin D, and 1,25-dihydroxyviatmin D[26] (**Figure 8.23**).

Congenital syphilis may present with osteochondritis, epiphysitis, and periostitis. These findings may mimic the metaphyseal fractures that are highly suspicious for abuse. The overall clinical presentation of the neonate with the classic associated findings, such as hepatomegaly, splenomegaly, rash, and adenopathy and possibly sniffles, should guide the evaluation with confirmation of the diagnosis made by serologic testing.[27]

Osteomyelitis may present with radiographic changes concerning periosteal reaction suspicious for inflicted bone trauma. Clinical finding and laboratory studies are usually apparent at the time of evaluation to support infections. Fever, swelling, tenderness to palpation of the affected bone as well as increased white count on the CBC, and increased erythrocyte sedimentation rate and C-reactive protein are usually present.[28]

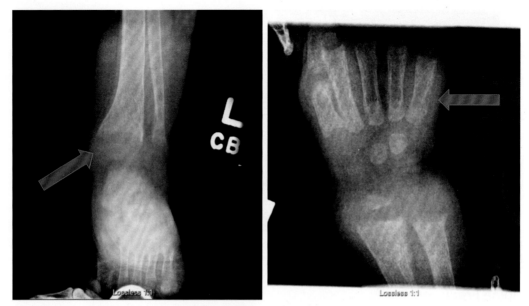

FIGURE 8.23 Nutritional rickets in a two-year-old with severe failure to thrive. Patient was primarily breastfed and had no medical care since birth. Bones are diffusely osteopenic and there is cupping and fraying of the metaphysis. There is also widening of the physis and periosteal reaction noted involving the metacarpals.

Osteogenesis imperfecta, OI, is a genetic condition characterized by bones that are predisposed to fractures due to a defect in the collagen resulting in fragile bones. Often referred to as "brittle bone disease," this disease has several different types with varying degrees of severity. Because OI affects other organ systems due to the abnormal collagen production, there are other clinical signs and symptoms of the disorder. Besides the fragile bones, the teeth may be affected, there may be hearing problems, respiratory problems, skin and joint laxity, and easy bruising. Wormian bones may be seen on skull X-rays. Visual problems may also be present, and "blue sclerae" is seen in patients with most types. Although genetic testing for mutations in the COL1A1 and COL1A2, CRTAP and P3H1 genes can be performed, the diagnosis is usually made clinically by a geneticist based on the history and physical examination. Mutations of the COL1A1 and COL1A2 genes are associated with 90% of the cases of OI. Prenatal diagnosis by ultrasound may also be made in severe forms of OI[29] (**Figure 8.24**).

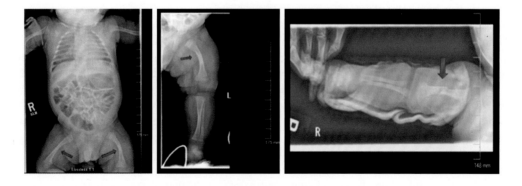

FIGURE 8.24 Seven-week-old with an acute humerus fracture. An skeletal survey showed complete oblique mid-diaphyseal acute fracture of the right humerus and bowing of the bilateral femurs. Bones are osteopenic. Remodeling and healing fractures most likely represent fractures that occurred *in utero*. Osteogenesis imperfecta Type IV was confirmed by genomic sequencing.

Infantile cortical hyperostosis, Caffey disease, is another genetic condition that results in multiple bone involvement, particularly the mandible and/or clavicle and ribs. There is usually fever, swelling, and subperiosteal new bone formation along the affected bones. It affects infants between 6 weeks and 6 months of age and may be misdiagnosed as multiple fractures from abuse. A mutation has been identified in the COL1A1 gene that may be inherited or sporadic[30] (**Figure 8.25**).

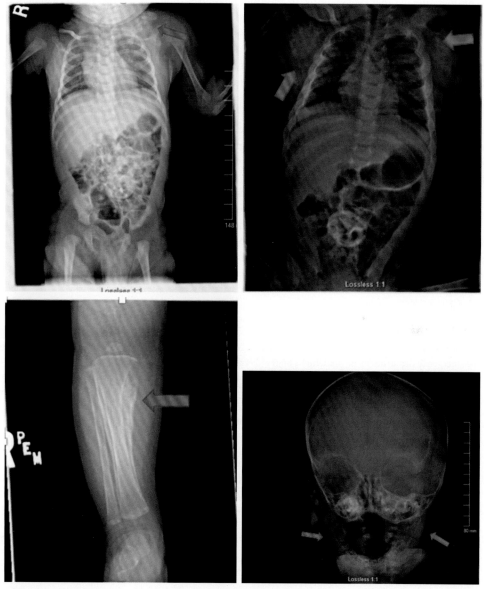

FIGURE 8.25 Caffey disease in a four-week-old with left chest swelling, fever, and irritability. Initially diagnosed and treated for suspected osteomyelitis. Follow-up osseous survey 6 weeks later showed periosteal reaction/hyperostosis involving the bilateral scapulae, bilateral ribs, right tibia, and mandible.

● Management of NAT

The first and foremost role of the physician is to manage the medical condition of the patient. If there is concern that the injury is the result of NAT, physicians are bound by mandatory reporting statutes in the United States and must file a report. Each jurisdiction has independent reporting requirements, and the physician should be aware of the local protocols for reporting suspected abuse. Physicians should inform caregivers of their concerns of NAT in an objective and nonjudgmental approach. The role of the physician is not to make a definitive determination or opinion as to whom is responsible for the injury, but to inform the authorities of a traumatic injury that is suspicious for abuse after careful evaluation and consideration of other explanations. In addition, physicians should be aware of their own biases and be mindful that abuse occurs in all racial, ethnic, and socioeconomic groups. Many children's hospitals have child abuse specialists on staff that may be consulted for assistance.

It can be difficult to explain to caregivers why NAT is being considered and the necessary steps required to fully evaluate the situation. Caregivers must consider the safety of the child as well as their own safety during these exchanges. The caregiver should consider having multiple team members present and have the ability for rapid egress from the examination room. It is mandatory to avoid any terms that are accusatory or imply casual mechanisms for NAT. It is helpful to frame the discussion on your sole concern to care for the child. It can also be helpful to state that you are required by law to go through these steps. "The law says that I have to stop when the light turns red. The law states I have to report this fracture if seen in any child including my own." "If I do not report this fracture pattern, I can lose my medical license or be criminally charged."

The child usually needs to be admitted and the appropriate specialists consulted to manage cranial, visceral, or soft tissue injuries. The orthopedic service is consulted to manage fractures, and it is important that full radiographic evaluation of the skeleton is performed before placement of casts or splints that could limit evaluation. Thankfully, most orthopedic injuries can be managed with short periods of immobilization (less than 4-5 weeks) and normal function is almost always the case without long-term skeletal problems. In cases where child abuse is suspected, make sure that follow-up plans are made and documented and that you are aware if follow-up visits are missed.

References

1. Naranje SM, Erali RA, Warner WC Jr, Sawyer JR, Kelly DM. Epidemiology of pediatric fractures presenting to emergency departments in the United States. *J Pediatr Orthop*. 2016;36(4):e45-e48.
2. U.S. Department of Health & Human Services; Administration for Children and Families, Administration on Children, Youth and Families, Children's Bureau. *Child Maltreatment 2017*. 2019. Available at https://www.acf.hhs.gov/cb/research-data-technology/statistics-research/child-maltreatment.
3. Puls HT, Anderst JD, Bettenhausen JL, et al. Newborn risk factors for subsequent physical abuse hospitalizations. *Pediatrics*. 2019;143(2):e20182108.
4. Jaudes PK, Mackey-Bilaver L. Do chronic conditions increase young children's risk of being maltreated? *Child Abuse Neglect*. 2008;32(7):671-681.
5. Schnitzer PG, Ewigman BG. Child deaths resulting from inflicted injuries: household risk factors and perpetrator characteristics. *Pediatrics*. 2005;116(5):e687-e693.
6. King J, Diefendorf D, Apthorp J, Negrete VF, Carlson M. Analysis of 429 fractures in 189 battered children. *J Pediatr Orthop*. 1988;8(5):585.
7. Maclean MJ, Sims S, Bower C, et al. Maltreatment risk among children with disabilities. *Pediatrics*. 2017;139(4):e20161817.
8. Eastwood D. Breaks without bruises. Are common and can't be said to rule out non-accidental injury. *BMJ*. 1998;317(7166):1095-1096.
9. Peters ML, Starling SP, Barnes-Eley ML, Heisler KW. The presence of bruising associated with fractures. *Arch Pediatr Adolesc Med*. 2008;162(9):877-881.
10. Kos L, Shwayder T. Cutaneous manifestations of child abuse. *Pediatr Dermatol*. 2006;23:311-320.

11. Maguire S, Mann MK, Sibert J, et al. Can you age bruises accurately in children? A systematic review. *Arch Dis Child.* 2005;90:187-189.

12. Sugar N, Taylor J, Feldman K. Bruises in infants and toddlers: those who don't cruise rarely bruise. Puget Sound Pediatric Research Network. *Arch Pediatr Adolesc Med.* 1999;153:399-403.

13. Keenan HT, Runyan DK, Marshall SW, Nocera MA, Merten DF, Sinal SH. A population-based study of inflicted traumatic brain injury in young children. *J Am Med Assoc.* 2003;290:621-626.

14. Narang S, Clarke J. Abusive head trauma: past, present, and future. *J Child Neurol.* 2014;29(12):1747-1756.

15. Jenny C, Hymel KP, Ritzén A, Reinert SE, Hay TC. Analysis of missed cases of abusive head trauma. *J Am Med Assoc.* 1999;281(7):621-626.

16. Krishnamoorthy V, Ramaiah R, Bhananker SM. Pediatric burn injuries. *Int J Crit Illn Inj Sci.* 2012;2(3):128-134. doi:10.4103/2229-5151.100889.

17. Maguire SA, Upadhyaya M, Evans A, et al. A systematic review of abusive visceral injuries in childhood-their range and recognition. *Child Abuse Negl.* 2013;37(7):430-445.

18. American Acadamy of Pediatrics; Section on Radiology. Diagnostic imaging of child abuse. *Pediatrics.* 2009;123(5):1430-1435.

19. Sanchez T, Stewart D, Walvick M, Swischuk L. Skull fracture vs. accessory sutures: how can we tell the difference? *Emerg Radiol.* 2010;17(5):413-418.

20. Kadom N, Khademian Z, Vezina G, Shalaby-Rana E, Rice A, Hinds T. Usefulness of MRI detection of cervical spine and brain injuries in the evaluation of abusive head trauma. *Pediatr Radiol.* 2014;44(7):839-848.

21. Kemp AM, Dunstan F, Harrison S, et al. Patterns of skeletal fractures in child abuse: systematic review. *BMJ.* 2008;337:a1518. Published October 2, 2008.

22. Xian CJ, Foster B. The biologic aspects of children's fractures. In Beaty JH, Kasser JR, eds. *Rockwood and Wilkins' Fractures in Children.* 7th ed. Philadelphia, PA: Lippincott Williams & Wilkins; 2010:18-44.

23. Nimkin K, Kleinman PK. Imaging of child abuse. *Radiol Clin North Am.* 2001;39(4):843-864.

24. Schwend RM, Werth C, Johnston A. Femur shaft fractures in toddlers and young children: rarely from child abuse. *J Pediatr Orthop.* 2000;20(4):475-481.

25. Zember JS, Rosenberg ZS, Kwong S, Kothary SP, Bedoya MA. Normal skeletal maturation and imaging pitfalls in the pediatric shoulder. *Radiographics.* 2015;35(4):1108-1122.

26. Rustico SE, Calabria AC, Garber SJ. Metabolic bone disease of prematurity. *J Clin Transl Endocrinol.* 2014;1(3):85-91.

27. Rasool MN, Govender S. The skeletal manifestations of congenital syphilis. A review of 197 cases. *J Bone Joint Surg Br.* 1989;71(5):752-755.

28. Ogden JA. Pediatric osteomyelitis and septic arthritis: the pathology of neonatal disease. *Yale J Biol Med.* 1979;52(5):423-448.

29. Dijk F, Cobben J, Kariminejad A, et al. Osteogenesis imperfecta: a review with clinical examples. *Mol Syndromol.* 2011;2:1-20.

30. Nistala H, Mäkitie O, Jüppner H. Caffey disease: new perspectives on old questions. *Bone.* 2014;60:246-251.

Examination of the Injured Child

Anthony I. Riccio and Shital N. Parikh

● Introduction

Although pediatric orthopedic injuries vary widely in severity, one must recall that even a seemingly innocuous musculoskeletal injury in a child can carry the potential for associated neurologic deficit, vascular compromise, or compartment syndrome or result from a nonaccidental etiology. As such associated issues cannot be detected with standard or advanced imaging, a carefully performed and skilled physical examination is essential in every child with an extremity or axial injury. In addition, higher energy extremity trauma often presents with concomitant visceral, cerebral, and thoracic injuries. While severe limb deformity and open fractures are often outwardly apparent, this may not be the case for trauma to other organ systems. One must therefore be cognizant of the potential for such life-threatening injuries and direct their initial examination of the child to detect such injuries prior to focusing on the musculoskeletal evaluation.

● Assessment of the Multiply Injured Child

Epidemiology

National data from the United States Center of Disease Control continues to demonstrate that unintentional injury remains the leading cause of death in children older than 1 year. Although most of these deaths result from intracranial, thoracic, and abdominal trauma, 63% of multiply injured children have associated extremity fractures.[1] It is therefore imperative that orthopedic surgeons are able to perform a thorough and systematic assessment of the polytraumatized pediatric patient.

Primary Survey

Initial evaluation of a traumatized child is directed at identifying life-threatening injuries while beginning resuscitative measures. The primary survey begins with a rapid compilation of the mechanism of injury, known medical problems, medication allergies, and any treatments initiated prior to arrival. Following this quick history, the patient is assessed for airway patency, breathing and ventilation, circulatory issues, and neurologic disability. This primary evaluation is commonly referred to as the ABCs of trauma care:

- Airway: Assure that the airway is patent. Talking and crying both require an open airway and usually indicate the absence of obstruction. Airway patency can be more difficult to assess in the unconscious patient. The presence of grunting, snorting, or choking may indicate a compromised airway obstruction that must be managed acutely with attempted removal of obstructing body fluids via suctioning, use of the jaw thrust maneuver, and intubation when necessary. It is critical to assume the presence of a cervical spine injury in all traumatized children. Therefore, airway management must be conducted using spinal precautions, including cervical stabilization with an appropriately sized rigid collar. Furthermore, because of the increased head size to body size ratio in younger children, flexion of the cervical spine should be avoided by placing the child on a backboard with a cutout for the head or by elevating the torso relative to the head.

- Breathing: Ventilation is assessed by inspection (looking), auscultation (listening), and palpation (feelings). Breath sounds should be present equally in both lung fields. Unilateral absence of breath sounds or diminished breath sounds may indicate a pneumothorax, hemothorax, or malpositioned endotracheal tube. The thorax should be inspected to assess for a flail segment or penetrating injury. Deviation of the trachea should be noted as this is indicative of a tension pneumothorax on the side opposite the direction of deviation. Palpation of the chest and neck may reveal the presence of subcutaneous emphysema that can be associated with a tension pneumothorax.
- Circulation: Elevated heart rate, diminished blood pressure, delayed capillary refill time (CRT), and coolness or mottling of the peripheral extremities may all be indicative of circulatory compromise. It is important to note that healthy pediatric patients can lose a considerable amount of blood volume prior to manifesting clinical signs of hypovolemic shock. In such instances, tachycardia usually precedes the onset of hypotension.
- Disability: Neurologic disability is frequently assessed by calculating the Glasgow Coma Scale (GCS) score (**Table 9.1**).
- Exposure: All clothing should be removed to allow for complete inspection of the patient. The patient should be kept warm with blankets, heat lamps, and/or warmed intravenous fluids following exposure.

Table 9.1	The Glasgow Coma Scale	
VARIABLE		**SCORE**
Eyes		
Open spontaneously		4
Open to verbal stimuli		3
Open to painful stimuli		2
Do not open		1
Verbal		
Smiles, follows objects, interacts, oriented		5
Crying but consolable with inappropriate interaction or confusion		4
Inconsistently consolable or using incoherent words		3
Incomprehensible sounds or moans		2
No response		1
Motor		
Spontaneous movement or obeys commands		6
Localizes to painful stimuli		5
Withdrawal from painful stimuli		4
Abnormal extremity flexion to painful stimuli		3
Abnormal extremity extension to painful stimuli		2
No movement		1

GCS, Glasgow Coma Scale.
The Glasgow Coma Scale score is calculated by adding the scores from each of the three variables
(GCS score = eyes + verbal + motor).

Secondary Survey

The secondary survey is conducted following initial resuscitation and management of any life-threatening injuries identified during the primary assessment. A complete history should be obtained along with a head-to-toe assessment of the entire patient. All extremities should be palpated including all digits, all joints without obvious deformity should be ranged, and an examination of the spine should be performed while maintaining spinal precautions. Radiographic evaluation includes a lateral cervical spine film, anteroposterior pelvis film, and an anteroposterior radiograph of the chest. Orthogonal radiographs are also obtained of any extremity that is deformed, swollen, or ecchymotic or demonstrates crepitus on examination. It is during the secondary survey that data can be gathered to classify injury severity via one of the numerous classification systems used to predict morbidity and mortality in the multiply injured patient (**Tables 9.2-9.4**). During the secondary survey, it is essential to continuously reassess the patient's airway, breathing, and circulation for deterioration that might warrant emergent intervention.

Tertiary Survey

The tertiary skeletal examination is a careful and more detailed assessment performed once vital signs have stabilized and emergent and urgent pathologies have been addressed. This examination is ideally performed once the patient is awake and alert enough to participate in the examination. The tertiary

---

Table 9.2	An Example of the Injury Severity Score in Use

INJURY SEVERITY SCORE

$$\text{ISS} = \text{sum of 3 highest}^2 \text{ AIS} = a^2 + b^2 + c^2$$

Region	Injury Description	AIS	Square Top Three
Head and neck	Cerebral contusion	3	9
Face	No injury	0	
Chest	Flail chest	4	16
Abdomen	Minor contusion of liver Complex rupture of spleen	2 5	25
Extremity	Fractured femur	3	
External	No injury	0	
Injury severity score:			**50**

ISS	
1–8	Minor
9–15	Moderate
16–24	Serious
25–49	Severe
50–74	Critical
75	Maximum

AIS, Abbreviated Injury Scale.

Table 9.3	The Revised Trauma Score		
		VARIABLES	
REVISED TRAUMA SCORE	**GLASGOW COMA SCALE SCORE**	**SYSTOLIC BLOOD PRESSURE (MM HG)**	**RESPIRATORY RATE (BREATHS/MIN)**
4	13-15	>89	>29
3	9-12	76-89	10-29
2	6-8	50-75	6-9
1	4-5	1-49	1-5
0	3	0	0

Table 9.4	The Pediatric Trauma Score		
		SCORE	
VARIABLE	**+2**	**+1**	**−1**
Airway	Patent	Maintainable	Unmaintainable
Weight (kg)	>20	10-20	<10
Systolic blood pressure (mm Hg)	>90	50-90	<50
Neurologic	Awake	Loss of consciousness	Unresponsive
Fractures	None	Closed	Open or multiple
Wounds	None	Minor	Major or penetrating

musculoskeletal examination involves palpation of all extremities, assessment of restriction, pain or crepitus with joint range of motion, a detailed neurologic examination, and a careful spinal examination. The goal of the tertiary survey is to identify missed injuries that have been reported to present in up to 12% of multiply injured patients.[2-5] In the presence of an uncooperative or unconscious patient, the tertiary survey should be repeated once the patient is extubated and awake.

Commonly Missed Injuries

While tertiary surveys and formalized tertiary survey protocols have been shown to decrease the incidence of missed injuries in polytrauma patients, delays in the detection of musculoskeletal injuries do occur.[2] Patients with lower GCS scores and more severe distracting trauma seem to be at higher risk for having a delay in diagnosis of a less obvious extremity or axial injury.[6] Although no high-level study or systematic literature review has characterized the distribution of missed injuries in children with multisystem injuries, the peripheral skeleton (hands, feet, and ankles) and the shoulder girdle region seem to be areas in which delayed diagnoses of fractures are frequently encountered[3] (**Figure 9.1**). These areas therefore deserve careful attention during the tertiary survey.

It is also important to note that the incidence of multilevel vertebral column injuries at both contiguous and noncontiguous levels has been reported to be as high as 47% in children.[7] Therefore, identification of a single spinal injury should prompt a careful physical and radiographic assessment of the entire spine to rule out a concomitant injury.

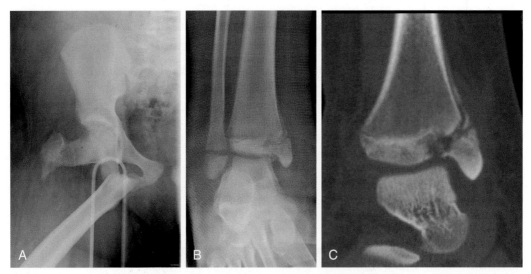

FIGURE 9.1 A, Right hip radiographs of a 12-year-old female unrestrained passenger in a motor vehicle collision demonstrate a displaced intertrochanteric hip fracture. The patient presented with a Glasgow Coma Scale (GCS) score of 7 and also sustained a closed head injury, a pneumothorax, a high-grade liver laceration requiring operative hemostasis, and multiple compression fractures of the thoracolumbar spine. B, Following a 2-week ICU stay during which the patient was intubated and sedated, she noted ankle pain with attempted mobilization. Right ankle films demonstrated a displaced healing medial malleolus fracture. C, CT scan of the ankle demonstrates abundant callus and significant joint diastasis.

Nonorthopedic System Evaluation

Modern level 1 trauma care delivery systems in the United States must adhere to strict criteria imposed by the American College of Surgeons to maintain accreditation, including the coordination of care for a multiply injured child by a trauma-trained pediatric surgeon. Nonetheless, it is important for the orthopedic specialist to be familiar with the basic assessment of nonorthopedic systems as the presence of visceral or thoracic trauma may raise awareness of orthopedic injuries and alter the timing or method of musculoskeletal care:

- Head injury: High rates of concomitant head trauma have been reported in the presence of pediatric cervical spine injuries.[7,8] Inspection and palpation of the skull for abrasions, depressions, and lacerations may heighten suspicion for intracranial trauma, especially in the setting of a known spinal injury.
- Thorax: The thorax should be carefully inspected. Paradoxical motion of a segment of the chest wall is defined as inward motion of the segment with inspiration while the remainder of the chest wall expands and outward movement of the segment with expiration as the remainder of the chest wall contracts. This is seen in the presence of a flail chest and usually indicates an associated pulmonary contusion as well. Palpation of the chest may reveal subcutaneous emphysema consistent with a tension pneumothorax. Absent or diminished breath sounds on auscultation of a hemithorax may result from a pneumothorax or hemothorax.
- Abdominal/genitourinary injury: An abdominal examination consists of palpation, percussion, and inspection of all our quadrants of the abdomen. Guarding, abdominal distention, and tympanic percussion are indicators of free air within the peritoneal cavity and possible bowel injury. An inspection of the abdomen may alert the examiner to possible axial trauma. Visual inspection of the abdomen of children involved in a motor vehicle collision may reveal transverse liner ecchymosis or abrasions across the abdomen commonly referred to as seatbelt sign (**Figure 9.2**). This finding has been associated with an underlying intra-abdominal injury, may be a predictor of the need for intra-abdominal surgery, and is frequently seen in the presence of a flexion-distraction injury of the thoracolumbar spine[9] (**Figure 9.2**). The presence of blood at the urethral meatus may indicate bladder rupture or urethral disruption, the latter of which can be secondary to an associated pelvic ring injury.

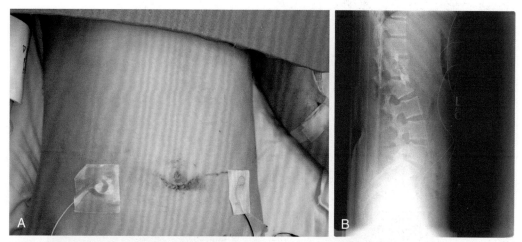

FIGURE 9.2 A, Clinical photograph of a 13-year-old female backseat passenger in a motor vehicle collision. The patient was restrained with a lap belt. Note the liner abrasions across the lower abdomen characteristic of a "seatbelt sign." **B,** The patient had a mesenteric hematoma and an L1-L2 flexion-distraction injury of the spine, both of which required surgical intervention.

Orthopedic Emergencies

Open Fractures

The accurate and prompt diagnosis of an open fracture is essential as the timely administration of antibiotics has been associated with diminished infection rates particularly in higher grade injuries.[10] The importance of the physical examination is underscored by the fact that antibiotic selection is usually guided by open injury classification, which is classically based on examination findings. While more severe open injuries are easily identified, the determination of whether smaller poke hole–type injuries are truly representative of an open fracture can be difficult. A careful examination is critical as identification that a pediatric fracture is open often times alters the treatment plan dramatically, frequently mandating operative intervention for an injury that might otherwise be managed closed in a splint or cast.

One tenet of open fracture management is that any unnecessary soft tissue and bony manipulation should be avoided during the initial physical examination. Repetitive and vigorous examinations may result in further dissemination of contamination within the wound, further injury, and devitalization to surrounding soft tissues from underlying fracture fragments as well as patient discomfort. Any wound over a fracture should therefore be visually inspected for size, integrity of the overlying skin, and the presence of gross contamination. Classification of open injuries is based on the size of the dermal laceration and the extent of underlying soft tissue injury (**Figure 9.3**). The former can be ascertained during initial examination, whereas the latter is often determined during intraoperative assessment. One should, however, note the presence of any obvious tendon or muscle disruption as well as exposure of any vascular or nervous structures when larger wounds are present.

As noted, small puncture wounds may be difficult to distinguish from abrasions. The presence of dark sanguineous drainage from a wound (representative of fracture hematoma) often indicates an open fracture. If sanguineous staining is present on a dressing that was applied prior to assessment and the wound is no longer draining, gentle manipulation of the extremity that yields such drainage should raise suspicion of an open fracture (**Figure 9.4**). Similarly, the presence of fatty tissue within any fluid extravagating from a wound is also concerning for an open injury.

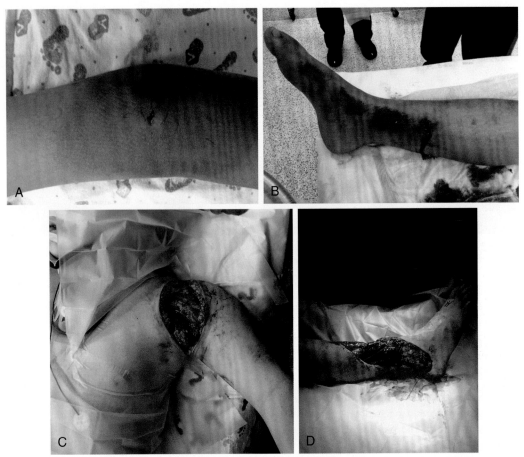

FIGURE 9.3 The Gustilo Anderson classification: A, A grade 1 open supracondylar humerus fracture. Grade 1 injuries have a wound less than 1 cm, minimal soft tissue injury, and intact periosteum. B, A grade 2 open tibia fracture. Grade 2 injuries have a wound that is greater than 1 cm, moderate soft tissue injury, and intact periosteum. C, A grade 3A open proximal humerus fracture. Grade 3A injuries have extensive soft tissue damage to the skin and underlying soft tissues with adequate tissue remaining for coverage of the wound. D, A grade 3B open tibia fracture. Grade 3B injuries have extensive soft tissue damage to the skin and underlying soft tissues, extensive periosteal striping, and do not have adequate tissue remaining for coverage of the wound.

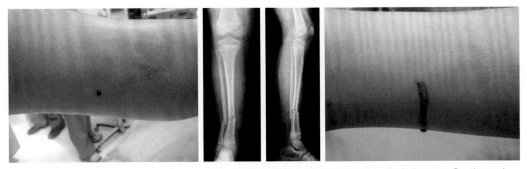

FIGURE 9.4 Innocuous-looking wound on the leg of an 8-year-old girl following tibia-fibula fracture. Gentle manipulation of the fracture led to a sanguineous discharge, suggesting an open fracture.

Compartment Syndrome

It is critical to understand that compartment syndrome is a clinical diagnosis, often based more on observation of a patient's pain level and analgesic needs than on objective physical examination findings. Consensus does exist as to the definition of compartment syndrome (elevated interstitial pressure within a closed fascial compartment resulting in microvascular compromise and tissue ischemia), the importance of making a timely diagnosis (preservation of limb function), and treatment (decompressive fasciotomies). On the other hand, no consensus exists with regard to diagnostic criteria. Moreover, as younger children are often incapable of understanding and verbalizing discomfort, the diagnosis in a child can be more difficult than in an alert adult. Consequently, few clinical entities pose as much consternation as a suspected compartment syndrome in a pediatric patient.

Signs and Symptoms

Classically, clinicians have been advised to seek out the five "P's" in their assessment of a patient with suspected compartment syndrome. These include pain with passive stretch, pallor, paresthesias, pulselessness, and paralysis. The utility of these signs and symptoms is questionable as the findings of pulselessness, pallor, and paralysis are all late findings that present after irreversible muscle ischemia has occurred. Furthermore, children are frequently unable to describe paresthesias, making this symptom of limited value in the pediatric setting.

The sentinel symptom of compartment syndrome is therefore pain, typically beyond what would be expected with the associated fracture or injury. Because pain can be sometimes difficult to measure in the young, assessing for anxiety and agitation out of proportion to what is expected for a given injury is advised. Pain in the pediatric patient is often better gauged by assessing analgesic pain medication requirements. In the setting of a fracture about the elbow, forearm, or tibia, increasing analgesic requirements should raise suspicion of a possible compartment syndrome. Together, these findings of agitation, anxiety, and increasing analgesic needs represent the three "A's" of compartment syndrome and are more useful for pediatric patients.

To complicate matters, painless or "silent" compartment syndrome has been well described in children and is reported in as many of 12% of pediatric patients.[11] One should not, therefore, exclude the diagnosis of pediatric compartment syndrome in the absence of the usual signs and symptoms.

Physical Examination

The examination for compartment syndrome often begins with palpation of the involved extremity to assess for fullness of the fascial compartments. Soft compressible compartments are often reassuring, while tight, firm, unyielding compartments should raise concern of a possible compartment syndrome in the setting of a characteristic fracture and the symptoms described previously. It should be understood, however, that the ability of orthopedic surgeons to manually detect elevated compartment pressures is far from perfect. A cadaveric study revealed a positive predictive value of only 19% and a negative predictive value of 24% for detection of leg compartment pressures above the commonly accepted threshold for a compartment syndrome. In addition, only 60% of examiners recommended fasciotomies when pressures of 80 mm Hg (greater than twice the commonly accepted threshold) were present.[12] Obviously, one cannot diagnose or exclude compartment syndrome by palpation alone.

The presence and symmetry of distal pulse strength should be noted as pressure elevation can result in diminished pulses. A complete neurologic examination is also essential to identify altered sensation and motor weakness resulting from nerve compression and/or muscle ischemia. Pain with passive stretch of the musculotendinous units within affected compartment by gentle flexion/extension of the digits has been classically associated with compartment syndrome of the leg and forearm. While part of an adequate examination for compartment syndrome, such pain with passive stretch may be present in the setting of normal compartment pressures in the presence of a displaced forearm or tibia fracture because of muscle contusion or motion across fracture spikes.

Compartment Measurements

Although not routinely performed in pediatric patients, compartment pressure measurements can be helpful when suspicion of a compartment syndrome exists in an obtunded patient or when the clinical scenario is suspicious. In children who are not obtunded, these measures are made under sedation or

Table 9.5	Suggested Compartment Pressures Diagnostic for Compartment Syndrome
Absolute pressure > 30 mm Hg	
(Diastolic blood pressure) – (compartment pressure) ≤ 20 mm Hg	
(Mean arterial pressure) – (compartment pressure) ≤ 30 mm Hg	

general anesthesia with a commercially available pressure monitor (▶ **Video 9.1**) or by using a needle attached to an arterial line pressure transducer. If using an arterial line, it is critical that the pressure transducer is placed level with the extremity being examined. In the leg, the needle should be introduced through the skin, subcutaneous tissue, and the fascia in the anterior, posterior, lateral, and deep posterior compartments. In the forearm, the volar, dorsal, and mobile wad compartments may be testing, although the volar compartment alone usually suffices.

Controversy exists as to the pressure that constitutes a compartment syndrome and whether an absolute pressure measurement alone is sufficient to make the diagnosis (**Table 9.5**). For instance, in an assessment of adult tibial shaft fractures in patients without clinical signs of compartment syndrome, one-time compartment pressure measurements were above these accepted thresholds in a high percentage of patients with a false-positive rate of 35%.[13] The use of catheter placement for continuous pressure monitoring has therefore been suggested as being more accurate.

In summary, pediatric compartment syndromes are a devastating complication that usually occurs in the leg or forearm after significant trauma or periods of avascularity greater than 6 hours (**Figure 9.5**). Most

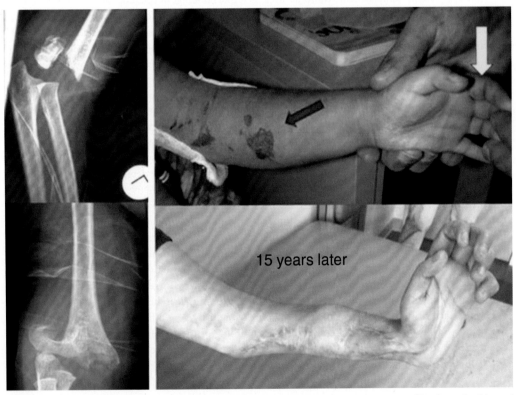

15 years later

FIGURE 9.5 A 3-year-old boy with a supracondylar humerus fracture undergoes treatment. After 3 weeks, his cast is removed and he has stiff fingers that do not extend (yellow arrow) and full-thickness skin lesions in the forearm are noted (red arrow). These skin lesions have been termed "sentinel lesions" and suggest an established compartment syndrome. Despite free muscles transfer, 15 years later, he has a scarred stiff and functionless arm.

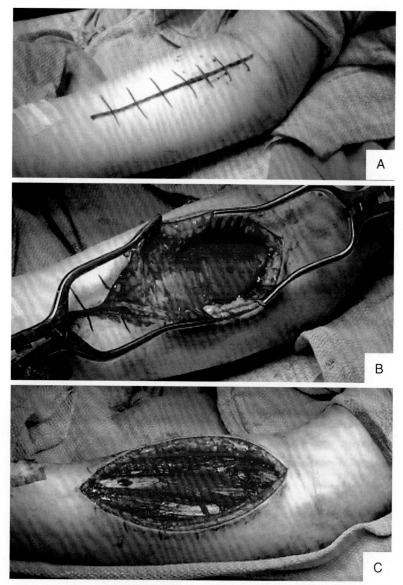

FIGURE 9.6 This boy has a very swollen and tense forearm after closed elbow injury, and there is clinical concern for a compartment syndrome (A). In the operating room, the pressure measures 40 mm Hg of mercury and a decision to release the forearm is made. After incision of the skin and subcutaneous tissue, the volar fascia is seen and is very tight (B). The superficial and deep fascia is cut and the muscles bulge out through the defect relieving the pressure (C).

importantly, compartment syndrome is a **clinical diagnosis** that should be suspected based on symptoms (the three "A's") and a swollen tense compartment that is extremely painful; although excessive compartment pressure measures are helpful to confirm diagnosis, they are not required to perform fasciotomy (**Figure 9.6**).

Vascular Injury

The importance of early detection of vascular compromise in the presence of an extremity injury cannot be understated. A prolonged tissue perfusion deficit can lead to irreversible ischemia, myonecrosis, fibrosis, severe functional loss, and nonviability of the involved extremity (**Figure 9.5**). Furthermore, the metabolic results (myoglobinuria and metabolic acidosis) of prolonged ischemia can be life threatening (renal failure). For these reasons, any vascular abnormality in the setting of extremity trauma should be considered an emergency and dealt with promptly and with the appropriate support of vascular surgeons or those trained in microvascular techniques when needed. One must also be aware of those fractures in children that are commonly associated with vascular disruption, occlusion, or spasm and be vigilant for any vascular differences on examination. Such fractures include displaced extension supracondylar humerus fractures (brachial artery injury) (**Figure 9.7**), fractures through the distal femur and proximal tibia (popliteal artery injury), and knee dislocations (popliteal artery injury) (**Figure 9.8**).

Physical Examination

Examination begins with inspection of the extremity for pallor and temperature. In the presence of arterial insufficiency, the skin is often cool, pale, and occasionally has a bluish hue or patchy areas of purple overlying otherwise white pale skin (mottling). In the setting of vascular congestion due to disruption of venous outflow, the extremity may appear swollen and dark purple in color, which may improve somewhat with elevation. In the setting of penetrating trauma, the presence of an expanding or pulsatile hematoma should raise concern about an active arterial bleed.

Capillary refill time (CRT) is easily assessed by manually compressing a distal phalanx to effectively exsanguinate the tip of the digit than observing for the duration of time before the end of the digit becomes pink and reperfused (▶ **Video 9.2**). This is oftentimes best observed through the nail plate. CRT of 2 seconds or less is commonly considered normal, although results should always be compared with the uninvolved extremity to identify differences.

The presence and quality of distal pulses must be documented and compared with the uninjured extremity. In the upper extremity, the radial pulse is usually easiest to assess. In the lower extremity, the posterior tibial artery (posterior to the medial malleolus) and the dorsalis pedis pulse (dorsum of the foot

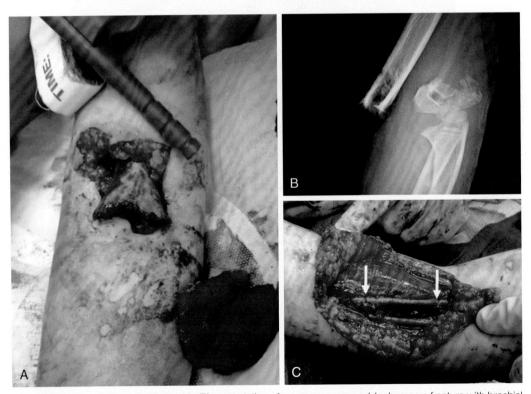

FIGURE 9.7 Clinical (A) and radiographic (B) presentation of an open supracondylar humerus fracture with brachial artery laceration. C, Arterial bypass grafting using saphenous vein (white arrows) was performed once the supracondylar humerus fracture was reduced. (Courtesy: Kevin Little, MD.)

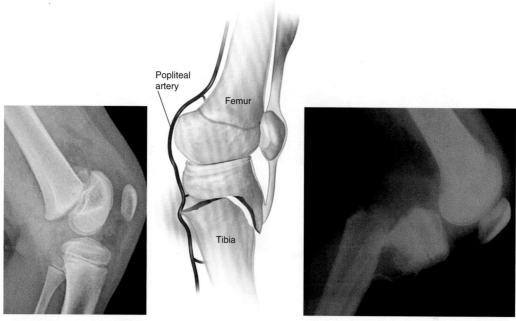

FIGURE 9.8 The popliteal artery is in close relationship to the posterior aspect of distal femur and proximal tibia. Displaced fractures of distal femur or proximal tibia can cause popliteal artery injury.

in the region of the medial midfoot) should be examined. A palpable pulse that is diminished in comparison with the contralateral extremity can be indicative of vascular compromise and merits concern. In the absence of a palpable pulse or in the setting of a barely palpable pulse, Doppler examination of the pulses is useful (▶ **Video 9.3A** and **B**). Dopplerable pulses are described as monophasic, biphasic, or triphasic (**Table 9.6**). Triphasic flow is normal (▶ **Video 9.4**), while a monophasic flow often represents partial occlusion of flow or even complete arterial occlusion with the signal resulting from retrograde flow.

In the setting of a side-to-side difference in the peripheral pulse examination, a more objective assessment can be obtained by determining the ankle brachial index (ABI) or arterial pressure index (API) (**Figure 9.9**). The ABI is obtained using a blood pressure cuff and stethoscope or Doppler to record the systolic pulse at the ankle and brachial artery (▶ **Video 9.5**). A patient's ABI is calculated by dividing the systolic blood pressure at the ankle by the pressure obtained at the arm. An ABI of less than 0.9 is considered abnormal and is commonly used as the threshold to perform more advanced diagnostics to assess for a vascular injury. The API is calculated by comparing the systolic pressure in the injured extremity with the systolic pressure in the contralateral uninjured extremity. As with the ABI, an API less than 0.9 should raise concern for a vascular insult and consideration of more advanced vascular assessment.

Table 9.6	Arterial Waveforms on Peripheral Pulse Doppler Examination
ARTERIAL WAVEFORM	**DESCRIPTION**
Triphasic	Forward flow (systole); reverse flow (early diastole); forward flow (late diastole)
Biphasic	Forward flow (systole); reverse flow (diastole)
Monophasic	Single phase with muted/absent acceleration or deceleration of flow

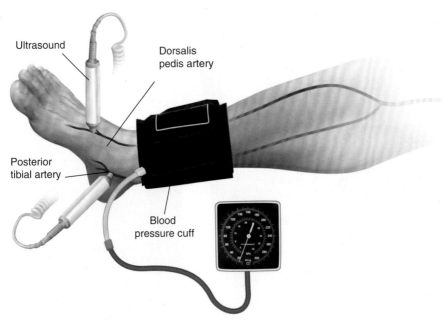

Ultrasound

Dorsalis
pedis artery

Posterior
tibial artery

Blood
pressure cuff

FIGURE 9.9 Determination the ankle brachial index (ABI).

Peripheral Neurologic Injury

A detailed peripheral nerve examination is essential in any assessment of an injured extremity. In children, neurologic deficits are commonly associated with supracondylar humerus fractures (**Figure 9.10**) and to a lesser degree physeal injuries about the knee.[14] Although many nerve injuries in children are neuropraxias that can be managed expectantly, the identification of a neurologic deficit **prior to** reduction or operative management of a fracture is critical to obviate concerns that intraoperative manipulation or implants might be the inciting cause if identified following treatment.

Upper Extremity Neurologic Examination

Motor Examination

Motor function of the anterior interosseous nerve is tested via active flexion at the interphalangeal (IP) joint of the thumb (indicating an innervated flexor pollicis longus) as well as active flexion of the distal interphalangeal (DIP) joint of the index finger (indicating an innervated flexor digitorum profundus) while manually maintaining extension at the proximal interphalangeal (PIP) joint and metacarpophalangeal (MP) joint. Asking younger children to make "an OK" sign allows for assessment of both the FDP and FPL simultaneously (**Figure 9.11**). Integrity of the posterior interosseous nerve is assessed via active extension of the MP joints of the fingers and the IP joint of the thumb, whereas DIP and PIP extension is an ulnar nerve function (**Figure 9.12**). A common pitfall, therefore, is trying to confirm posterior interosseous function by watching the child extend his or her fingers (**Figure 9.13**). The ability to abduct and adduct the fingers indicates innervated interosseous muscles and thus a functioning ulnar nerve. Asking a child to cross their fingers is an easy method to check ulnar nerve function (**Figure 9.14**). Active wrist extension indicates an intact radial nerve and motor function. The median nerve can be isolated by asking a child to touch their thumb to their little finger, thereby testing function of the opponens pollucis (▶ **Video 9.6**).

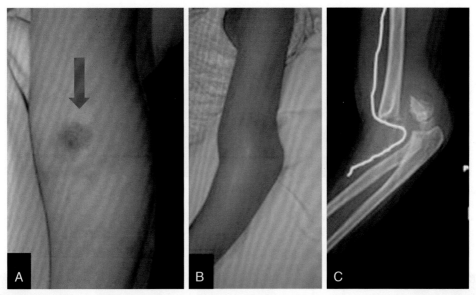

FIGURE 9.10 A 9-year-old girl with severe extension-type supracondylar humerus fracture. A, The child has ecchymosis (red arrow) over the brachialis, and this implies significant trauma and displacement. B and C, The distal humerus is displaced posteriorly, and one could imagine that the median nerve (yellow line) would be at risk for stretch and compromise over the spike of bone.

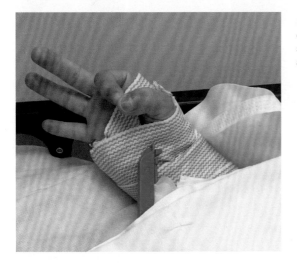

FIGURE 9.11 The anterior interosseous nerve is the commonest nerve affected following extension-type supracondylar humerus fracture. It can be tested by asking the child to make an OK sign.

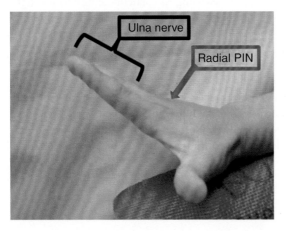

FIGURE 9.12 When a child extends their fingers, the distal interphalangeal (DIP) and proximal interphalangeal (PIP) joints are extended by the interossei, which is predominantly ulnar function; metacarpophalangeal (MP) extension is controlled by the radial and posterior interosseous nerves (PIN).

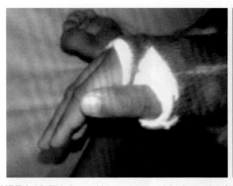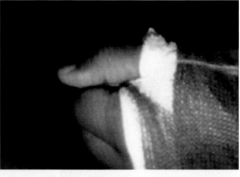

FIGURE 9.13 This boy with a supracondylar humerus fracture was "able to wiggle his fingers," and the second-year resident assumed the nerves were working. Careful examination demonstrated the ability to extend his distal interphalangeal (DIP) and proximal interphalangeal (PIP) joints but no active extension of his thumb interphalangeal (IP) joint or his finger metacarpophalangeal (MP) joints: he had a posterior interosseous nerve palsy.

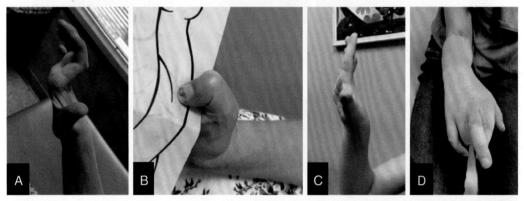

FIGURE 9.14 This young girl has an ulnar nerve injury after her flexion style supracondylar humerus fracture. A, She has developed a claw hand posture as she uses her extensor digitorum communis tendons (radial nerve) to hyperextend her metacarpophalangeal (MP) joints as her distal interphalangeal (DIP) and proximal interphalangeal (PIP) joints cannot extend. B, To generate a weak pinch, she has to flex her thumb interphalangeal (IP) joint and use the flexor pollicis longus (FPL) muscle (median nerve) as her adductor pollicis muscle is not able to generate a powerful key pinch. After 5 months, she has return of ulnar nerve function (C) with the ability to cross her fingers (D).

Sensory Examination

In older children, sensation is most easily documented by assessing the patient's ability to feel light touch along the autonomous neurologic zones of the main sensory nerves of the upper extremity (**Figure 9.15**). These include the volar tip of the index finger for the median nerve, the volar tip of the little finger for the ulnar nerve, and the first dorsal webspace for the radial nerve. For younger or obtunded children, the sweat patterns along the tips of the index and small fingers can be compared with the uninjured extremity. Frank dryness or diminished moisture in these areas commonly accompanies injuries to the median and ulnar nerves, respectively (**Figure 9.16**). Another indirect method of assessing the sensory component of a suspected nerve injury in the young or uncooperative patient is to submerge the hand in water for several minutes. Normal skin wrinkling following submersion relies on normal innervation and thus does not occur in the distribution of an injured nerve (**Figure 9.17**).

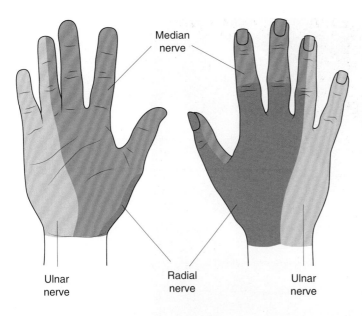

FIGURE 9.15 Autonomous neurologic zones of the main sensory nerves of the upper extremity.

Lower Extremity Examination

Motor Examination

Motor function of the deep peroneal nerve is assessed by eliciting active ankle dorsiflexion indicating a functioning anterior tibialis tendon. The remainder of the anterior compartment muscles is innervated by the deep peroneal nerve as well. Thus, lack of extension of the great toe and lesser digits may indicate a peroneal nerve deficit. Tibial nerve function is assessed via active plantar flexion of the digits and ankle. The superficial peroneal nerve innervates the peroneal muscles in the lateral compartment of the leg and may be assessed by isolating active ankle eversion, although this can sometimes be challenging in the traumatized patient (▶ **Video 9.7**).

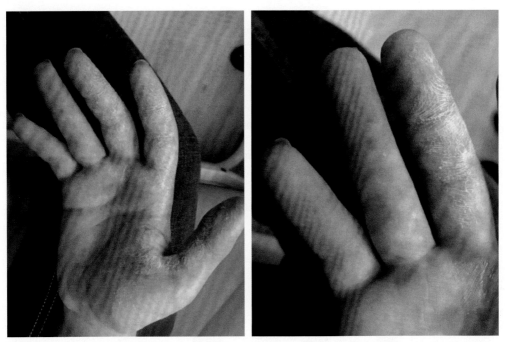

FIGURE 9.16 This boy with a median nerve palsy has altered sweat pattern with dry skin in the thumb index and long and radial side of the ring finger.

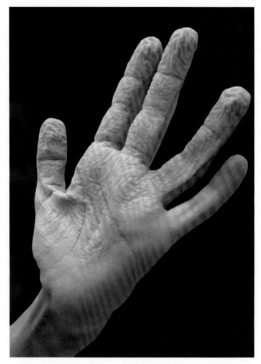

FIGURE 9.17 Because of the presence of an ulnar neuropraxia, no skin wrinkling is present in the ulnar sensory distribution of this child's left hand following submersion in water.

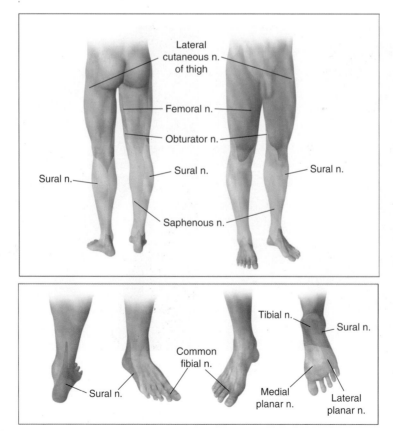

FIGURE 9.18 Autonomous neurologic zones of the main sensory nerves of the lower extremity.

Sensory Examination

As with the upper extremity, testing the patient's ability to detect light touch is an easy method of performing a basic sensory examination following trauma (**Figure 9.18**). Sensation should be assessed along the plantar aspect of the foot (tibial nerve), dorsolateral foot (superficial peroneal nerve), and at the dorsal webspace between the great and second toes (deep peroneal nerve).

Spinal Cord Injury

The vast majority of spinal cord injuries are traumatic in etiology, with motor vehicle collisions, falls, and penetrating trauma accounting for upward of 80% of all new cases of spinal cord injury in the United States. The consequences of spinal cord injury are severe and include loss of independence, depression, multiple hospitalizations, and premature death. A careful initial examination is essential to documenting neurologic progression or decline during the course of treatment.

Repeat examinations are critical to assess progress. In addition, it is important to recall that a complete understanding of the extent of the deficit cannot often be made until the resolution of spinal shock (temporary loss of reflexes below the injured level), which can range from 24 to 72 hours from the time of injury. The resolution of spinal shock is best determined by return of the bulbocavernosus reflex, which is the presence of involuntary contraction of the anal sphincter during manual compression of the glans penis or clitoris.

For standardization and completeness, neurologic evaluation in the setting of a spinal cord injury should follow the guidelines established by the International Standards for the Neurological Classification of Spinal Cord Injury (ISNCSCI).[15,16]

Motor Examination

Five upper extremity and five lower extremity myotomes are graded for strength ranging from complete paralysis to normal motor function (**Tables 9.7** and **9.8**). A complete motor examination must also include the presence or absence of voluntary anal sphincter contraction. The presence of voluntary anal contraction indicates intact motor function of the S2-4 levels.

Table 9.7	International Standards for the Neurological Classification of Spinal Cord Injury Motor Examination Components: Muscle Functions and Corresponding Myotomes	
	MYOTOME	**NERVE ROOT**
Upper Extremity		
	Elbow flexors	C5
	Wrist extensors	C6
	Elbow extensors	C7
	Finger flexors	C8
	Finger abductors	T1
Lower Extremity		
	Hip flexors	L2
	Knee extensors	L3
	Ankle dorsiflexors	L4
	Long toe extensors	L5
	Ankle plantar flexors	S1

Table 9.8	Motor Function Grading
GRADE	**DEFINITION**
0	Complete paralysis
1	Palpable or visible muscle contraction
2	Active movement with gravity eliminated
3	Active movement against gravity
4	Active movement against moderate resistance
5	Normal active movement a gainst full resistance in an unimpaired patient
5*	*Movement against sufficient resistance to be considered normal if impairing factors were not present
NT	Not testable due to immobilization, pain, contracture, or amputation

Sensory Examination

Sensory examination consists of testing sensation to light touch and pin prick along 28 dermatomes including the S4-5 dermatome via assessment of perianal sensation (**Figure 9.19**). For both pin prick and light touch, sensation is graded as absent (0), impaired (1), or normal (2).

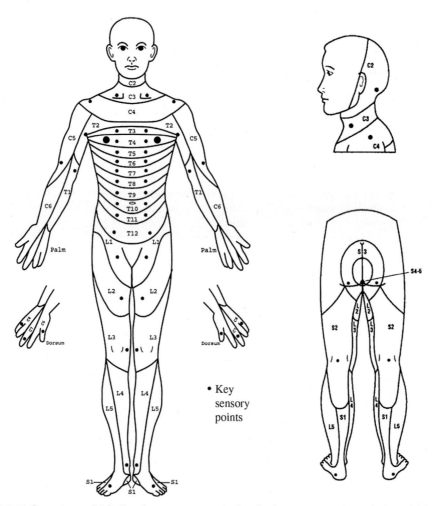

FIGURE 9.19 Dermatome distribution for sensory examination in the presence of a spinal cord injury. (From Kirshblum SC, Burns SP, Biering-Sorensen F, et al. International standards for neurological classification of spinal cord injury (revised 2011). *J Spinal Cord Med.* 2011;34(6):535-546.)

Table 9.9	The American Spinal Cord Injury Association Impairment Scale	
ASIA GRADE	**DESCRIPTOR**	**DEFINITION**
A	Complete	No motor or sensory function in sacral segments S4-5
B	Sensory incomplete	Sensory function present below the level of injury (LI) and No motor function present >3 levels below the motor LI bilaterally
C	Motor incomplete	Voluntary anal contraction present or Sensory function present below the LI with some motor function > 3 levels below the motor LI and Less than half the muscle functions below the LI have a grade ≥ 3
D	Motor incomplete	Sensory function present below the LI with some motor function > 3 levels below the motor LI and Half or more of the muscle functions below the LI have a grade ≥ 3
E	Normal	Normal motor and sensory function in all segments in a patient with a prior deficit

Classification

Spinal cord injuries are characterized as complete or incomplete. In a complete injury, no sensory or motor function exists below the level of injury. When an incomplete injury is present, some sensory or motor function is retained below the level of injury even if this only consists of preservation of some sensory or motor function at the S4-5 level. The American Spinal Cord Injury Association Impairment Scale (ASIA) is derived from the results of the motor and sensory examinations (**Table 9.9**).

● *Regional Assessment of the Traumatized Child*

General Principles

In the setting of high-velocity injury, the general assessment, as mentioned previously, should be completed before focusing on a specific area or an obvious fracture. Displaced fractures with associated pain, deformity, swelling, ecchymosis, or crepitus are difficult to miss, but they should not distract the examiner from evaluation for other associated injuries. In a clinic setting, physical assessment of an injured extremity should be performed after proper exposure of both limbs up to the joint above the injury, and not simply by pulling the sleeves or pants up on one side. The contralateral side should be checked first, so that an anxious child would understand what to expect during physical assessment of the involved side and comparison between both sides could be made. Asking the patient to localize the point of maximum pain using a finger frequently helps with the diagnosis. Neurovascular assessment is critical and their findings should be documented. In children, ligaments are stronger than bone and hence ligamentous injuries are less common. In addition, the physis represents an area of structural weakness with most physeal injuries demonstrating predictable fracture patterns that are quite different from adult fracture counterparts (**Figure 9.20**).

Because casts and splints are frequently used as definitive treatment in children, it is important to be aware of cast-related complications and their varied presentation (**Figure 9.21**). After treatment of any fracture, muscle wasting, stiffness of the joint, and deconditioning are expected. Family should be counseled at the time of injury that reluctance to use the involved arm or persistent limp is common for few weeks to few months after fracture healing. Most young children (younger than 8-10 years) do not require formal physical therapy. Issues specific to high-risk fractures, including growth

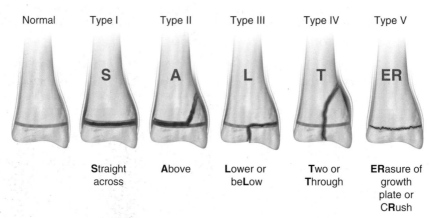

FIGURE 9.20 The Salter-Harris classification of physeal fractures.

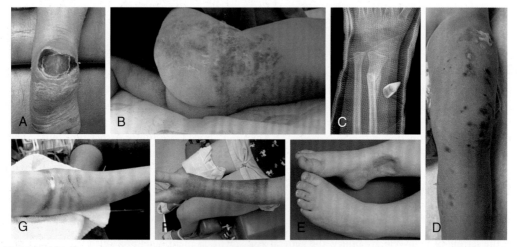

FIGURE 9.21 Cast-related complications include (A) pressure sore, (B) dermatitis from soiling of cast, (C) foreign body in the cast, (D) fungal infection from prolonged wet cast, (E) full-thickness skin loss requiring skin grafting, (F) allergic reaction or sensitivity to cast material, and (G) cellulitis.

disturbances, deformity, and limb length discrepancy, should be explained to the family beforehand. These patients should be followed after fracture healing till adequate growth of the extremity is confirmed or till skeletal maturity.

Clavicle and Scapula

In newborns, clavicle fractures or neonatal brachial plexus palsy may be difficult to differentiate as both may present as a flail arm. Risk factors for these injuries include large birth weight (>4.5 kg) and shoulder dystocia.[17] Asymmetric Moro reflexes and radiographs can help to diagnose each injury, but both may coexist (▶ **Video 9.8**). Once a clavicle fracture is healed (approximately 3 weeks), then definite diagnosis of brachial plexus palsy can be made.

In older children, swelling, tenderness, bruising, or a palpable bony prominence are often present in the setting of a clavicle fracture. When severely displaced, a fracture spike can protrude through the soft tissues and result in skin tenting, skin erosion, or ultimate conversion of a closed injury to an open

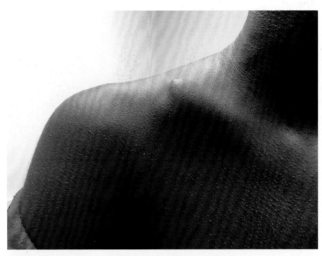

FIGURE 9.22 Displaced clavicle fracture leading to skin tenting. Persistent tenting can cause skin necrosis and conversion to an open fracture.

fracture (**Figure 9.22**). In rare instances, with inferior or posterior displacement, limb-threatening injuries to subclavian vessels, brachial plexus, and mediastinal structures (with medial-sided injuries) can occur (**Figure 9.23**). Bilateral vascular examinations assessing for pulse asymmetry are therefore imperative.

Although most clavicle fractures heal well in children, bony bumps from displacement and callus formation can be unsightly and bothersome. As 80% of clavicle growth is complete by the age of 9 years in girls and 12 years in boys, the limited remodeling potential after this age and the possibility of a permanent bump should be discussed with the family during the initial encounter.[18] Symptomatic nonunion or malunion is uncommon in children, but the rate increases with age and can lead to pain, deformity, restricted motion, discomfort with athletic activities, difficulty carrying backpack, and brachial plexus irritation.[19] The possibility of supraclavicular nerve injury and resultant paresthesia or numbness over the anterior chest wall should be discussed (**Figure 9.24**). This may be a concern, especially for girls, when they wear shoulder straps.

In high-velocity injuries around the shoulder, the sternoclavicular joint should be carefully examined. Such injuries are missed 25% of time (▶ **Video 9.9**). Most medial-sided injuries represent physeal fractures rather than true dislocations. Subtle swelling and tenderness around the sternoclavicular joint should raise suspicion of an injury, which can be confirmed with a computed tomography. Prominence over the sternoclavicular joint is often found in anteriorly displaced sternoclavicular injury. Because of the possibility of a posteriorly displaced sternoclavicular injury compressing the subclavian vasculature, trachea, and esophagus, a vascular examination is critical, as well as an assessment for stridor (**Figure 9.25**).

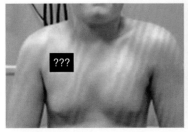
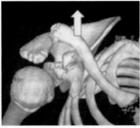
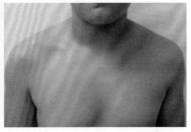

FIGURE 9.23 This 13-year-old boy has a shoulder injury. His father wanted to know where his collarbone went. CT scan demonstrates posterior displacement (yellow arrow), and after surgical repair, his collarbone "reappeared".

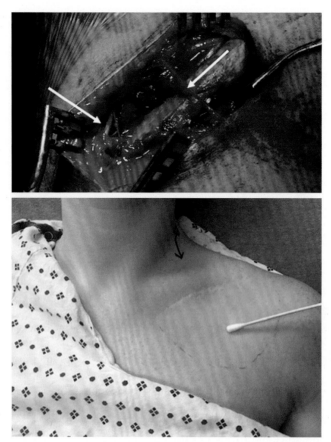

FIGURE 9.24 The major branches of supraclavicular nerves (white arrows) should be identified and protected during surgery. Inadvertent injury can cause numbness along a variable area below the incision.

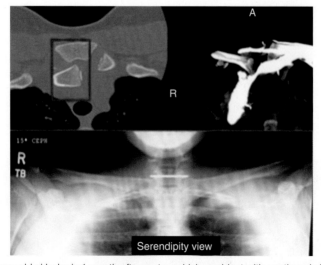

FIGURE 9.25 A 16-year-old girl who is 1 month after motor vehicle accident with continued chest pain and difficulty swallowing. The original trauma CT scan read missed the posteriorly displaced clavicle (red box). CT angiogram demonstrated its precarious location with the great vessels. After open reduction, the serendipity view demonstrates stable reduction.

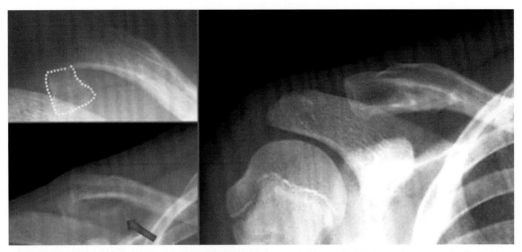

FIGURE 9.26 This 12-year-old boy with a distal clavicle fracture (white outline) is treated nonoperatively, and new bone from periosteum rapidly forms (red arrow). Eventually full remodeling is present.

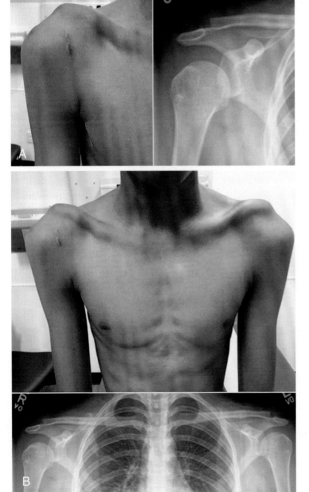

Lateral-sided clavicle injuries also represent physeal fractures rather than true acromioclavicular dislocations. Despite significant deformity, the thick periosteum in children typically remains intact and helps with fracture healing (**Figure 9.26**). The normal prominence of acromioclavicular joint is variable across individuals; hence, it should be compared with the contralateral side (**Figure 9.27**). Because the lateral end of clavicle and acromion are not completely ossified in children, erroneous diagnosis of acromioclavicular joint separation on radiographs is not uncommon. Comparison with the contralateral shoulder radiograph should help establish diagnosis. Tenderness, swelling, bruising, and asymmetric prominence of acromioclavicular joint would indicate joint separation (**Figure 9.28**).

FIGURE 9.27 A, A 16-year-old boy sustained an injury after a direct fall on to his right shoulder. The patient was referred from the emergency department (ED) after clinical assessment and radiographs suggested acromioclavicular joint separation. The opposite shoulder was not examined. B, Evaluation of contralateral acromioclavicular joint in the clinic and comparison radiograph suggests that there was no joint separation and that the prominence on clinical assessment and radiographs was physiologic.

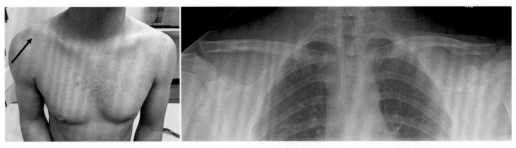

FIGURE 9.28 Clinical and radiographic assessment of right acromioclavicular joint separation in a 15-year-old boy. Compared with the normal left side, the injured side demonstrates swelling, prominence, and bruising (black arrow).

Scapular fractures seldom need treatment, but their diagnosis is important because they are frequently the result of high-velocity trauma and have associated injuries to the head, chest, or spine. Acromion fractures may have to be differentiated from os acromiale by direct palpation and contralateral radiographs. Displaced glenoid fractures or fractures of scapular neck with associated fracture of clavicle or acromioclavicular joint (floating shoulder) are serious injuries and frequently require surgical intervention.

Proximal Humerus and Humerus Shaft

Separation of proximal humerus epiphysis in newborn would have clinical features similar to clavicle fracture at birth with a flail limb and asymmetric Moro reflex (▶ **Video 9.8**). As 80% of humeral growth is from the proximal physis, significant angulation and displacement usually remodels in children up to around 11 years of age. The thick muscle envelope of the shoulder typically masks the presence of any malunion. In those older than 11 years, inadequate fracture reduction may lead to deformity or restricted shoulder, motion which may not improve with time[20] (**Figure 9.29**). Brachial plexus injury is rare but has been reported when the distal metaphyseal fragment is displaced in the axilla.[21] The axillary nerve should therefore be examined by testing the sensation over the deltoid.

Displaced humeral shaft fractures present with gross deformity of the arm. Examination of the radial nerve is critical because of the intimate relationship of the nerve and humeral diaphysis at the junction of middle and lower thirds of the shaft.[22] Nerve injuries are more common in older patients with distal third fractures (▶ **Video 9.10**). In younger children, the nerve is protected by the thick periosteum around the fracture. When a radial nerve injury is identified, observation is recommended as most are neuropraxias with maintained continuity of the nerve. The earliest sign of nerve recovery is active firing of the brachioradialis and extensor carpi radialis muscles.

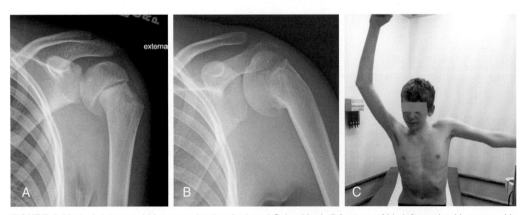

FIGURE 9.29 A, A 14-year-old boy sustained a displaced Salter-Harris II fracture of his left proximal humerus. He was treated conservative. B, At 1-year follow-up, the fracture has healed, but there is humerus varus which is unlikely to remodel. C, The patient did not have pain or deformity but had restricted shoulder abduction.

Fractures Around the Elbow

As the elbow joint is cartilaginous in the very young and several ossification centers appear during childhood, the diagnosis of elbow fractures and the true extent of injury may be challenging to determine. In case of an acutely swollen elbow, the anxious child will keep the arm adducted and supported. Asking the child to point to the area of maximum pain can help localize the site of injury.

Supracondylar Humerus Fractures

Extension-type supracondylar fractures are the most common, leading to typical deformity at the elbow (**Figure 9.30**). The deformity may be inappropriately referred to as an elbow dislocation by the novice. If the proximal fragment has buttonholed through the brachialis muscle or subcutaneous tissues, significant ecchymosis (brachialis sign) or puckering of the skin may be present (**Figure 9.31**).

Although a complete neurologic evaluation of all nerves may be difficult to perform in an anxious child in an acute setting, all attempts should be made to perform as thorough of an examination as possible. All findings, including inability to perform neurologic evaluation, should be documented. Injuries of the anterior interosseous nerve predominate in extension-type fractures where the distal segment is displaced posteriorly (**Figure 9.10**). The ulnar nerve is the most commonly injured with flexion-type fractures (**Figure 9.32**).

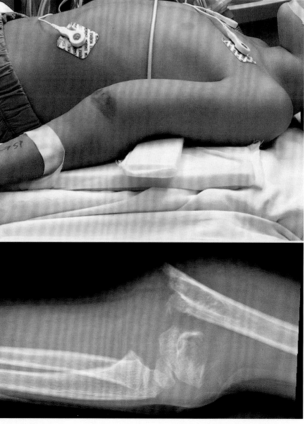

FIGURE 9.30 Clinical and radiographic presentation of the typical deformity of completely displaced supracondylar humerus fracture in a 5-year-old boy. The ecchymosis in the cubital fossa suggests disruption of brachialis muscle. This classic deformity is frequently misdiagnosed as elbow dislocation, which is uncommon in this each group.

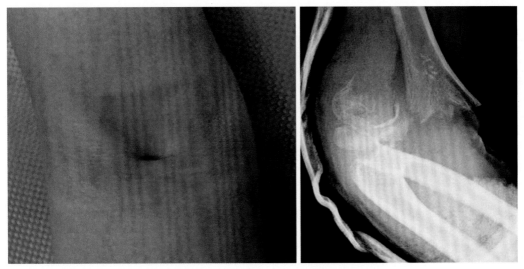

FIGURE 9.31 Pucker sign in a 6-year-old boy with displaced supracondylar humerus fracture. The proximal metaphyseal spike buttonholes through the muscle and pierces the subcutaneous tissues to lie just under the skin.

7-year-old… "pinky asleep"

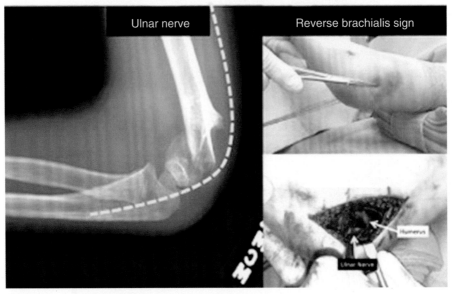

FIGURE 9.32 This 7-year-old female has a flexion-style supracondylar humerus fracture where the distal segment is displaced anteriorly. One can imagine why she has a numb small finger with possible traction on the ulnar nerve. Her skin shows ecchymosis posteriorly over the proximal spike of bone. Open incision confirms the ulnar nerve is draped across the fracture.

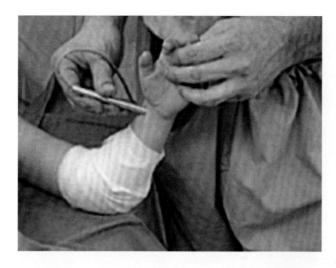

FIGURE 9.33 Doppler examination after elbow fixation.

Vascular assessment should include an examination of both radial pulses and testing of CRT to document hand perfusion. An assessment of swelling and tightness of the forearm compartments is also important. Lack of perfusion after fracture reduction (white hand) is an emergency that mandates brachial artery exploration (**Figure 9.5**). Lack of palpable pulsations but a pink hand with dopplerable pulses after fracture reduction may be observed in the hospital for 24 to 48 hours (**Figure 9.33**). Swelling around the elbow may continue to increase during this time, even after fracture fixation. In the presence of increased swelling or when swelling is expected (difficult reduction or pink pulseless hand), casting and elbow flexion beyond 90° should be avoided. Beware of the presence of high (complete) median nerve injury and resultant sensory loss, which can accompany brachial artery injury and can lead to "silent" compartment syndrome.[11]

The most common deformity following inadequate treatment of a supracondylar humerus fracture is a combination of varus, extension, and internal rotation of the distal fragment: the so-called gunstock deformity (**Figure 9.34**). This results from a failure to recognize medial collapse or comminution in minimally displaced fractures, inadequate reduction, or loss of reduction after fixation. Besides being of cosmetic concerns, this deformity can lead to future fractures (often of the lateral condyle), elbow instability, or morphologic changes to the elbow joint. It does not remodel with time; hence, corrective surgery may be required.

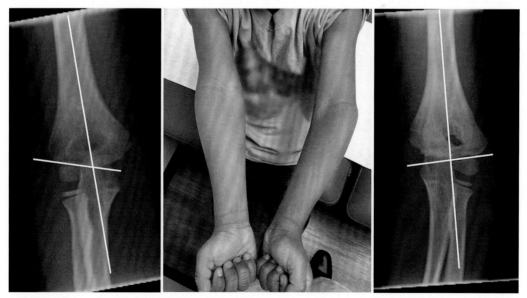

FIGURE 9.34 Malunion of supracondylar humerus fracture on the left side, causing cubitus varus with internal rotation and hyperextension deformity. On radiographs, a decrease in Bauman angle is noted on the left side as compared to the right side.

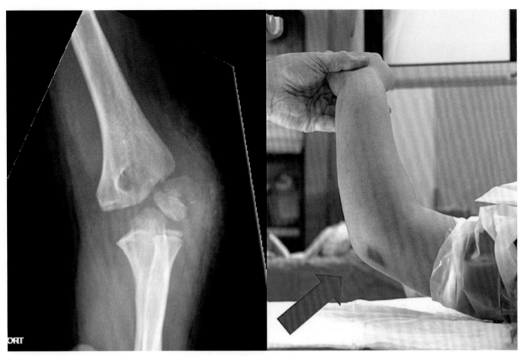

FIGURE 9.35 This 6-year-old boy suffered a completely displaced lateral condyle fracture 3 days prior to fixation. Lateral ecchymosis and swelling (red arrow) are noted.

Lateral Condyle Humerus Fractures

These intra-articular distal humerus fractures present clinically with tenderness, swelling, and often ecchymosis over the lateral aspect of the elbow (**Figure 9.35**). While vascular and neurologic examinations are important, nerve and vascular injuries are much less commonly encountered than with supracondylar humerus fractures.

It can be challenging to distinguish between a lateral condyle fracture with elbow joint displacement versus a transphyseal supracondylar humerus fracture in the very young patient. Physical examination can be helpful. When palpating the elbow, the child with the transphyseal fracture will have normal anatomic relationship between the medial epicondyle and olecranon (**Figure 9.36**). In addition, the fracture line of a transphyseal fracture may traverse the physis and exit on the medial aspect of the elbow (**Figure 9.37**) and can be identified by the presence of swelling or ecchymosis on the medial side of the elbow.

The healing of both nondisplaced and displaced lateral condyle fractures, irrespective of treatment, is frequently accompanied by lateral bony spur formation along the metaphyseal extent of the fracture, which can often be palpated on examination and give the illusion of a varus deformity of the elbow (pseudovarus) (**Figure 9.38**). Radiographically, the ossification leading to lateral spur formation can be confused with lateral displacement of the fracture (**Figure 9.39**).

Even after internal fixation, lateral condyle fractures take longer to heal than supracondylar fractures. Delayed union and nonunion are not uncommon. Nonunion can lead to a progressive cubitus valgus deformity with a resultant tardy ulnar nerve palsy and elbow instability (**Figure 9.40**). Cubitus valgus can also result from premature physeal closure, especially when the fracture line traverses the capitellum.

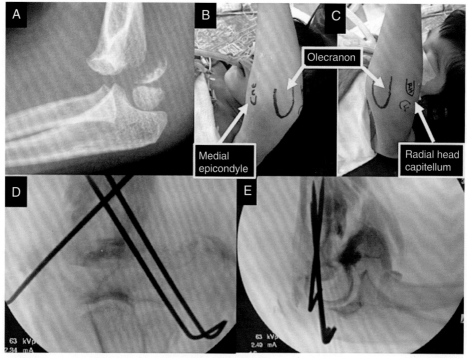

FIGURE 9.36 A, This 4-year-old with a possible lateral condyle fracture is examined in the operating room. B and C, The medial epicondyle and olecranon are in normal anatomic proximity. If this was a fracture dislocation of the elbow, this would not be the case. D and E, The child underwent arthrogram and closed reduction and pinning of a transphyseal supracondylar humerus fracture.

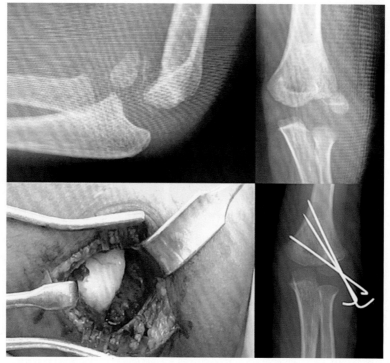

FIGURE 9.37 Although radiographs suggest a lateral condyle fracture. After opening the elbow joint, it became apparent that this is actually a flexion-style transphyseal supracondylar humerus fracture.

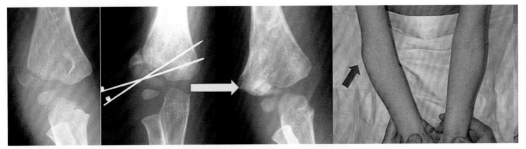

FIGURE 9.38 This 5-year-old boy has a history of a lateral condyle fracture that underwent pin fixation with good healing. His mom is convinced his arm did not heal correctly. The apparent varus positioning (red arrow) is most likely due to the prominent healing bone (yellow arrow).

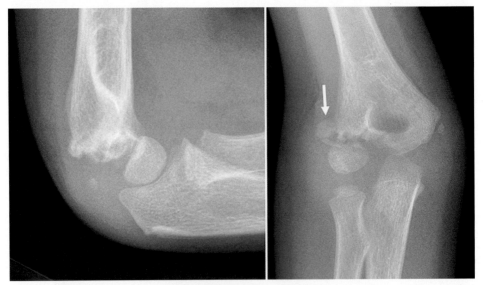

FIGURE 9.39 During healing of lateral condyle fracture of distal humerus, it may be difficult to distinguish the lateral displacement of fracture fragment from a developing lateral spur (arrow). This 5-year-old boy actually developed a malunion of lateral condyle fracture with lateral displacement of fracture and a 2 mm intra-articular gap, although he remains asymptomatic 3 years after injury.

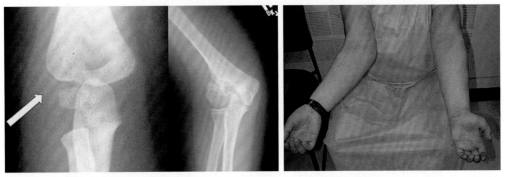

FIGURE 9.40 This 3-year-old had a lateral condyle fracture that was undiagnosed and untreated (arrow). After 8 years, she comes to clinic with pain and a deformed arm as a result of a long standing nonunion.

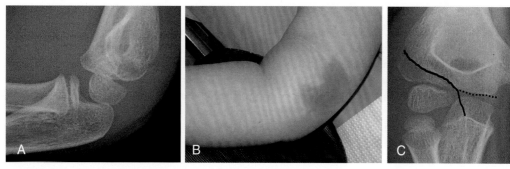

FIGURE 9.41 Minimally displaced lateral condyle fracture (A) with medial-sided ecchymosis (B). C, Although most lateral condyle fractures follow the typical intra-articular pattern (black line), some fractures do extend medially (dashed line). Because these fracture lines are not visualized across the unossified cartilage, medial-sided swelling or ecchymosis aids in diagnosis.

Rarely, the fracture line of a typical appearing lateral condyle fracture may traverse the physis and exit on the medial aspect of the elbow. These represent SH2 fractures of the distal humerus and can be identified by the presence of swelling or ecchymosis on the medial side of the elbow (**Figure 9.41**). Although rare, physeal closure on medial side can lead to cubitus varus deformity. Therefore, an assessment for symmetry of carrying angles of the upper extremities is important.

Medial Epicondyle Fractures

Medial epicondyle fractures are avulsion injures that can occur in isolation from a valgus force applied to the elbow or with a posterior elbow dislocation. Isolated medial epicondyle fractures will demonstrate more focal medial-sided swelling and tenderness on examination. Those associated with an elbow dislocation will have more generalized elbow swelling and tenderness. When identified acutely in the setting of a dislocated elbow, the examiner must be cognizant of the possibility of entrapment of the epicondyle within the elbow joint following closed reduction. After reduction, the elbow should be ranged to document for stability and identify crepitus. It is important that postreduction radiographs be scrutinized to ensure concentric reduction and identify an entrapped medial epicondylar fragment (**Figure 9.42**).

Medial epicondyle fractures have a propensity for nonunion and in some cases can lead to symptomatic joint instability (▶ **Video 9.11**).

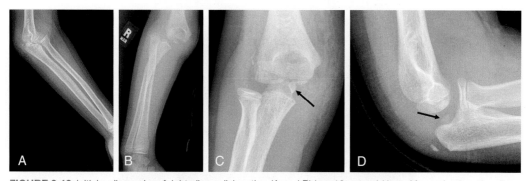

FIGURE 9.42 Initial radiographs of right elbow dislocation (A and B) in a 13-year-old boy. After reduction, the elbow radiographs (C and D) demonstrate entrapped medial epicondyle fracture fragment (arrows). Clinical assessment and radiographs are critical to make the diagnosis of incarcerated medial epicondyle fracture fragment because missed diagnosis can lead to significant degeneration of the joint.

Radial Neck Fracture

Although most radial neck fractures are minimally displaced, presenting only with tenderness laterally just dorsal to the mobile wad, displacement is not uncommon. When left untreated, displacement can result in a limitation of forearm rotation and loss of congruity of the radiocapitellar joint. After reduction of displaced or angulated radial neck fracture, forearm rotation should be assessed to identify any block to supination or pronation. The most common pattern of displacement involves lateral translation or angulation of the radial head. Although difficult to identify by clinical examination, any ulnar displacement of the radial shaft should be identified radiographically as it may increase the risk of proximal radioulnar synostosis or cause difficulty in obtaining adequate reduction of the radial head (**Figure 9.43**).

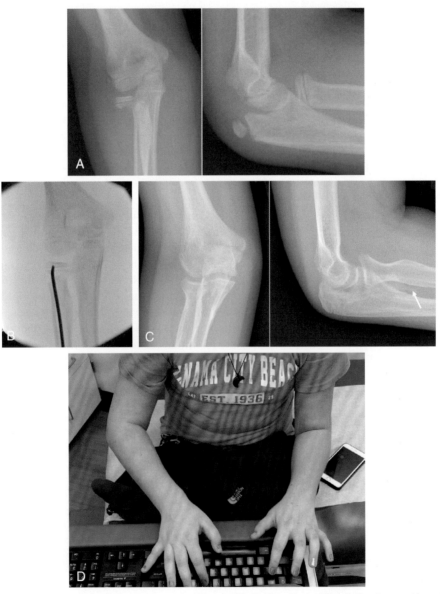

FIGURE 9.43 A, Right-sided radial neck fracture in a 9-year-old girl where the radiocapitellar alignment is maintained but the radial shaft is displaced ulnarward. An associated olecranon fracture is visualized. B, The radial neck fracture was treated with closed reduction using flexible nail. C, The fracture healed with mild residual deformity. Heterotrophic ossification is seen (arrow). D, Clinically, the patient had restricted pronation, which is typically compensated by shoulder abduction and internal rotation.

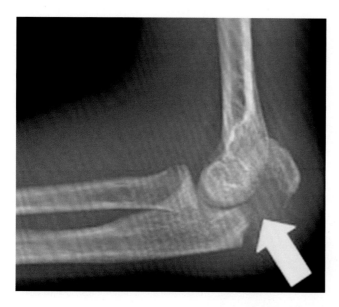

FIGURE 9.44 This boy with an olecranon fracture has palpable defect in the olecranon (yellow arrow) and no active elbow extension after minimal trauma. This fracture can be a sign of osteogenesis imperfecta; genetic testing confirmed this diagnosis in this case.

Patients with proximal radial ulnar synostosis (whether posttraumatic or congenital) will have decreased pronation and supination on physical examination. It is important to test forearm rotation by attempting passive rotation proximal to the wrist joint. One can be fooled that rotation exists if one tries to rotate the forearm by using the hand; in the case, the apparent forearm rotation comes from the wrist joint (▶ **Video 9.12**).

Olecranon Fracture

Nondisplaced or occult olecranon fractures can be differentiated from an elbow contusion in the presence of normal apophyseal irregularity by the presence of point tenderness, swelling, and weakness or excessive pain with elbow extension (▶ **Video 9.13**). Displaced olecranon fractures usually present with swelling and an inability to extend the elbow (**Figure 9.44**). Often, a palpable bony gap can be identified over the proximal ulna. These fractures are rarely isolated, so complete elbow assessment is important.

Nursemaids Elbow

This injury often occurs when the arm or wrist of a preschool child is pulled axially causing partial subluxation of the radial head under the annular ligament. Children with a nursemaids elbow present with pain and refusal to use the involved arm. On examination, the extremity is held in mild elbow flexion with the forearm in pronation. If gentle forearm rotation exerted just proximal to the wrist reveals resistance or a block to supination, the diagnosis is essentially confirmed. This is a truly clinical diagnosis. Although radiographs are not helpful in making the diagnosis of a nursemaids elbow, they are important to exclude other potential elbow fractures. A "click" felt during full elbow flexion and supination indicates reduction of the radial head (▶ **Video 9.14**). Following reduction, the children rapidly regain comfort and start using the extremity.

Forearm Fractures

Examination of the injured forearm focuses on an assessment of deformity, skin integrity, and swelling (**Figure 9.45**). Motor, sensory, and vascular examinations should be documented. Particular attention should be pain to sensory differences or paresthesias in the median nerve distribution as these may be indicative of acute carpal tunnel syndrome in the presence of displaced distal forearm fracture. While compartment syndrome can be associated with isolated forearm fractures, excessive swelling and firmness of the compartments should be noted (**Figure 9.46**). Open injuries are not infrequent, and skin wounds often do not seem to correlate with the location of bony spikes seen radiographically. Inadequate treatment of forearm fracture can lead to malunion and resultant deformity (**Figure 9.47**) or loss of forearm rotation (**Figure 9.48**). Clinical evaluation of elbow and wrist joint is important so as to avoid missing Monteggia or Galeazzi fracture-dislocation patterns, respectively (**Figure 9.49**).

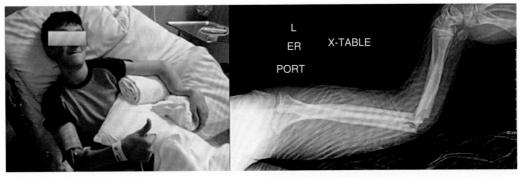

FIGURE 9.45 Forearm fractures are usually easy to diagnosis.

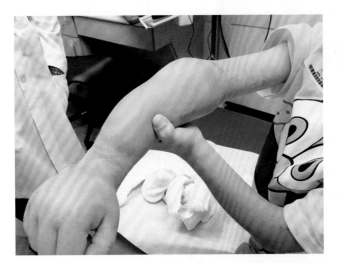

FIGURE 9.46 A 7-year-old boy, 2 days after a complex injury to his right elbow and proximal forearm. He was treated with a splint and an elastic wrap at an outside emergency department (ED) before being seen in clinic. Fortunately, patient did not have compartment syndrome. Swelling may not be present at the time of initial presentation but should be anticipated based on injury patterns.

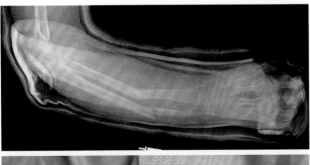

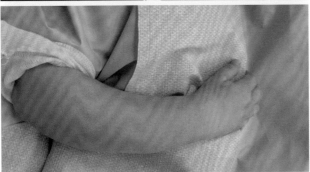

FIGURE 9.47 Loss of reduction and resultant deformity following closed reduction and cast immobilization of both-bone forearm fracture. The splint and overwrapped cast are ill-fitting and of poor quality. The apex ulnar deformity is the typical deformity expected in a maluniting both-bone forearm fracture.

Fractures of the distal radius are the commonest injuries seen in children. Most fractures are buckle or incomplete fractures, with or without physeal involvement. Tenderness is present over the distal radius, but there is no significant deformity or swelling. High-energy injuries to the distal radius, such as after fall from height, would present with significant swelling and deformity and could lead to growth disturbances (**Figure 9.50**).

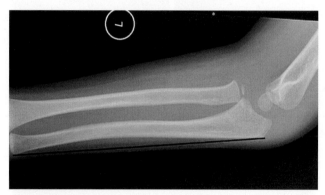

FIGURE 9.48 Malunion of both-bone forearm fracture can lead to restricted forearm rotation. This 15-year-old girl has symmetric 70° of pronation but lacks about 80° of supination on the right side.

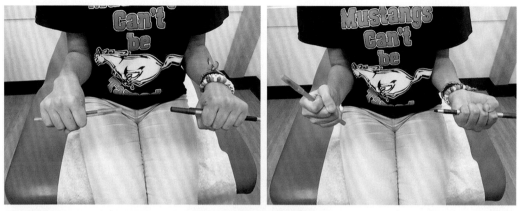

FIGURE 9.49 The Monteggia type I variant with ulnar bowing (black line) and anterior dislocation of radial head was missed in the emergency department (ED) and by the radiologist. Clinical assessment revealed mild deformity of the forearm but, more importantly, pain and swelling of the left elbow.

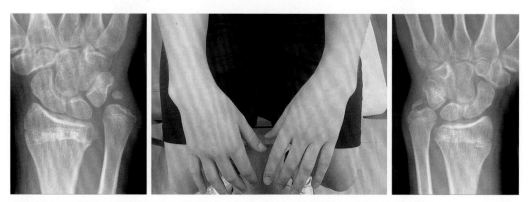

FIGURE 9.50 Bilateral distal radius and ulnar styloid fractures after fall from height at age of 14 years. 4 years after of injury, he presented with bilateral wrist deformities and new onset of ulnar-sided wrist pain. The radial and volar deviation at the wrist joint are typical deformities after distal radius growth arrest with continued growth of ulna, leading to ulnocarpal impaction.

Hip Dislocations and Fractures

Hip dislocations are more common than proximal femoral fractures in young children. These can occur following a simple fall in a younger child with increasing amount of force often necessary to cause a dislocation as age increases. The more common posterior hip dislocation would cause the hip to be shortened, flexed, adducted, and internally rotated (**Figure 9.51**). Anterior hip dislocation would cause the limb to be in an extended, abducted, and externally rotated position (**Figure 9.52**). Inferior or obturator dislocation is extremely rare and could have varied presentation. The sciatic nerve, especially its peroneal division, may be affected by a posterior dislocation, especially in adolescents with high energy trauma. Radiographs should be assessed to diagnose any associated fractures.

Femoral neck and intertrochanteric hip fractures comprise less than 1% of all pediatric fractures. As they result from high-energy trauma in the absence of any underlying bony pathology, a comprehensive trauma examination is essential to avoid missing other injuries. Clinically, the involved extremity is shortened and externally rotated (**Figure 9.53**). Examination of the hip must be done gently and frog leg positioning during radiographic evaluation should be avoided to prevent further vascular disruption to the femoral head.

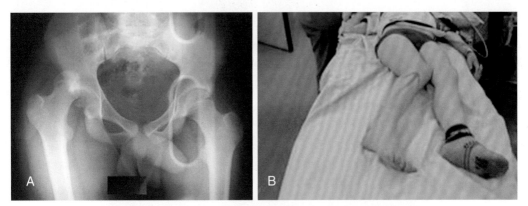

FIGURE 9.51 A, Posterior hip dislocation. B, This injury results in a shortened, flexed, and adducted extremity.

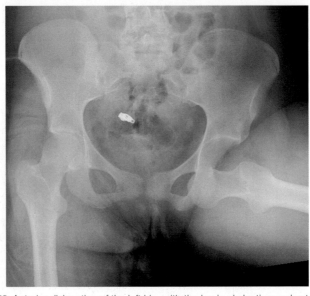

FIGURE 9.52 Anterior dislocation of the left hip, with the leg in abduction and external rotation.

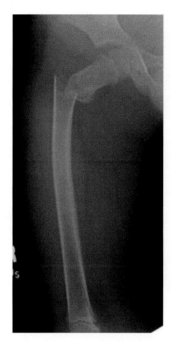

FIGURE 9.53 This displaced femoral neck fracture will result in the leg appearing shorter and externally rotated.

Femoral Shaft Fractures

Femoral shaft fractures are common in children and adolescents, and unlike adults, these fractures in children seldom lead to hypovolemic shock. Nonetheless, vital signs and distal neurovascular status should still be monitored. Although open fractures are extremely rare, the integrity of the skin, particularly for higher energy injures, should be assessed (**Figure 9.54**). The examiner will note gross deformity in the presence of a displaced injury along with swelling of the thigh (**Figure 9.55**). While reactive knee effusions can be encountered after a femoral shaft fracture, the presence of a swollen knee demands an intraoperative physical examination to assess for intra-articular pathology. This is ideally performed at the time of fracture management under anesthesia. For those patients undergoing operative intervention, preoperative examination of the hip rotational profile of the uninvolved extremity may assist in determining proper rotational alignment of the fracture prior to fixation.

Femoral shaft fractures are frequent sources of litigation because of limb length discrepancy, deformity, or persistently abnormal gait (**Figure 9.56**). The family should be counseled early on about potential complications and that it may take several weeks to months to regain normal gait and function once the fracture is healed. Follow-up assessment should include documentation of rotational profiles of both hips to detect rotational malalignment as well as an assessment for femoral segment length differences via Galeazzi testing (**Figure 9.57**).

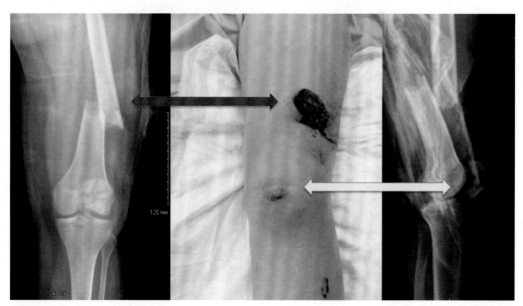

FIGURE 9.54 This 16-year-old girl fell from a cliff. Her thigh is swollen, and an open wound corresponds with the location of the femur fracture (red arrow). Ecchymosis and swelling over the knee are signs pointing to a comminuted patella fracture (yellow arrow).

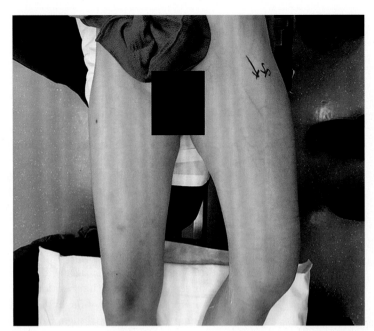

FIGURE 9.55 Typical presentation of displaced femoral shaft fracture with thigh swelling and external rotation and shortening of the leg.

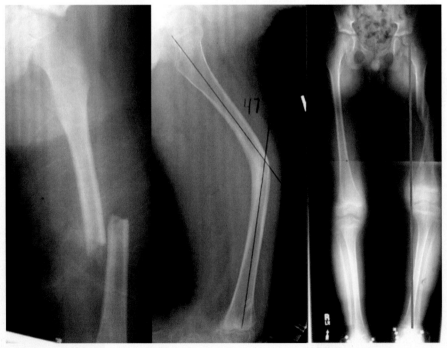

FIGURE 9.56 This 9-year-old boy with a femur fracture was treated with a cast and developed a significant malunion with a 2.5-cm discrepancy in length.

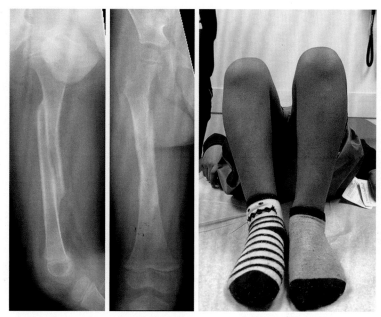

FIGURE 9.57 A 5-year-old boy with femoral shaft fracture that healed with about 2 cm of shortening as noted on the radiographs. Galeazzi test can be used for approximate measurements of length differences of the femoral and tibial segment by comparing with the contralateral side.

Fractures About the Knee

Physeal injuries around the knee (distal femur and proximal tibia) are more common than injuries to collateral ligaments in children. The initial radiograph may look innocuous if the fracture had spontaneously reduced after initial displacement. Swelling, pain, inability to bear weight, inability to move the knee, and ecchymosis should point toward a more serious injury that would warrant careful vascular and neurologic assessment (**Figure 9.58**). The popliteal artery is tethered on the posterior aspect of proximal tibia as it bifurcates and as

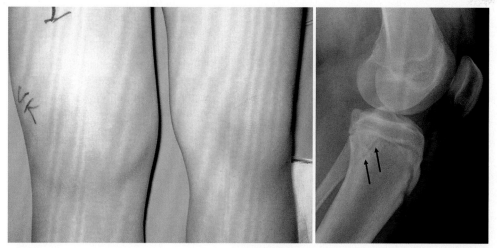

FIGURE 9.58 A 12-year-old boy who presented with injury to his right knee. At presentation, he had significant swelling and was unable to bear weight or move his knee. Radiographs show the metaphyseal extension of the fracture line (arrows). Such fractures around the knee could have been displaced and spontaneously reduced following the injury. Suspicion for neurovascular injuries and compartment syndrome should be high for such knee injuries even though the radiographs are not too impressive.

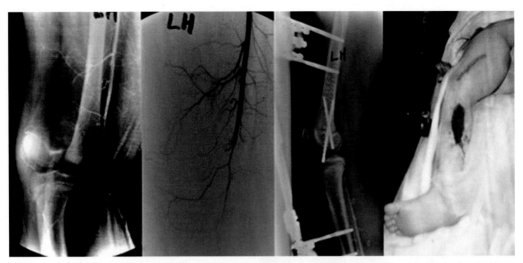

FIGURE 9.59 This 12-year-old girl was in a motor vehicle crash with a distal femoral physeal injury and with no pulses. Angiogram demonstrates complete occlusion. The child underwent fracture fixation, vascular repair, and then prophylactic fasciotomy to prevent reperfusion compartment syndrome.

the anterior tibial artery traverses to the anterior compartment (**Figure 9.8**). Any disruption around the knee (knee dislocation, tibial tuberosity fracture, displaced fracture of distal femur, or proximal tibia) could stretch or disrupt these vessels (**Figure 9.59**). The classic signs of vascular compromise including cold, pale, and pulseless leg may be absent. ABI should be performed when in doubt (▶ **Video 9.4**).

Patellar sleeve fractures are a unique subset of knee fractures seen in children (**Figure 9.60**). The disrupted sleeve from the inferior (and less commonly, superior) pole of patella comprises little bone, articular surface cartilage, and periosteum from the dorsum of patella. These fractures may be missed on radiographs as major components of the fractured patella are soft tissues. Clinically, there may be a palpable gap in the extensor mechanism, inability to do straight leg raise (or an extensor lag), and/or a high riding patella (▶ **Video 9.15**).

Traumatic knee hemarthrosis could be from intra-articular fracture, ligament injury, meniscus injury, or patellar dislocation (**Figure 9.61**). Physical assessment of an acutely swollen knee may be limited, and MRI may be justified, once radiographs rule out a fracture. These intra-articular injuries are commonly sports-related injuries. Stiffness of knee is common following intra-articular injuries and early diagnosis is important to prevent arthrofibrosis (**Figure 9.62**).

Any laceration or wound around the knee may be associated with an underlying traumatic knee arthrotomy. When in doubt, a traumatic knee arthrotomy can be confirmed with a saline load test (▶ **Video 9.16**).

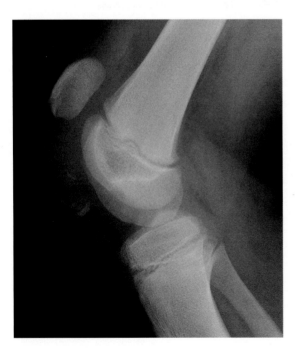

FIGURE 9.60 Patellar sleeve fractures are unique to children and could be missed if clinical assessment and careful evaluation of radiographs are not performed. An extensor lag or inability to perform straight leg raise is a hallmark of extensor mechanism disruption. The radiographs show the inferior avulsed fragment to which the patellar tendon is attached.

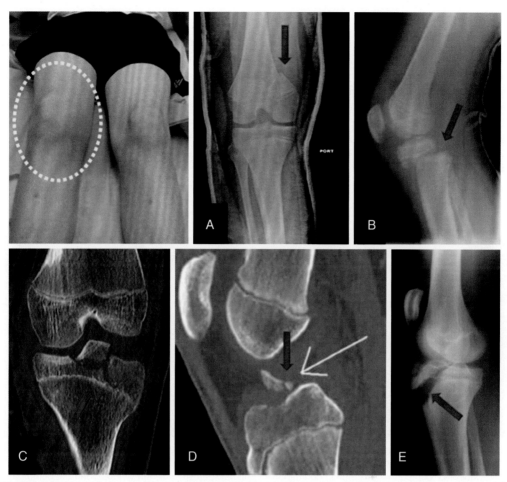

FIGURE 9.61 This child has significant joint effusion (yellow circle). A variety of different knee injuries could result in this appearance. A, Distal femoral physeal fracture (Red Arrow). B, Proximal tibial physeal fracture (Red Arrow). These are more prone to popliteal injury. C, Tibial plateau fractures are usually a result of significant trauma (Red Arrow). D, Tibial spine fractures are the pediatric equivalent of an anterior cruciate ligament (ACL) tear (Red/White Arrow). E, Tibial tubercle fractures occur with forced rapid quadriceps contracture often seen in basketball players (Red Arrow). These fractures are known to develop a compartment syndrome.

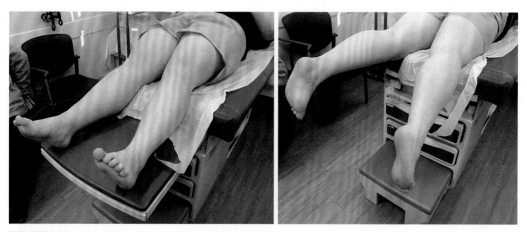

FIGURE 9.62 Knee stiffness, especially lack of full knee extension, is common after intra-articular knee injuries. The fixed flexion contracture, if minimal, could be missed on examination in a supine position but would be readily apparent in a prone position, as seen on the left side in this 15-year-old girl. Even minimal degrees of flexion contracture could lead to long-term morbidity and should be promptly addressed.

Tibial Shaft Fractures

A nondisplaced spiral fracture of the distal third of the tibia (commonly referred to as a "toddler's fracture") should be suspected in a toddler with a limp or refusal to bear weight. Gentle examination by palpation along both legs may reveal focal tenderness over the distal half of tibia. Watching the child's face for a grimace while palpating is often helpful. Radiographs may or may not show a subtle long oblique fracture line. An infectious process should be ruled out when fractures cannot be seen on radiographs. High-energy fractures of tibia and fibula may be associated with open fractures and compartment syndrome (**Figure 9.4**). Careful neurologic and vascular examinations are essential, and vigilance should be maintained for signs and symptoms of compartment syndrome (**Figure 9.63**).

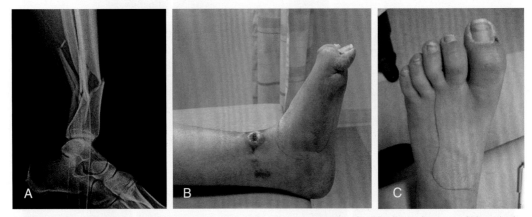

FIGURE 9.63 Missed compartment syndrome in this 16-year-old girl with tibia-fibula fracture. Although the anterior leg compartment is most commonly involved, the sequelae of missed compartment syndrome is usually due to posterior compartment ischemic contractures. She had paresthesias in the foot along the demarcated areas. She required multiple subsequent surgical procedures to address infection, fracture union, and claw toe deformities.

Ankle Fractures

Fractures in younger children following a twisting or inversion injury to the ankle tend to propagate through the physes of the distal tibia or fibula, while older adolescents typically sustain adult-type rotational ankle fractures and sprains. Nondisplaced fractures of the distal fibula physis are common and largely diagnosed by physical examination. Swelling may be present, and focal tenderness in the region of the distal fibular physis is nearly always identified. Surgical intervention is frequently warranted for displaced triplane, tillaux, and adult-type rotational ankle fractures. Surgery should be performed either before significant swelling develops (within the first 24 hours following the injury) or after the swelling subsides to allow for healing of surgical incisions (**Figure 9.64**). The "wrinkle test" is helpful to determine if swelling has resolved sufficiently to proceed with surgery. This test is performed by inspecting the skin for evidence of wrinkling or noting skin wrinkling as the skin is gentle pinched together or the ankle is gently dorsiflexed (**Figure 9.65**).

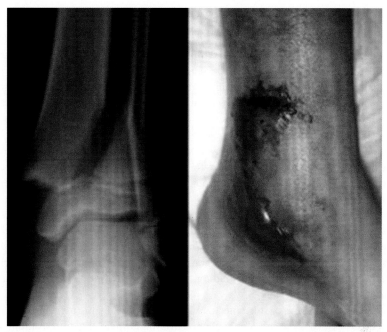

FIGURE 9.64 This 12-year-old girl was stepped on by a horse. Surgery is best performed after the swelling goes down.

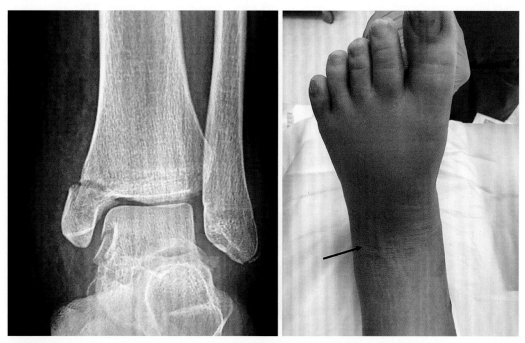

FIGURE 9.65 Ankle injuries are frequently associated with significant swelling. Unless the joint is dislocated, it is better to wait for a few days before definitive treatment is performed. As the swelling subsides, skin wrinkles (arrow) are visible, which indicates a safe time to proceed with planned treatment.

Foot Fractures

When a preschool child presents with a vague history and a limp, foot injuries should be ruled out when evaluation of spine and the more proximal limb are unremarkable. Cuboid compression fractures are often sustained following a jump from a low height (such as a bed or couch) and can be diagnosed by identifying point tenderness over the lateral border of the midfoot. Radiographs may be normal or show proximal cuboid sclerosis (**Figure 9.66**). Another commonly missed injury is a retained foreign body or puncture wound that can be diagnosed by careful inspection of the plantar aspect of the foot (**Figure 9.67**).

Hindfoot injuries in children are frequently missed. These include fracture of the lateral process of the talus (diagnosed by tenderness anterior to lateral malleolus) and osteochondral fractures of the talar dome. The latter are diagnosed radiographically, but examination can identify joint line tenderness and an ankle effusion which can be relatively subtle.

High-energy injuries with axial loading of the midfoot that present with pain, swelling, and/or plantar ecchymosis should raise the suspicion for a tarsometatarsal fracture dislocation (Lisfranc injury). Injury radiographs can be normal as they are rarely taken in weight-bearing position because of patient discomfort. If missed, these fractures can lead to significant long-term morbidity and foot pain. Weight-bearing films, stress radiographs (if tolerated), or a CT/MRI scan can help to diagnose subtle injuries (**Figure 9.68**).

Stress fractures of the second or third metatarsals are diagnosed by history, limp, and point tenderness along the metatarsal shaft, as initial radiographs may be normal. In contrast, multiple metatarsal fractures from high-energy injuries can result in significant swelling and rarely compartment syndrome of the foot (**Figure 9.69**).

Although a stubbed great toe is frequently an innocuous injury, plantar flexion of the hallux can result in a physeal fracture of the distal phalanx with apex-dorsal angulation (**Figure 9.70**). The fracture angulation itself does not cause significant deformity, but the associated injury to the nail bed and matrix creates an open fracture with the associated risks of infection and osteomyelitis. The examiner should

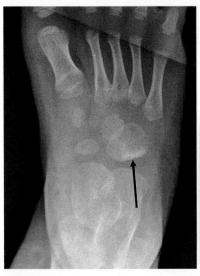
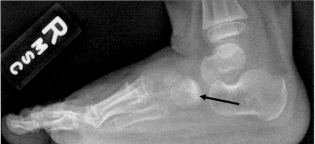

FIGURE 9.66 When a toddler presents with a limp after a trivial fall or jump from a couch, cuboid fracture should be suspected. These fractures are diagnosed by clinical evaluation of tenderness along the lateral border of the foot and proximal sclerosis in the cuboid (arrows) on radiographs.

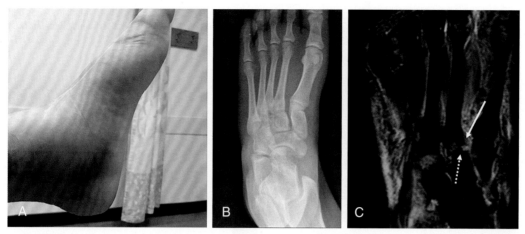

FIGURE 9.68 A, Swelling, ecchymosis, inability to bear weight, and tenderness along the midfoot in this 15-year-old girl following soccer injury should raise suspicion for a Lisfranc injury, even though radiographs may be negative (B). Further imaging with MRI (C) shows tear of the Lisfranc ligament (solid arrow) and incongruity at the second metatar-sal–middle cuneiform joint (dashed arrow).

assess for evidence of a subungual hematoma. In addition, in such injuries, the nail plate can come to lie dorsal to the nail fold giving the appearance of a longer nail on the involved side when compared with the contralateral side. Identification of nail bed disruption is important as these injuries require meticulous fracture debridement, repositioning of the nail matrix and nail plate, possible reduction and pinning of the fracture, and antibiotics (**Figure 9.71**).

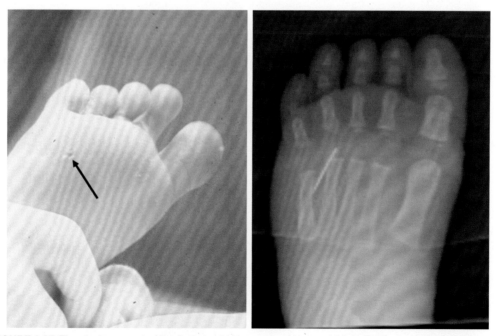

FIGURE 9.67 The plantar aspect of the foot should be examined in any child presenting with a limp of uncertain etiology. A poke hole (arrow) may be the only positive clinical finding and may indicate a foreign body (a needle in this case), which can be diagnosed on appropriate imaging studies.

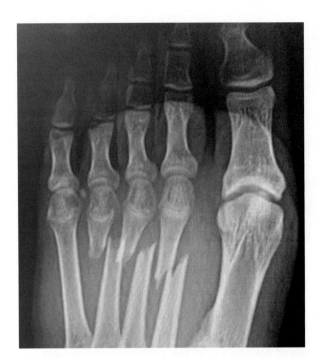

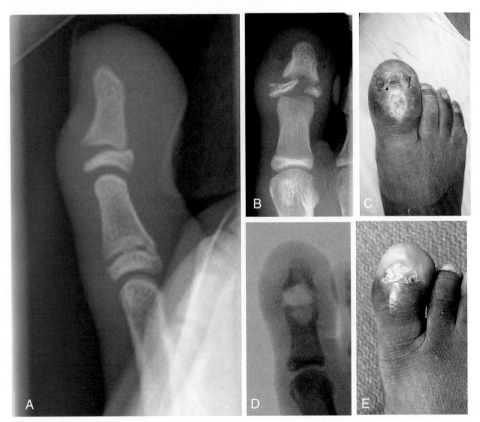

FIGURE 9.70 A, Fracture through the physis of the distal phalanx of great toe should be approached as an open fracture unless proven otherwise. This 15-year-old boy had initial treatment in the emergency department (ED) but did not follow-up for further care till about 6 weeks after injury. B and C, Fulminant infection and osteomyelitis affecting the distal phalanx and interphalangeal joint. D and E, Final outcome after two surgical debridements, removal of sequestered epiphysis, removal of nail plate and wound management.

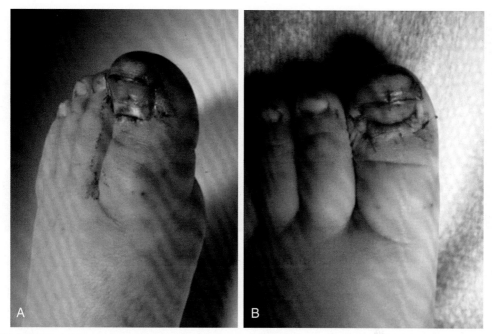

FIGURE 9.71 A, Inappropriate suturing of the nail plate on the eponychium of the great toe, which can be diagnosed by comparing the length of the nail to the contralateral toe nail length. B, The nail plate was repositioned underneath the eponychium to prevent inadvertent adhesions.

Pelvis Fractures

Avulsion fractures of pelvis are frequently seen in teenage athletes with open apophysis. Anterior superior iliac spine, anterior inferior iliac spine, and ischial tuberosity avulsion injuries are all common due to the pull of sartorius, rectus femoris, and hamstring muscles, respectively (**Figure 9.72**). Suspicion should be raised for such injuries in adolescents who report a sudden painful pop during an athletic activity. Physical examination reveals tenderness around the fracture site and increased pain with active firing of the involved muscle. Patients will often have weakness due to pain with active straight leg raise against gravity.

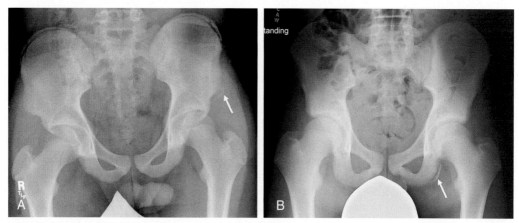

FIGURE 9.72 Pelvic radiograph aid in diagnosis of avulsion fractures that are common in adolescent athletes. A, Avulsion of anterior inferior iliac spine (arrow) through the pull of rectus femoris. B, Avulsion of ischial tuberosity (arrow) through the pull of hamstring tendons.

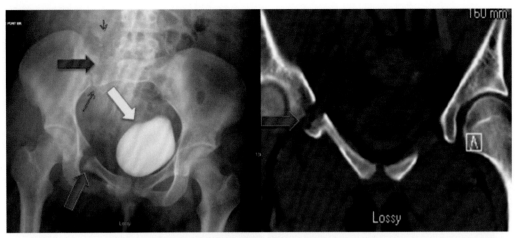

FIGURE 9.73 This 14-year-old was in a severe motor vehicle accident and has an unstable pelvis injury (red arrows). She has deviation of her bladder (yellow arrow), which is indicative of pelvic hematoma.

Because of open triradiate cartilage and increased plasticity of the immature pelvis, most pelvic ring injuries in children are biomechanically stable. Fractures of the pubic rami, iliac wing, or ischium are often single-break injuries of the pelvic ring that do not involve the acetabulum, sacroiliac joint, or pelvic viscera. In contrast, displaced fractures of pelvic ring from high-velocity mechanisms in older children frequently mimic adult patterns and involve two or more breaks within the pelvic ring that create an biomechanical instability (**Figure 9.73**). Pelvic stability tests including the spring test and the pelvic compression test are not used frequently because of patient discomfort, fear of dislodging an organizing hematoma, and the potential to increase pelvic instability. Tenderness, perineal hematoma, ecchymosis, swelling, laceration, degloving injuries (Moral-Lavallee lesion), and open fractures should be recognized. Neurologic, urogenital, and rectal examination should be completed. Asymmetric rotation of the leg or limb shortening could suggest rotationally and vertically unstable hemipelvis. Associated skeletal, visceral, and vascular injuries are common and may be life threatening.

Spine Fracture

Any child complaining of neck or back pain or neurologic symptoms following an injury should be suspected of a spine injury. Similarly, a child who cannot communicate or cooperate should be suspected of a spinal injury. The common mechanism of spine injury are motor vehicle accident (MVA), falls, or sports-related injuries. Spine injury encompasses spine fracture, ligamentous injury, or spinal cord injury. Early immobilization using a spine or any rigid board would prevent further insult to a potentially unstable injury. Because of the relatively large size of the child's head, a head recess in the board or elevation of the trunk using padding support would prevent neck flexion. A pediatric cervical orthosis would help limit neck motion. Movement of the patient should only be performed with in-line traction and a logroll technique (▶ **Video 9.17**).

If the child was involved in an MVA, inspection of the abdominal wall ecchymosis or abrasions, suggestive of a lap belt injury, can help discern the spectrum of injury (**Figure 9.2**). Pain or step-off along the spinous process should raise the suspicion of a flexion-distraction injury. Other pertinent examination findings, including tenderness, swelling, bruising, or subtle deformity of the spine, should be noted.

The cervical spine orthosis should be maintained until cervical spine clearance is obtained. An asymptomatic patient can be cleared on clinical grounds without advanced imaging. For symptomatic or obtunded patients, CT scan evaluation is recommended. If the CT scan is negative, it is controversial if the patient should be cleared or if an MRI should be performed; the decision is based on institutional guidelines.[23]

References

1. Loder RT. Pediatric polytrauma: orthopaedic care and hospital course. *J Orthop Trauma*. 1987;1(1):48-54.
2. Enderson BL, Reath DB, Meadors J, Dallas W, DeBoo JM, Maull KI. The tertiary trauma survey: a prospective study of missed injury. *J Trauma*. 1990;30(6):666-669, discussion 669-670.
3. Furnival RA, Woodward GA, Schunk JE. Delayed diagnosis of injury in pediatric trauma. *Pediatrics*. 1996;98(1):56-62.
4. Laasonen EM, Kivioja A. Delayed diagnosis of extremity injuries in patients with multiple injuries. *J Trauma*. 1991;31(2):257-260.
5. Metak G, Scherer MA, Dannohl C. [Missed injuries of the musculoskeletal system in multiple trauma – A retrospective study]. *Zentralbl Chir*. 1994;119(2):88-94.
6. Pfeifer R, Pape HC. Missed injuries in trauma patients: a literature review. *Patient Saf Surg*. 2008;2:20.
7. Knox JB, Schneider JE, Cage JM, Wimberly RL, Riccio AI. Spine trauma in very young children: a retrospective study of 206 patients presenting to a level 1 pediatric trauma center. *J Pediatr Orthop*. 2014;34(7):698-702.
8. Knox J, Schneider J, Wimberly RL, Riccio AI. Characteristics of spinal injuries secondary to nonaccidental trauma. *J Pediatr Orthop*. 2014;34(4):376-381.
9. Drucker NA, McDuffie L, Groh E, Hackworth J, Bell TM, Markel TA. Physical examination is the best predictor of the need for abdominal surgery in children following motor vehicle collision. *J Emerg Med*. 2018;54(1):1-7.
10. Lack WD, Karunakar MA, Angerame MR, et al. Type III open tibia fractures: immediate antibiotic prophylaxis minimizes infection. *J Orthop Trauma*. 2015;29(1):1-6.
11. Bae DS, Kadiyala RK, Waters PM. Acute compartment syndrome in children: contemporary diagnosis, treatment, and outcome. *J Pediatr Orthop*. 2001;21(5):680-688.
12. Shuler FD, Dietz MJ. Physicians' ability to manually detect isolated elevations in leg intracompartmental pressure. *J Bone Joint Surg Am*. 2010;92(2):361-367.
13. Whitney A, O'Toole RV, Hui E, et al. Do one-time intracompartmental pressure measurements have a high false-positive rate in diagnosing compartment syndrome?. *J Trauma Acute Care Surg*. 2014;76(2):479-483.
14. Muchow RD, Riccio AI, Garg S, Ho CA, Wimberly RL. Neurological and vascular injury associated with supracondylar humerus fractures and ipsilateral forearm fractures in children. *J Pediatr Orthop*. 2015;35(2):121-125.
15. Kirshblum SC, Burns SP, Biering-Sorensen F, et al. International standards for neurological classification of spinal cord injury (revised 2011). *J Spinal Cord Med*. 2011;34(6):535-546.
16. Waring WP III, Biering-Sorensen F, Burns S, et al. 2009 review and revisions of the International Standards for the Neurological Classification of Spinal Cord Injury. *J Spinal Cord Med*. 2010;33(4):346-352.
17. Foad SL, Mehlman CT, Ying J. The epidemiology of neonatal brachial plexus palsy in the United States. *J Bone Joint Surg Am*. 2008;90(6):1258-1264.
18. McGraw MA, Mehlman CT, Lindsell CJ, Kirby CL, et al. Postnatal growth of the clavicle: birth to 18 years of age. *J Pediatr Orthop*. 2009;29(8):937-943.
19. Hill JM, McGuire MH, Crosby LA. Closed treatment of displaced middle-third fractures of the clavicle gives poor results. *J Bone Joint Surg Br*. 1997;79(4):537-539.
20. Neer CS II, Horwitz BS. Fractures of the proximal humeral epiphysial plate. *Clin Orthop Relat Res*. 1965;41:24-31.
21. Hwang RW, Bae DS, Waters PM. Brachial plexus palsy following proximal humerus fracture in patients who are skeletally immature. *J Orthop Trauma*. 2008;22(4):286-290.
22. Holstein A, Lewis GM. Fractures of the humerus with radial-nerve paralysis. *J Bone Joint Surg Am*. 1963;45:1382-1388.
23. Anderson PA, Gugala Z, Lindsey RW, Schoenfeld AJ, Harris MB. Clearing the cervical spine in the blunt trauma patient. *J Am Acad Orthop Surg*. 2010;18(3):149-159.

10

Evaluation of the Concussed Child/Adolescent

Naomi Brown, Eileen P. Storey, William P. Meehan III, Corina Martinez, and Christina L. Master

● Introduction

Concussion is a common injury among active young athletes. According to the parent-reported National Health Interview Survey conducted in 2016, 8.3% of boys and 5.6% of girls aged 3 to 17 years have experienced at least one significant head injury. Among children 15 to 17 years of age, 11.7% experienced at least one head injury.[1] A recent epidemiological study in a large-scale pediatric network reported that most pediatric concussions occur during sports, especially in children older than 5 years.[2] Although 30% of pediatric and adolescent concussions occur outside of sports, an increasing proportion of concussions occur during sports as children get older. Timely recognition and diagnosis of concussion is important, especially because continuing to play is associated with delay in recovery.[3] It is critical for coaches, team physicians, athletic trainers, and other clinicians responsible for the care of athletes to be knowledgeable in the diagnosis, acute management, and ongoing care of the concussed child.

Each year, hundreds of thousands of children and young adults are diagnosed with concussion. According to the Centers for Disease Control and Prevention (CDC), an estimated 2.6 million children aged 19 years or younger were treated annually for sports- and recreation-related injuries. Of those, approximately 6.5% were traumatic brain injuries and 70.5% were among persons aged 10 to 19 years.[4] The incidence of concussion is higher for contact and collision sports, particularly those male athletes playing American football, ice hockey, rugby, and lacrosse. For female athletes, soccer, lacrosse, and field hockey have the highest incidences of concussion.[5-7] The most recent High School Reporting Information Online (RIO) data from the 2016 to 2017 school year found that concussions accounted for 24.8% of all injuries sustained during 1.18 million athletic exposures.[8]

A concussion, by definition, is a traumatic brain injury that affects brain function. However, concussion remains a heterogeneous injury that affects individuals in different ways. There are a wide variety of mechanisms of injury, with the most common involving a direct blow to the head, face, or neck, as often occurs in sport. An injury can also occur from forces that are transmitted to the head, such as a whiplash injury during a motor vehicle accident or a blow delivered to another part of the body.[9]

After an injury, there is a neurometabolic disturbance that can result in a variety of symptoms.[10] Symptoms can be organized into four domains: physical, sleep, thinking/remembering, and mood disruption. Symptoms often worsen when the brain is required to perform more metabolically demanding activities such as physical activity or higher level cognitive processing involved with schoolwork.[11] However, the diagnosis and management of concussion remains challenging because symptoms are nonspecific and overlap with several other possible etiologies, including depression, lack of sleep, primary headaches, autonomic dysfunction, viral illness, dehydration, and many others. In fact, uninjured teenagers also report concussion-like symptoms even when they are healthy (**Figures 10.1** and **10.2**).[12]

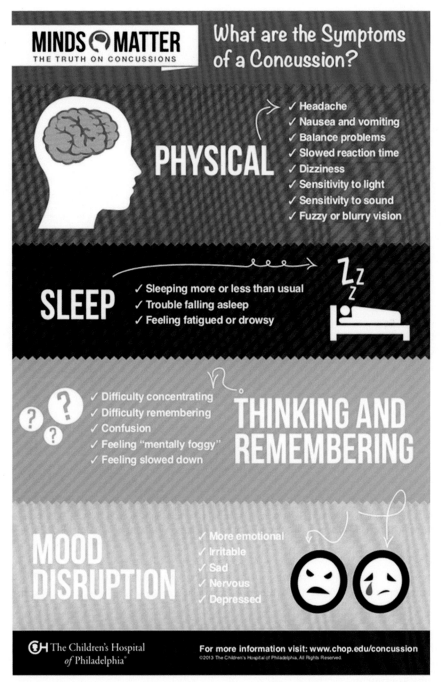

FIGURE 10.1 Symptoms of concussion. (Image courtesy and © The Childrens's Hospital of Philadelphia.)

● *Acute On-Field Evaluation*

Acute on-field evaluation is directed at excluding a more emergent injury, recognizing concussion, and removing injured athletes from play and the possibility of additional injury. In evaluating a child who has been injured on the field, one should first ensure that the child is stable and does not need

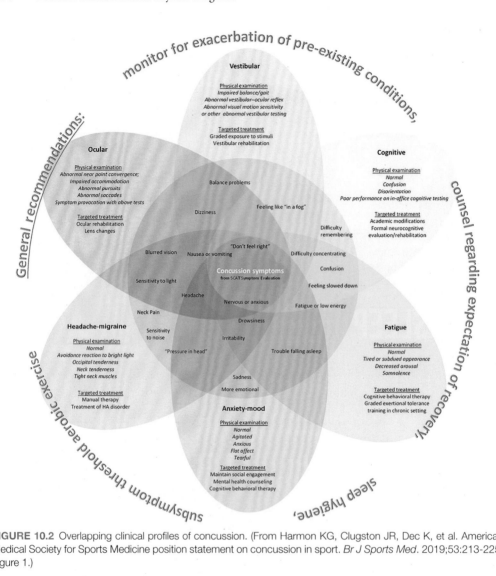

FIGURE 10.2 Overlapping clinical profiles of concussion. (From Harmon KG, Clugston JR, Dec K, et al. American Medical Society for Sports Medicine position statement on concussion in sport. *Br J Sports Med*. 2019;53:213-225: Figure 1.)

emergency resuscitation by performing a primary survey. The primary survey, ABCDE, consists of the following steps to ensure that a provider does not miss a more severe head, cervical spine, or other injury:

1. Airway assessment and protection
2. Breathing and ventilation assessment
3. Circulation assessment
4. Disability assessment
5. Exposure assessment

Airway

As part of the airway assessment, one must first determine if the child is conscious or unconscious. If the child is conscious, asking the patient a simple question, such as "what is your name?" determines if the person is conscious and able to speak, indicating that the patient is aware and able to protect the airway. For those sports that require helmets, the face mask and chin strap are designed to be removed quickly to enable access to the athlete's airway. It is important for anyone providing medical coverage for such sports to be familiar with the required protective equipment and to have the knowledge and the tools to be able to safely and quickly remove equipment (eg, facemask) in the setting of serious injury. In the unconscious child, the airway must be protected immediately and a mouth guard should be removed so it does not block the airway. One should also recognize the possibility that an injury to the cervical spine has occurred until proven otherwise. Maintaining cervical spine stabilization is critical, because an unconscious child may also have a cervical spine injury.[13]

Breathing

Once airway patency is assessed, the adequacy of oxygenation and ventilation should be determined and steps should be taken to ensure that adequate oxygenation is maintained by the injured party or if further support of the airway is urgently needed.

Circulation

The provider should evaluate circulation by palpating central pulses, and if needed, steps should be taken to control any hemorrhage and maintain adequate end-organ perfusion. Emergency response should be activated to call for an ambulance and an automated external defibrillator (AED). Chest compressions should be initiated, if no pulse is detected, and AED applied for defibrillation if indicated.

Disability

A general neurologic evaluation is performed, including determining the Glasgow Coma Scale (GCS) score assessing the pupillary size and reactivity, gross motor function, and sensation. During the assessment on the field, one should immediately evaluate for signs of more serious head trauma, such as a skull hematoma or a scalp defect. If there are signs of a skull fracture, such as hematoma, scalp step off or depression, crepitus, or significant soft-tissue swelling, there is increased concern for elevated intracranial pressure. Any concerning signs should prompt emergent transportation to an emergency facility for evaluation and advanced imaging (**Figure 10.3**).

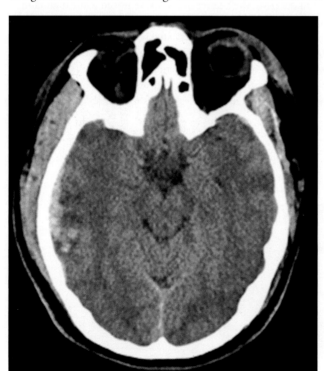

Any athlete suspected of having a concussion should be immediately removed from play. If the athlete is conscious and it has been determined that he or she does not need immediate emergency care, sideline screening assessments for concussion, such as the SCAT5 or Child SCAT5, could be considered. These tests, however, are brief and not intended to replace a more comprehensive office clinical concussion evaluation as described below.

FIGURE 10.3 Axial CT shows the right temporal scalp hematoma with underlying subdural hematoma and parenchymal contusions. (From Castillo M. *Neuroradiology Companion.* 4th ed. Philadelphia, PA: Wolters Kluwer; 2011: Figures 8-27, with permission.)

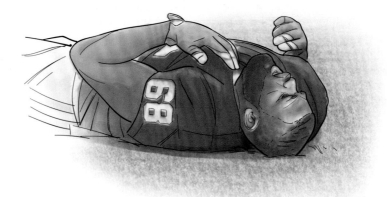

FIGURE 10.4 If a neck injury is suspected in an athlete wearing shoulder pads and a helmet, the equipment should be left in place to maintain a neutral spine position. Note in this picture that the athlete's neck is in an unsafe hyperextended position because shoulder pads are in place and helmet has been removed.

Exposure

Depending on the sport, the sideline evaluation can be difficult because of the equipment worn. Many sports have equipment that can either be easily removed or is designed to be left on during an emergency. In football, lacrosse, and ice hockey, shoulder pads, helmets, and chin strap should be left in place when possible to keep an injured neck in a neutral position (**Figure 10.4**). The helmet also prevents head movement, and towel rolls, foam head blocks, and/or tape can be used to stabilize the head if needed. If the helmet or the shoulder pads are to be removed, they both need to be removed (**Figure 10.5**). Removing just the helmet will force the neck into extension by shoulder pads. Conversely, removing just the shoulder pads would flex the neck out of a neutral position due to the helmet. If the athlete with a neck injury is wearing a helmet without shoulder pads, the helmet should be removed while maintaining the cervical spine in a neutral position in a controlled manner by an experienced clinical provider with experience in helmet removal, such as a certified athletic trainer.[14] Repeated rehearsal of these procedures is highly recommended for those covering athletic events. Site-specific emergency action plans should also be reviewed to ensure efficient access to athletic venues for emergency responders.

Emergent injuries identified during the primary survey should be addressed and prompt transfer to an appropriate medical facility should be arranged. A trained professional should stabilize the athlete's

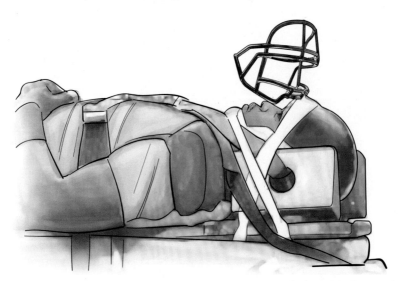

FIGURE 10.5 Before emergency transport, the head and neck should be stabilized and the face mask removed to allow for access to the airway if emergency management is required.

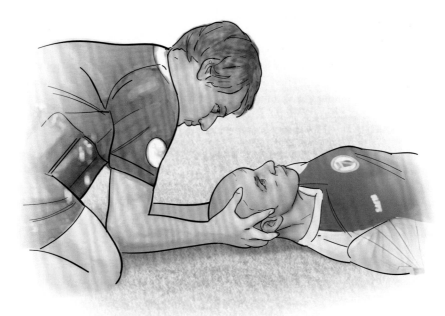

FIGURE 10.6 Stabilization of neck while patient is being moved

neck in a neutral position and ensure there is no added injury when moving the patient (**Figure 10.6**). The log-roll maneuver is used to move a patient without flexing the spinal column. At least three, ideally more, people are required to perform the log-roll technique properly (**Figure 10.7**). If trained personnel are available, the six-person lift may be utilized. With the legs stretched, the head is immobilized and the

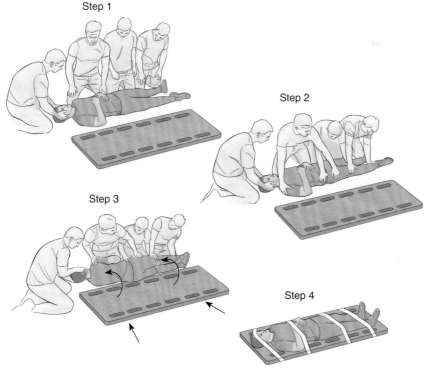

Step 1

Step 2

Step 3

Step 4

FIGURE 10.7 Logroll method.

patient moved in a secure manner typically in order to examine the patient or move the athlete from the field to a stretcher. The arms should be placed palms inward, extended by the athlete's side, unless an arm is injured. If the arm is injured, the backboard should be placed on the injured side, so the athlete rolls onto his/her uninjured side. One rescuer is placed at the head of the athlete and the other two kneeling opposite the board; one at the mid-chest and one at the upper legs. When the patient is logrolled, the posterior side of the body should be examined by an additional rescuer.[15]

Sideline Evaluation

The concussion examination and assessment may vary somewhat when performed in the emergency department, the office setting, or from the sideline. This is due, in part, to the pressures and constraints of the setting, as well as the ultimate goals of the assessment. Yet in each location, assessment of consciousness, awareness, and orientation should occur immediately. Potential intracranial pathologies should be considered if there is any alteration in loss of consciousness, presence of amnesia, seizures, weakness or paralysis, or other concerning signs or symptoms, such as severe worsening of headache or vomiting or level of consciousness.

If the general neurologic examination is normal (eg, the pupillary size and reactivity, gross motor function and sensation are normal), then the goal is to determine if there is a sports-related concussion. It is important to note that the diagnosis of a concussion remains a clinical judgment made by a medical professional. There are tests that have been created specifically for sideline use, such as the SCAT5 which includes the Maddocks questions, a cervical assessment, the Post-Concussion Symptom Scale (PCSS), Standardized Assessment of Concussion (SAC), and modified Balance Error Scoring System (BESS). Preinjury baseline tests may be helpful but are not essential for use of these tools following injury (▶ **Video 10.1-10.9**).

SCAT5

The SCAT5 is a tool used for evaluating athletes aged 13 years and older to aid in the diagnosis of concussion, but a normal SCAT5 does not necessarily exclude the possibility of a concussion as signs and symptoms may evolve early after the injury (**Appendix 10.1**). While the SCAT5 is currently the mainstay for acute sideline assessment,[11,16,17] its utility decreases over time and does not seem to be as helpful 3 to 5 days out from injury.

While Maddocks questions are helpful in the immediate assessment, they do not need to be performed serially. In his original description, Maddocks found that if these questions were answered correctly, the athlete was unlikely to have a concussion with high specificity (86%-100%), but the sensitivity of the test was variable (32%-75%).

The PCSS is helpful in both diagnosis and serial tracking of symptom recovery, keeping in mind that many of the included symptoms are nonspecific and many athletes will report symptoms even in the absence of a concussion. If a baseline PCSS is not available, then the goal for the clinician is to have the patient return to their preconcussion conditions, and it may be helpful for the injured athlete to report a preinjury symptom level for comparison if an actual preinjury scale was not obtained because not all adolescents are asymptomatic prior to concussion.

The SAC is included as part of the SCAT5 and includes an age-appropriate cognitive screen including immediate and delayed recall, reverse digit recall, and reverse months of the year.[18-20] Normative values of the SAC in nonconcussed individuals have been reported to be between 26.12 and 27.17 out of a total of 30 points.[18]

Modified BESS has been used in the SCAT5 including three stances: narrow double-leg, single-leg, and tandem stance, and each stance is held with hands on hips and eyes closed for 20 seconds. A maximum of 30 points can be given (10 for each stance), with error point deduction for opening of the eyes, lifting hands off the hips, stepping, stumbling, or falling. The BESS is most sensitive at the time of injury. Studies have demonstrated concern with interrater and intrarater reliability.[21,22]

Child SCAT5

The Child SCAT5 is a variation of the SCAT5 to test children aged 5 to 12 years with age-specific modifications (**Appendix 10.2**). The test initially used modified pediatric Maddocks questions which were eventually removed from the Child SCAT for the fifth version due to questionable reliability and usefulness in young.[16] Symptom reports are performed by both the child and the parent as children may not be able to communicate or recognize symptoms. Normative values of the SAC are age-dependent ranging from 19.5 to 26.1 out of a total of 30.[20] Additional differences in the Child SCAT5 include fewer numbers for reverse digit recall and reverse days of the week instead of months of the year.

King-Devick Test

The King-Devick Test (**Figure 10.8**), a rapid test that assesses saccadic eye movements, is another tool that takes approximately 2 minutes to complete and may be helpful in the sideline evaluation to determine if a concussion has occurred. Each card increases progressively in difficulty with eye tracking. The total number of errors are noted during the timed test and is then compared to an individual's preinjury score which is the currently recommended use of this test. As a straightforward and brief tool, it holds promise for sideline use in determining the presence of a concussion, especially in comparison to an uninjured test score. Thus far, however, studies have involved only small sample sizes and further investigation is warranted before recommending its use universally as a sideline concussion tool.[23]

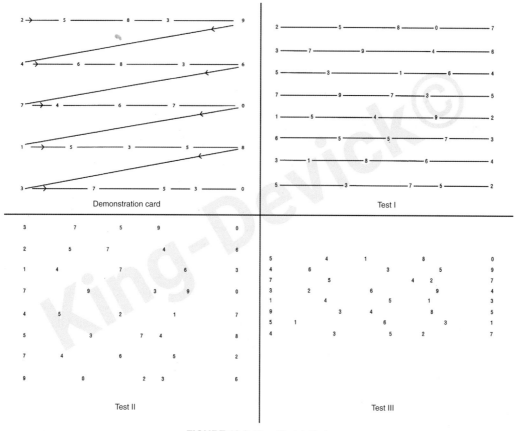

FIGURE 10.8 King-Devick Test.

● In-Office Clinical Evaluation

If a concussion is suspected or diagnosed in an individual, a clinical concussion evaluation should be performed to provide education on postconcussion management including return to school and sport recommendations, identify the presence of risk factors for prolonged recovery, and determine need for additional treatment referrals. An initial concussion examination should assess cognitive function, neck pain, vision, and the vestibular system. Additional assessments of activity tolerance, sleep disturbance, and behavioral changes should also be incorporated to provide comprehensive guidance on appropriate care recommendations.

Cognitive Screen

Cognitive impairments, such as confusion and memory issues, are common symptoms after a concussion and should be assessed with a standardized tool. The SAC component of the SCAT5 is a readily available cognitive screen that can be used during an initial office assessment. Additional questions regarding school performance, memory and recall, and social interactions can help identify cognitive dysfunctions.

Cervical Screen

A cervical screen should be performed to identify potential cervicogenic-related symptoms of concussion such as headache and dizziness. Components of the cervical screen include postural assessment, palpation, range of motion, strength testing, and cervical instability tests. Poor posture can place the neck in an extended position and contribute to muscular tightness. Altered neck postures such as rotation or tilting may indicate avoidance of painful positions. Palpation along the spinous processes and cervical musculature can help localize involved regions of the neck that may be contributing to pain and symptoms. Range of motion and strength in the three cardinal planes should be assessed. Cervical instability testing such as the Sharp-Purser and alar ligament test should also be performed. If positive cervical findings are identified, standard cervical spine radiographs should be ordered and treatment should be initiated to restore motion, strength, and pain-free function.

Visio-Vestibular Assessment

The concussion physical examination includes a targeted assessment of balance and the visio-vestibular system (https://www.chop.edu/video/pediatric-exams-concussion-evaluation).

The visio-vestibular examination involves assessing both vestibular-oculomotor function and vision (**Figure 10.9**). One such screening examination, the vestibular-oculomotor screen (VOMS), includes assessing smooth pursuits, horizontal and vertical saccades, horizontal and vertical gaze stability/vestibular-ocular reflex (VOR), and visual motion sensitivity (VMS).[24] The visio-vestibular assessment additionally includes an assessment of convergence and accommodation and balance using tandem gait, forward and backward with eyes open and closed.[25] Balance may also be assessed with single leg stance, with both eyes open and closed.[26] Smooth pursuits assess the ability to follow a moving target and is performed by the patient focusing on the examiner's moving finger and keeping the head still. The examiner moves the pointer finger slowly at first and then increases speed in a horizontal direction. The examiner notes if there is excessive blinking, eyes watering, eye redness, or if the patient complains of headache, dizziness, nausea, eye fatigue, or eye pain. Of note, a few beats of nystagmus at end-gaze is normal, but is generally not seen at the midline.

Next, saccades are performed where the patient keeps the head still and moves eyes between targets (the examiner's fingers are held approximately 1.5 ft apart and the patient looks at the fingertips back and forth until it elicits symptoms or the examiner tells the patient to stop, up to 30 repetitions). The examination is repeated in the vertical direction. Again, it is noted if there are physical signs such as excessive blinking, eyes watering, eye redness, or symptom provocation, complaining of headache, dizziness, nausea, eye fatigue, or eye pain.

Smooth pursuits horizontal

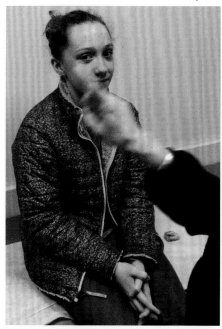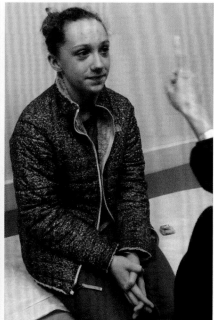

Smooth pursuits vertical

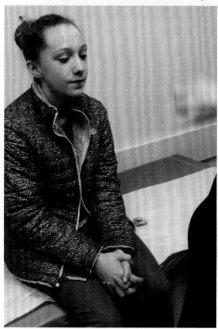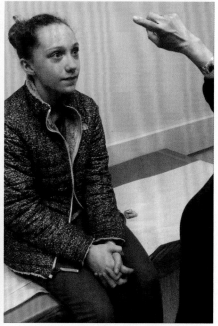

FIGURE 10.9 Visio-vestibular examination pictures.

Saccades horizontal

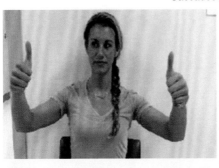
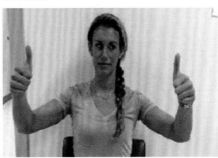

Saccades vertical

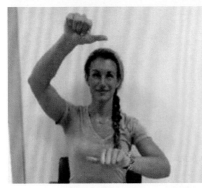
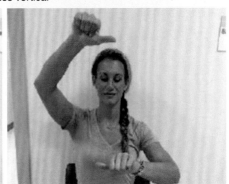

Gaze stability horizontal

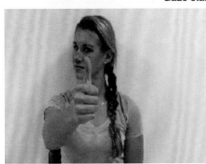
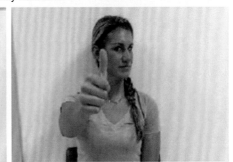

Gaze stability vertical

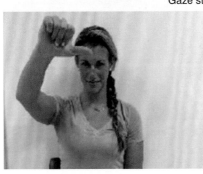
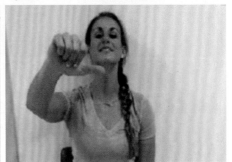

FIGURE 10.9 cont'd

Visual motion sensitivity

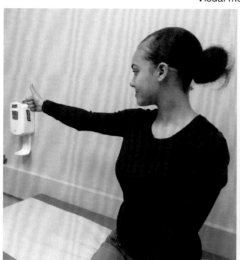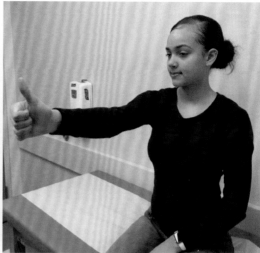

Balance testing
Vestibular spinal reflex-tandem gait

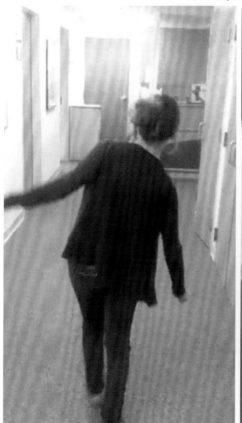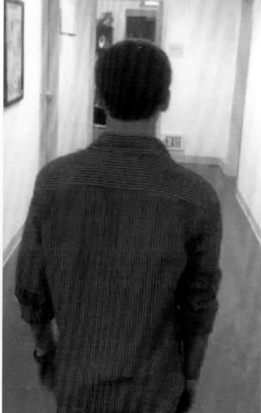

FIGURE 10.9 cont'd

Near point of convergence

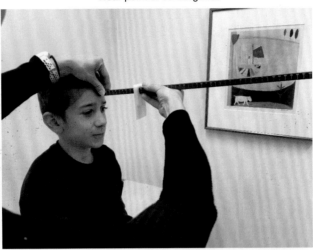

Accommodative amplitude

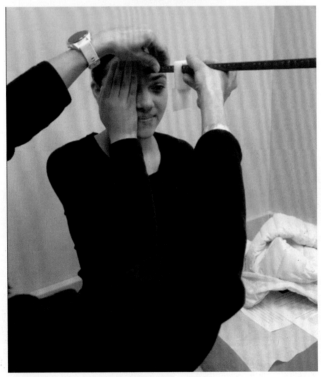

FIGURE 10.9 cont'd

   Gaze stability/VOR assessment occurs next in both the horizontal and the vertical directions. The examiner holds their thumb in front of the patient, and the patient is asked to rotate their head first horizontally (shaking head) then vertically (nodding head) while maintaining focus on the target (thumb) up to 10 to 15 repetitions or when the patient has symptom provocation or manifests excessive blinking, eyes watering, or eye redness.

The VMS test is next assessed by having the patient extend their arm in an outstretched position with their thumb up, rotating their arm across their trunk back and forth for a total of five repetitions while maintaining visual fixation on their thumb, again observing for subjective symptoms or provocable physical signs.[27]

Visual Screen

The vision examination beyond visual acuity includes an assessment of near point of convergence and accommodation.[25] Vision problems such as abnormal near point of convergence or accommodative amplitude appear to represent a subset of patients who also present with vestibular deficits after injury.

Near point of convergence is the ability to maintain a single visual target at near distance with both eyes which should be less than or equal to 6 cm. This is best assessed with a special tool called a convergence rule (http://www.guldenophthalmics.com/products/index.php/near-point-rule.html), but can be estimated by using a pen and a tape measure. Binocular convergence break (where the visual target becomes double) and subsequent recovery (where the visual target becomes single again) are measured. The patient is seated and wearing corrective lenses (if needed). The patient focuses on a small card with writing (approximately 14 point font size), and the card is slowly brought closer to the patient until the patient states that the letters have split in two. The examiner then moves the card outward until the patient state the letters single again. The measurement on the ruler in centimeters is recorded for each step (**Figure 10.9**).

Monocular accommodation is next assessed in a similar manner. The left eye is covered, and the right eye's accommodative amplitude is assessed with the convergence rule. The patient states when the letters on the card become blurry. The same is done for the left eye while looking for symptom or physical sign provocation. Normal accommodative amplitude for adolescents and children should be less than 10 cm.[28]

Visio-vestibular deficits are common after concussion, and targeted assessment should be included in a comprehensive evaluation of concussion.[25] These deficits are often related to one another and can have substantial impact on day-to-day function. Balance and oculomotor saccadic deficits are associated such that anyone presenting with a balance deficit after concussion should also be assessed for oculomotor and vision deficits.

Balance Assessment

The modified BESS is performed as part of the SCAT5. The complete BESS can be performed during clinical assessment and differs from the modified BESS by the inclusion of a foam pad surface for the three test stance positions. The scoring remains the same with counting of errors over a 20-second period.

Balance can also be assessed via a progressively more challenging tandem gait task. The patient is instructed to walk heel to toe, like on a tight rope. The patient walks both forward and backward and with eyes open and closed. Each condition is a bit more challenging, in order to minimize a ceiling effect. Those who have a concussion may have very poor balance, so it is important to be nearby so the examiner can help steady the patient if necessary. The test is failed if athletes step off the line, have a separation between their heel and toe, or touch or grab the examiner or another object. The patient is again asked about any symptom provocation.[26] Visio-vestibular deficits are common after concussion, and targeted assessment should be included in a comprehensive evaluation of concussion.[25] These deficits are often related to one another and can have substantial impact on day-to-day function. Vision problems such as abnormal near point of convergence or accommodative amplitude appear to represent a subset of patients who also present with vestibular deficits after injury. Balance and oculomotor saccadic deficits are associated such that anyone presenting with a balance deficit after concussion should also be assessed for oculomotor and vision deficits. Abnormal accommodative amplitude, balance, smooth pursuit, and VOR function are important predictors of prolonged concussion recovery in certain populations and have been associated with persisting symptoms lasting longer than 28 days.[28]

Neurocognitive Testing

In addition to performing a physical examination, neurocognitive testing is often part of the concussion office assessment.[29] The utility of neurocognitive testing, either by a neuropsychologist or a brief computerized assessment, has been debated. Gaudet and Weyandt in 2017 concluded there is a high incidence of invalid results in those with a learning disability, attention-deficit hyperactivity disorder, or if administered in a large group setting, which frequently occurs when a baseline is given in a school setting and[30] there are limited options for preinjury computerized neurocognitive testing in preadolescent children. The fifth international consensus on concussion in sport, while acknowledging that such testing may contribute to the overall evaluation, does not formally recommend universal neurocognitive testing in the treatment of concussion.

A recent study by Alsalaheen et al in 2015 concluded that ImPACT testing should be implemented on a case-by-case scenario and its benefit was unclear.[31] Neurocognitive testing may be particularly useful in high-risk athletes who are at risk of symptom nondisclosure in order to return to play before recovered or to provide additional information to patients, employers, school teachers, or others. Results, however, must be interpreted within the clinical context by someone experienced in the use of the test. Under these conditions, neurocognitive testing has been shown to have moderate sensitivity in the detection of postconcussive cognitive deficits,[32] which may persist beyond the point at which athletes become asymptomatic.[33] Neurocognitive testing may be used as an adjunct tool in the clinical assessment of concussion but should not be used alone for the diagnosis or management of a concussion.[21]

Exercise Tolerance Testing

Following concussion, autonomic dysfunction may cause exercise intolerance and inhibit an individual's ability to return back to physical activity. The Buffalo Concussion Treadmill Test and the Buffalo Concussion Bike Test are exercise tolerance tests that can be performed to determine if the individual has a physiologic concussion. The exercise tolerance testing also identifies exercise prescription parameters that the individual can begin to improve autonomic function. If an individual is able to complete the exercise tolerance testing without provocation of symptoms, then it is likely that the symptoms are resulting from cervical injury, vestibular/ocular dysfunction, and/or headache or migraine syndrome.[34]

● Conclusion

In summary, the physical examination of the child with an acute concussion must exclude more serious brain or cervical spine injury. Emergency evaluation may be warranted to assess for the possibility of intracranial hemorrhage or other potential or associated injuries.

Upon outpatient follow-up for concussion, a more comprehensive examination should be undertaken including assessment of the visio-vestibular system, because these deficits commonly occur after concussion and predict prolonged recovery of concussion. Neurocognitive testing is also another adjunctive tool that may be helpful in the assessment and management of concussion when interpreted by a qualified provider in the context of the patient and injury.

Identifiable visio-vestibular deficits in functioning on physical examination support the diagnosis of concussion after trauma to the head followed by new-onset symptoms. Abnormal accommodative amplitude, balance, smooth pursuit, and VOR function are important predictors of prolonged concussion recovery in certain populations and have been associated with persisting symptoms lasting longer than 28 days.[28] In addition, such findings can be used to track recovery and estimate, to some extent, duration of symptoms. Thus, an appropriately targeted physical examination is now an essential component of the assessment of a child with suspected concussion.

BJSM Online First, published on April 26, 2017 as 10.1136/bjsports-2017-097506SCAT5

To download a clean version of the SCAT tools please visit the journal online (http://dx.doi.org/10.1136/bjsports-2017-097506SCAT5)

SCAT5©

SPORT CONCUSSION ASSESSMENT TOOL — 5TH EDITION
DEVELOPED BY THE CONCUSSION IN SPORT GROUP
FOR USE BY MEDICAL PROFESSIONALS ONLY

supported by

FIFA®   ○○○   ⚽   *FEI*

Patient details

Name: _____

DOB: _____

Address: _____

ID number: _____

Examiner: _____

Date of Injury: _____   Time: _____

WHAT IS THE SCAT5?

The SCAT5 is a standardized tool for evaluating concussions designed for use by physicians and licensed healthcare professionals[1]. The SCAT5 cannot be performed correctly in less than 10 minutes.

If you are not a physician or licensed healthcare professional, please use the Concussion Recognition Tool 5 (CRT5). The SCAT5 is to be used for evaluating athletes aged 13 years and older. For children aged 12 years or younger, please use the Child SCAT5.

Preseason SCAT5 baseline testing can be useful for interpreting post-injury test scores, but is not required for that purpose. Detailed instructions for use of the SCAT5 are provided on page 7. Please read through these instructions carefully before testing the athlete. Brief verbal instructions for each test are given in italics. The only equipment required for the tester is a watch or timer.

This tool may be freely copied in its current form for distribution to individuals, teams, groups and organizations. It should not be altered in any way, re-branded or sold for commercial gain. Any revision, translation or reproduction in a digital form requires specific approval by the Concussion in Sport Group.

Recognise and Remove

A head impact by either a direct blow or indirect transmission of force can be associated with a serious and potentially fatal brain injury. If there are significant concerns, including any of the red flags listed in Box 1, then activation of emergency procedures and urgent transport to the nearest hospital should be arranged.

Key points

- Any athlete with suspected concussion should be REMOVED FROM PLAY, medically assessed and monitored for deterioration. No athlete diagnosed with concussion should be returned to play on the day of injury.

- If an athlete is suspected of having a concussion and medical personnel are not immediately available, the athlete should be referred to a medical facility for urgent assessment.

- Athletes with suspected concussion should not drink alcohol, use recreational drugs and should not drive a motor vehicle until cleared to do so by a medical professional.

- Concussion signs and symptoms evolve over time and it is important to consider repeat evaluation in the assessment of concussion.

- The diagnosis of a concussion is a clinical judgment, made by a medical professional. The SCAT5 should NOT be used by itself to make, or exclude, the diagnosis of concussion. An athlete may have a concussion even if their SCAT5 is "normal".

Remember:

- The basic principles of first aid (danger, response, airway, breathing, circulation) should be followed.

- Do not attempt to move the athlete (other than that required for airway management) unless trained to do so.

- Assessment for a spinal cord injury is a critical part of the initial on-field assessment.

- Do not remove a helmet or any other equipment unless trained to do so safely.

APPENDIX 10.1 SCAT5.

1

IMMEDIATE OR ON-FIELD ASSESSMENT

The following elements should be assessed for all athletes who are suspected of having a concussion prior to proceeding to the neurocognitive assessment and ideally should be done on-field after the first first aid / emergency care priorities are completed.

If any of the "Red Flags" or observable signs are noted after a direct or indirect blow to the head, the athlete should be immediately and safely removed from participation and evaluated by a physician or licensed healthcare professional.

Consideration of transportation to a medical facility should be at the discretion of the physician or licensed healthcare professional.

The GCS is important as a standard measure for all patients and can be done serially if necessary in the event of deterioration in conscious state. The Maddocks questions and cervical spine exam are critical steps of the immediate assessment; however, these do not need to be done serially.

STEP 1: RED FLAGS

RED FLAGS:	
• Neck pain or tenderness	• Seizure or convulsion
• Double vision	• Loss of consciousness
• Weakness or tingling/ burning in arms or legs	• Deteriorating conscious state
	• Vomiting
• Severe or increasing headache	• Increasingly restless, agitated or combative

STEP 2: OBSERVABLE SIGNS

Witnessed ☐   Observed on Video ☐

Lying motionless on the playing surface	Y	N
Balance / gait difficulties / motor incoordination: stumbling, slow / laboured movements	Y	N
Disorientation or confusion, or an inability to respond appropriately to questions	Y	N
Blank or vacant look	Y	N
Facial injury after head trauma	Y	N

STEP 3: MEMORY ASSESSMENT
MADDOCKS QUESTIONS[2]

"I am going to ask you a few questions, please listen carefully and give your best effort. First, tell me what happened?"

Mark Y for correct answer / N for incorrect

What venue are we at today?	Y	N
Which half is it now?	Y	N
Who scored last in this match?	Y	N
What team did you play last week / game?	Y	N
Did your team win the last game?	Y	N

Note: Appropriate sport-specific questions may be substituted.

Name: _____

DOB: _____

Address: _____

ID number: _____

Examiner: _____

Date: _____

STEP 4: EXAMINATION
GLASGOW COMA SCALE (GCS)[3]

Time of assessment			
Date of assessment			
Best eye response (E)			
No eye opening	1	1	1
Eye opening in response to pain	2	2	2
Eye opening to speech	3	3	3
Eyes opening spontaneously	4	4	4
Best verbal response (V)			
No verbal response	1	1	1
Incomprehensible sounds	2	2	2
Inappropriate words	3	3	3
Confused	4	4	4
Oriented	5	5	5
Best motor response (M)			
No motor response	1	1	1
Extension to pain	2	2	2
Abnormal flexion to pain	3	3	3
Flexion / Withdrawal to pain	4	4	4
Localizes to pain	5	5	5
Obeys commands	6	6	6
Glasgow Coma score (E + V + M)			

CERVICAL SPINE ASSESSMENT

Does the athlete report that their neck is pain free at rest?	Y	N
If there is NO neck pain at rest, does the athlete have a full range of ACTIVE pain free movement?	Y	N
Is the limb strength and sensation normal?	Y	N

In a patient who is not lucid or fully conscious, a cervical spine injury should be assumed until proven otherwise.

© Concussion in Sport Group 2017

Davis GA, *et al. Br J Sports Med* 2017;**0**:1–8. doi:10.1136/bjsports-2017-097506SCAT5

APPENDIX 10.1 cont'd

OFFICE OR OFF-FIELD ASSESSMENT

Please note that the neurocognitive assessment should be done in a distraction-free environment with the athlete in a resting state.

STEP 1: ATHLETE BACKGROUND

Sport / team / school: _____

Date / time of injury: _____

Years of education completed: _____

Age: _____

Gender: M / F / Other

Dominant hand: left / neither / right

How many diagnosed concussions has the
athlete had in the past?: _____

When was the most recent concussion?: _____

How long was the recovery (time to being cleared to play)
from the most recent concussion?: _____ (days)

Has the athlete ever been:

Hospitalized for a head injury?	Yes	No
Diagnosed / treated for headache disorder or migraines?	Yes	No
Diagnosed with a learning disability / dyslexia?	Yes	No
Diagnosed with ADD / ADHD?	Yes	No
Diagnosed with depression, anxiety or other psychiatric disorder?	Yes	No

Current medications? If yes, please list:

_____

_____

_____

_____

_____

_____

Name: _____

DOB: _____

Address: _____

ID number: _____

Examiner: _____

Date: _____

2

STEP 2: SYMPTOM EVALUATION

The athlete should be given the symptom form and asked to read this instruction paragraph out loud then complete the symptom scale. For the baseline assessment, the athlete should rate his/her symptoms based on how he/she typically feels and for the post injury assessment the athlete should rate their symptoms at this point in time.

Please Check: ☐ Baseline ☐ Post-Injury

Please hand the form to the athlete

	none	mild		moderate		severe	
Headache	0	1	2	3	4	5	6
"Pressure in head"	0	1	2	3	4	5	6
Neck Pain	0	1	2	3	4	5	6
Nausea or vomiting	0	1	2	3	4	5	6
Dizziness	0	1	2	3	4	5	6
Blurred vision	0	1	2	3	4	5	6
Balance problems	0	1	2	3	4	5	6
Sensitivity to light	0	1	2	3	4	5	6
Sensitivity to noise	0	1	2	3	4	5	6
Feeling slowed down	0	1	2	3	4	5	6
Feeling like "in a fog"	0	1	2	3	4	5	6
"Don't feel right"	0	1	2	3	4	5	6
Difficulty concentrating	0	1	2	3	4	5	6
Difficulty remembering	0	1	2	3	4	5	6
Fatigue or low energy	0	1	2	3	4	5	6
Confusion	0	1	2	3	4	5	6
Drowsiness	0	1	2	3	4	5	6
More emotional	0	1	2	3	4	5	6
Irritability	0	1	2	3	4	5	6
Sadness	0	1	2	3	4	5	6
Nervous or Anxious	0	1	2	3	4	5	6
Trouble falling asleep (if applicable)	0	1	2	3	4	5	6

Total number of symptoms:	of 22
Symptom severity score:	of 132
Do your symptoms get worse with physical activity?	Y N
Do your symptoms get worse with mental activity?	Y N
If 100% is feeling perfectly normal, what percent of normal do you feel?	
If not 100%, why?	

_____

_____

_____

Please hand form back to examiner

© Concussion in Sport Group 2017

Davis GA, *et al. Br J Sports Med* 2017;**0**:1–8. doi:10.1136/bjsports-2017-097506SCAT5   3   3

APPENDIX 10.1 cont'd

3

STEP 3: COGNITIVE SCREENING
Standardised Assessment of Concussion (SAC)[4]

ORIENTATION

What month is it?	0	1
What is the date today?	0	1
What is the day of the week?	0	1
What year is it?	0	1
What time is it right now? (within 1 hour)	0	1
Orientation score		of 5

Name:	
DOB:	
Address:	
ID number:	
Examiner:	
Date:	

IMMEDIATE MEMORY

The Immediate Memory component can be completed using the traditional 5-word per trial list or optionally using 10-words per trial to minimise any ceiling effect. All 3 trials must be administered irrespective of the number correct on the first trial. Administer at the rate of one word per second.

Please choose EITHER the 5 or 10 word list groups and circle the specific word list chosen for this test.

I am going to test your memory. I will read you a list of words and when I am done, repeat back as many words as you can remember, in any order. For Trials 2 & 3: I am going to repeat the same list again. Repeat back as many words as you can remember in any order, even if you said the word before.

List	Alternate 5 word lists					Score (of 5) Trial 1 Trial 2 Trial 3
A	Finger	Penny	Blanket	Lemon	Insect	
B	Candle	Paper	Sugar	Sandwich	Wagon	
C	Baby	Monkey	Perfume	Sunset	Iron	
D	Elbow	Apple	Carpet	Saddle	Bubble	
E	Jacket	Arrow	Pepper	Cotton	Movie	
F	Dollar	Honey	Mirror	Saddle	Anchor	
	Immediate Memory Score					of 15
	Time that last trial was completed					

List	Alternate 10 word lists					Score (of 10) Trial 1 Trial 2 Trial 3
G	Finger	Penny	Blanket	Lemon	Insect	
	Candle	Paper	Sugar	Sandwich	Wagon	
H	Baby	Monkey	Perfume	Sunset	Iron	
	Elbow	Apple	Carpet	Saddle	Bubble	
I	Jacket	Arrow	Pepper	Cotton	Movie	
	Dollar	Honey	Mirror	Saddle	Anchor	
	Immediate Memory Score					of 30
	Time that last trial was completed					

CONCENTRATION

DIGITS BACKWARDS

Please circle the Digit list chosen (A, B, C, D, E, F). Administer at the rate of one digit per second reading DOWN the selected column.

I am going to read a string of numbers and when I am done, you repeat them back to me in reverse order of how I read them to you. For example, if I say 7-1-9, you would say 9-1-7.

Concentration Number Lists (circle one)					
List A	List B	List C			
4-9-3	5-2-6	1-4-2	Y	N	0
6-2-9	4-1-5	6-5-8	Y	N	1
3-8-1-4	1-7-9-5	6-8-3-1	Y	N	0
3-2-7-9	4-9-6-8	3-4-8-1	Y	N	1
6-2-9-7-1	4-8-5-2-7	4-9-1-5-3	Y	N	0
1-5-2-8-6	6-1-8-4-3	6-8-2-5-1	Y	N	1
7-1-8-4-6-2	8-3-1-9-6-4	3-7-6-5-1-9	Y	N	0
5-3-9-1-4-8	7-2-4-8-5-6	9-2-6-5-1-4	Y	N	1
List D	List E	List F			
7-8-2	3-8-2	2-7-1	Y	N	0
9-2-6	5-1-8	4-7-9	Y	N	1
4-1-8-3	2-7-9-3	1-6-8-3	Y	N	0
9-7-2-3	2-1-6-9	3-9-2-4	Y	N	1
1-7-9-2-6	4-1-8-6-9	2-4-7-5-8	Y	N	0
4-1-7-5-2	9-4-1-7-5	8-3-9-6-4	Y	N	1
2-6-4-8-1-7	6-9-7-3-8-2	5-8-6-2-4-9	Y	N	0
8-4-1-9-3-5	4-2-7-9-3-8	3-1-7-8-2-6	Y	N	1
		Digits Score:			of 4

MONTHS IN REVERSE ORDER

Now tell me the months of the year in reverse order. Start with the last month and go backward. So you'll say December, November. Go ahead.

Dec - Nov - Oct - Sept - Aug - Jul - Jun - May - Apr - Mar - Feb - Jan   0   1

Months Score	of 1
Concentration Total Score (Digits + Months)	of 5

© Concussion in Sport Group 2017

Davis GA, *et al. Br J Sports Med* 2017;**0**:1–8. doi:10.1136/bjsports-2017-097506SCAT5

4   4

APPENDIX 10.1 cont'd

4

STEP 4: NEUROLOGICAL SCREEN

See the instruction sheet (page 7) for details of test administration and scoring of the tests.

Can the patient read aloud (e.g. symptom checklist) and follow instructions without difficulty?	Y	N
Does the patient have a full range of pain-free PASSIVE cervical spine movement?	Y	N
Without moving their head or neck, can the patient look side-to-side and up-and-down without double vision?	Y	N
Can the patient perform the finger nose coordination test normally?	Y	N
Can the patient perform tandem gait normally?	Y	N

BALANCE EXAMINATION

Modified Balance Error Scoring System (mBESS) testing[5]

Which foot was tested (i.e. which is the non-dominant foot)	☐ Left ☐ Right

Testing surface (hard floor, field, etc.) _____

Footwear (shoes, barefoot, braces, tape, etc.) _____

Condition	Errors
Double leg stance	of 10
Single leg stance (non-dominant foot)	of 10
Tandem stance (non-dominant foot at the back)	of 10
Total Errors	of 30

Name:	_____
DOB:	_____
Address:	_____
ID number:	_____
Examiner:	_____
Date:	_____

5

STEP 5: DELAYED RECALL:

The delayed recall should be performed after 5 minutes have elapsed since the end of the Immediate Recall section. Score 1 pt. for each correct response.

Do you remember that list of words I read a few times earlier? Tell me as many words from the list as you can remember in any order.

Time Started ▩▩▩▩▩

Please record each word correctly recalled. Total score equals number of words recalled.

_____
_____
_____
_____

Total number of words recalled accurately:	of 5	or	of 10

6

STEP 6: DECISION

Domain	Date & time of assessment:		
Symptom number (of 22)			
Symptom severity score (of 132)			
Orientation (of 5)			
Immediate memory	of 15 / of 30	of 15 / of 30	of 15 / of 30
Concentration (of 5)			
Neuro exam	Normal / Abnormal	Normal / Abnormal	Normal / Abnormal
Balance errors (of 30)			
Delayed Recall	of 5 / of 10	of 5 / of 10	of 5 / of 10

Date and time of injury: _____

If the athlete is known to you prior to their injury, are they different from their usual self?
☐ Yes ☐ No ☐ Unsure ☐ Not Applicable
(If different, describe why in the clinical notes section)

Concussion Diagnosed?
☐ Yes ☐ No ☐ Unsure ☐ Not Applicable

If re-testing, has the athlete improved?
☐ Yes ☐ No ☐ Unsure ☐ Not Applicable

I am a physician or licensed healthcare professional and I have personally administered or supervised the administration of this SCAT5.

Signature: _____

Name: _____

Title: _____

Registration number (if applicable): _____

Date: _____

SCORING ON THE SCAT5 SHOULD NOT BE USED AS A STAND-ALONE METHOD TO DIAGNOSE CONCUSSION, MEASURE RECOVERY OR MAKE DECISIONS ABOUT AN ATHLETE'S READINESS TO RETURN TO COMPETITION AFTER CONCUSSION.

© Concussion in Sport Group 2017

Davis GA, *et al. Br J Sports Med* 2017;**0**:1–8. doi:10.1136/bjsports-2017-097506SCAT5

5   5

APPENDIX 10.1 cont'd

CLINICAL NOTES:

Name: _____

DOB: _____

Address: _____

ID number: _____

Examiner: _____

Date: _____

✂ . . . .

CONCUSSION INJURY ADVICE

(To be given to the person monitoring the concussed athlete)

This patient has received an injury to the head. A careful medical examination has been carried out and no sign of any serious complications has been found. Recovery time is variable across individuals and the patient will need monitoring for a further period by a responsible adult. Your treating physician will provide guidance as to this timeframe.

If you notice any change in behaviour, vomiting, worsening headache, double vision or excessive drowsiness, please telephone your doctor or the nearest hospital emergency department immediately.

Other important points:

Initial rest: Limit physical activity to routine daily activities (avoid exercise, training, sports) and limit activities such as school, work, and screen time to a level that does not worsen symptoms.

1) Avoid alcohol

2) Avoid prescription or non-prescription drugs without medical supervision. Specifically:

   a) Avoid sleeping tablets

   b) Do not use aspirin, anti-inflammatory medication or stronger pain medications such as narcotics

3) Do not drive until cleared by a healthcare professional.

4) Return to play/sport requires clearance by a healthcare professional.

Clinic phone number: _____

Patient's name: _____

Date / time of injury: _____

Date / time of medical review: _____

Healthcare Provider: _____

© Concussion in Sport Group 2017

Contact details or stamp

Davis GA, *et al. Br J Sports Med* 2017;**0**:1–8. doi:10.1136/bjsports-2017-097506SCAT5

APPENDIX 10.1 cont'd

INSTRUCTIONS

Words in *Italics* throughout the SCAT5 are the instructions given to the athlete by the clinician

Symptom Scale

The time frame for symptoms should be based on the type of test being administered. At baseline it is advantageous to assess how an athlete "typically" feels whereas during the acute/post-acute stage it is best to ask how the athlete feels at the time of testing.

The symptom scale should be completed by the athlete, not by the examiner. In situations where the symptom scale is being completed after exercise, it should be done in a resting state, generally by approximating his/her resting heart rate.

For total number of symptoms, maximum possible is 22 except immediately post injury, if sleep item is omitted, which then creates a maximum of 21.

For Symptom severity score, add all scores in table, maximum possible is 22 x 6 = 132, except immediately post injury if sleep item is omitted, which then creates a maximum of 21x6=126.

Immediate Memory

The Immediate Memory component can be completed using the traditional 5-word per trial list or, optionally, using 10-words per trial. The literature suggests that the Immediate Memory has a notable ceiling effect when a 5-word list is used. In settings where this ceiling is prominent, the examiner may wish to make the task more difficult by incorporating two 5–word groups for a total of 10 words per trial. In this case, the maximum score per trial is 10 with a total trial maximum of 30.

Choose one of the word lists (either 5 or 10). Then perform 3 trials of immediate memory using this list.

Complete all 3 trials regardless of score on previous trials.

"I am going to test your memory. I will read you a list of words and when I am done, repeat back as many words as you can remember, in any order." The words must be read at a rate of one word per second.

Trials 2 & 3 MUST be completed regardless of score on trial 1 & 2.

Trials 2 & 3:

"I am going to repeat the same list again. Repeat back as many words as you can remember in any order, even if you said the word before."

Score 1 pt. for each correct response. Total score equals sum across all 3 trials. Do NOT inform the athlete that delayed recall will be tested.

Concentration

Digits backward

Choose one column of digits from lists A, B, C, D, E or F and administer those digits as follows:

Say: *"I am going to read a string of numbers and when I am done, you repeat them back to me in reverse order of how I read them to you. For example, if I say 7-1-9, you would say 9-1-7."*

Begin with first 3 digit string.

If correct, circle "Y" for correct and go to next string length. If incorrect, circle "N" for the first string length and read trial 2 in the same string length. One point possible for each string length. Stop after incorrect on both trials (2 N's) in a string length. The digits should be read at the rate of one per second.

Months in reverse order

"Now tell me the months of the year in reverse order. Start with the last month and go backward. So you'll say December, November ... Go ahead"

1 pt. for entire sequence correct

Delayed Recall

The delayed recall should be performed after 5 minutes have elapsed since the end of the Immediate Recall section.

"Do you remember that list of words I read a few times earlier? Tell me as many words from the list as you can remember in any order."

Score 1 pt. for each correct response

Modified Balance Error Scoring System (mBESS)[5] testing

This balance testing is based on a modified version of the Balance Error Scoring System (BESS)[5]. A timing device is required for this testing.

Each of 20-second trial/stance is scored by counting the number of errors. The examiner will begin counting errors only after the athlete has assumed the proper start position. The modified BESS is calculated by adding one error point for each error during the three 20-second tests. The maximum number of errors for any single condition is 10. If the athlete commits multiple errors simultaneously, only

one error is recorded but the athlete should quickly return to the testing position, and counting should resume once the athlete is set. Athletes that are unable to maintain the testing procedure for a minimum of five seconds at the start are assigned the highest possible score, ten, for that testing condition.

OPTION: For further assessment, the same 3 stances can be performed on a surface of medium density foam (e.g., approximately 50cm x 40cm x 6cm).

Balance testing – types of errors

1. Hands lifted off iliac crest	3. Step, stumble, or fall	5. Lifting forefoot or heel
2. Opening eyes	4. Moving hip into > 30 degrees abduction	6. Remaining out of test position > 5 sec

"I am now going to test your balance. Please take your shoes off (if applicable), roll up your pant legs above ankle (if applicable), and remove any ankle taping (if applicable). This test will consist of three twenty second tests with different stances."

(a) Double leg stance:

"The first stance is standing with your feet together with your hands on your hips and with your eyes closed. You should try to maintain stability in that position for 20 seconds. I will be counting the number of times you move out of this position. I will start timing when you are set and have closed your eyes."

(b) Single leg stance:

"If you were to kick a ball, which foot would you use? [This will be the dominant foot] Now stand on your non-dominant foot. The dominant leg should be held in approximately 30 degrees of hip flexion and 45 degrees of knee flexion. Again, you should try to maintain stability for 20 seconds with your hands on your hips and your eyes closed. I will be counting the number of times you move out of this position. If you stumble out of this position, open your eyes and return to the start position and continue balancing. I will start timing when you are set and have closed your eyes."

(c) Tandem stance:

"Now stand heel-to-toe with your non-dominant foot in back. Your weight should be evenly distributed across both feet. Again, you should try to maintain stability for 20 seconds with your hands on your hips and your eyes closed. I will be counting the number of times you move out of this position. If you stumble out of this position, open your eyes and return to the start position and continue balancing. I will start timing when you are set and have closed your eyes."

Tandem Gait

Participants are instructed to stand with their feet together behind a starting line (the test is best done with footwear removed). Then, they walk in a forward direction as quickly and as accurately as possible along a 38mm wide (sports tape), 3 metre line with an alternate foot heel-to-toe gait ensuring that they approximate their heel and toe on each step. Once they cross the end of the 3m line, they turn 180 degrees and return to the starting point using the same gait. Athletes fail the test if they step off the line, have a separation between their heel and toe, or if they touch or grab the examiner or an object.

Finger to Nose

"I am going to test your coordination now. Please sit comfortably on the chair with your eyes open and your arm (either right or left) outstretched (shoulder flexed to 90 degrees and elbow and fingers extended), pointing in front of you. When I give a start signal, I would like you to perform five successive finger to nose repetitions using your index finger to touch the tip of the nose, and then return to the starting position, as quickly and as accurately as possible."

References

1. McCrory et al. Consensus Statement On Concussion In Sport – The 5th International Conference On Concussion In Sport Held In Berlin, October 2016. British Journal of Sports Medicine 2017 (available at www.bjsm.bmj.com)

2. Maddocks, DL; Dicker, GD; Saling, MM. The assessment of orientation following concussion in athletes. Clinical Journal of Sport Medicine 1995; 5: 32-33

3. Jennett, B., Bond, M. Assessment of outcome after severe brain damage: a practical scale. Lancet 1975; i: 480-484

4. McCrea M. Standardized mental status testing of acute concussion. Clinical Journal of Sport Medicine. 2001; 11: 176-181

5. Guskiewicz KM. Assessment of postural stability following sport-related concussion. Current Sports Medicine Reports. 2003; 2: 24-30

APPENDIX 10.1 cont'd

CONCUSSION INFORMATION

Any athlete suspected of having a concussion should be removed from play and seek medical evaluation.

Signs to watch for

Problems could arise over the first 24-48 hours. The athlete should not be left alone and must go to a hospital at once if they experience:

- Worsening headache
- Repeated vomiting
- Weakness or numbness in arms or legs
- Drowsiness or inability to be awakened
- Unusual behaviour or confusion or irritable
- Unsteadiness on their feet.
- Inability to recognize people or places
- Seizures (arms and legs jerk uncontrollably)
- Slurred speech

Consult your physician or licensed healthcare professional after a suspected concussion. **Remember, it is better to be safe.**

Rest & Rehabilitation

After a concussion, the athlete should have physical rest and relative cognitive rest for a few days to allow their symptoms to improve. In most cases, after no more than a few days of rest, the athlete should gradually increase their daily activity level as long as their symptoms do not worsen. Once the athlete is able to complete their usual daily activities without concussion-related symptoms, the second step of the return to play/sport progression can be started. The athlete should not return to play/sport until their concussion-related symptoms have resolved and the athlete has successfully returned to full school/learning activities.

When returning to play/sport, the athlete should follow a stepwise, **medically managed exercise progression, with increasing amounts of exercise.** For example:

Graduated Return to Sport Strategy

Exercise step	Functional exercise at each step	Goal of each step
1. Symptom-limited activity	Daily activities that do not provoke symptoms.	Gradual reintroduction of work/school activities.
2. Light aerobic exercise	Walking or stationary cycling at slow to medium pace. No resistance training.	Increase heart rate.
3. Sport-specific exercise	Running or skating drills. No head impact activities.	Add movement.
4. Non-contact training drills	Harder training drills, e.g., passing drills. May start progressive resistance training.	Exercise, coordination, and increased thinking.
5. Full contact practice	Following medical clearance, participate in normal training activities.	Restore confidence and assess functional skills by coaching staff.
6. Return to play/sport	Normal game play.	

In this example, it would be typical to have 24 hours (or longer) for each step of the progression. If any symptoms worsen while exercising, the athlete should go back to the previous step. Resistance training should be added only in the later stages (Stage 3 or 4 at the earliest).

Written clearance should be provided by a healthcare professional before return to play/sport as directed by local laws and regulations.

Graduated Return to School Strategy

Concussion may affect the ability to learn at school. The athlete may need to miss a few days of school after a concussion. When going back to school, some athletes may need to go back gradually and may need to have some changes made to their schedule so that concussion symptoms do not get worse. If a particular activity makes symptoms worse, then the athlete should stop that activity and rest until symptoms get better. To make sure that the athlete can get back to school without problems, it is important that the healthcare provider, parents, caregivers and teachers talk to each other so that everyone knows what the plan is for the athlete to go back to school.

Note: If mental activity does not cause any symptoms, the athlete may be able to skip step 2 and return to school part-time before doing school activities at home first.

Mental Activity	Activity at each step	Goal of each step
1. Daily activities that do not give the athlete symptoms	Typical activities that the athlete does during the day as long as they do not increase symptoms (e.g. reading, texting, screen time). Start with 5-15 minutes at a time and gradually build up.	Gradual return to typical activities.
2. School activities	Homework, reading or other cognitive activities outside of the classroom.	Increase tolerance to cognitive work.
3. Return to school part-time	Gradual introduction of school-work. May need to start with a partial school day or with increased breaks during the day.	Increase academic activities.
4. Return to school full-time	Gradually progress school activities until a full day can be tolerated.	Return to full academic activities and catch up on missed work.

If the athlete continues to have symptoms with mental activity, some other accomodations that can help with return to school may include:

- Starting school later, only going for half days, or going only to certain classes
- More time to finish assignments/tests
- Quiet room to finish assignments/tests
- Not going to noisy areas like the cafeteria, assembly halls, sporting events, music class, shop class, etc.
- Taking lots of breaks during class, homework, tests
- No more than one exam/day
- Shorter assignments
- Repetition/memory cues
- Use of a student helper/tutor
- Reassurance from teachers that the child will be supported while getting better

The athlete should not go back to sports until they are back to school/learning, without symptoms getting significantly worse and no longer needing any changes to their schedule.

Davis GA, *et al. Br J Sports Med* 2017;**0**:1–8. doi:10.1136/bjsports-2017-097506SCAT5

APPENDIX 10.1 cont'd

BJSM Online First, published on April 26, 2017 as 10.1136/bjsports-2017-097492childscat5

To download a clean version of the SCAT tools please visit the journal online (http://dx.doi.org/10.1136/bjsports-2017-097492childscat5)

Child SCAT5©

SPORT CONCUSSION ASSESSMENT TOOL
FOR CHILDREN AGES 5 TO 12 YEARS
FOR USE BY MEDICAL PROFESSIONALS ONLY

supported by

Patient details

Name: _____

DOB: _____

Address: _____

ID number: _____

Examiner: _____

Date of Injury: _____ Time: _____

WHAT IS THE CHILD SCAT5?

The Child SCAT5 is a standardized tool for evaluating concussions designed for use by physicians and licensed healthcare professionals[1].

If you are not a physician or licensed healthcare professional, please use the Concussion Recognition Tool 5 (CRT5). The Child SCAT5 is to be used for evaluating Children aged 5 to 12 years. For athletes aged 13 years and older, please use the SCAT5.

Preseason Child SCAT5 baseline testing can be useful for interpreting post-injury test scores, but not required for that purpose. Detailed instructions for use of the Child SCAT5 are provided on page 7. Please read through these instructions carefully before testing the athlete. Brief verbal instructions for each test are given in italics. The only equipment required for the tester is a watch or timer.

This tool may be freely copied in its current form for distribution to individuals, teams, groups and organizations. It should not be altered in any way, re-branded or sold for commercial gain. Any revision, translation or reproduction in a digital form requires specific approval by the Concussion in Sport Group.

Recognise and Remove

A head impact by either a direct blow or indirect transmission of force can be associated with a serious and potentially fatal brain injury. If there are significant concerns, including any of the red flags listed in Box 1, then activation of emergency procedures and urgent transport to the nearest hospital should be arranged.

Key points

- Any athlete with suspected concussion should be REMOVED FROM PLAY, medically assessed and monitored for deterioration. No athlete diagnosed with concussion should be returned to play on the day of injury.

- If the child is suspected of having a concussion and medical personnel are not immediately available, the child should be referred to a medical facility for urgent assessment.

- Concussion signs and symptoms evolve over time and it is important to consider repeat evaluation in the assessment of concussion.

- The diagnosis of a concussion is a clinical judgment, made by a medical professional. The Child SCAT5 should NOT be used by itself to make, or exclude, the diagnosis of concussion. An athlete may have a a concussion even if their Child SCAT5 is "normal".

Remember:

- The basic principles of first aid (danger, response, airway, breathing, circulation) should be followed.

- Do not attempt to move the athlete (other than that required for airway management) unless trained to do so.

- Assessment for a spinal cord injury is a critical part of the initial on-field assessment.

- Do not remove a helmet or any other equipment unless trained to do so safely.

APPENDIX 10.2 Child SCAT5.

1

IMMEDIATE OR ON-FIELD ASSESSMENT

The following elements should be assessed for all athletes who are suspected of having a concussion prior to proceeding to the neurocognitive assessment and ideally should be done on-field after the first first aid / emergency care priorities are completed.

If any of the "Red Flags" or observable signs are noted after a direct or indirect blow to the head, the athlete should be immediately and safely removed from participation and evaluated by a physician or licensed healthcare professional.

Consideration of transportation to a medical facility should be at the discretion of the physician or licensed healthcare professional.

The GCS is important as a standard measure for all patients and can be done serially if necessary in the event of deterioration in conscious state. The cervical spine exam is a critical step of the immediate assessment, however, it does not need to be done serially.

STEP 1: RED FLAGS

RED FLAGS:

- Neck pain or tenderness
- Double vision
- Weakness or tingling/ burning in arms or legs
- Severe or increasing headache
- Seizure or convulsion
- Loss of consciousness
- Deteriorating conscious state
- Vomiting
- Increasingly restless, agitated or combative

STEP 2: OBSERVABLE SIGNS

Witnessed ☐   Observed on Video ☐

Lying motionless on the playing surface	Y	N
Balance / gait difficulties / motor incoordination: stumbling, slow / laboured movements	Y	N
Disorientation or confusion, or an inability to respond appropriately to questions	Y	N
Blank or vacant look	Y	N
Facial injury after head trauma	Y	N

STEP 3: EXAMINATION
GLASGOW COMA SCALE (GCS)[2]

Time of assessment			
Date of assessment			
Best eye response (E)			
No eye opening	1	1	1
Eye opening in response to pain	2	2	2
Eye opening to speech	3	3	3
Eyes opening spontaneously	4	4	4
Best verbal response (V)			
No verbal response	1	1	1

Name:	
DOB:	
Address:	
ID number:	
Examiner:	
Date:	

Incomprehensible sounds	2	2	2
Inappropriate words	3	3	3
Confused	4	4	4
Oriented	5	5	5
Best motor response (M)			
No motor response	1	1	1
Extension to pain	2	2	2
Abnormal flexion to pain	3	3	3
Flexion / Withdrawal to pain	4	4	4
Localizes to pain	5	5	5
Obeys commands	6	6	6
Glasgow Coma score (E + V + M)			

CERVICAL SPINE ASSESSMENT

Does the athlete report that their neck is pain free at rest?	Y	N
If there is NO neck pain at rest, does the athlete have a full range of ACTIVE pain free movement?	Y	N
Is the limb strength and sensation normal?	Y	N

In a patient who is not lucid or fully conscious, a cervical spine injury should be assumed until proven otherwise.

OFFICE OR OFF-FIELD ASSESSMENT
STEP 1: ATHLETE BACKGROUND

Please note that the neurocognitive assessment should be done in a distraction-free environment with the athlete in a resting state.

Sport / team / school: _____

Date / time of injury: _____

Years of education completed: _____

Age: _____

Gender: M / F / Other

Dominant hand: left / neither / right

How many diagnosed concussions has the athlete had in the past?: _____

When was the most recent concussion?: _____

How long was the recovery (time to being cleared to play) from the most recent concussion?: _____ (days)

Has the athlete ever been:

Hospitalized for a head injury?	Yes	No
Diagnosed / treated for headache disorder or migraines?	Yes	No
Diagnosed with a learning disability / dyslexia?	Yes	No
Diagnosed with ADD / ADHD?	Yes	No
Diagnosed with depression, anxiety or other psychiatric disorder?	Yes	No

Current medications? If yes, please list: _____

© Concussion in Sport Group 2017

Davis GA, et al. Br J Sports Med 2017;**0**:1–8. doi:10.1136/bjsports-2017-097492childscat5

APPENDIX 10.2 cont'd

STEP 2: SYMPTOM EVALUATION

The athlete should be given the symptom form and asked to read this instruction paragraph out loud then complete the symptom scale. For the baseline assessment, the athlete should rate his/ her symptoms based on how he/she typically feels and for the post injury assessment the athlete should rate their symptoms at this point in time.

To be done in a resting state

Please Check: ☐ **Baseline** ☐ **Post-Injury**

Name: _____
DOB: _____
Address: _____
ID number: _____
Examiner: _____
Date: _____

2

Child Report[3]

	Not at all/ Never	A little/ Rarely	Somewhat/ Sometimes	A lot/ Often
I have headaches	0	1	2	3
I feel dizzy	0	1	2	3
I feel like the room is spinning	0	1	2	3
I feel like I'm going to faint	0	1	2	3
Things are blurry when I look at them	0	1	2	3
I see double	0	1	2	3
I feel sick to my stomach	0	1	2	3
My neck hurts	0	1	2	3
I get tired a lot	0	1	2	3
I get tired easily	0	1	2	3
I have trouble paying attention	0	1	2	3
I get distracted easily	0	1	2	3
I have a hard time concentrating	0	1	2	3
I have problems remembering what people tell me	0	1	2	3
I have problems following directions	0	1	2	3
I daydream too much	0	1	2	3
I get confused	0	1	2	3
I forget things	0	1	2	3
I have problems finishing things	0	1	2	3
I have trouble figuring things out	0	1	2	3
It's hard for me to learn new things	0	1	2	3
Total number of symptoms:				of 21
Symptom severity score:				of 63
Do the symptoms get worse with physical activity?		Y		N
Do the symptoms get worse with trying to think?		Y		N

Overall rating for child to answer:

	Very bad									Very good	
On a scale of 0 to 10 (where 10 is normal), how do you feel now?	0	1	2	3	4	5	6	7	8	9	10

If not 10, in way do you feel different?:

Parent Report

The child:

	Not at all/ Never	A little/ Rarely	Somewhat/ Sometimes	A lot/ Often
has headaches	0	1	2	3
feels dizzy	0	1	2	3
has a feeling that the room is spinning	0	1	2	3
feels faint	0	1	2	3
has blurred vision	0	1	2	3
has double vision	0	1	2	3
experiences nausea	0	1	2	3
has a sore neck	0	1	2	3
gets tired a lot	0	1	2	3
gets tired easily	0	1	2	3
has trouble sustaining attention	0	1	2	3
is easily distracted	0	1	2	3
has difficulty concentrating	0	1	2	3
has problems remembering what he/she is told	0	1	2	3
has difficulty following directions	0	1	2	3
tends to daydream	0	1	2	3
gets confused	0	1	2	3
is forgetful	0	1	2	3
has difficulty completing tasks	0	1	2	3
has poor problem solving skills	0	1	2	3
has problems learning	0	1	2	3
Total number of symptoms:				of 21
Symptom severity score:				of 63
Do the symptoms get worse with physical activity?		Y		N
Do the symptoms get worse with mental activity?		Y		N

Overall rating for parent/teacher/ coach/carer to answer

On a scale of 0 to 100% (where 100% is normal), how would you rate the child now?

If not 100%, in what way does the child seem different?

Davis GA, *et al. Br J Sports Med* 2017;**0**:1–8. doi:10.1136/bjsports-2017-097492childscat5

3

3

APPENDIX 10.2 cont'd

3

STEP 3: COGNITIVE SCREENING
Standardized Assessment of Concussion - Child Version (SAC-C)[4]

IMMEDIATE MEMORY

The Immediate Memory component can be completed using the traditional 5-word per trial list or optionally using 10-words per trial to minimise any ceiling effect. All 3 trials must be administered irrespective of the number correct on the first trial. Administer at the rate of one word per second.

Please choose EITHER the 5 or 10 word list groups and circle the specific word list chosen for this test.

I am going to test your memory. I will read you a list of words and when I am done, repeat back as many words as you can remember, in any order. For Trials 2 & 3: I am going to repeat the same list again. Repeat back as many words as you can remember in any order, even if you said the word before.

List	Alternate 5 word lists					Trial 1	Trial 2	Trial 3
A	Finger	Penny	Blanket	Lemon	Insect			
B	Candle	Paper	Sugar	Sandwich	Wagon			
C	Baby	Monkey	Perfume	Sunset	Iron			
D	Elbow	Apple	Carpet	Saddle	Bubble			
E	Jacket	Arrow	Pepper	Cotton	Movie			
F	Dollar	Honey	Mirror	Saddle	Anchor			
				Immediate Memory Score			of 15	
				Time that last trial was completed				

Score (of 5)

List	Alternate 10 word lists					Trial 1	Trial 2	Trial 3
G	Finger	Penny	Blanket	Lemon	Insect			
	Candle	Paper	Sugar	Sandwich	Wagon			
H	Baby	Monkey	Perfume	Sunset	Iron			
	Elbow	Apple	Carpet	Saddle	Bubble			
I	Jacket	Arrow	Pepper	Cotton	Movie			
	Dollar	Honey	Mirror	Saddle	Anchor			
				Immediate Memory Score			of 30	
				Time that last trial was completed				

Score (of 10)

CONCENTRATION

DIGITS BACKWARDS

Please circle the Digit list chosen (A, B, C, D, E, F). Administer at the rate of one digit per second reading DOWN the selected column.

I am going to read a string of numbers and when I am done, you repeat them back to me in reverse order of how I read them to you. For example, if I say 7-1-9, you would say 9-1-7.

Concentration Number Lists (circle one)

List A	List B	List C			
5-2	4-1	4-9	Y	N	0
4-1	9-4	6-2	Y	N	1
4-9-3	5-2-6	1-4-2	Y	N	0
6-2-9	4-1-5	6-5-8	Y	N	1
3-8-1-4	1-7-9-5	6-8-3-1	Y	N	0
3-2-7-9	4-9-6-8	3-4-8-1	Y	N	1
6-2-9-7-1	4-8-5-2-7	4-9-1-5-3	Y	N	0
1-5-2-8-6	6-1-8-4-3	6-8-2-5-1	Y	N	1
7-1-8-4-6-2	8-3-1-9-6-4	3-7-6-5-1-9	Y	N	0
5-3-9-1-4-8	7-2-4-8-5-6	9-2-6-5-1-4	Y	N	1

List D	List E	List F			
2-7	9-2	7-8	Y	N	0
5-9	6-1	5-1	Y	N	1
7-8-2	3-8-2	2-7-1	Y	N	0
9-2-6	5-1-8	4-7-9	Y	N	1
4-1-8-3	2-7-9-3	1-6-8-3	Y	N	0
9-7-2-3	2-1-6-9-	3-9-2-4	Y	N	1
1-7-9-2-6	4-1-8-6-9	2-4-7-5-8	Y	N	0
4-1-7-5-2	9-4-1-7-5	8-3-9-6-4	Y	N	1
2-6-4-8-1-7	6-9-7-3-8-2	5-8-6-2-4-9	Y	N	0
8-4-1-9-3-5	4-2-7-3-9-8	3-1-7-8-2-6	Y	N	1
		Digits Score:			of 5

DAYS IN REVERSE ORDER

Now tell me the days of the week in reverse order. Start with the last day and go backward. So you'll say Sunday, Saturday. Go ahead.

Sunday - Saturday - Friday - Thursday - Wednesday - Tuesday - Monday	0 1
Days Score	of 1
Concentration Total Score (Digits + Days)	of 6

Davis GA, *et al. Br J Sports Med* 2017;**0**:1–8. doi:10.1136/bjsports-2017-097492childscat5

APPENDIX 10.2 cont'd

4

STEP 4: NEUROLOGICAL SCREEN

See the instruction sheet (page 7) for details of
test administration and scoring of the tests.

Can the patient read aloud (e.g. symptom check-list) and follow instructions without difficulty?	Y	N
Does the patient have a full range of pain-free PASSIVE cervical spine movement?	Y	N
Without moving their head or neck, can the patient look side-to-side and up-and-down without double vision?	Y	N
Can the patient perform the finger nose coordination test normally?	Y	N
Can the patient perform tandem gait normally?	Y	N

BALANCE EXAMINATION
Modified Balance Error Scoring System (BESS) testing[5]

Which foot was tested   ☐ Left
(i.e. which is the non-dominant foot)   ☐ Right

Testing surface (hard floor, field, etc.) _____

Footwear (shoes, barefoot, braces, tape, etc.) _____

Condition	Errors
Double leg stance	of 10
Single leg stance (non-dominant foot, 10-12 y/o only)	of 10
Tandem stance (non-dominant foot at back)	of 10
Total Errors	5-9 y/o of 20 10-12 y/o of 30

Name: _____
DOB: _____
Address: _____
ID number: _____
Examiner: _____
Date: _____

5

STEP 5: DELAYED RECALL:

The delayed recall should be performed after 5 minutes have
elapsed since the end of the Immediate Recall section. Score 1
pt. for each correct response.

Do you remember that list of words I read a few times earlier? Tell me as many words from the list as you can remember in any order.

Time Started

Please record each word correctly recalled. Total score equals number of words recalled.

_____
_____
_____

Total number of words recalled accurately: of 5 or of 10

6

STEP 6: DECISION

Domain	Date & time of assessment:		
Symptom number Child report (of 21) Parent report (of 21)			
Symptom severity score Child report (of 63) Parent report (of 63)			
Immediate memory	of 15 of 30	of 15 of 30	of 15 of 30
Concentration (of 6)			
Neuro exam	Normal Abnormal	Normal Abnormal	Normal Abnormal
Balance errors (5-9 y/o of 20) (10-12 y/o of 30)			
Delayed Recall	of 5 of 10	of 5 of 10	of 5 of 10

Date and time of injury: _____

If the athlete is known to you prior to their injury, are they different from their usual self?
☐ Yes ☐ No ☐ Unsure ☐ Not Applicable
(If different, describe why in the clinical notes section)

Concussion Diagnosed?
☐ Yes ☐ No ☐ Unsure ☐ Not Applicable

If re-testing, has the athlete improved?
☐ Yes ☐ No ☐ Unsure ☐ Not Applicable

I am a physician or licensed healthcare professional and I have personally administered or supervised the administration of this Child SCAT5.

Signature: _____
Name: _____
Title: _____
Registration number (if applicable): _____
Date: _____

SCORING ON THE CHILD SCAT5 SHOULD NOT BE USED AS A STAND-ALONE METHOD TO DIAGNOSE CONCUSSION, MEASURE RECOVERY OR MAKE DECISIONS ABOUT AN ATHLETE'S READINESS TO RETURN TO COMPETITION AFTER CONCUSSION.

Davis GA, *et al. Br J Sports Med* 2017;**0**:1–8. doi:10.1136/bjsports-2017-097492childscat5   5

APPENDIX 10.2 cont'd

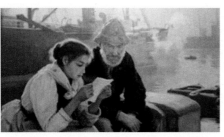

Name:	_____
DOB:	_____
Address:	_____
ID number:	_____
Examiner:	_____
Date:	_____

For the Neurological Screen (page 5), if the child cannot read, ask him/her to describe what they see in this picture.

CLINICAL NOTES:

_____

_____

_____

_____

_____

_____

✂ ·

Concussion injury advice for the child and parents/carergivers

(To be given to the person monitoring the concussed child)

This child has had an injury to the head and needs to be carefully watched for the next 24 hours by a responsible adult.

If you notice any change in behavior, vomiting, dizziness, worsening headache, double vision or excessive drowsiness, please call an ambulance to take the child to hospital immediately.

Other important points:

Following concussion, the child should rest for at least 24 hours.

- The child should not use a computer, internet or play video games if these activities make symptoms worse.

- The child should not be given any medications, including pain killers, unless prescribed by a medical doctor.

- The child should not go back to school until symptoms are improving.

- The child should not go back to sport or play until a doctor gives permission.

Clinic phone number: _____

Patient's name: _____

Date / time of injury: _____

Date / time of medical review: _____

Healthcare Provider: _____

© Concussion in Sport Group 2017

Contact details or stamp

APPENDIX 10.2 cont'd

INSTRUCTIONS

Words in *Italics* throughout the Child SCAT5 are the instructions given to the athlete by the clinician

Symptom Scale

In situations where the symptom scale is being completed after exercise, it should still be done in a resting state, at least 10 minutes post exercise.

At Baseline	On the day of injury	On all subsequent days
• The child is to complete the Child Report, according to how he/she feels today, and	• The child is to complete the Child Report, according to how he/she feels now.	• The child is to complete the Child Report, according to how he/she feels today, and
• The parent/carer is to complete the Parent Report according to how the child has been over the previous week.	• If the parent is present, and has had time to assess the child on the day of injury, the parent completes the Parent Report according to how the child appears now.	• The parent/carer is to complete the Parent Report according to how the child has been over the previous 24 hours.

For Total number of symptoms, maximum possible is 21

For Symptom severity score, add all scores in table, maximum possible is 21 x 3 = 63

Standardized Assessment of Concussion Child Version (SAC-C)

Immediate Memory

Choose one of the 5-word lists. Then perform 3 trials of immediate memory using this list. Complete all 3 trials regardless of score on previous trials.

"I am going to test your memory. I will read you a list of words and when I am done, repeat back as many words as you can remember, in any order." The words must be read at a rate of one word per second.

OPTION: The literature suggests that the Immediate Memory has a notable ceiling effect when a 5-word list is used. (In younger children, use the 5-word list). In settings where this ceiling is prominent the examiner may wish to make the task more difficult by incorporating two 5-word groups for a total of 10 words per trial. In this case the maximum score per trial is 10 with a total trial maximum of 30.

Trials 2 & 3 MUST be completed regardless of score on trial 1 & 2.

Trials 2 & 3: *"I am going to repeat the same list again. Repeat back as many words as you can remember in any order, even if you said the word before."*

Score 1 pt. for each correct response. Total score equals sum across all 3 trials. Do NOT inform the athlete that delayed recall will be tested.

Concentration

Digits backward

Choose one column only, from List A, B, C, D, E or F, and administer those digits as follows:

"I am going to read you some numbers and when I am done, you say them back to me backwards, in reverse order of how I read them to you. For example, if I say 7-1, you would say 1-7."

If correct, circle "Y" for correct and go to next string length. If incorrect, circle "N" for the first string length and read trial 2 in the same string length. One point possible for each string length. Stop after incorrect on both trials (2 N's) in a string length. The digits should be read at the rate of one per second.

Days of the week in reverse order

"Now tell me the days of the week in reverse order. Start with Sunday and go backward. So you'll say Sunday, Saturday ... Go ahead"

1 pt. for entire sequence correct

Delayed Recall

The delayed recall should be performed after at least 5 minutes have elapsed since the end of the Immediate Recall section.

"Do you remember that list of words I read a few times earlier? Tell me as many words from the list as you can remember in any order."

Circle each word correctly recalled. Total score equals number of words recalled.

Neurological Screen

Reading

The child is asked to read a paragraph of text from the instructions in the Child SCAT5. For children who can not read, they are asked to describe what they see in a photograph or picture, such as that on page 6 of the Child SCAT5.

Modified Balance Error Scoring System (mBESS)[5] testing

These instructions are to be read by the person administering the Child SCAT5, and each balance task should be demonstrated to the child. The child should then be asked to copy what the examiner demonstrated.

Each of 20-second trial/stance is scored by counting the number of errors. The This balance testing is based on a modified version of the Balance Error Scoring System (BESS)[5].

A stopwatch or watch with a second hand is required for this testing.

"I am now going to test your balance. Please take your shoes off, roll up your pants above your ankle (if applicable), and remove any ankle taping (if applicable). This test will consist of two different parts."

OPTION: For further assessment, the same 3 stances can be performed on a surface of medium density foam (e.g., approximately 50cm x 40cm x 6cm).

(a) Double leg stance:

The first stance is standing with the feet together with hands on hips and with eyes closed. The child should try to maintain stability in that position for 20 seconds. You should inform the child that you will be counting the number of times the child moves out of this position. You should start timing when the child is set and the eyes are closed.

(b) Tandem stance:

Instruct or show the child how to stand heel-to-toe with the non-dominant foot in the back. Weight should be evenly distributed across both feet. Again, the child should try to maintain stability for 20 seconds with hands on hips and eyes closed. You should inform the child that you will be counting the number of times the child moves out of this position. If the child stumbles out of this position, instruct him/her to open the eyes and return to the start position and continue balancing. You should start timing when the child is set and the eyes are closed.

(c) Single leg stance (10-12 year olds only):

"If you were to kick a ball, which foot would you use? [This will be the dominant foot] Now stand on your other foot. You should bend your other leg and hold it up (show the child). Again, try to stay in that position for 20 seconds with your hands on your hips and your eyes closed. I will be counting the number of times you move out of this position. If you move out of this position, open your eyes and return to the start position and keep balancing. I will start timing when you are set and have closed your eyes."

Balance testing – types of errors

1. Hands lifted off iliac crest
2. Opening eyes
3. Step, stumble, or fall
4. Moving hip into > 30 degrees abduction
5. Lifting forefoot or heel
6. Remaining out of test position > 5 sec

Each of the 20-second trials is scored by counting the errors, or deviations from the proper stance, accumulated by the child. The examiner will begin counting errors only after the child has assumed the proper start position. The modified BESS is calculated by adding one error point for each error during the 20-second tests. The maximum total number of errors for any single condition is 10. If a child commits multiple errors simultaneously, only one error is recorded but the child should quickly return to the testing position, and counting should resume once subject is set. Children who are unable to maintain the testing procedure for a minimum of five seconds at the start are assigned the highest possible score, ten, for that testing condition.

Tandem Gait

Instruction for the examiner - Demonstrate the following to the child:

The child is instructed to stand with their feet together behind a starting line (the test is best done with footwear removed). Then, they walk in a forward direction as quickly and as accurately as possible along a 38mm wide (sports tape), 3 metre line with an alternate foot heel-to-toe gait ensuring that they approximate their heel and toe on each step. Once they cross the end of the 3m line, they turn 180 degrees and return to the starting point using the same gait. Children fail the test if they step off the line, have a separation between their heel and toe, or if they touch or grab the examiner or an object.

Finger to Nose

The tester should demonstrate it to the child.

"I am going to test your coordination now. Please sit comfortably on the chair with your eyes open and your arm (either right or left) outstretched (shoulder flexed to 90 degrees and elbow and fingers extended). When I give a start signal, I would like you to perform five successive finger to nose repetitions using your index finger to touch the tip of the nose as quickly and as accurately as possible."

Scoring: 5 correct repetitions in < 4 seconds = 1

Note for testers: Children fail the test if they do not touch their nose, do not fully extend their elbow or do not perform five repetitions.

References

1. McCrory et al. Consensus Statement On Concussion In Sport – The 5th International Conference On Concussion In Sport Held In Berlin, October 2016. British Journal of Sports Medicine 2017 (available at www.bjsm.bmj.com)

2. Jennett, B., Bond, M. Assessment of outcome after severe brain damage: a practical scale. Lancet 1975; i: 480-484

3. Ayr, L.K., Yeates, K.O., Taylor, H.G., Brown, M. Dimensions of postconcussive symptoms in children with mild traumatic brain injuries. Journal of the International Neuropsychological Society. 2009; 15:19–30

4. McCrea M. Standardized mental status testing of acute concussion. Clinical Journal of Sports Medicine. 2001; 11: 176-181

5. Guskiewicz KM. Assessment of postural stability following sport-related concussion. Current Sports Medicine Reports. 2003; 2: 24-30

APPENDIX 10.2 cont'd

CONCUSSION INFORMATION

If you think you or a teammate has a concussion, tell your coach/trainer/parent right away so that you can be taken out of the game. You or your teammate should be seen by a doctor as soon as possible. YOU OR YOUR TEAMMATE SHOULD NOT GO BACK TO PLAY/SPORT THAT DAY.

Signs to watch for

Problems can happen over the first 24-48 hours. You or your teammate should not be left alone and must go to a hospital right away if any of the following happens:

- New headache, or headache gets worse
- Neck pain that gets worse
- Becomes sleepy/drowsy or can't be woken up
- Cannot recognise people or places

- Feeling sick to your stomach or vomiting
- Acting weird/strange, seems/feels confused, or is irritable
- Has any seizures (arms and/or legs jerk uncontrollably)

- Has weakness, numbness or tingling (arms, legs or face)
- Is unsteady walking or standing
- Talking is slurred
- Cannot understand what someone is saying or directions

Consult your physician or licensed healthcare professional after a suspected concussion. **Remember, it is better to be safe.**

Graduated Return to Sport Strategy

After a concussion, the child should rest physically and mentally for a few days to allow symptoms to get better. In most cases, after a few days of rest, they can gradually increase their daily activity level as long as symptoms don't get worse. Once they are able to do their usual daily activities without symptoms, the child should gradually increase exercise in steps, guided by the healthcare professional (see below).

The athlete should not return to play/sport the day of injury.

NOTE: An initial period of a few days of both cognitive ("thinking") and physical rest is recommended before beginning the Return to Sport progression.

Exercise step	Functional exercise at each step	Goal of each step
1. Symptom-limited activity	Daily activities that do not provoke symptoms.	Gradual reintroduction of work/school activities.
2. Light aerobic exercise	Walking or stationary cycling at slow to medium pace. No resistance training.	Increase heart rate.
3. Sport-specific exercise	Running or skating drills. No head impact activities.	Add movement.
4. Non-contact training drills	Harder training drills, e.g., passing drills. May start progressive resistance training.	Exercise, coordination, and increased thinking.
5. Full contact practice	Following medical clearance, participate in normal training activities.	Restore confidence and assess functional skills by coaching staff.
6. Return to play/sport	Normal game play.	

There should be at least 24 hours (or longer) for each step of the progression. If any symptoms worsen while exercising, the athlete should go back to the previous step. Resistance training should be added only in the later stages (Stage 3 or 4 at the earliest). The athlete should not return to sport until the concussion symptoms have gone, they have successfully returned to full school/learning activities, and the healthcare professional has given the child written permission to return to sport.

If the child has symptoms for more than a month, they should ask to be referred to a healthcare professional who is an expert in the management of concussion.

Graduated Return to School Strategy

Concussion may affect the ability to learn at school. The child may need to miss a few days of school after a concussion, but the child's doctor should help them get back to school after a few days. When going back to school, some children may need to go back gradually and may need to have some changes made to their schedule so that concussion symptoms don't get a lot worse. If a particular activity makes symptoms a lot worse, then the child should stop that activity and rest until symptoms get better. To make sure that the child can get back to school without problems, it is important that the health care provider, parents/caregivers and teachers talk to each other so that everyone knows what the plan is for the child to go back to school.

Note: If mental activity does not cause any symptoms, the child may be able to return to school part-time without doing school activities at home first.

Mental Activity	Activity at each step	Goal of each step
1. Daily activities that do not give the child symptoms	Typical activities that the child does during the day as long as they do not increase symptoms (e.g. reading, texting, screen time). Start with 5-15 minutes at a time and gradually build up.	Gradual return to typical activities.
2. School activities	Homework, reading or other cognitive activities outside of the classroom.	Increase tolerance to cognitive work.
3. Return to school part-time	Gradual introduction of schoolwork. May need to start with a partial school day or with increased breaks during the day.	Increase academic activities.
4. Return to school full-time	Gradually progress school activities until a full day can be tolerated.	Return to full academic activities and catch up on missed work.

If the child continues to have symptoms with mental activity, some other things that can be done to help with return to school may include:

- Starting school later, only going for half days, or going only to certain classes
- More time to finish assignments/tests
- Quiet room to finish assignments/tests
- Not going to noisy areas like the cafeteria, assembly halls, sporting events, music class, shop class, etc.

- Taking lots of breaks during class, homework, tests
- No more than one exam/day
- Shorter assignments
- Repetition/memory cues
- Use of a student helper/tutor
- Reassurance from teachers that the child will be supported while getting better

The child should not go back to sports until they are back to school/learning, without symptoms getting significantly worse and no longer needing any changes to their schedule.

APPENDIX 10.2 cont'd

References

1. Black LI, Zammitti EP, Hoffman HJ, Li C-M. *Parental Report of Significant Head Injuries in Children Aged 3–17 Years: United States, 2016.* Hyattsville, MD: National Center for Health Statistics; 2018.

2. Haarbauer-Krupa J, Arbogast KB, Metzger KB, et al. Variations in mecahnisms of injury for youth with concusison. *J Pediatr.* 2018;197:241-248.e1.

3. Brown NJ, Mannix RC, O'Brien MJ, Gostine D, Collins MW, Meehan WP III. Effect of cognitive activity level on duration of post-concussion symptoms. *Pediatrics.* 2014;133(2):e299-e304.

4. Gilchrist J, Thomase K, Xu L, McGuire L, Coronado V. Nonfatal traumatic brain injuries related to sports and recreation activities among persons aged <19 years – United States 2001-2009. *MMWR Morb Mortal Wkly Rep.* 2011;60:1337-1342.

5. Pfister T, Pfister K, Hagel B, Ghali WA, Ronksley PE. The incidence of concussion in youth sports: a systematic review and meta-analysis. *Br J Sports Med.* 2016;50(5):292-297.

6. Meehan WP III, d'Hemecourt P, Collins CL, Comstock RD. Assessment and management of sport-related concussions in United States high schools. *Am J Sports Med.* 2011;39(11):2304-2310.

7. Halstead ME, Walter KD, Council on Sports Medicine and Fitness. American Academy of Pediatrics. Clinical report – Sport-related concussion in children and adolescents. *Pediatrics.* 2010;126(3):597-615.

8. Comstock R, Pierpoint L, Erkenbeck A, Bihl J. *National High School Sports-Related Injury Surveillance Study: 2016-2017 School Year.* Aurora, CO: Colorado School of Public Health; 2018.

9. McCrory P, Feddermann-Demont N, Dvorak J, et al. What is the definition of sports-related concussion: a systematic review. *Br J Sports Med.* 2017;51(11):877-887.

10. Giza CC, Hovda DA. The new neurometabolic cascade of concussion. *Neurosurgery.* 2014;75(suppl 4):S24-S33.

11. McCrory P, Meeuwisse W, Dvorak J, et al. Consensus statement on concussion in sport – The 5th international conference on concussion in sport held in Berlin, October 2016. *Br J Sports Med.* 2017;51:838-847. doi:10.1136/bjsports-2017-097699.

12. Iverson GL, Silverberg ND, Mannix R, et al. Factors associated with concussion-like symptom reporting in high school athletes. *JAMA Pediatr.* 2015;169(12):1132-1140.

13. McGinley AD, Master CL, Zonfrillo MR. Sports-related head injuries in adolescents: a comprehensive update. *Adolesc Med State Art Rev.* 2015;26(3):491-506.

14. Waninger KN, Swartz EE. Cervical spine injury management in the helmeted athlete. *Curr Sports Med Rep.* 2011;10(1):45-49.

15. Spine and Spinal Cord Trauma. *Manual of Advanced Trauma Life Support.* 7 ed. Chicago, IL: American College of Surgeons; 2004:177.

16. Davis GA, Purcell L, Schneider KJ, et al. The child sport concussion assessment tool 5th edition (child SCAT5): background and rationale. *Br J Sports Med.* 2017;51(11):859-861.

17. Echemendia RJ, Meeuwisse W, McCrory P, et al. The sport concussion assessment tool 5th edition (SCAT5): background and rationale. *Br J Sports Med.* 2017;51(11):848-850.

18. Brooks A, MacDonald K, Wasylyk N, et al. Normative values for the SCAT3 IN adolescent athletes. *Br J Sports Med* 2014;48:573-574.

19. Adam Z, Marcinak J, Stuart H, Frank W. Normative values of major SCAT2 and SCAT3 components for a College athlete population, *Appl Neuropsychol Adult.* 2015;22(2):132-140. doi:10.1080/23279095.2013.867265.

20. Brooks MA, Snedden TR, Mixis B, Hetzel S, McGuine TA. Establishing baseline normative values for the child sport concussion assessment tool. *JAMA Pediatr.* 2017;171(7):670-677. doi:10.1001/jamapediatrics.2017.0592.

21. Harmon KG, Drezner JA, Gammons M, et al. American Medical Society for Sports Medicine position statement: concussion in sport. *Br J Sports Med.* 2013;47(1):15-26.

22. Bell DR, Guskiewicz KM, Clark MA, Padua DA. Systematic review of the balance error scoring system. *Sports Health.* 2011;3(3):287-295.

23. Committee on Sports-Related Concussions in Youth; Board on Children, Youth, and Families; Institute of Medicine; National Research Council; Graham R, Rivara FP, Ford MA, Mason Spicer C. *Sports-Related Concussions in Youth: Improving the Science, Changing the Culture.* Washington, DC: National Academies Press; 2014.

24. Mucha A, Collins MW, Elbin RJ, et al. A brief vestibular/ocular motor screening (VOMS) assessment to evaluate concussions: preliminary findings. *Am J Sports Med.* 2014;42:2479-2486.

25. Master CL, Scheiman M, Gallaway M, et al. Vision diagnoses are common after concussion in adolescents. *Clin Pediatr (Phila)*. 2016;55(3):260-267.
26. Corwin DJ, Wiebe DJ, Zonfrillo MR, et al. Vestibular deficits following youth concussion. *J Pediatr*. 2015;166(5):1221-1225.
27. Mayer AR, Wertz C, Ryman SG, et al. Neurosensory deficits vary as a function of point of care in pediatric mild traumatic brain injury. *J Neurotrauma*. 2018;35(10):1178-1184.
28. Master CL, Master SR, Wiebe DJ, et al. Vision and vestibular system dysfunction predicts prolonged concussion recovery in children. *Clin J Sport Med*. 2018;28(2):139-145.
29. Darby DG, Master CL, Grady MF. Computerized neurocognitive testing in the medical evaluation of sports concussion. *Pediatr Ann*. 2012;41(9):371-376.
30. Gaudet CE, Weyandt LL. Immediate Post-Concussion and Cognitive Testing (ImPACT): a systematic review of the prevalence and assessment of invalid performance. *Clin Neuropsychol*. 2017;31(1):43-58.
31. Alsalaheen B, Stockdale K, Pechumer D, Broglio SP. Validity of the immediate post concussion assessment and cognitive testing (ImPACT). *Sports Med*. 2016;46:1487-1501.
32. Broglio SP, Macciocchi SN, Ferrara MS. Sensitivity of the concussion assessment battery. *Neurosurgery*. 2007;60(6):1050-1057; discussion 1057-1058.
33. Kriz PK, Mannix R, Taylor AM, Ruggieri D, Meehan WP III. Neurocognitive deficits of concussed adolescent athletes at self-reported symptom resolution in the Zurich guidelines era. *Orthop J Sports Med*. 2017;5(11):2325967117737307.
34. Leddy JJ, Haider MN, Ellis M, Willer BS. Exercise is medicine for concussion. *Curr Sports Med Rep*. 2018;17(8):262-270. doi:10.1249/JSR.0000000000000505.

11

Spine and Spinal Conditions

Amy L. McIntosh and Bryan Tompkins

Overview

Spinal conditions in growing children are varied and include a variety of disorders. These may present with deformity, pain, physical limitations, and neurological compromise. A good understanding of the basic growth and development of the spine is necessary to diagnose this vast array of spinal conditions in pediatric patients. In this chapter, we discuss the most common conditions affecting the pediatric population.

Torticollis

Torticollis is derived from Latin, meaning twisted neck and is most often associated with conditions involving the cervical spine. The condition may be congenital or present shortly after birth (usually not painful) or can be late onset (often associated with pain from infection, tumor, inflammation, or trauma). Plagiocephaly, an asymmetric head, might also develop in congenital torticollis due to abnormal pressure on the immature skull from the fixed head position of the infant (**Figure 11.1**). Plagiocephaly usually does not occur in those patients who have late onset torticollis as the skull is usually matured by then.

Over time, the skull can be permanently altered as a result of its persistent positioning (**Figure 11.2**).

There are several causes of nonpainful congenital torticollis. The most common is known as congenital muscular torticollis (CMT) and is due to tightness of the sternocleidomastoid muscle (SCM) (**Figure 11.3**) and may be a result of perinatal trauma to the muscle that causes it to become fibrotic.

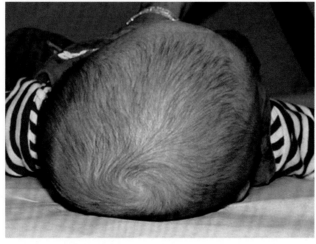

FIGURE 11.1 Flattening of the skull (plagiocephaly) can result from positioning of the immature skull (with open cranial sutures) as a result of tight sternocleidomastoid muscle (SCM).

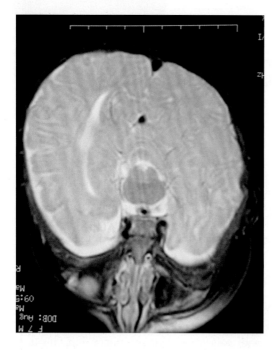

FIGURE 11.2 An MRI of the brain was obtained in a child with long-standing torticollis. There was no sign of tumor but the skull was obviously misshaped.

CMT becomes apparent within the first few months after birth. Other causes for congenital torticollis can be related to vertebral bone abnormalities such as failure of formation and segmentation. These bony abnormalities can be complex involving osseous fusions and can be seen in Klippel-Feil syndrome, which is known as a triad of findings (webbed neck, low hairline, and cervical spine fusions) (**Figure 11.4**). The fixed tilted position of the head and lack of neck rotation are a result of varying degrees of synostosis between the cervical vertebrae.

Late onset torticollis can be painful or nonpainful. Atlantoaxial rotatory displacement (AARD) is the most common cause of painful acquired torticollis and can follow trauma or infection of the neck and pharynx. Torticollis with oropharyngeal infection is felt to be a result of tissue laxity from associated inflammation in the surrounding neck tissues and is commonly referred to as Grisel syndrome. More unusual causes for acquired torticollis include juvenile idiopathic arthritis, tumors of the neck or brain, ligament laxity (eg, Down syndrome), and other neurological conditions (**Figure 11.5**).

Physical Examination for Torticollis

As these conditions often involve newborns, a calm and relaxed environment is preferred to best assess the full extent of the child's cervical motion. A crying or upset baby may resist the examiner when attempting to range the child's neck. It can be incredibly hard to determine if a tight SCM is

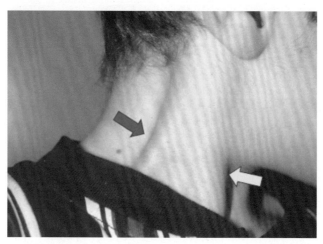

FIGURE 11.3 The sternocleidomastoid muscle (SCM) originates from the mastoid and has two insertions on the medial clavicle (blue arrow) and the sternum (yellow arrow).

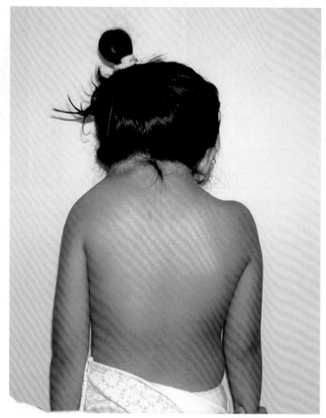

FIGURE 11.4 This child with Klippel-Feil syndrome has classic webbing of the neck with a low hairline.

due to fibrosis or is merely a normal muscle that is contracted by an irritated infant. Palpation of the neck can also give clues as to the cause. In CMT, a knot may be palpated in the SCM muscle (**Figure 11.6**).

It is important to remember that the absence of the mass does not rule out a muscular cause for the torticollis. A good examination of the throat and neck is important to detect swelling in the neck or palpable lymph nodes, which might be a clue of an infectious cause for the torticollis as in the case of Grisel syndrome.

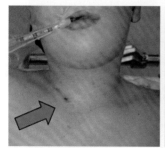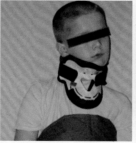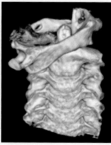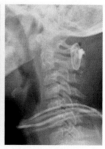

FIGURE 11.5 This eight-year-old boy was in a motor vehicle accident and had a severe laceration to his right neck platysma and deeper muscles (blue arrow). His initial trauma X-rays and CT scan were normal. Six weeks later, he developed AARD (note rotation of C1 on C2) that persisted despite cervical collar and cervical traction. Eventually, he needed posterior spine fusion.

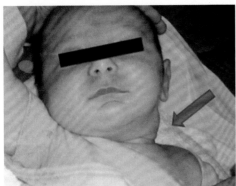
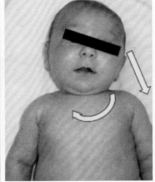
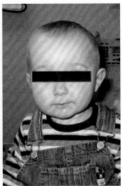

FIGURE 11.6 This newborn was delivered with forceps and 2 months after delivery, he was noted to have torticollis with tilt toward the affected side (yellow arrow) and rotation to the contralateral side (curved yellow arrow). Palpation of his sternocleidomastoid muscle (SCM) demonstrated a small mass (red arrow) and swelling which some have called a pseudotumor. After a year of therapy, his torticollis had resolved but mild plagiocephaly persisted.

As children get older, it can be easier to examine the child and detect the tightened SCM (**Figure 11.7**).

It is important to note the direction in which the head is tilted. In CMT, the head always tilts toward the affected side and is rotated away from the involved SCM (**Figure 11.8**).

The next step is to determine the range of motion of the neck, which may not be possible in late onset torticollis, as a result of pain from inflammation or trauma. When examining an infant, place the parent or favorite toy opposite the side of the resting neck position. The child will want to turn toward the parent or object, which may help determine the amount of rotation opposite the deformity. Serial measurements at each visit of the amount of motion in each plane are important to determine the amount of improvement and ultimately the success of treatment.

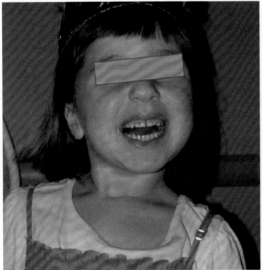
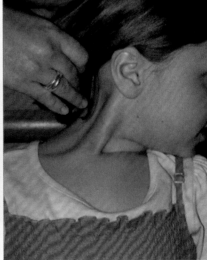

FIGURE 11.7 This child with long-standing congenital muscular torticollis (CMT) has a very tight sternocleidomastoid muscle (SCM) that becomes apparent as the head is tilted to the opposite side.

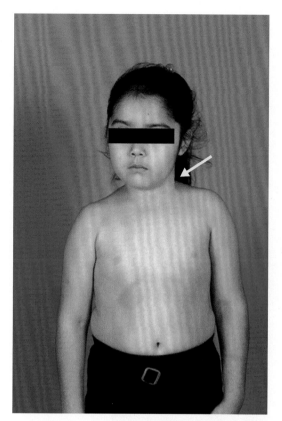

FIGURE 11.8 This child has obvious sternocleido-mastoid muscle (SCM) contracture that tilts the head toward the affected side with rotation away.

Older patients may be able to follow directions allowing determination of active range of motion but in the younger patients, only a passive examination of motion will be possible. Cervical motion is measured in terms of neck flexion, extension, left and right rotation, and side-to-side bending (**Figure 11.9**).

Depending on the age of the patient, a more thorough neurological examination should be performed as well. Deficits in upper and lower extremity strength and sensory examinations can point to an underlying neurological cause for the torticollis. It is important to remember that late-onset torticollis can be the initial finding for intraspinal neoplasia. Ocular and visual testing may be appropriate in certain settings as well (**Figure 11.10**).

Children with congenital cervical spine fusions usually do not have classic rotation in one direction with tilt in the other. More often, they have tilt with symmetric limitation of motion without any muscle tightness. When evaluating a child with congenital cervical fusions, it is

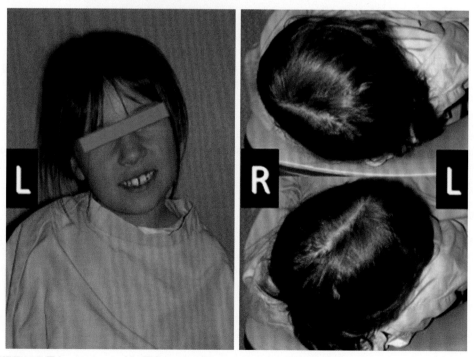

FIGURE 11.9 This seven-year-old with long-standing conmuscular torticollis (CMT) has a tight left sternocleidomastoid muscle (SCM) muscle, which limits rotation to the left.

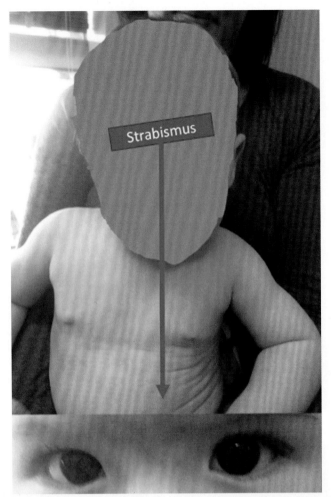

FIGURE 11.10 Part of the differential diagnosis for torticollis includes strabismus as a result of ocular nerve palsies. This child with subtle strabismus and torticollis is referred to ophthalmology for confirmation and treatment if needed.

important to remember the association with Klippel-Feil deformity as well as the possibility of vertebral abnormalities in the thoracic and lumbar spine. These children can occasionally have an associated small, elevated scapula (Sprengel anomaly) which then limits their ability to fully abduct their arm due to abnormal scapula-thoracic mechanics (**Figure 11.11**).

Additional Testing and Treatment

As mentioned, infants with a congenital torticollis can be difficult to examine and it can be challenging to confirm that it is a tight SCM from CMT or is a result of congenital cervical fusions. A tight SCM can respond to treatment with physical therapy where head tilt from bony fusions do not. It is a good idea to order cervical spine X-rays as well as a lateral skull X-ray. The later film is needed to properly visualize the upper cervical spine.

In later onset torticollis, the differential diagnosis can include neoplasia in the brain or spinal cord and AARD from infection or trauma. X-rays are ordered to look for fractures, displacement, and

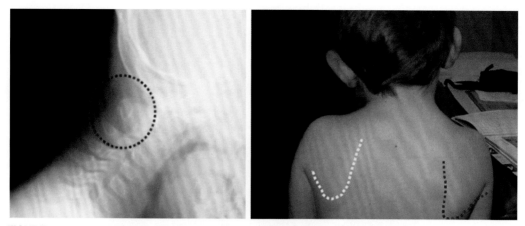

FIGURE 11.11 This child with congenital cervical fusion (red circle) has head tilt without rotation and a mild left Sprengel deformity is noted. The left scapula (outlined in yellow) is smaller and elevated when compared to the normal scapula outlined in red.

soft tissue swelling. Laboratory markers for infection may be needed if an infectious cause is considered. Advanced imaging such as an MRI is needed if neoplasia is suspected. Dynamic CT scan can be obtained to document rotatory subluxation (**Figure 11.12**).

Treatment depends on the cause of the torticollis. For CMT, a program of physical therapy is initially started to stretch the tightened SCM (**Figure 11.7**). Occasionally, surgical release of the SCM is needed if torticollis does not resolve with more conservative methods (**Figure 11.13**).

Treatment for Klippel-Feil syndrome and congenital bony abnormalities is often observation. Surgical treatment is rarely needed and only for progressive deformities. In terms of AARD, supportive treatment with a soft collar is sometimes all that is needed in the acute presentation. More chronic or resistive presentations may result in surgical stabilization (**Figure 11.5**).

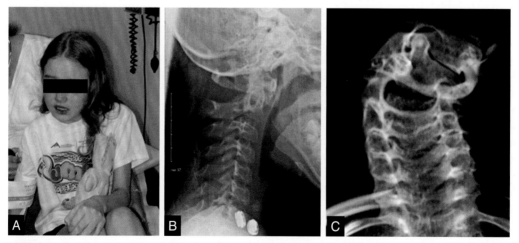

FIGURE 11.12 This child with acute Grisel syndrome has radiographs (B) which suggest rotatory subluxation that is confirmed via CT scan (C).

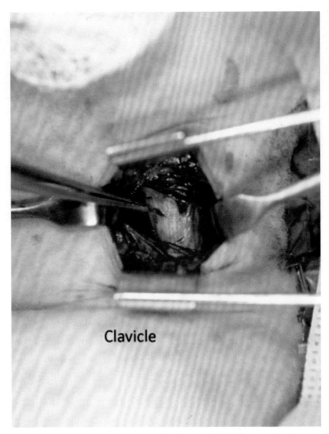

Clavicle

FIGURE 11.13 Fibrotic sternocleidomastoid muscle (SCM) muscle prior to release.

● *Scoliosis*

Scoliosis is a curvature in the spinal column that creates a "C"-shaped single curve or "S"-shaped double curve, when viewed from behind (**Figure 11.14**).

It is important to remember that "*scoliosis*" is not a diagnosis per se; it is a term that describes a curved spine detected on physical examination and that measures more than 10° on radiographs. Many different conditions can cause scoliosis and the first task in the treatment is a detailed history and physical examination to detect the cause and to understand the natural history. Some cases worsen with time and can result in problems such as abnormal appearance in posture, increasing back pain as one ages, and in the worst cases, interference with heart and lung function. Idiopathic (no underlying cause) scoliosis is the most common type of scoliosis, and it occurs in 2% to 3% of the adolescent population, usually affecting young people between the ages of 10 and 16. Scoliosis detection is usually earlier in girls than in boys—generally, ages 10 to 14 for girls and 12 to 16 for boys.

Clinical Features—Initial Signs and Symptoms

Adolescents with scoliosis do not usually seek medical evaluation because of back discomfort but rather because of some physical aspect of their deformity, such as a high shoulder, one-sided prominence of a scapula or breast, elevated or protuberant iliac crest, or asymmetry in flank creases and the trunk (**Figure 11.15**). Except for being noticed personally by the adolescent, these findings are often first appreciated during school screening programs for scoliosis or during back-to-school and sports physical examinations by the family physician.

Similar to the incidence of back pain in adolescents without scoliosis, back pain can occur in individuals with idiopathic scoliosis. Nearly 32% of adolescents with idiopathic scoliosis complain of back discomfort at some point (23% at initial evaluation and 9% during the period of observation).[1] When an adolescent with presumed idiopathic scoliosis has back pain, a careful history should be obtained, a thorough physical examination performed, and plain radiographs ordered. If findings on this initial evaluation are normal, a diagnosis of idiopathic scoliosis can be made, the scoliosis can be treated appropriately, and nonsurgical treatment of the back pain can be initiated. It is not necessary to perform extensive diagnostic studies in every adolescent with scoliosis and occasional mild back pain. Simply educating the family that just because their child has scoliosis does not mean they are related may be all that is required. Further evaluation with an MRI of the spine and spinal cord may be useful if the patient's back pain becomes a dominant feature (night pain, pain at rest, pain that radiates down the leg) and significantly restricts normal activities, if they have systemic changes in health (fatigue, weight loss, fever), or if they have findings on physical examination that are abnormal (foot deformity, abnormal reflexes, spine imbalance, weakness).

While respiratory symptoms are uncommon in patients with adolescent idiopathic scoliosis (AIS), pulmonary assessments have identified subclinical yet measurable mild restrictive lung disease in one-third of patients with idiopathic scoliosis. When the breathing kinematics of the chest wall and spine is evaluated, individuals with AIS have decreased motion in comparison to healthy individuals. The effect on lung function is dependent on the magnitude of deformity. Studies have shown that clinically significant cardiopulmonary compromise does not usually occur until the magnitude of the curve approaches 80° to 100°. When thoracic lordosis (exceeding 20°) significantly narrows the anteroposterior dimensions of the chest, vital capacity becomes less than 45%.

In summary, AIS has a small measurable effect on lung function that patients do not notice in all but the largest of curves. Problems with respiration do not exist unless the curves reach 100° (**Figure 11.15**) or unless there is significant pulmonary comorbid conditions.

Neurologic deficits are also rare in individuals with AIS, yet a detailed physical examination can yield findings that can identify structural spinal cord abnormalities that can be present in what appears to be idiopathic scoliosis in an apparently normal child. An adolescent with a large Chiari malformation (**Figure 11.16**) may describe symptoms such as persistent neck pain, frequent headaches, difficulty swallowing, ataxia, or weakness. Unilateral foot deformities may be associated with tethering of the spinal cord (**Figure 11.17**). In addition, the convexity of thoracic curves in AIS is normally directed to the right; abnormal left thoracic curves are more common in those with an underlying syrinx (**Figure 11.18**). In addition, if any neurologic deficits are found on examination, appropriate imaging of the neural axis is undertaken.

Physical Examination for Scoliosis

Physical examination of an adolescent with idiopathic scoliosis should be performed with the patient properly draped. The patient may be dressed in underpants and an examination gown open at the back. The patient's entire back, including the shoulders and iliac crests, must be visible. The skin is inspected closely for abnormalities such as café-au-lait spots (**Figure 11.19**).

Other cutaneous aspects include midline hemangiomas, hair tufts, and dimpling in the lumbosacral region. Any of these surface findings may indicate the presence of an underlying spinal cord abnormality such as a tethered cord or diastematomyelia (this term describes a spinal cord that is split by fibrous, cartilaginous, or bony tissue). The spinous processes are palpated from the cervical region to the sacrum for any deficiencies or areas of discomfort. Occasionally, absence of a spinous process is noted, which usually corresponds to spina bifida occulta seen on a spinal radiograph.

With the patient standing, the examiner should determine whether the iliac crests are level (**Figure 11.20**). If they are not, a lower limb length discrepancy is likely, and which can be quantified by placing measured blocks under the short extremity until the iliac crests are level. Leg length discrepancy can be responsible for the appearance of lumbar scoliosis, and the condition must not be overlooked as timely treatment is available for those children who are growing. In these cases, one can confirm that the scoliosis is postural and compensatory by having the child stand on blocks

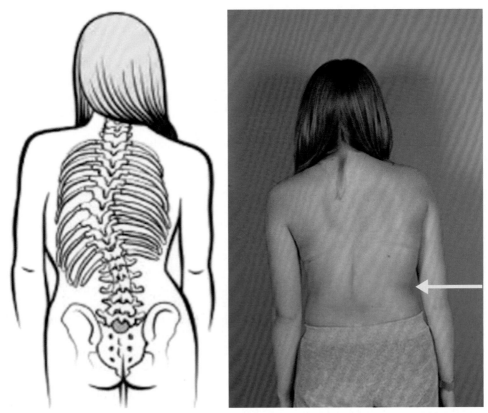

FIGURE 11.14 This child has a scoliosis which can be detected on physical examination that demonstrates trunk shift as well as prominences in the trunk with a forward bend.

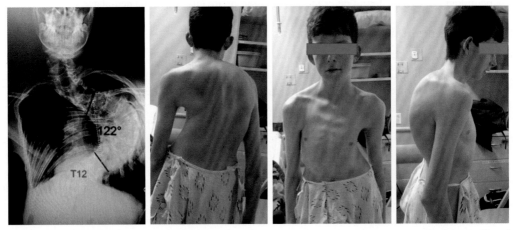

FIGURE 11.15 This 11-year-old boy has absolutely no back pain, but has a curve well over 100° that significantly alters his body habitus and decreases his lung function.

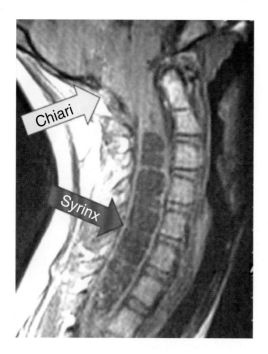

FIGURE 11.16 This child has a large Chiari malformation (displacement of the cerebellar tonsils into the foramen magnum) (yellow arrow). Many of these children will have a syrinx (red arrow) as a result of altered CSF flow.

or simply sit on the examination table and examining the now straightened lumbar spine from the back.

While examining the back, any asymmetry should be noted:

- asymmetry of the shoulders
- unequal scapular prominence
- prominent iliac crest
- increased space between the arm and body on one side with respect to the other with the arms hanging loosely at the side

Although these findings are consistent with scoliosis, the best noninvasive clinical test for evaluating spinal curvature is the Adams forward-bending test. With this test, the degree and direction of associated rotation of the vertebrae are clearly demonstrated. The examiner observes the adolescent from behind as the patient bends forward at the waist until the spine is horizontal. The patient's knees should be straight, the feet together, the arms dependent, and the palms in opposition. Vertebral rotation causes one side of the back to appear higher. This is noted as rib prominence in the thoracic region or as paraspinal fullness in the lumbar region (**Figure 11.21**).

One can assess the spine deformity from the back and a rib prominence will herald the presence of a thoracic curve (**Figure 11.22A**). The amount of rotation (apical trunk rotation) can be quantified with a scoliometer and when the degree of rotation is greater than 7°, the child has a scoliosis curve that is 20° to 30° and may require treatment based on skeletal maturity (**Figure 11.22B**).

If any of these signs are present, then the child should be referred to a pediatric orthopedic surgeon. The orthopedic surgeon will obtain standing full-length (posterior-anterior and lateral) spine X-rays to measure the Cobb angle in both the frontal and sagittal planes. The Cobb angle measurement and the skeletal maturity of the child will determine the treatment.

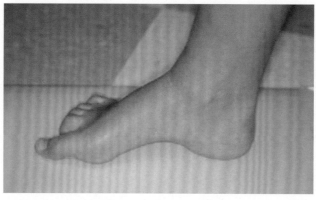

FIGURE 11.17 A unilateral cavovarus foot with claw toes should raise suspicion of intraspinal abnormalities such as tethered cord or other spinal cord abnormalities and necessitate an MRI of the entire neuroaxis.

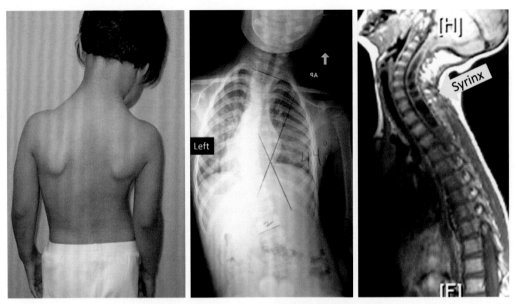

FIGURE 11.18 Left-sided thoracic curves are associated with intraspinal pathology in about 20% of cases. This boy has a 44° left-sided scoliosis with a long sweeping curve without rotation and his head is not centered over his pelvis. All three aspects (left-sided thoracic curve, lack of rotation, and imbalance) can be associated with intraspinal pathology. (Case courtesy of Chad Price MD.)

Frequently, if the patient is inspected from the front, asymmetry of the pectoral regions, breasts, or rib cage may be evident and could be a sign of patient with Marfan syndrome (**Figure 11.23**). Although these asymmetries are probably related to the spinal curvature, they may also occur in individuals without scoliosis. Occasionally, breast asymmetry is the primary concern of the patient and parents. Families should be informed that correcting the scoliosis will improve but not completely correct this asymmetry.

Because idiopathic scoliosis is basically a diagnosis of exclusion, a thorough evaluation is necessary to rule out a neurologic cause of the deformity. The neurologic examination begins by assessing spinal balance, a normal neurologic examination demonstrates that the head likes to be centered over the pelvis from the frontal and side views (**Figure 11.24**).

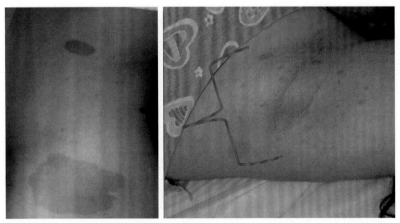

FIGURE 11.19 A child with café-au-lait spots and axillary or inguinal freckling (red bracket) (freckles where the sun does not shine is not normal) may be a sign of neurofibromatosis. Children with NF-1 can have a dystrophic form of scoliosis that can be difficult to treat.

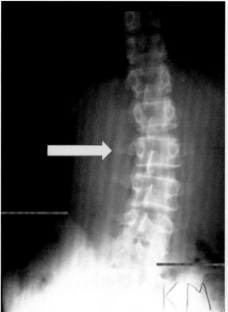
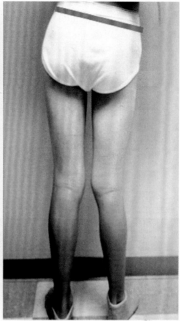

FIGURE 11.20 This 14-year-old boy was referred for a 20° lumbar scoliosis, which was really a compensation for his 4-cm limb length discrepancy. One can suspect that the lumbar curve is postural due to pelvic obliquity (red lines) and the fact that the curve has no rotation of the pedicles (yellow arrow). Thoracic curves usually cannot be ascribed to a limb length discrepancy.

An important part of the neurological examination is assessing the patient's reflexes. Examination of the superficial abdominal reflexes is useful for determining which patients should undergo MRI to rule out syringomyelia. This child (▶ **Video 11.1**) from **Figure 11.17** has asymmetric abdominal reflex. The abdominal reflex examination is performed with the patient supine on an examination table and the arms relaxed along the side of the body. An area approximately 10 cm above and below the umbilicus and to each anterior axillary line is exposed. With the patient relaxed, the bluntly pointed handle of a reflex hammer or other edged device (ruler) is used to lightly stroke the skin in each quadrant over a distance of 10 cm. The stroke starts lateral to the umbilicus near the anterior axillary line and is directed diagonally toward the umbilicus in each quadrant. The umbilicus is observed for deviation toward the side on which the test is performed. If these reflexes are consistently present on one side and absent on the other side, further evaluation is warranted because this finding does not occur in neurologically normal patients with scoliosis. However, other variations might occur, such as absent reflexes in all quadrants (▶ **Video 11.2**).

The patellar and Achilles tendon reflexes should also be tested, with the expectation that they will be symmetric and not too brisk. This child (▶ **Video 11.3**) has increased reflexes and sustained clonus that requires an MRI and neurologic referral. Muscle

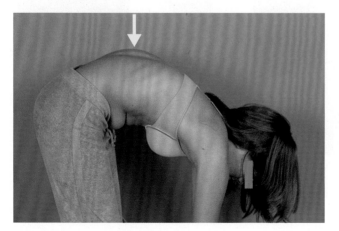

FIGURE 11.21 This adolescent has a lumbar curve that is detected by prominence in the lumbar spine (yellow arrow).

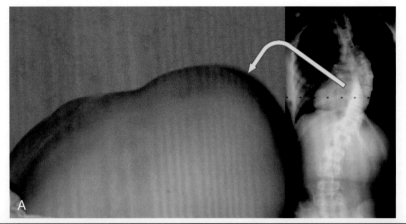

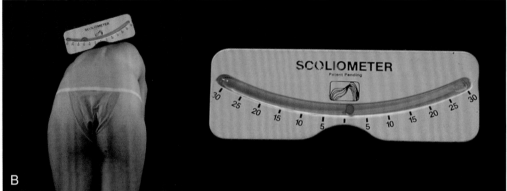

ATR > 5 to 7° = Cobb Angle 20 − 25°

FIGURE 11.22 A, Because the spine is rotated, the ribs which attach to the spine at that level result in a rib prominence. B, The scoliometer can be placed at the apex of the deformity and a measurement greater than 7° may indicate a scoliosis that could require treatment.

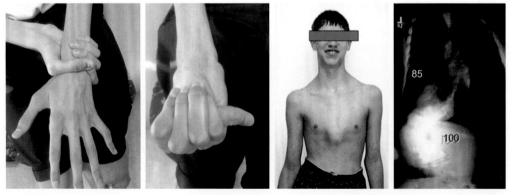

FIGURE 11.23 A child with Marfan syndrome may have pectus deformities and will have long extremities and long fingers. The Walker-Murdoch sign is positive for possible Marfan syndrome, if thumb and ring finger overlap on contralateral wrist and the Steinberg test is positive if the thumb sticks out with a clenched fist.

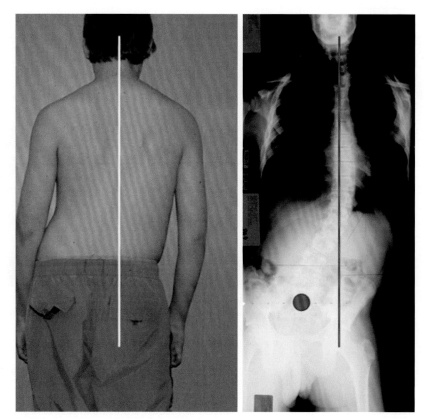

FIGURE 11.24 This boy with a scoliosis is significantly out of balance and was found to have an altered craniocervical junction.

testing and examination of the range of motion of all four extremities should always be conducted. The hands and feet should be examined for abnormal posture (**Figure 11.25**) and for evidence of abnormal sensation (excessive callus formation or nail bed irregularities). Abnormal findings may be the only clinical evidence of underlying pathology of the neural axis, such as syringomyelia or tethered cord.

Treatment of Idiopathic Scoliosis

- **Observation:**

    Routine rescreening or observation by the physician is a form of treatment for mild curves (<20°). This observation period consists of regular clinical examinations and spine X-rays throughout the rapid growth years of adolescence until the spine is mature. It is important to note that more than 90% of patients with scoliosis require no treatment other than observation.

- **Bracing:**

    For curves greater than 25° in patients that are still growing rapidly, a brace is prescribed. The brace can prevent the curve from progressing and may eliminate the need for spinal surgery. However, the brace cannot correct the curve that already exists. Bracing is generally recommended for curves between 25° and 40° in adolescent patients with significant growth remaining. The main factor in achieving a high rate of bracing success is the number of hours a day that the brace is worn. Various spinal orthoses are available, with the most common being a custom thoracolumbar sacral orthosis (TLSO) (**Figure 11.26**). Getting into a daily routine of wearing the brace while participating in activities helps with compliance, which is key to successful treatment.

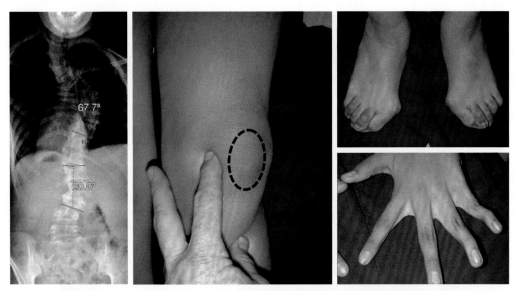

FIGURE 11.25 Another diagnosis that can be present with scoliosis and may go undetected can be Ehlers-Danlos syndrome. This child with Type VI EDS has an unusual scoliosis pattern and has severe joint laxity manifest with very flat feet and hyperlaxity of fingers and other instability such as the elbow and patella (dashed circle).

- **Surgery:**

    Some patients present with severe spinal deformity, and in other patients, scoliosis worsens despite compliant brace wear. In these specific patients, surgery can reduce a portion of the curve and prevent it from increasing in the future. Usually surgery is reserved for adolescents and preadolescents who already have a curve of 45° to 50° or more. The most common surgical procedure is a posterior spinal fusion with instrumentation and bone graft (**Figure 11.27**). This type of surgery involves attaching rods to the spinal column to help straighten it. The bone graft between the affected vertebrae encourages fusion to prevent further progression of the curve.

Congenital Scoliosis

Just as there are congenital abnormalities in bone formation that can cause torticollis, there are bone abnormalities, which can lead to structural scoliosis. Normally, vertebral bodies are rectangular in shape, some can be wedged (hemivertebra), which causes imbalance from asymmetric growth, and some can be partially fused (bony bar) which can lead to decreased growth (**Figure 11.28**). These are referred to as failure of formation or segmentation more generally referred to as congenital scoliosis.

Many times, these are incidentally found on screening radiographs for children with multiple congenital anomalies such as Klippel-Feil and VATER or Vacterl syndrome. In general, the natural history is specific for each individual patient and the treatment is different from that for idiopathic scoliosis. For instance, some children can have multiple offsetting hemivertebra or bony bars, which lead to a short but balanced spine and thus treatment is not needed. Brace treatment is not uniformly considered effective for congenital scoliosis and surgery may be considered for those rare patients with progressive deformity (**Figure 11.29**).

Physical findings are different in congenital scoliosis where there is more often trunk shifts as opposed to the rotational characteristics seen in AIS (**Figure 11.30**). It is critical to perform detailed neurologic examinations as cavus feet and progressive spinal imbalance can accompany spinal cord abnormalities, which are present in 20% of these children. These spinal cord abnormalities such as tethered cord or diastematomyelia can be suspected with cutaneous abnormalities in the lumbar sacral spine (**Figure 11.31**).

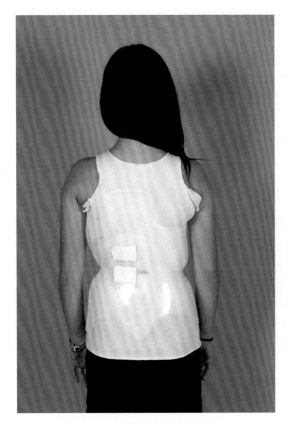

FIGURE 11.26 The TLSO is named by the areas it is designed to stabilize: the thoracic, lumbar, and sacral parts of the spine. It is cosmetically acceptable as it can be covered well by clothing. Wearing a brace is not an easy treatment for an adolescent. Even covered by clothing, it is hot, hard, and can make the student feel self-conscious.

Kyphosis

Kyphosis is a term that relates to relative roundness of the back. While coronal plane curvature greater than 10° (scoliosis) is considered abnormal, we all have some degree of thoracic kyphosis. A good understanding of the normal alignment of the back is necessary to determine pathological conditions. In an adult, the normal sagittal alignment of the spine is cervical lordosis, thoracic kyphosis, and lumbar lordosis. In general, normal thoracic kyphosis from T1 to T12 is 20° to 40° while the lumbar spine is 30° to 50° of lordosis from L1 to L5. Conditions affecting one segment of the spine often create alignment alterations in other parts of the spine. Children who are in sagittal balance, but who have excessive thoracic kyphosis, must have a large amount of compensatory lordosis in the lumbar spine in order to remain compensated. Sagittal alignment of the spine also changes with growth and development. Studies have shown that in children, the thoracic kyphosis (T1-T12) was larger than adult measurements and lumbar lordosis was smaller than adult measurements.[2] This suggests a lessening of thoracic kyphosis as we grow from children to adults.

Abnormal kyphosis can affect the quality of life due to increases in back pain, poor self-esteem, and, in rare progressive cases, neurological compromise. Extreme kyphosis does not lead to decreased lung and cardiovascular function as seen in severe scoliosis. Postural kyphosis is a common benign presentation with a flexible deformity of the thoracic spine and is a common cause of parental haranguing for adolescent slouching. Rigid excessive kyphosis of the thoracic spine is often referred to as Scheuermann kyphosis and is defined as a fixed angular kyphosis in which there is anterior wedging of 5° or more on at least three adjacent vertebral bodies[3] (**Figure 11.32**). This is typically seen in the adolescent population ranging from 0.4% to 10% of teenagers.[4] Originally, Scheuermann kyphosis was considered to be a type of osteochondritis due to the associated radiographic abnormalities seen on the vertebral end plates but more recent literature suggests a genetic cause much like adolescent idiopathic scoliosis.[5]

Similar to coronal plane deformity where there are congenital causes of scoliosis such as hemivertebra and bone fusions, fixed kyphosis or other fixed sagittal imbalances may also be caused by congenital abnormalities of the spine such as failure of formation or failure of segmentation (**Figure 11.33**). These are present at birth but are often not noticed until later in childhood when the curve becomes visually obvious. These congenital defects may be also associated with structural abnormalities of the heart, spinal cord, and urinary system and require additional imaging of the body systems. Other less common causes of kyphosis include association with genetic disorders (achondroplasia, mucopolysaccharidosis, Marfan syndrome), postinfectious causes, neoplasm, and trauma.

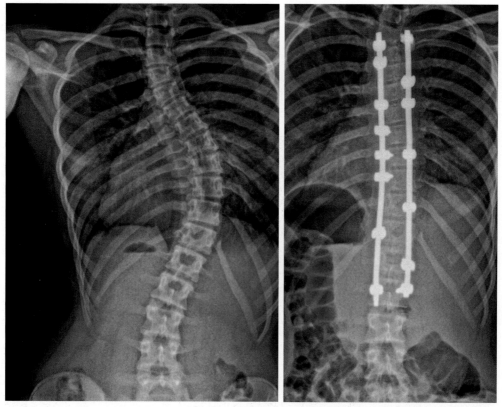

FIGURE 11.27 This child with scoliosis undergoes posterior instrumentation (designed to correct and stabilize the spine) and spine fusion. Instrumentation refers to the various rods, screws, hooks, or wires that are used to hold the spine in the corrected position while the bone fusion occurs. Following surgery, the fused section is no longer flexible. (Provided by A.L. McIntosh, MD.)

Physical Examination for Kyphosis

Many of the same physical examination tests described above for scoliosis are equally important for kyphosis. Most patients presenting with a complaint of kyphosis will be adolescents (**Figure 11.34**).

All patients should be properly draped to allow for visualization of the entire back, including the shoulders and iliac crests. All good examinations start with observation. An assessment of how the patient stands at rest can give clues to the underlying cause of the deformity. Patients that are out of balance (eg, head not centered over the pelvis) may be attributed to intraspinal pathology or some underlying neurological cause for the kyphosis (**Figure 11.35**).

Inspection of the back is necessary to look for surface findings such as midline hemangiomas, hair tufts, and dimpling that may indicate the presence of an underlying spinal cord abnormality such as a tethered cord or diastematomyelia (**Figure 11.31**). The spinous processes are palpated from the cervical region to the sacrum for any deficiencies or areas of discomfort. Pain in a localized area may necessitate the need for imaging to evaluate for trauma or neoplasm.

Range of motion of the entire spine is next completed to determine if the curve is flexible or rigid. The amount of forward flexion and extension should be recorded. A kyphosis that completely resolves with activation of the patient's paraspinal muscles is most likely postural. More rigid curves are more likely associated with Scheuermann or congenital causes (**Figure 11.34**). An Adams forward bend test can also be completed at this time to check for scoliosis. The presence of a kyphoscoliosis should warrant a detailed neurological examination and MRI of the neuroaxis as this finding can be associated with spinal cord abnormalities such as syringomyelia.

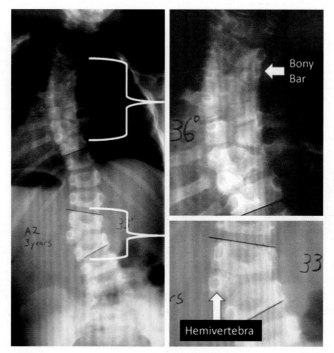

FIGURE 11.28 This child with congenital scoliosis has multiple hemivertebra and bony fusions which overall lead to a relatively balanced spine.

Similar to adolescent idiopathic scoliosis, a thorough neurological physical evaluation is necessary to rule out a neurologic cause of the deformity. Patient's gait and balance can be evaluated by making them walk a short distance down a hallway. Strength and sensation testing should be performed on both upper and lower extremities to determine any asymmetry or deficits. Both deep tendon reflexes and abdominal reflexes should be performed and asymmetry or deficits noted. Spasticity or clonus in the extremities should also be evaluated. Patients with postural kyphosis or Scheuermann kyphosis should have a normal neurological examination. Abnormal findings during the neurological examination should warrant further workup such as advanced imaging of the spinal cord or brain.

Additional Testing and Treatment

Most patients with a painless flexible deformity have a benign postural cause and do not require imaging. If the kyphosis is more rigid or significantly painful, plain standing radiographs of the entire spine in both the frontal and sagittal planes are helpful. Rigid thoracic kyphosis that measures in excess of 45° with associated vertebral body wedging and vertebral end plates changes in an adolescent patient with no neurological complaints or findings is consistent with Scheuermann kyphosis. Congenital, post infectious, or traumatic causes for kyphosis often are easily diagnosed on plain radiographs (**Figure 11.36**). Neoplastic or infection causes may require necessary laboratory markers to be obtained. Abnormal neurological findings on examination require further workup with advanced imaging of the spine (eg, neuroaxis MRI).

Treatment of postural kyphosis involves patient and parent education and nonsurgical management. A program of therapy that focuses on back and core muscle strengthening and stretching is typically all that is needed. Orthotic management such as use of a lumbar corset can be useful in patients with more excessive pain in combination with a physical therapy program.

Treatment of Scheuermann kyphosis is similar to adolescent idiopathic scoliosis. Most patients with smaller degrees of curvature can simply be observed using serial radiography over time to determine

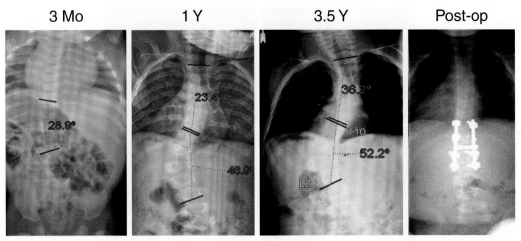

FIGURE 11.29 This child with congenital scoliosis has rapid curve progression, which required surgical correction.

progression. Associated pain in patients with Scheuermann kyphosis is most commonly muscular in origin and responds well to a back and core physical therapy strengthening program. Progression of the deformity is highly correlated with growth potential as younger patients have a higher likelihood of progression. Progressive curves may be treated with bracing, but this is often poorly tolerated, and compliance is poor[6] (**Figure 11.37**).

The natural history of mild to moderate curves (<70°) is benign resulting in only an increased incidence of mild back pain but no measurable functional limitations into adulthood.[7] Surgical management of Scheuermann kyphosis is often reserved for curves greater than 75°, significant cosmetic patient concerns, and restrictive back pain recalcitrant to nonoperative treatment (eg, bracing and physical therapy). Surgery involves fusion of the involved area of the spine through a posterior approach similar to the techniques used for AIS (**Figure 11.38**). Congenital forms of kyphosis are managed similarly to Scheuermann kyphosis with serial radiographic observation and surgery reserved for large progressive curves.

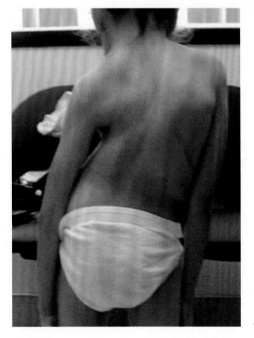

Back Pain/Spondylolysis/ Spondylolisthesis

Back pain in the adolescent population is frequent and studies have shown that up to half of all teenagers will experience back pain.[8] The majority of these patients have no identifiable cause for their pain. Many of these patients likely have benign muscular discomfort, which is self-limiting and responds well to back and core physical therapy programs. However, some adolescents can have serious conditions such as tumor, infection, and trauma, which cannot be overlooked. In younger children (<10 years), back pain is uncommon and should involve a complete workup for a cause.

FIGURE 11.30 This child with congenital scoliosis has significant trunk shift.

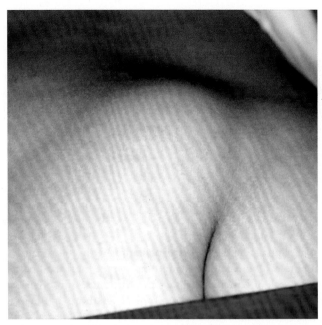

FIGURE 11.31 A sacral lipoma can herald spinal cord dysraphism such as this child with congenital scoliosis and a tethered cord.

While Scheuermann kyphosis tends to be the most common cause of thoracic back pain, the most common cause of lumbar pain is spondylolysis, which is defined as a unilateral or bilateral bony defect in the pars interarticularis (most commonly at L5). Most believe that stress fractures are related to repetitive hyperextension activities such as swimming and diving, gymnastics and

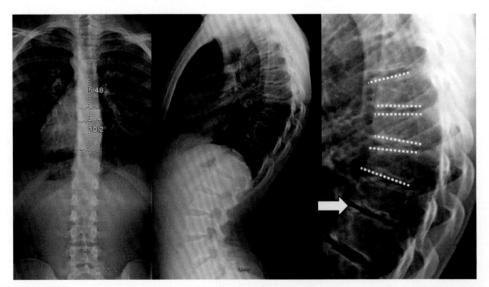

FIGURE 11.32 Scheuermann kyphosis is a result of wedging in the sagittal plane that increases the thoracic kyphosis. Wedging is not always perfectly in the sagittal plane and thus some slight scoliosis is occasionally seen. Unlike AIS where the spine is rotated, in Scheuermann kyphosis, the coronal plane scoliosis is more of a tilt from wedging. In order to make the diagnosis of Scheuermann kyphosis, there must be three adjacent vertebrae with more than 5° of wedging (white lines). In addition, end-plate irregularities (yellow arrow) and disk space narrowing are noted.

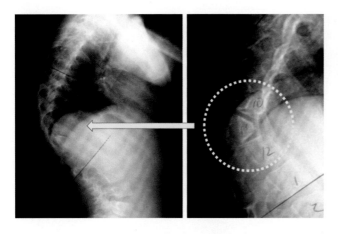

FIGURE 11.33 Congenital kyphosis (yellow circle) can present as Scheuermann kyphosis.

volleyball. When the vertebral body translates forward of the adjacent vertebral body, the patient is described as having spondylolisthesis. Spondylolisthesis can be congenital or acquired and is often classified into five types by the Wiltse-Newman classification[9]; only Types I or II are seen in growing patients. **Type I—Dysplastic** is much less common and is characterized by congenital slippage at the L5-S1 articulation with abnormalities in the facet joints themselves. A special note is required about symptoms seen in the Type I or the dysplastic type. In these cases, the posterior arch of L5 remains intact and with increasing anterior translation can lead to sacral nerve root irritation and radicular pain. **Type II—Isthmic** is a defect in the pars interarticularis that is acquired from trauma associated with repetitive hyperextension of the lumbar spine. Patients with spondylolysis and Type II spondylolisthesis typically present with activity-related low back pain localized to the base of the lumbar spine, which is nonradiating as the arch of L5 does not impinge nerve roots. Classically, patients will report that hyperextension of lower back will worsen symptoms.

Patient Evaluation

As in other aspects of medicine, a detailed history and review of systems is important in making a diagnosis in pediatric back pain and guiding next steps. Patients should be asked about the onset, duration, and character of their pain. Night pain, progressive pain, and constant pain are all worrisome symptoms that are associated with infection and tumors and warrant a more aggressive workup. Alleviating and aggravating factors should also be asked of the patient. Typical nonorganic muscular back pain typically is worse with activity but is quick to resolve the following day. Dramatic pain relief from the use of NSAIDs might point toward osteoid osteoma as a cause. Participation in sports and activities that require repetitive hyperextension motions (swimming or gymnastics) can often correlate with spondylolysis or spondylolisthesis.

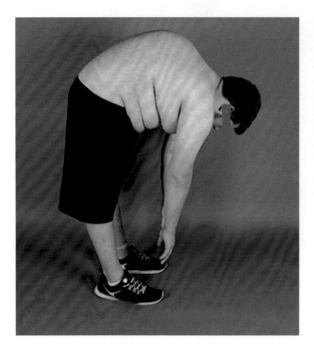

FIGURE 11.34 This adolescent boy has fairly large angular kyphosis (often termed a "gibbus") that is consistent with Scheuermann kyphosis.

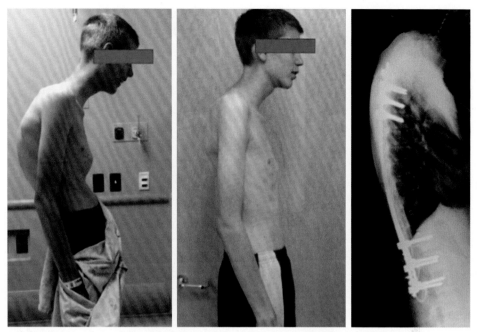

FIGURE 11.35 This 17-year-old boy with autistic spectrum disorder and developmental delay is severely out of balance preoperatively; his head is positioned well forward of his pelvis. After surgery, his balance is better, yet he still has a propensity to pitch forward.

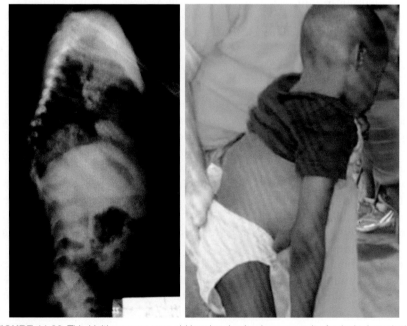

FIGURE 11.36 This Haitian seven-year-old boy has kyphosis as a result of spinal tuberculosis.

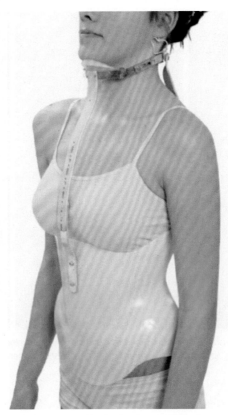

FIGURE 11.37 In order to effectively brace some kyphosis, the cervical spine needs to be included. Compliance is low for obvious reasons.

In growing individuals with back pain, it is important to discern "pathologic pain" versus nonorganic pain. Clinicians should worry about patients who have a high preponderance of pathologic pain and symptoms. These patients may benefit from further investigation and advanced imaging (**Table 11.1**).

Physical Examination for Back Pain

Although the history is often paramount for guiding next steps, physical examination is also relevant and is similar to that which was mentioned above when evaluating spinal deformity. Inspection of the back region is necessary in all patients presenting for back pain. All patients should be properly draped to allow for visualization of the entire back, including the shoulders and iliac crests. Obesity should be noted and is often a factor in patients complaining of back pain.

As previously discussed, some large spinal deformities can have some back pain as a result of the deformity. Importantly, some painful process can lead to mild temporary spinal deformity such as a nonstructural scoliosis (**Figure 11.39**).

In many cases, the painful process can be found in the concavity of the scoliotic curve (**Figure 11.40**).

Besides looking for spinal deformity on physical examination, a thorough neurological examination is also warranted in patients with back pain. This should include strength, sensory, and reflex testing in both upper and lower extremities. Observational gait analysis should be performed and is often helpful in finding subtle neurological defects. Younger patients may not complain of specific pain but will limit their movements to avoid aggravating their back or spine. This can be tested by having the child pick up

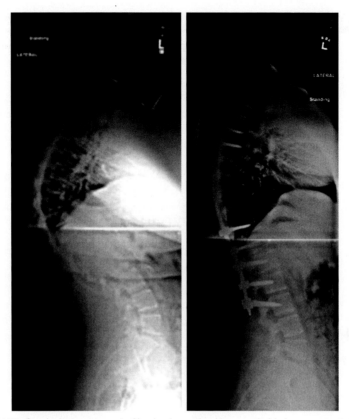

FIGURE 11.38 Surgical management of kyphosis can lead to remarkable improvements in posture.

an object off the floor from a standing position. Children with back pain will use a variety of compensatory motions to grab the object avoiding spinal motion. Additional workup may be indicated if the child has abnormal reflexes, if the child stands out of balance, or has foot deformity, muscle weakness, or cutaneous manifestations of spinal dysraphism (lumbosacral hairy patch, lumbar dimples, hemangioma, etc.). In addition, it is important to determine how well they move and if motion is limited by pain. In general, patients with pathology in the vertebral body and the intervertebral disc have pain with flexion (**Figure 11.41**), while pathology in the posterior elements (spondylolysis/spondylolisthesis) will have pain with hyperextension. Many patients with spondylolysis or spondylolisthesis will have tight hamstrings.

The standing position of the patient should also be examined with careful attention to abnormal contours of the spine. In spondylolysis and low-grade spondylolisthesis, the spinal contour will be normal. However, in high-grade spondylolisthesis (eg, greater than 50% forward slippage), postural disturbances might be noted. These include a sacral prominence and lumbar hyperlordosis (**Figure 11.42**).

Additional Evaluation and Treatment

Most back pain in the adolescent with a normal physical examination and benign clinical presentation does not require additional imaging. Typical muscular back pain is often improved with a back and core physical therapy regimen or observation and time. If there is a concern for structural causes, plain radiographs of the spine are often helpful in the initial workup. Laboratory markers should be performed if there is a suspicion of an infectious cause for the pain. Neurological findings often require advanced imaging such as an MRI of the neural axis and soft tissues (eg, herniation of a disk).

Table 11.1	Historical Features as They Relate to Organic Causes of Back Pain	
	ORGANIC CAUSES OF PAIN PATHOLOGICAL SYMPTOMS	**NONORGANIC SYMPTOMS**
Onset of pain	Recent (weeks to months ago) Recent trauma or activity change	Presence for years
Character	Deep, boring, localized, constant, and progressive pain. Pain that self-limits activity[a]	Generalized nonspecific pain that comes and goes, relieved with homeopathic measures
Night pain	Yes	No
Radicular pain	Lower extremity pain that follows dermatomes	All four extremity or whole extremity (nondermatomal)
ROS	Fever, weight loss, fatigue, leg weakness, perineal numbness, change in bowel and bladder function, pain with Valsalva	Nonspecific, nonsensical symptoms Multiple joint symptoms
Past history	History of cancer, immune suppression	History of irritable bowel syndrome, nonspecific pelvic pain, migraines, complex regional pain syndrome Depression, anxiety, family stress, pending legal action
Family history	Not related	High incidence of back pain and disability in the family

[a]It is always concerning when a child will not do activities that they love because of pain.

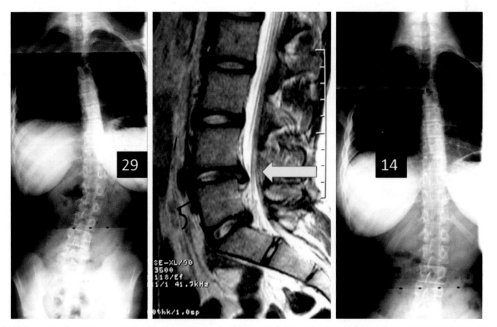

FIGURE 11.39 This 15-year-old girl has severe back pain and left leg pain that radiates down to her foot. Her X-ray reveals a 29° non-AIS curve pattern (a long-sweeping curve with little rotation). An MRI demonstrates a large L5 disc herniation. After 6 months of conservative treatment, her pain has largely resolved and her scoliosis has improved.

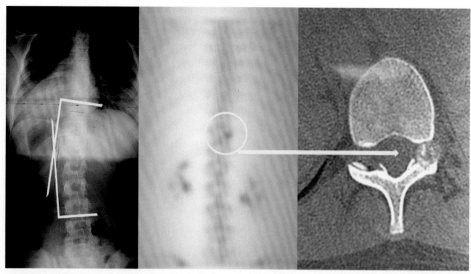

FIGURE 11.40 This 16-year-old girl has right-sided thoracolumbar pain that wakes her up from a sound sleep and plain radiographs show a mild scoliosis to the left. A bone scan demonstrates uptake at the T11 level on the right (yellow circle) and a CT scan of this area reveals a lesion that after removal was confirmed as an osteoid osteoma.

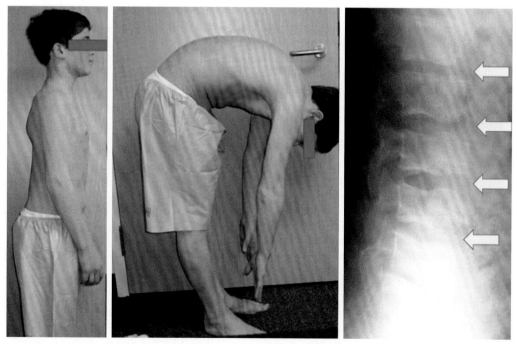

FIGURE 11.41 This 13-year-old boy has activity-related back pain and tends to stand with decreased lordosis. His pain is worse with forward flexion. Plain radiographs, multiple Schmorl nodes, and endplate irregularities are consistent with thoracolumbar ("atypical") Scheuermann disease. Children with atypical Scheuermann disease do not have the wedging and kyphotic deformity seen in the thoracic variety, but they do tend to have more pain.

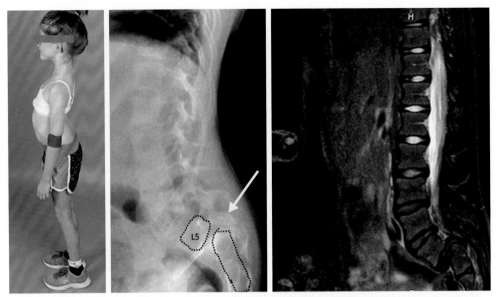

FIGURE 11.42 This girl with dysplastic spondylolisthesis has a prominent sacrum and the kyphosis at L5-S1 must be compensated by hyperlordosis above it. As opposed to isthmic type, the posterior arch of L5 is still intact (yellow arrow) and thus she is more susceptible to radicular pain.

In terms of spondylolysis and spondylolisthesis, plain radiographs of the lumbar spine are supportive in confirming the diagnosis. A defect in the pars area is often best seen on the lateral or oblique radiographs. MRI can be used as well but is often less sensitive in visualizing the defect for fracture. An MRI will often show T2 edema in the associated pedicle, facet or pars region. In spondylolisthesis, the amount of slippage can be determined from the lateral film. CT is very sensitive for the detection of a spondylolysis but does carry the risk of additional radiation.

Treatment for back pain depends on the cause of the pain. In most cases of spondylolysis and spondylolisthesis, nonsurgical treatment is successful. Operative management is reserved for patients with a symptomatic spondylolysis or low-grade spondylolisthesis that failed a long course (>6 months) of conservative therapy.

References

1. Ramirez N, Johnston CE, Browne RH. The prevalence of back pain in children who have idiopathic scoliosis. *J Bone Joint Surg Am.* 1997;79(3):364-368.
2. Kamaci S, Yucekul A, Demirkiran G, Berktas M, Yazici M. The evolution of the sagittal spinal alignment in sitting position during childhood. *Spine.* 2015;40(13):E787-E793.
3. Scheuermann HW. Deforming osteochondritis of the spine. *Ugeskr Leaeger.* 1920;(82):385.
4. Robin GC. *The Etiology of Scheuermann's Kyhosis: The Textbook Of Spinal Surgery.* Philadelphia, PA: Lippincott-Raven; 1977.
5. Gustavel M, Beals RK. Scheuermann;s disease of the lumbar spine in identical twins. *AJR Am J Roentgenol.* 2002;179:1078-1079.
6. Tsirikos AI, Jain AK. Scheuermann's kyphosis: current controversies. *J Bone Joint Surg Br.* 2011;93(7):857-864.
7. Murry PM, Weintein SL, Spratt KF. The natural history and long-term follow-up of Scheuermann kyphosis. *J Bone Joint Surg Am.* 1993;75(2):236-248.
8. Aartun E, Hartvigsen J, Wedderkopp N, Hestbaek L. Spinal pain in adolescents: prevalence, incidence and course. A school-based two-year prospective cohort study in 1,300 Danes aged 11-13. *BMC Musculoskelet Disord.* 2014;15:187.
9. Wiltse LL, Newman PH, Macnab I. Classification of spondylolysis and spondylolisthesis. *Clin Orthop Relat Res.* 1957;10:48-60.

12

Foot and Ankle Deformity

Benjamin Shore and Megan E. Johnson

● Introduction

Foot and ankle concerns are a common cause for evaluation in the pediatric patient. Fortunately, the majority of pediatric foot deformities are asymptomatic and do not require treatment or surgical intervention. This chapter will outline the clinically relevant congenital and physiologic conditions, which are common causes for orthopedic referral. Careful examination of the three segments of the foot (hindfoot, midfoot, and forefoot) is critical to help guide diagnosis and treatment. When it comes to describing the hindfoot, orthopedists will describe the hindfoot as being in varus (always abnormal) or valgus. Normal feet are in some degree of valgus, yet excessive valgus is abnormal (**Figure 12.1**).

● Congenital and Infantile Foot Deformities

Clubfoot

Introduction

Clubfoot (talipes equinovarus) occurs in approximately one of every 1000 live births and is a common cause for consultation in the nursery. Clubfoot is also one of the most common congenital deformities of the lower extremity. The ratio of idiopathic clubfoot among males to females is 2:1 and is consistent across ethnic groups. The majority of clubfoot cases are sporadic, indicating a complex multigene etiology. A careful examination of the three segments of the foot will help confirm the diagnosis of talipes equinovarus (**Figure 12.2**).

While the Ponseti method of correction was first developed in the early 1940s, the wide dissemination of this method has spread over the past two decades, whereby almost 95% of clubfeet are now initially corrected by the Ponseti method of serial casting[1] (**Figure 12.3**).

Clinical Significance and Natural History

Approximately 80% of clubfeet are considered idiopathic, while the remaining 20% are associated with neuromuscular conditions, genetic disorders, or syndromes. Left untreated, the idiopathic clubfoot is a significant disability. In many cultures, affected individuals will be

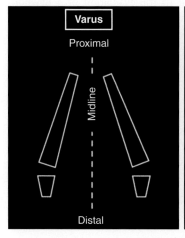
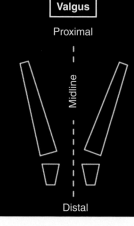

FIGURE 12.1 This figure demonstrates the difference between varus and valgus. The small trapezoid represents the foot while the longer one represents the shank of the tibia.

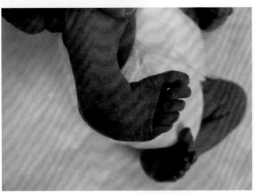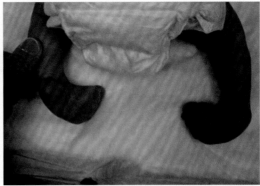

FIGURE 12.2 This newborn has bilateral clubfoot deformity.

ostracized and restricted to a lifetime of poverty. The affected individual ends up walking on the dorsum of their feet and develops severe callosities. Their gastrocnemius muscle becomes very atrophic as there is little meaningful power at toe off (**Figure 12.4**).

History and Physical Examination

Clubfoot can often be detected during routine second trimester prenatal ultrasounds; ultrasounds in the third trimester may not be specific for clubfeet as isolated metatarsus adductus can be detected by ultrasound (**Figure 12.5**).

Clubfoot has a distinct clinical appearance at birth, consisting of midfoot cavus and forefoot adduction as well as hindfoot equinus and varus. This foot position is often accompanied by internal tibial rotation with abnormalities existing at the midtarsal and subtalar joints. One can appreciate and describe the unique clinical appearance at birth with the anacronym "CAVE" (**Figure 12.6**).

Hindfoot equinus can be difficult to appreciate in clubfoot as well as in other conditions with a tight heel cord such as congenital vertical talus. In cases of hindfoot equinus, the examiner will notice that when the heel pad is palpated, there is no palpable bone as a result of the tight tendo-Achilles that pulls the calcaneus up and the calcaneus is pitched plantarly (**Figure 12.7**).

The term plantarflexed implies that the long toe flexors are also tight. In the normal foot, the calcaneus is not elevated and the pitch points dorsal.

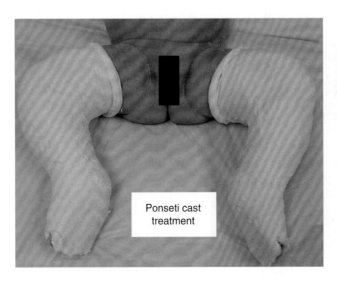

Ponseti cast treatment

Pitfalls in Diagnosis

General physical examination is critical in the evaluation of a newborn child with clubfoot. A detailed head and neck examination should look for the presence of torticollis. Spinal examination involves ruling out the presence of scoliosis (with shoulder asymmetry) or spinal dysraphism such as a hairy tuft or sacral dimple. Focused examination of the lower extremities should confirm normal hip and knee examination. The

FIGURE 12.3 The Ponseti method of casting obtains initial correction in greater than 95% of idiopathic clubfeet.

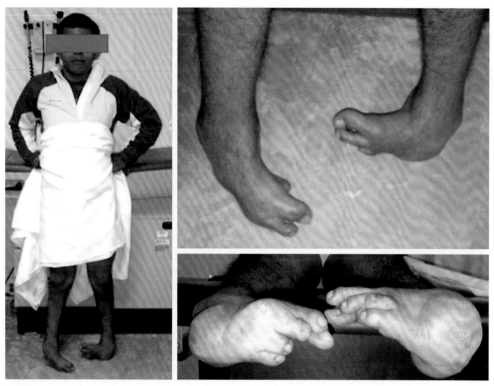

FIGURE 12.4 This 19-year-old Honduran man has uncorrected clubfeet. He walks on the tops of his feet and has extensive calluses and tough dorsal skin.

FIGURE 12.5 Prenatal ultrasound of a child later born with clubfoot deformity.

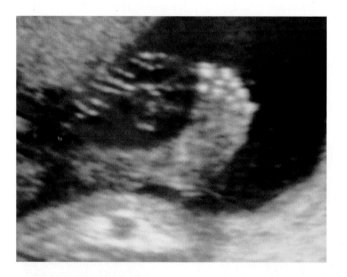

Four features of clubfoot
"CAVE"

C= Midfoot **cavus**
A= Forefoot **adductus**
V= Hindfoot **varus**
E= Hindfoot **equinus**

FIGURE 12.6 Clubfeet have four features consisting of **cavus**, which is a high arched midfoot with a plantar crease. **Adductus** is medial deviation of the forefoot, which results in a curved lateral border of the foot (yellow line). **Varus** is noted when the foot is rolled in and the plantar aspect of the foot faces medial. **Equinus** is noted when the foot is not easily dorsiflexed to 90° (red line).

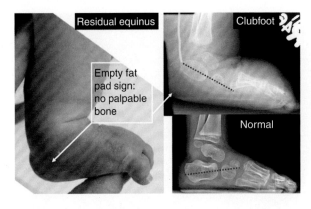

FIGURE 12.7 This treated clubfoot appears to be fully corrected. Yet if the examiner were to carefully palpate the heel pad, they would notice the calcaneus is not present at the point of the heel. This is due to the tight tendo-Achilles (yellow line) which elevates the calcaneus (dashed red line). In addition, one will notice the toes are plantarflexed implying the long toe flexors are also tight. In the normal foot, the calcaneus is not elevated and the pitch points dorsal.

practitioner will examine both legs and perform a detailed neurologic examination, testing for active muscle control, especially ankle and toe dorsiflexion. Patients with inability to dorsiflex the toes may have a neurologic clubfoot (▶ **Video 12.1**).

The diagnosis of clubfoot is made clinically and is fairly reliable based on the clinical examination noted above. It is important to realize anatomic variants associated with clubfoot such as an increased prevalence of an absent dorsalis pedis artery. Reduced muscle mass has been seen in the affected lower leg of children with clubfeet and may be the result of genetic induced fibrosis of the muscle-tendon units.

Differential Diagnosis

Metatarsus adductus should not be confused with talipes equinovarus. In metatarsus adductus, there is isolated adductus of the midfoot without evidence of cavus, varus, or equinus. The deformity is typically flexible where a clubfoot tends to be more rigid.

Syndromic clubfoot (arthrogryposis) should not be confused with the idiopathic clubfoot. Atypical clubfeet appear fat with short metatarsals, and severe rigid cavus with a hallmark deep transverse plantar crease. Often, these atypical feet require a different casting technique for manipulation (**Figure 12.8**).

Diagnostic Tests or Advanced Imaging

Clubfoot diagnosis is based on physical examination and radiographs are not routinely indicated. If a syndromic clubfoot is suspected, then genetic testing and neurological consultation are indicated.

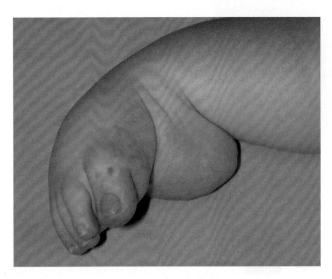

Treatment

The Ponseti casting method has become recognized over the last several decades as the treatment of choice for idiopathic clubfoot. This method involves serial casting of the foot over successive weeks, gradually stretching and correcting the foot in a stepwise sequence. The deformities are corrected in the CAVE sequence: cavus is corrected first, adductus and varus are corrected simultaneously, and

FIGURE 12.8 This child with arthrogryposis has severe clubfoot that is stiff and difficult to treat with standard casting.

equinus is the last deformity. To prevent recurrence, the child is then placed in an abduction orthosis for nighttime use over the next 2 to 4 years of life. Final success with the treatment is directly related to compliance of brace wear.

When to Refer

If a clubfoot is suspected, it is best to refer early. Ideally, treatment for clubfoot typically begins in the first several weeks of life. Yet even if the child is older, the Ponseti method is indicated; colleagues have successfully casted children with untreated idiopathic scoliosis as old as 9 years of age.

Metatarsus Adductus

Introduction

Metatarsus adductus is a common foot deformity in the newborn. Some have confused this with "clubbed feet"; yet, the informed practitioner knows that metatarsus adductus is just one of four deformities seen in clubfeet. The incidence of isolated metatarsus adductus is similar to clubfeet—one in 1000 live births with 50% being bilateral. While clubfeet are suspected to have a genetic etiology with some effect from external factors, the etiology of isolated metatarsus adductus is thought to be related to increased intrauterine crowding.[2] The deformity consists of medial deviation of the infant forefoot leading to a "bean"-shaped foot. Toddlers who present with metatarsus adductus walk with an internal foot progression angle, and "intoeing" may have been the reason for the original referral. It is important to evaluate for other causes of intoeing, such as internal tibial torsion which is a common cause for intoeing in older toddlers.

Clinical Significance and Natural History

Metatarsus adductus is thought to be caused by foot deformation due to intrauterine positioning. Most cases will resolve at least partially on their own without intervention. If the metatarsus adductus is flexible, resolution may be facilitated with parental stretching (**Figure 12.9A**). Surgery is rarely indicated unless the deformity is severe and rigid.[2]

History and Physical Examination

Metatarsus adductus can be associated with other "packaging disorders," such as torticollis and developmental dysplasia of the hip (DDH). The incidence of DDH in children with metatarsus adductus may be as high as 1 in 25. Given the association with DDH, a thorough examination of the hips should be performed.

The foot will generally be "bean" shaped, with the forefoot medially deviated on the hindfoot. The medial border of the foot is concave. The base of the fifth metatarsal may be prominent and there may be a wider than normal space between the first and second toes. The arch of the foot often appears higher than normal.

The heel bisector line can be used to document the severity of the metatarsus adductus. With the patient prone, a line drawn from the middle of the heel down the foot should land between the second and third toes. With metatarsus adductus, the line will fall lateral to this with greater deviation implying greater deformity.

The flexibility of the deformity can be assessed and may be prognostic. In mild cases, the deformity will correct when the lateral border of the foot is stimulated. In intermediate cases, the foot will not spontaneously correct when stimulated, but the deformity is passively correctable by the examiner. Rigid cases will not correct at all and may have a soft tissue crease along the medial border and/or a noticeable medial soft tissue contracture.

Pitfalls in Diagnosis

Metatarsus adductus can be a feature of other foot deformities, such as clubfoot (hindfoot in varus) or skewfoot (hindfoot in excessive valgus). It is important to recognize these other pathologies if present. In clubfoot, there will also be hindfoot varus and equinus with cavus in the midfoot. The deformity will not be flexible. Skewfoot will demonstrate hindfoot valgus along with forefoot adductus.

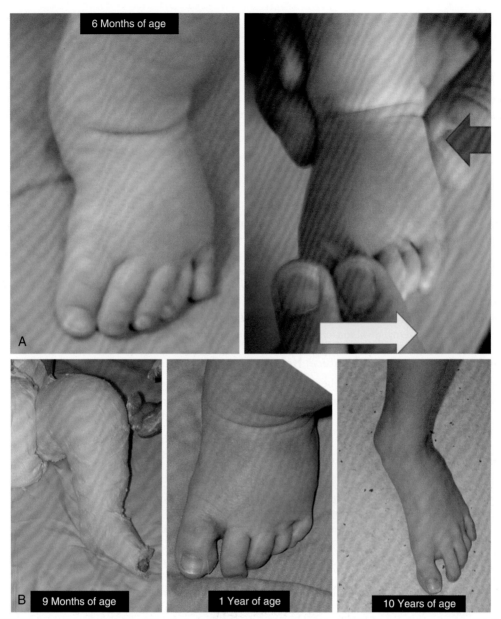

FIGURE 12.9 A, This 6-month-old boy has moderate stiff metatarsus adductus. The family is taught to stretch the forefoot by abducting the forefoot (yellow arrow) against a fulcrum against the cuboid (red arrow). B, Despite the use of home stretching, the family wanted to try casting to obtain improvement. At 10 years of age, he is doing well despite residual mild adductus.

Differential Diagnosis

Whenever evaluating a child with metatarsus adductus, one should consider whether or not a more complex foot deformity is present, such as clubfoot or skewfoot. Patients with metatarsus adductus will often present with the chief complaint of intoeing. It is therefore important to rule out other causes of intoeing, such as femoral anteversion and tibial torsion.

Diagnostic Tests or Advanced Imaging

Radiographs are generally not indicated in cases of mild, flexible metatarsus adductus. If the deformity is severe, rigid, or persists past 2 to 3 years of age, and/or surgery is planned, radiographs of the affected foot/feet may be indicated.

Treatment

Most cases of mild, flexible metatarsus adductus will correct spontaneously before 6 months. The family can be instructed to perform serial stretching during this time. Another significant portion will resolve as the child starts to walk. If the deformity is more rigid, serial casting can be done to obtain a straight lateral border of the foot (**Figure 12.9B**).

An orthosis may be utilized to maintain correction, including reverse-last and straight-last shoes, as well as other off-the-shelf orthoses. For refractory cases with severe deformity that persists after 3 years of age, surgical treatment may be considered.[3]

When to Refer

If the deformity is flexible, it is reasonable to treat metatarsus adductus with observation with or without serial stretching for the first 6 months, as most cases will resolve on their own without further treatment. If the deformity persists past 6 months, or the foot is rigid, referral to a pediatric orthopedic surgeon for further evaluation is indicated.

Skewfoot

Introduction

Skewfoot is defined as a congenital or acquired valgus deformity of the hindfoot with concomitant adductus of the forefoot. Clinically, it appears similar to the name with the hindfoot going in one direction and the forefoot going in the opposite direction.

Clinical Significance and Natural History

Early on in childhood, skewfoot is frequently confused with metatarsus adductus, and some consider it a more significant variant of metatarsus adductus. There can be many etiologies associated with skewfoot, the most common is idiopathic, followed by iatrogenic (from previous casting or bracing) and associated with an underlying neuromuscular condition or chromosomal abnormality. The natural history is not well documented, but most people function well without pain or arthrosis. On occasion, shoe wear can be difficult.

History and Physical Examination

On clinical examination, one should look for a medial midfoot concavity (navicular/midfoot) and the adjacent lateral convexity (head of the talus). It is important to break the foot down into segments for examination. The hindfoot is in valgus and everted. The midfoot is adducted and the forefoot is pronated. The longitudinal arch may be variable in presentation depending on the underlying etiology. Typically, the ankle is in neutral position (**Figure 12.10**).

Diagnostic Tests or Advanced Imaging

Radiographs demonstrate a medial deviated talar head on the anteroposterior (AP) view, but on the lateral view, the talus is not plantarflexed. As the child ages, the midfoot deformities accentuate and the longitudinal arch drops leading to hindfoot valgus and equinus in some children. The adolescent skewfoot looks very close to a flat foot to the unexperienced examiner (**Figure 12.11**).

Treatment

One can consider serial casting early in a similar fashion to metatarsus adductus. In older children with symptomatic pain or callosities a lateral calcaneal lengthening, osteotomy coupled with a medial opening wedge osteotomy can help correct the hindfoot valgus and midfoot adductus (**Figure 12.12A** and **B**).

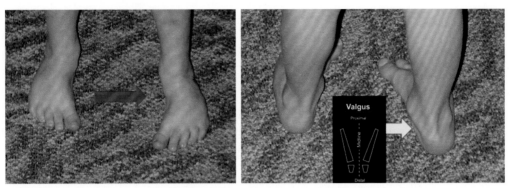

FIGURE 12.10 This 4-year-old girl has a skewfoot. It has the same forefoot adduction (red arrow) seen in metatarsus adductus. Yet, the hindfoot has significantly more valgus than usual (yellow arrow).

When to Refer

Skewfoot is a relatively uncommon foot condition and should be referred to a pediatric orthopedic surgeon. As a general practitioner, the skewfoot diagnosis is elusive and is often confused with typical pes planus (flatfoot). A foot that seems severe in its clinical appearance or a young child who appears to have more than one foot deformity should trigger the referral.

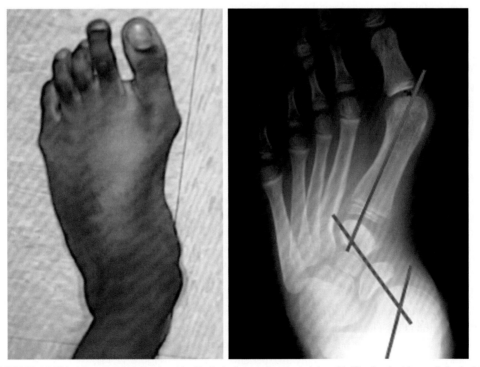

FIGURE 12.11 This 15-year-old high school football star has a skewfoot deformity. The forefoot is medially deviated on the midfoot, and the midfoot is laterally deviated on the hindfoot. Some have termed this a "serpentine foot"; despite the ominous name, the boy is asymptomatic and is the fastest runner on his team.

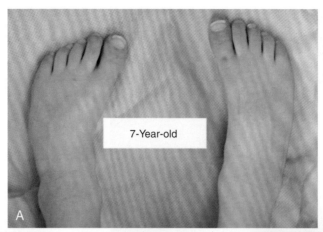

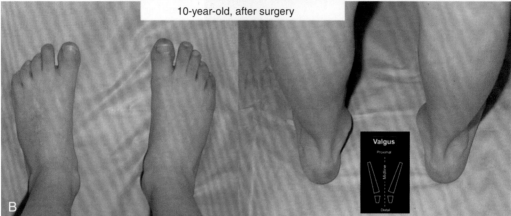

FIGURE 12.12 A, The child in **Figure 12.10** is having difficulty with shoe wear and the family desires correction. Midfoot osteotomy was suggested. B, Three years after surgery, shoe wear has improved and the patient is asymptomatic despite persistent hindfoot valgus that was not corrected.

Congenital Vertical Talus

Introduction

Congenital vertical talus (CVT) is a rare foot deformity, with an estimated prevalence of 1 in 10,000 live births. Anatomically both clubfoot and CVT have a tight heel cord; but the CVT foot is flat with dorsal dislocation of the navicular on the talus with the hindfoot in valgus, while a clubfoot is a cavus foot with the navicular medially displaced on the talus head and the hindfoot is in varus. It is important to remember that the navicular is the last bone in the foot to ossify (3-4 years); thus it is impossible to see on radiographs prior to this period. In CVT the displacement of the navicular is confirmed it when the first metatarsal axis and the talus axis is displaced (the talus-first metatarsal axis is normally colinear). Fifty percent of cases are bilateral. The condition occurs equally in males and females. While major reconstructive surgery was once the mainstay of treatment, like clubfoot, CVT can now be treated successfully with serial manipulation/casting and minimally invasive surgery.[4,5]

Clinical Significance and Natural History

The etiology of CVT is considered idiopathic in half of cases and associated with neuromuscular or genetic conditions in the other half. Therefore, it is essential that a thorough history and physical examination be performed to rule out the presence of any associated conditions. It is important to recognize CVT as this can cause disability if left untreated.

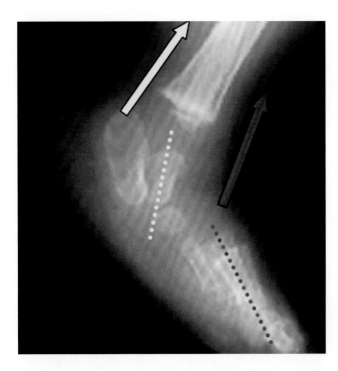

FIGURE 12.13 Pathophysiology of congenital vertical talus. The talus is vertically positioned (dashed yellow line) and is not colinear with first metatarsal (dashed red line). This is due to contracture of the Achilles tendon (yellow arrow) and the dorsal tendons of the foot (red arrow).

History and Physical Examination

The physical appearance and anatomic orientation are a result of two forces pitted against each other and resulting in midfoot dislocation at the talonavicular joint. The anterior tendons (toe extensors and tibialis anterior tendons) are contracted leading to a dorsiflexed navicular and an abducted/everted forefoot, while the hindfoot is being pulled into equinus and valgus by the Achilles and peroneal tendons (**Figure 12.13**).

The CVT foot has a distinct "rocker-bottom" appearance due to the dorsal dislocation of the navicular on the talus. This causes a convex appearance to the plantar surface of the foot; age-old descriptions have compared this foot to a Persian slipper (**Figure 12.14**).

The head of the talus is palpable along the plantar medial aspect of the midfoot, contributing to the rocker-bottom appearance of the foot. The key factor that determines the difference between CVT and other flat feet (calcaneovalgus foot, oblique talus, or flexible flat foot) is the presence of Achilles contracture in CVT.[5]

Features to Confirm

A thorough physical examination should be performed to rule out an associated neuromuscular or genetic condition. Particular attention should be paid to the presence of abnormal appearing facies and other congenital anomalies, such as upper extremity deformities, multiple joint contractures, limb deficiencies, etc. Examination of the hips should be done to evaluate for hip dysplasia. Spinal examination should also be done to rule out the presence of scoliosis and a hairy tuft or a presacral dimple can signify spinal dysraphism such as a tethered cord.

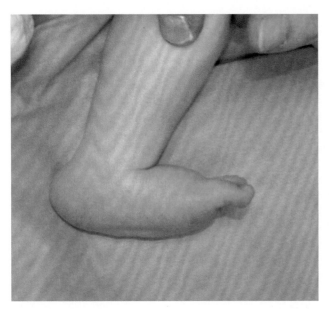

FIGURE 12.14 Clinical appearance of congenital vertical talus.

Pitfalls in Diagnosis

Most cases of CVT can be diagnosed by clinical examination based on the appearance of a "rocker-bottom" foot that is usually rigid and with an empty heel pad signifying an equinus contracture. There is a less severe variant of CVT, known as an oblique talus, which can have a similar appearance, but is less rigid. With an oblique talus, the navicular will reduce (Noted by reduction of the talus-first metatarsus axis on a plantarflexion lateral radiograph of the foot.) with plantar flexion, while it remains rigidly dislocated in a foot with CVT. This can be determined both on clinical examination and also with radiographs. Practitioners must also consider an underlying neuromuscular diagnosis in children presenting with CVT.

Differential Diagnosis

A calcaneovalgus foot can be easily mistaken for CVT. A foot with calcaneovalgus deformity is severely dorsiflexed with the dorsal surface of the foot resting on the anterior surface of the lower leg. The calcaneovalgus foot will be much more flexible than one with a CVT due to the absence of any true equinus contractures. The calcaneovalgus deformity almost always corrects on its own in the first 6 months of life, while a foot with a CVT requires special treatment.

Diagnostic Tests or Advanced Imaging

When the diagnosis of CVT is not clearly based on the physical examination, radiographs (AP and lateral views in maximum plantar and dorsiflexion) can be used to help make the diagnosis. It is important to remember that the navicular does not ossify until 2 to 3 years of age; thus, the position of the cartilaginous navicular is inferred by using the longitudinal axis of the first metatarsal. In calcaneovalgus and oblique talus, the first metatarsal axis is not colinear with the axis of the talus on the forced dorsiflexion lateral radiograph. Yet with the oblique talus, this will reduce on the maximum plantar flexion lateral radiograph (**Figure 12.15**).

In CVT, the first metatarsal axis (and the navicular) will remain dorsally displaced and not aligned with talus on the forced plantar flexion lateral (**Figure 12.16**).

Treatment

Treatment of CVT has shifted away from extensive soft tissue releases to a more minimally invasive method utilizing serial casting, called the "reverse Ponseti method." Weekly manipulation of the foot is performed with the goal of stretching the foot into plantar flexion and adduction, while pushing the talus dorsally and laterally. A long leg cast, similar to the Ponseti type used for clubfoot, is applied while the foot is being stretched. Casting is initiated in the first few months of life and continued weekly until reduction of the talonavicular joint has been achieved. In the final cast, the foot is positioned into

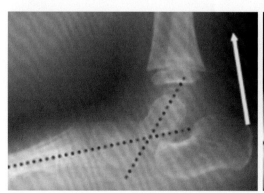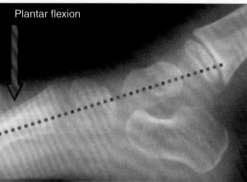

FIGURE 12.15 This child with an oblique talus has a vertically positioned talus as a result of Achilles contracture (yellow arrow). In plantar flexion, the talus and the first metatarsal are colinear.

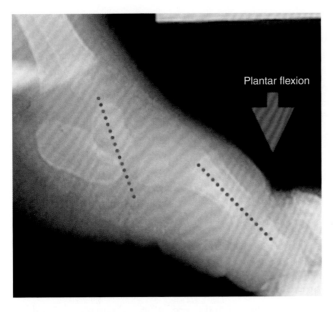

Plantar flexion

FIGURE 12.16 This child has congenital vertical talus as the talus and the first metatarsal do not align with a forced plantarflexion lateral.

extreme equinovarus, resembling a clubfoot. After application of the final cast, the patient is scheduled for surgical stabilization of the talonavicular joint with a k-wire and a percutaneous tenotomy of the Achilles tendon. The patient then uses a shoe and bar brace system, similar to that used to treat club foot, full time for several months and then at night only for several years[4] (**Figure 12.17**).

When to Refer

A patient with suspected CVT should be referred as early as possible. Evaluation and treatment are best performed by a fellowship trained pediatric orthopedic surgeon. While awaiting evaluation, gentle stretching and manipulation of the foot by the child's family members can be done.

Calcaneal Valgus Foot

Introduction

A calcaneovalgus foot is another common diagnosis made in the newborn nursery or during the first couple of pediatrician visits. Clinically, a calcaneovalgus foot is associated with hyperdorsiflexion with valgus deformity of the hindfoot; the foot itself can almost appear to touch the anterior aspect of the tibia. The deformity is likely related to positioning in the womb.

Clinical Significance and Natural History

Thankfully, 100% of these feet correct without any intervention and reassurance to the family is necessary (**Figure 12.18**).

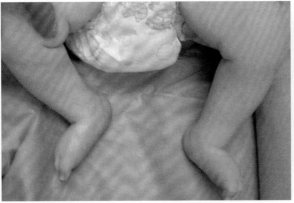
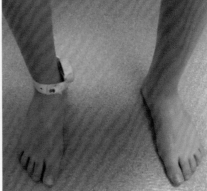

FIGURE 12.17 This boy with bilateral congenital vertical talus underwent the reverse Ponseti method as described by Dr Matt Dobbs. At 9 years, he has an excellent clinical result.

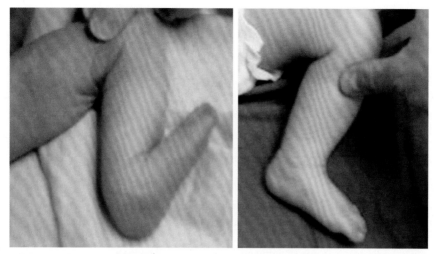

FIGURE 12.18 This newborn has a calcaneal valgus foot, which corrects in 6 weeks of observation.

The calcaneovalgus foot can be associated with a posteromedial bow of the tibia, which in combination makes the deformity quite striking. Even though the foot deformity gets better, the tibial deformity is associated with a limb length discrepancy at maturity and may require orthopedic intervention in adolescence.

History and Physical Examination

The deformity is limited to the hindfoot, which is in valgus or everted, with hyper dorsiflexion of the ankle such that the anterior aspect of the foot can touch the tibia. Typically, the forefoot and midfoot are in a neutral position.

Pitfalls in Diagnosis

One must not mistake a CVT foot for a calcaneovalgus foot as the treatment is quite different with different outcomes. A calcaneovalgus foot is very flexible, while a CVT foot demonstrates a typical rocker-bottom deformity with more rigidity that does not resolve. Radiographs described above will determine which foot has CVT and which is more benign (**Figure 12.19**).

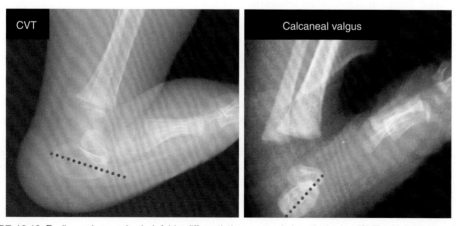

FIGURE 12.19 Radiographs can be helpful in differentiating congenital vertical talus (CVT) which has an elevated calcaneus with a depressed calcaneal pitch (dashed line) while the calcaneal valgus foot has a normally positioned calcaneus.

Treatment

No operative techniques are necessary. Parents can be instructed to perform daily plantar flexion exercises if they feel they need to do something. Formal physical therapy is typically not indicated.

When to Refer

A typical calcaneovalgus foot can be safely watched by a child's pediatrician. If there are concerns regarding the rigidity of the foot or the presence of a posteromedial bow, it is important to refer to a pediatric orthopedic surgeon.

Macrodactyly

Introduction

Macrodactyly is a rare form of local gigantism that is usually isolated to the hand and feet. In the feet, the condition is characterized by enlargement of both the soft tissue and bony structures of the foot. It can be progressive. Unlike macrodactyly of the hand, there is generally less involvement of neural elements.[6] Treatment is typically required due to pain and difficulty with shoe wear.

Clinical Significance and Natural History

Macrodactyly is significant because it can impede foot development and affect normal function and gait.[7] There is a static type in which the digit or digits are already enlarged at birth and their growth remains proportionate with the growth of the rest of the limb. In the progressive type, the involved digit grows disproportionately.[7]

History and Physical Examination

There will be enlargement of a single digit or multiple digits of the foot. The enlargement can also be appreciated into the forefoot.

Features to Confirm

Evaluate the limb for any associated findings that may be indicative of an underlying condition, such as a port-wine stain or arteriovenous malformation in Klippel-Trenaunay-Weber or café-au-lait spots that are indicative of neurofibromatosis (**Figure 12.20**). It is also important to look for the presence of a tumor. In most cases, however, macrodactyly is an isolated feature without other findings or systemic involvement.

Diagnostic Tests or Advanced Imaging

Radiographs of the affected foot should be obtained to evaluate the underlying bony structure. If surgery is planned, magnetic resonance imaging (MRI) may be helpful to understand the soft tissue component of the disease and to assist with surgical planning.

Treatment

In most cases, macrodactyly requires surgical treatment. The goal of surgery is to create a cosmetically acceptable foot that will allow for a normal gait and facilitate shoe wear.[6,7] Macrodactyly is the enlargement of the length, width, and height of the forefoot and toes, with involvement of both bone and soft tissue. Soft tissue debulking alone may be successful in the short term, but is not considered a long-term solution. Specific surgical treatment depends on the area of involvement (lesser vs great toe). For lesser toes with metatarsal involvement, the best results are obtained with ray resection (**Figure 12.21**).

When the metatarsal is not involved, phalangeal amputation, epiphysiodesis, and shortening can be considered. Many surgeons have gone away from epiphysiodesis, however, because the timing of surgery is difficult to assess. When the great toe is involved, ray resection is not an option, as this would alter normal gait substantially. For macrodactyly in this location, a combination of shortening, epiphysiodesis, and soft tissue debulking may be required. There is debate as to the timing of surgical

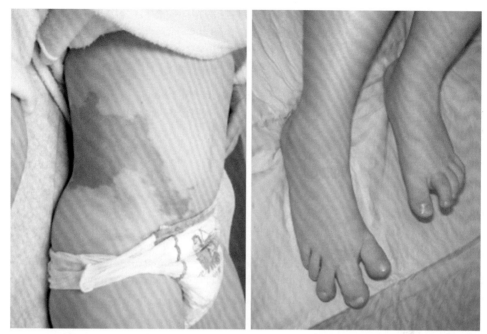

FIGURE 12.20 This 5-year-old girl has macrodactyly of her right foot involving the second and third rays. Her right flank has a large port-wine stain consistent with Klippel-Trenauney-Weber (KTW) syndrome.

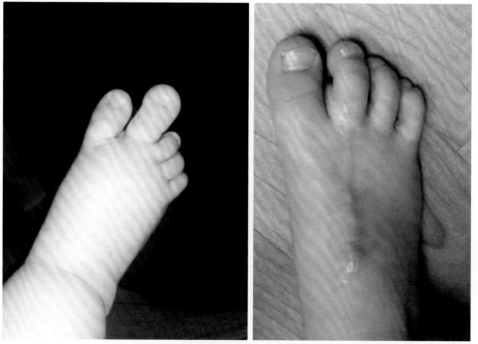

FIGURE 12.21 This 2-year-old with macrodactyly underwent second ray amputation and has a foot that is painless and fits in a standard shoe at age 5. She will continue to be followed to determine if this will be a progressive form of enlargement.

intervention; however, most practitioners feel it is best to intervene before walking age. This allows for assessment of the extent and type of growth pattern of the macrodactyly and corrects the shape of the foot to facilitate shoe wear when the child is ready to start walking.[6]

When to Refer

Children with macrodactyly should be referred as soon as the condition is diagnosed. This will allow for assessment of the extent and growth pattern of the macrodactyly to facilitate surgical planning and not delay walking.

● Lesser Toe Deformities

Congenital Curly Toe

Introduction

Curly toe is a common congenital deformity, which is usually bilateral. It typically involves the lateral three toes, yet it can involve just the third toe and rarely all four lesser toes to varying degrees. This flexion and varus deformity of the interphalangeal joint results from contracture of flexor digitorum longus (FDL). Surgical treatment can be recommended if the deformity becomes symptomatic and persists beyond 6 years of age.

Clinical Significance and Natural History

The natural history demonstrates that about 20% of curly toes will resolve spontaneously and conservative initial treatment is a reasonable first treatment option. In many cases of resolution, the flexion will resolve leaving a residual external rotation and adduction deformity, which are not of clinical significance.[8]

History and Physical Examination

On examination, look for ***flexion, adduction, and external rotation*** of one or more toes with contracture of FDL. The proximal interphalangeal joint will rest in flexion with or without a flexion deformity of the distal interphalangeal joint. It is important to examine the toes in neutral ankle dorsiflexion, which will put the tendons on stretch and illustrate the affected toe. Look for callosities on the plantar aspect of the toe and associated skin and nail irritation on the affected toes.

Pitfalls in Diagnosis

Patients are often referred for overlapping second toe and parents think the problem is with this toe; therefore, it is important to explain that the overlapping is compensation for the contracted third toe (**Figure 12.22**).

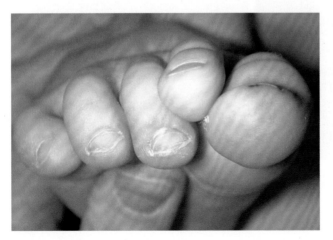

Diagnostic Tests or Advanced Imaging

Radiographs are not indicated to make the diagnosis of a curly toe.

Treatment

Taping can temporarily improve the position of the toes but the deformity typically recurs when taping has been discontinued. Typically, no treatment

FIGURE 12.22 This 3-year-old boy was referred for a second toe problem. In fact, the second toe is merely accommodating for curly toes 3, 4, and 5.

should be performed before the age of 6, due to the likelihood of resolution. If still symptomatic at age 6, tenotomy of the toe flexors should be considered.

When to Refer

Conservative watchful waiting and accommodative shoes are a very reasonable first step. Children who demonstrate skin-related issues such as ingrown nails, bleeding, pain, or callosities should be referred to a pediatric orthopedic surgeon.

Overriding Fifth Toe

Introduction

Congenital deformity affects males and females equally and is typically bilateral in presentation. It is believed to occur from a capsular contraction and tightness of the extensor digitorum longus. There can be a familial component to the deformity.

Clinical Significance and Natural History

Less common than curly toe, the deformity is rarely disabling and the indication for surgical intervention is to improve function and relieve foot pain, which is recalcitrant to shoe modification.

History and Physical Examination

On examination, there is dorsomedial angulation of the fifth toe at the MTP joint with concomitant extensor tendon contracture, and the web space skin between the fourth and fifth toe can be abnormal.

Diagnostic Tests or Advanced Imaging

The diagnosis of an overriding fifth toe is made clinically and there is no indication for radiographs to confirm the diagnosis.

Treatment

Approximately 50% of those with an overriding fifth toe can be treated conservatively with shoe modification. Surgical reconstruction can be considered for those feet with severe pain and callosities, yet the recurrence is high (**Figure 12.23**).

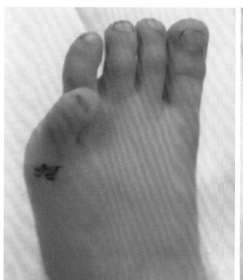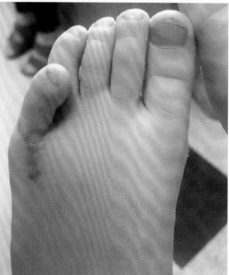

FIGURE 12.23 This child had a painful congenital overriding fifth toe that underwent Butler procedure with only minor improvement in position.

When to Refer

Since 50% of overriding fifth toes do not require surgical intervention, it is reasonable for referring provider to initially prescribe accommodative shoes and conservative interventions to alleviate symptoms. If the toe remains persistently symptomatic, then referral to an orthopedic surgeon is appropriate.

Polydactyly

Introduction

Polydactyly is a condition where extra digits of the toe are present at birth. Incidence is 1 in 500 births. The condition is more common in African-Americans. There is usually a family history of polydactyly, and it can be inherited as an autosomal dominant trait.[9] The most common location of the extra digit is on the lateral side of the foot (postaxial), an extra digit on the medial side of the foot is considered preaxial. While postaxial polydactyly is usually an isolated finding, preaxial polydactyly may be seen with other disorders such as tibial hemimelia (**Figure 12.24**).

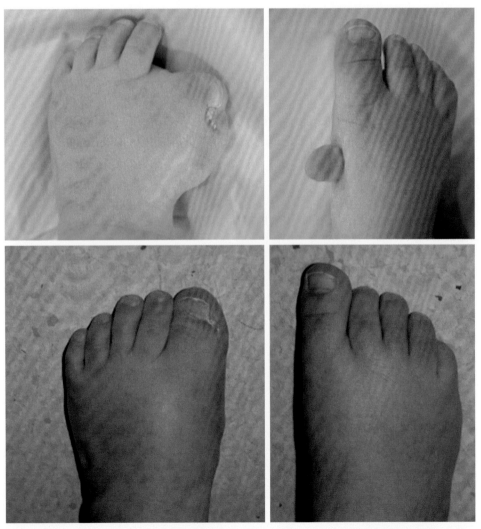

FIGURE 12.24 This 5-year-old boy with Dandy Walker syndrome, agenesis of the corpus callosum, and hand polydactyly has preaxial polysyndactyly on the left and polydactyly on the right foot. Surgical reconstruction was useful for improving shoe wear.

Clinical Significance and Natural History

Postaxial polydactyly is the most common presentation; however, there can be a central duplication of the second, third, or fourth ray or preaxial duplication of the first ray. Postaxial polydactyly is divided into Type A and B. Type A postaxial polydactyly is a fully developed extra digit on the lateral border of foot with a fully or partially duplicated (bifid) metatarsal. Type B postaxial polydactyly is a rudimentary digit attached to the lateral aspect of the foot by a narrow neurovascular pedicle at the level of the metatarsal-phalangeal joint.[10] The extra digit is smaller than the fifth digit and often contains a small phalanx and toenail. Besides issues with cosmesis, polydactyly can lead to problems with shoe wear and angular deformities of the toes.

History and Physical Examination

The examiner should note the location of the duplicated digit—preaxial (medial border), central, or postaxial (lateral border)—and whether or not the postaxial digit is Type B or Type A. The patient may also have polydactyly of the hand and thus it is important to do a thorough physical examination of both the upper and lower extremities.

Diagnostic Tests or Advanced Imaging

It is helpful to obtain a radiograph of the involved forefoot to evaluate the underlying bony structure of the extra digit prior to any surgical treatment.

Treatment

Polydactyly can be treated by observation if the digit is well aligned and the patient does not have issues with shoe wear due to the forefoot being widened. This is more often done in cases of postaxial or central polydactyly. Surgical treatment involves amputation of the extra digit at around 9 to 12 months of age (**Figure 12.25**).

When to Refer

If the family desires surgical treatment, it is appropriate to refer the patient to a pediatric orthopedist.

Syndactyly

Introduction

Syndactyly is a relatively common presentation and can involve fusion of the soft tissue of toes and sometimes bony fusion of the phalanges of the foot. The epidemiology is about 1 in 2000 births. Most frequently, it is found between the second and third toe and is felt to be the result of incomplete apoptosis during gestation. It is believed to follow an autosomal dominance pattern of inheritance (**Figure 12.26**).

If there is more than one syndactyly per foot, they are often manifestations of a syndrome such as Apert syndrome. Thorough clinical examination and radiographic review will help to recognize and differentiate acrosyndactyly (fusion of the tip, associated with amniotic band syndrome or Streeter dysplasia) from syndactyly.

Clinical Significance and Natural History

There are two types of syndactyly; simple syndactyly involves soft tissue fusion and complex syndactyly involves both skin and bone fusion. Simple syndactyly can be classified as partial to complete from proximal to distal with each toe having normal bones, ligaments, joints, and neurovascular structures. Typically, simple syndactyly does not require surgical intervention as the two joined toes grow at a similar rate. Complex syndactyly relates to failure of segmentation of soft tissue as well as bone between adjacent toes. In complex situations, the bones are typically abnormal and conjoined. Joints are typically fused and neurovascular structures on adjacent sides of the toes are absent or malformed. Toenails are frequently unsegmented and conjoined.

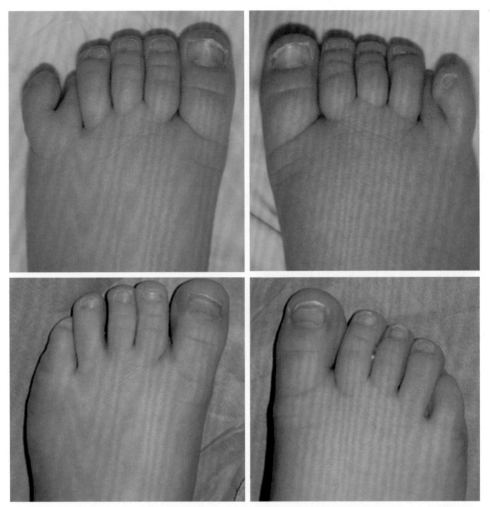

FIGURE 12.25 Postaxial polydactyly is usually bilateral and is an isolated finding. This healthy boy underwent amputation of the lateral digits at 18 months of age.

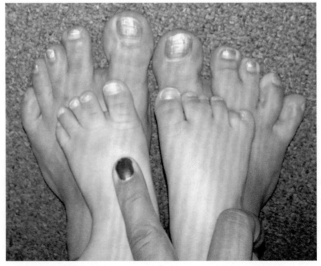

FIGURE 12.26 A 2-year-old girl rests her feet on her mothers, both have syndactyly of their second and third toes. Mother has been asymptomatic her whole life and likely, so will her daughter.

History and Physical Examination

The diagnosis of syndactyly is relatively straightforward; however, what is challenging is the differentiation between simple and complex syndactyly. Often radiographs are used to help confirm the diagnosis. It is important to identify where the syndactyly is occurring and rule out the presence of acrosyndactyly, if present, as the etiology and treatment are different.

Diagnostic Tests or Advanced Imaging

No imaging is necessary for simple syndactyly, but simulated weight-bearing AP and lateral radiographs of the forefoot are helpful for surgical planning in cases of complex syndactyly.

Treatment

Simple syndactyly rarely requires surgical intervention as the only affect is cosmetic. Surgical separation, while commonly performed in the hand to improve finger function, is reasonable, in the foot, potential complications do not justify surgical separation in most parent's minds. Operative management of complex syndactyly is usually indicated in the setting of pain, due to abnormal position/fusion of conjoined bones or joints (**Figure 12.27**).

When to Refer

It is reasonable to refer all complex syndactyly patients to a pediatric orthopedic surgeon to establish care and facilitate surveillance. Simple syndactyly cases may not warrant referral but many families demand referral even though eventual treatment is unlikely.

Bunionette Deformity

Introduction

Bunionette is a prominence on the lateral aspect of the fifth metatarsal head. The deformity is more common in women and is frequently bilateral. It is caused by compression of the forefoot, generally from tight shoes or abnormal forces on the lateral side of the foot.[11] Bunionette can also be a component of other congenital foot deformities and can be seen with some inflammatory arthropathies.

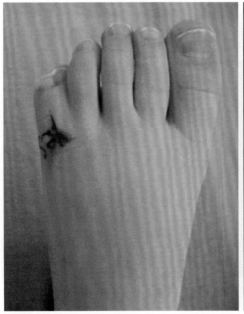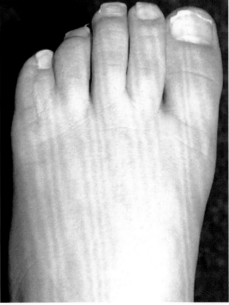

FIGURE 12.27 Polysyndactyly in the foot is treated with amputation of the lateral toe in order to improve shoe wear.

Clinical Significance and Natural History

More often than not, this is just a cosmetic finding, yet the deformity can cause pain over the fifth metatarsal head with callousing and can interfere with shoe wear, which can lead to difficulty with weight-bearing activity.

History and Physical Examination

The deformity mimics a traditional bunion deformity of the great toe. There will be medial deviation of the fifth toe with a prominence of the fifth metatarsal head. The patient may have redness and callousing over the fifth toe where the bunionette is located. There may also be concomitant pes planovalgus (flat foot) and hallux valgus (bunion).[11]

Diagnostic Tests or Advanced Imaging

Weight-bearing radiographs of the affected foot/feet are recommended to plan surgical reconstruction. These will show an increased 4 to 5 intermetatarsal angle, increased lateral deviation angle, and increased width of the metatarsal head.[11]

Treatment

Most cases of bunionette deformity can be treated nonoperatively with anti-inflammatories, shoe modification, and padding. If there is concomitant flat foot deformity, inserts can help to off load the lateral side of the foot. Surgery for symptomatic bunionette deformity can be considered for the patient with painful shoe wear that is limiting activities (**Figure 12.28**).

When to Refer

Patients with mild symptoms can be managed nonoperatively as directed above. If a patient presents with significant pain and disability, or has failed conservative treatment, referral to a pediatric orthopedic surgeon is reasonable.

Juvenile Hallux Valgus

Introduction

A juvenile bunion (hallux valgus with open growth plates) is lateral deviation of the first toe at the MTP joint. The condition occurs most often in females and there is frequently a family history. Some think that up to half of adult bunions have their onset in childhood.[12] Hallux valgus is frequently encountered

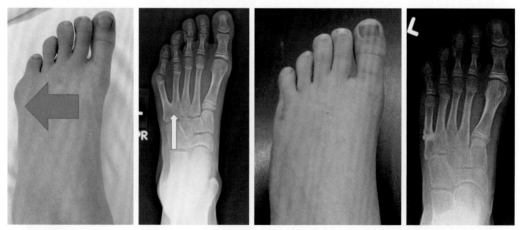

FIGURE 12.28 A 10-year-old boy with a painful bunionette deformity (blue arrow) as a result of congenital fusion of the fourth and fifth metatarsal (yellow arrow). Surgical correction was performed to improve symptoms.

in the neuromuscular population due to spasticity. In the non-neuromuscular population, hallux valgus may be associated with ligamentous laxity and flat foot. As the hallux valgus progresses, the great toe starts to pronate, and the sesamoids move laterally due to the pull of the short toe flexor and adductor tendons.

Clinical Significance and Natural History

Hallux valgus deformity is a concerning deformity for patients because it can lead to dissatisfaction with cosmesis and occasional difficulty with shoe wear. The main complaint is pain over the bunion, which can become debilitating and can lead to problems with weight bearing and activity.

History and Physical Examination

The great toe is laterally deviated with prominence of the medial MTP joint (**Figure 12.29**). There may be callousing with skin irritation/inflammation over the bunion. There can be associated flexible flat foot with forefoot widening. One should also look for valgus interphalangeus, which is valgus deformity present in the IP joint of the great toe.

Pitfalls in Diagnosis

There is really no other condition that mimics a bunion. Patients with neuromuscular disease commonly develop a dorsal bunion. In these cases, the great toe is laterally deviated and flexed, creating callousing on the dorsal-medial aspect of the MP joint rather than the medial aspect.

Diagnostic Tests or Advanced Imaging

When considering surgery, the orthopedist will order weight-bearing radiographs of the involved foot/feet necessary for evaluation (**Figure 12.29**) and for measurement of the hallux valgus angle, 1-2 intermetatarsal angle, distal metatarsal articular angle, and hallux valgus interphalangeus angle. These measurements are helpful for surgical planning.

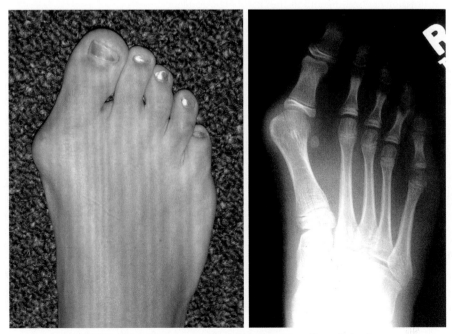

FIGURE 12.29 Clinical and radiographic examples of juvenile bunion.

Treatment

If the patient is not symptomatic, no treatment is necessary. If the patient is having pain over the bunion, shoe modification, nighttime bracing/splinting, padding of the bony prominence, and anti-inflammatory medication can be helpful. If there is associated flexible flat foot, an orthotic can be used. Surgery "can be" considered if the patient still has pain that is activity limiting after conservative treatment; yet surgical correction of juvenile bunions with open growth plates has a high rate of recurrence. For patients with painful dorsal bunions associated with neuromuscular disease, a first MTP joint fusion is the treatment of choice.[12]

When to Refer

Bunions can be managed initially with conservative/symptomatic treatment. It would be reasonable to refer a patient when those measures have failed and the patient is having significant disability due to pain.

Disorders of Walking Children and Adolescents

Flexible Flatfoot

Introduction

Most infants have feet that appear flat, and the normal arch may not fully develop until approximately 7 to 10 years of age. Flat feet are typically a result of generalized ligamentous laxity without underlying pathology. In a series of 835 children, flexible flat feet were noted in 54% of those aged 3 years, decreasing to 24% of those aged 6 years.[13] The male to female ratio is 2:1 and obese children are three times more likely to develop acquired flexible flatfoot than those with a healthy weight.[14.]

Clinical Significance and Natural History

Extrapolating into adulthood, only 15% to 20% of adults have some degree of flexible pes planus, and most of these are asymptomatic. Overall, only 1% of flat feet in children end up being painful, becoming stiff or functionally limiting and in the "pathologic" category.

History and Physical Examination

The diagnosis of flexible pes planus can be suspected with the return of a normal-appearing medial longitudinal arch as the patient goes from stance to toe raise (**Figure 12.30**).

The diagnosis of flexible pes planus can be confirmed with this maneuver by observing the hindfoot. In stance, the hindfoot of the flexible flat feet will be in valgus, which changes to a varus hindfoot when the child stands on his or her toes.[15] Tarsal coalition or other cause of rigid pes planus should be considered for the foot in which the heel does not change to varus during toe rise (**Figure 12.31**).

A tight gastrocnemius can be associated with adolescent pes planus that is characterized by restricted ankle dorsiflexion.[14] It is important to examine the calf length with the knee flexed and extended (Silfverskiold test) with care to maintain the foot supinated. This ensures the talonavicular joint is in a reduced position rather than with abduction of forefoot and midfoot break.[15]

If a child is complaining of pain, it is typically under the plantar-medial midfoot and occasionally in the sinus tarsi (more common with concomitant Achilles contracture).

Diagnostic Tests or Advanced Imaging

If the child is asymptomatic, no further consideration for evaluation or treatment is indicated. There is little utility in evaluating a foot that does not require treatment, and it is hard to make an asymptomatic patient better. Radiographic imaging is only indicated when the child has pain or functional problems. In this case, standing radiographs in both AP and lateral planes and nonstanding oblique views are necessary (**Figure 12.32**).

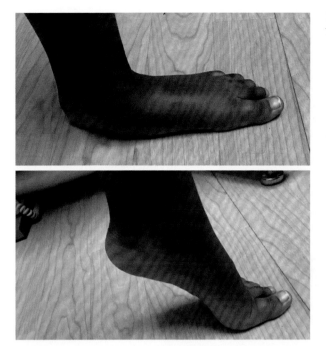

FIGURE 12.30 This flexible flatfoot reconstitutes an arch when standing on tip toes.

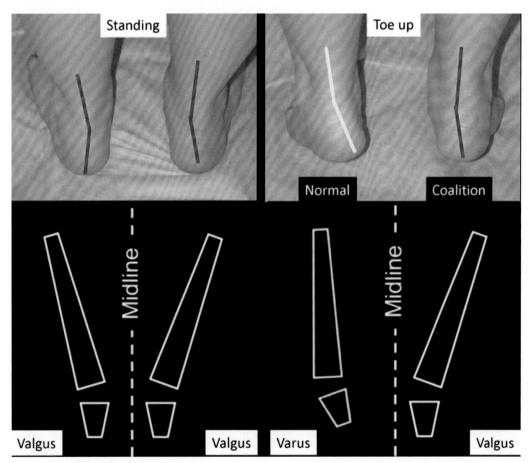

FIGURE 12.31 This figure demonstrates that when standing both hindfeet are in valgus as indicated by red lines (top left). When the child stands on his toes, the normal flexible foot goes into varus (yellow lines) while the foot with the rigid flat foot secondary to a coalition stays in valgus.

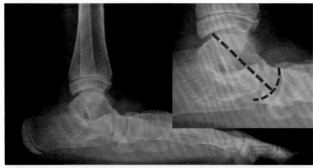

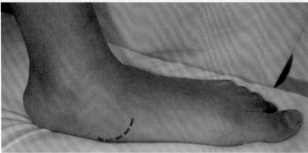

FIGURE 12.32 This child with a flat foot deformity has radiographic collapse of the midfoot with verticality of the talus and a plantar-oriented talar head (curved red line) which is also palpable clinically.

The relationship between the talus and calcaneus should be examined in both planes. On the AP view of the ankle, the coronal alignment of the ankle is assessed and ankle valgus is identified. On the lateral view, typically talonavicular "sag or plantarflexion" can be appreciated (**Figure 12.32**). The oblique view is helpful to identify a calcaneonavicular tarsal coalition. MRI or CT scan can be considered for the painful flat foot with normal radiographs.

Pitfalls in Diagnosis

Although rare, initially flexible flat feet can become painful and appear to be more rigid with time. Other causes of painful flat feet include untreated CVT, severe skewfoot, tarsal coalition and subtalar inflammation, or neoplasia. Pes planus can be the primary sign for syndromes such as Ehlers-Danlos, Marfan syndrome, or fragile X.

Treatment

It is important to reinforce that painless flat feet (flexible or rigid) do not require treatment. In younger children presenting with flexible pes planus, no treatment is indicated apart from reassurance. If the growing child has pain, then conservative measures such as orthotic use may be helpful (**Figure 12.33**).

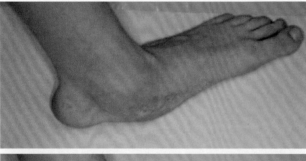

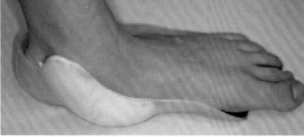

If a child has tightness of the Achilles, then a stretching program may be useful especially for parents who want something done.[15] Surgical treatment to correct pes planus is indicated in children with pain and dysfunction, who have failed conservative therapy. Most described procedures to correct pes planus are extensive and involve soft tissue reefing, tendon transfers or lengthenings, and bony osteotomies.

FIGURE 12.33 An adolescent boy with Marfanoid characteristics has a painful flat foot managed by this UCBL orthosis.

When to Refer

Pes planus is common and the majority can be initially managed in the office of the general practitioner. If a child has persistent pain recalcitrant to therapy and shoe modifications, then he or she should be seen by a pediatric orthopedic specialist.

Tarsal Coalition

Introduction

Tarsal coalition is a congenital fibrous, cartilaginous, or bony connection between two bones in the foot.[16] The most common coalitions in the foot occur between the talus and calcaneus (called talocalcaneal or subtalar) and between the calcaneus and navicular (calcaneonavicular). It is thought to be caused by failure of the normal joint to separate at these locations due to lack of differentiation of mesenchymal tissue.[16] The overall incidence is 1% and coalitions are bilateral in 60% of cases.[16]

Clinical Significance and Natural History

Many tarsal coalitions remain asymptomatic, and in bilateral cases, only one side may present with pain.[16] Unlike flexible flat foot, the foot with a tarsal coalition will be more rigid. This is an important characteristic to distinguish when evaluating these patients because symptomatic tarsal coalitions generally require surgical treatment.[16]

History and Physical Examination

Patients with tarsal coalition present with painful flat feet and/or frequent ankle sprains. The increased incidence of ankle sprains is due to decreased subtalar motion, which, when normal, generally accommodates normal inversion and eversion stresses to the hindfoot. When the subtalar motion is decreased due to fusion, those stresses are imparted up to the ankle, which is not designed for inversion and eversion (**Figure 12.34**).

Painful tarsal coalitions most often present between the ages of 10 and 14, as the coalition begins to ossify. Patients may complain of diffuse ankle pain or point to the sinus tarsi and around the fibula with a calcaneonavicular coalition and around the medial malleolus for a talocalcaneal coalition. A key factor is that the pain is usually activity related. In more severe cases, the foot may be in a rigid everted position, for which arose the classic descriptor "peroneal spastic flat foot." This finding is caused by pain, decrease in subtalar motion, and spasm in the peroneus brevis and longus leading to eversion of the foot.

A thorough examination of the foot must be performed when considering the diagnosis of tarsal coalition. The foot will demonstrate mild to moderate flattening of the arch, with the hindfoot in valgus and the forefoot abducted. It is critical to distinguish whether or not the subtalar joint is flexible. This is done by asking the child to stand on his or her tiptoes. The heel should be in varus when the patient raises up on his or her toe. A stiff subtalar joint will remain in the valgus position while the patient is toe-standing (▶ **Video 12.2**).

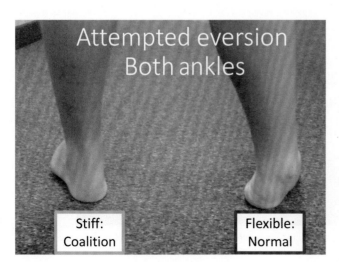

FIGURE 12.34 This boy complains of frequent ankle sprains on the left side. In the clinic, he cannot evert his subtalar joint while his normal flexible side can evert fully. The inability of his left subtalar joint to move from the coalition makes him prone to ankle sprains on uneven ground.

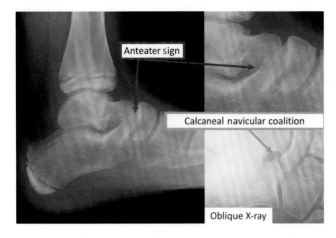

FIGURE 12.35 A calcaneal navicular coalition can be suspected when the anterior process of the calcaneus appears elongated "anteater sign" (red arrow). A bony coalition is confirmed on the internal oblique radiograph (blue arrow).

Subtalar motion and the amount of inversion/eversion will be limited and can be assessed by holding the tibiotalar joint steady while inverting and everting the patient's heel. There may also be a concomitant heel cord contracture. It is important to examine both feet, as tarsal coalition is bilateral in 60% of cases.

Pitfalls in Diagnosis

Most tarsal coalitions become symptomatic between ages 10 and 14 perhaps due to the timing of ossification of the coalition. When a patient presents with a rigid flat foot before the age of 10, other diagnoses must be considered. The most common cause of rigid flat foot in this age group is juvenile idiopathic arthritis. This diagnosis requires referral to a pediatric rheumatologist.[16]

Diagnostic Tests or Advanced Imaging

Weight-bearing radiographs of the affected foot should be obtained when considering the diagnosis of tarsal coalition. With a calcaneonavicular coalition, the lateral ankle radiograph may show an "anteater sign" which is an elongated anterior process of the calcaneus. A 45° internal oblique view of the foot may show an abnormal articulation between the calcaneus and navicular bones (**Figure 12.35**).

Patients with a subtalar or talocalcaneal coalition often have a "c-sign" on the lateral ankle radiograph, which is formed by the medial outline of the talar dome and the posteroinferior aspect of the sustentaculum tali (**Figure 12.36**).

There may also be talar beaking present due to abnormal motion of the subtalar joint. A Harris heel view may reveal an irregular middle facet joint.[16] While tarsal coalition can often (but not always) be visualized on standard radiographs, advanced imaging is necessary to evaluate the painful foot with

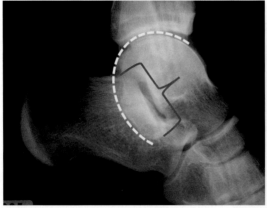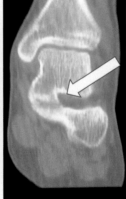

FIGURE 12.36 A subtalar coalition may be suspected on a lateral radiograph by noticing the C-sign (yellow line) which is due to the bony coalition (red bracket). A CT scan is needed to confirm the bony coalition (white arrow).

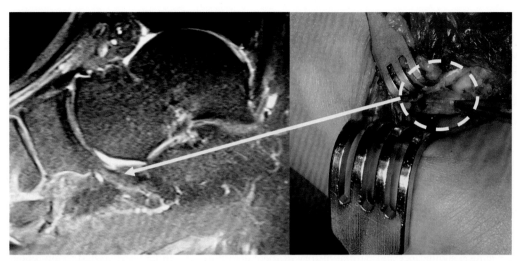

FIGURE 12.37 This child has a fibrous calcaneonavicular coalition detected on MRI scan (yellow arrow). Diagnostic injection relieved her pain and surgical approach confirmed the band (yellow circle) which when removed, relieved her pain.

decreased subtalar motion or to confirm a suspected coalition. It is required for preoperative planning to assist with surgical resection. Some practitioners prefer MRI over CT due to the fact that MRI can also visualize a fibrous or cartilaginous coalition (**Figure 12.37**).

Treatment

Treatment for symptomatic coalitions starts with conservative measures including rest, activity modification, physical therapy, and anti-inflammatories. A walking boot or cast may be used for a short period of time to immobilize the foot/ankle. Orthotics may also be helpful once immobilization is discontinued.[16]

When nonoperative management fails, surgery treatment consists of coalition resection with interposition of fat or muscle to prevent recurrence (**Figure 12.38**).

If the coalition involves more than 50% of the joint surface area, fusion of that joint or osteotomy of the calcaneus can be considered. In cases with severe flat foot deformity, coalition resection may be combined with deformity correction, such as lateral column lengthening, or medial calcaneal slide.

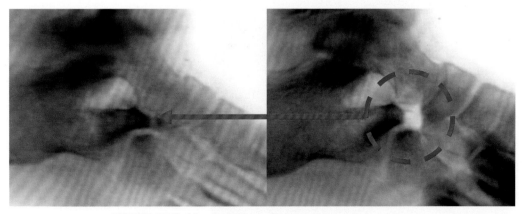

FIGURE 12.38 A bony coalition before and after surgical resection.

When to Refer

Tarsal coalitions can initially be treated by the referring provider with the conservative measures described above. Some patients achieve pain relief with a short period of immobilization. If nonoperative management fails, the patient should be referred to a pediatric orthopedist for surgical treatment.

Cavus and Cavovarus Feet

Introduction

A cavus foot relates to a high arch appreciated within the midfoot.[17] The arch elevation may be due to variable degrees of plantar-flexion deformity of the forefoot and dorsiflexion of the calcaneus (**Figure 12.39**).

When the cavus foot is extreme and fixed, it can lead to varus deformity of the hindfoot. Cavus and cavovarus feet have a high chance of a neurologic etiology, and the astute practitioner should perform a careful neurologic examination and consider ordering an MRI of the spine to rule out intraspinal pathology.

Clinical Significance and Natural History

The clinical significance and natural history of these deformities are more likely related to any underlying etiology such as Charcot-Marie-Tooth or other hereditary motor sensory neuropathies (HMSN), Friedreich ataxia, muscular dystrophy, spina bifida, or cerebral palsy. Most of these patients have bilateral (though not necessarily symmetric) deformities. Patients with unilateral deformities are more likely to have structural abnormalities within the brain or spinal column. Cavus feet are typically more symptomatic than pes planus and can present with a history of ankle sprains and lateral column overloaded with callosities (**Figure 12.40**).

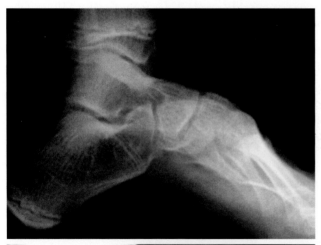

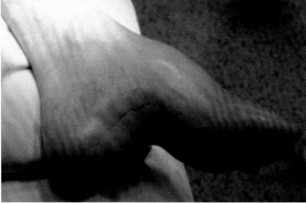

Physical History and Physical Examination

It is important to determine when the deformity was noted, if it is progressive, and if it is bilateral. Has there been a history of trauma that has resulted in peripheral nerve dysfunction or scaring from a compartment syndrome? (See **Figure 12.41**.)

The family history is important as many of these underlying disorders are hereditary with more severity in later generations.

It is important to perform a detailed general neurologic examination looking for ataxic gait, presence, or absence of reflexes; examination of the upper extremities can confirm a more systemic disorder such as HMSN. Careful inspection of the back is needed to detect scoliosis and to identify signs (lipoma, hairy patches, presacral dimples, or fistulas) of spinal dysraphism.

FIGURE 12.39 This boy has fixed cavus without hindfoot varus.

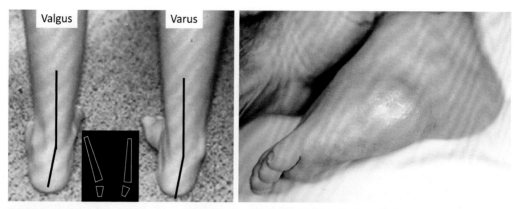

FIGURE 12.40 This child with cavovarus foot bears most of the weight on the lateral column of the foot and has a callus over the base of the fifth metatarsal head.

On examination, the forefoot is pronated, the hindfoot is in varus, and the ankle can be in a variable position. Often the ankle is not in equinus but the apparent equinus appreciated is related to the fixed cavus position of the forefoot. Clawing of the toes can lead to skin irritation over the dorsal IP joints and is highly suspected for neurologic disorders (**Figure 12.42**).

Typical muscle imbalances are present (weak tibialis anterior and peroneus brevis with relative overpull of the peroneus longus and posterior tibialis) and one should confirm if the foot is flexible or rigid as this affects treatment. A flexible or dynamic deformity indicates that the present deformities will correct with soft tissue release or transfers. A rigid deformity is one that will not correct during the clinical examination and is therefore an indication for osteotomies to realign the foot. A Coleman block test can be used to assess the flexibility of the hindfoot in a cavus foot.[18] Here the patient stands with a block under the lateral aspect of the forefoot to see if with standing pressure the hindfoot will move out of the varus position into a more neutral position (**Figure 12.43**). Look for callosities on the plantar aspect of the foot, at the lateral border and base of the fifth metatarsal.

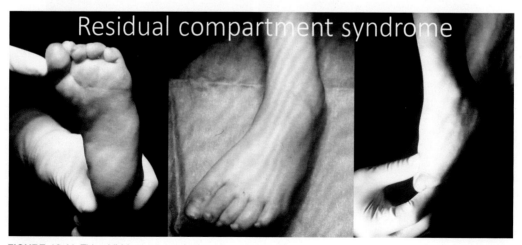

FIGURE 12.41 This child has an acquired equinocavovarus foot as a result of old compartment syndrome with contracted muscles.

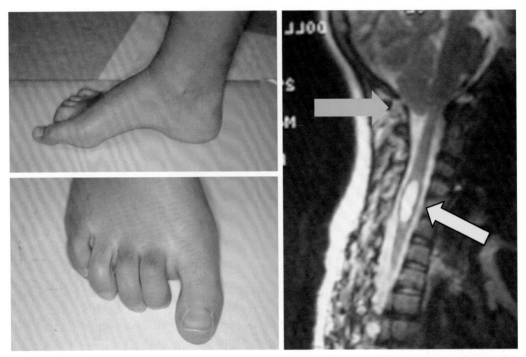

FIGURE 12.42 This child with a unilateral cavovarus foot has clawing of the toes. MRI scan reveals a Chiari malformation (green arrow) with a cervical spinal cord syrinx (yellow arrow).

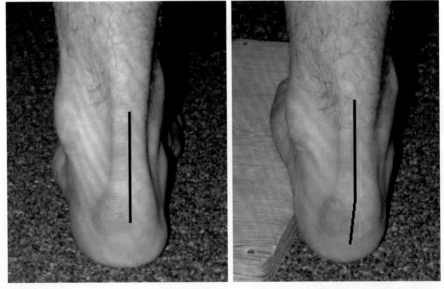

FIGURE 12.43 Coleman block test: This young man has a neutral to varus hindfoot as a result of forefoot cavus (left panel). When a wooden block is placed under the fifth ray, it allows the flexible hindfoot to correct to normal valgus.

Diagnostic Tests or Advanced Imaging

When a unilateral foot deformity or an asymmetric deformity is present, an MRI of the entire spinal column is needed to rule out Chiari malformation, spinal cord tumor, tethered cord, or syrinx (**Figure 12.42**). Bilateral cavus deformities without a known diagnosis should prompt referral to a pediatric neurologist who can orchestrate evaluation that may consist of genetic testing and neuro-conduction studies. These evaluations should be done BEFORE any surgical treatment is attempted.

Standing radiographs of the foot are helpful to evaluate the deformity and plan for surgical treatment. On the lateral view, the lateral talo-first metatarsal (Meary) angle and calcaneal pitch should be assessed[19] (**Figure 12.44**). Both angles will be increased. There may also be a sinus tarsi "see-through" sign to confirm hindfoot varus.

If CMT is suspected, a standing AP view of the pelvis should be performed to evaluate for acetabular dysplasia, which is commonly seen in CMT.[20] A scoliosis series should also be considered to evaluate for scoliosis, spinal dysraphism, or other spinal abnormality.

Treatment

Nonoperative management is most effective with mild and flexible deformities. This includes physical therapy, orthotics, supramalleolar orthoses, or ankle-foot orthoses bracing. Progressive increase in the deformity and lateral column overload across increasingly rigid foot segments leads to pain and potential for skin breakdown and infection. This and a propensity for ankle instability and associated gait instability often indicate the need for surgery. Typically, surgical intervention involves a combination of soft tissue and bony surgical procedures.

When to Refer

A cavus foot is a fairly uncommon presentation to a general practitioner's office, and due to the neurologic association with the deformity, early referral to a pediatric orthopedist and a pediatric neurologist is reasonable.

Accessory Navicular

Introduction

Accessory navicular is considered a normal variant, and it develops from a secondary ossification center that does not unite during childhood. This leads to enlargement of the plantar-medial aspect of the navicular (**Figure 12.45**).

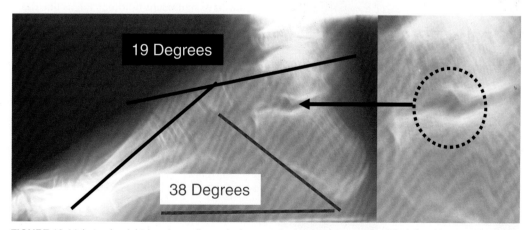

FIGURE 12.44 Lateral weight-bearing radiograph shows an increase in Meary angle (black lines) beyond the normal 10°. Another measure of cavus is an increase in the calcaneal pitch (red lines) above 30°. The "see-through" sign (black circle) allows one to look across the sinus tarsi and is indicative of hindfoot varus.

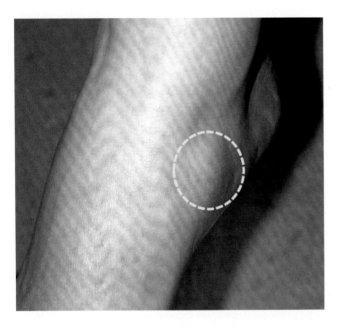

FIGURE 12.45 The yellow circle high-lights the location of tenderness and swelling seen in this girl with a painful accessory navicular.

The incidence is 12% and occurs more often in females. The tibialis posterior tendon inserts along the medial navicular and the synchondrosis can become inflamed with this condition leading to pain. While many patients respond to nonoperative treatment, some may require resection if they continue to have pain despite these measures.

Clinical Significance and Natural History

Accessory navicular is considered a normal variant of development of the navicular, and while the majority of children with this are asymptomatic, some may have significant pain and disability.

History and Physical Examination

Patients often present with arch pain along the medial border of the foot. They will have a medial prominence that may be inflamed or have callousing. There is usually point tenderness along the plantar-medial aspect of the navicular. Patients with accessory navicular may also have pain along the course of the posterior tibialis tendon with palpation and resisted inversion. Many patients with accessory navicular also have flat feet. A severe flat foot can mimic the appearance of an accessory navicular due to the prominence of the talar head. Typically, patients with accessory navicular do not have significant hindfoot valgus like those who have severe flat feet.

Diagnostic Tests or Advanced Imaging

The diagnosis of accessory navicular can be made on plain radiographs (**Figure 12.46**).

A standing AP, lateral, and external oblique view of the affected foot should be obtained. The accessory bone is best seen on the external oblique view. Advanced imaging is rarely required in this condition.

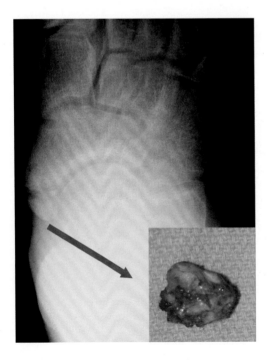

FIGURE 12.46 Radiographs confirm an accessory navicular, and the excised navicular is presented here.

Treatment

Nonoperative treatment includes activity restriction, orthotics, and anti-inflammatories. If these measures fail, practitioners may consider a short course of cast immobilization. Excision of the accessory navicular bone is considered when nonoperative measures fail. Surgical treatment consists of resecting the accessory bone through the synchondrosis as well as some of the native navicular bone to remove any medial prominence.

When to Refer

It is appropriate for general practitioners to start with nonoperative management. Patients who fail this type of treatment can be referred to a pediatric orthopedist to discuss resection of the accessory navicular bone.

References

1. Cooper DM, Dietz FR. Treatment of idiopathic clubfoot. A thirty-year follow-up note. *J Bone Joint Surg Am.* 1995;77(10):1477-1489.
2. Sankar WN, Weiss J, Skaggs DL. Othopaedic conditions in the newborn. *J Am Acad Orthop Surg.* 2009;17(2):112-122.
3. Feng L, Sussman M. Combined medial cuneiform osteotomy and multiple metatarsal osteotomies for correction of persistent metatarsus adductus in children. *J Pediatr Orthop.* 2016;36(7):730-735.
4. Miller M, Dobbs MB. Congenital vertical talus: etiology and management. *J Am Acad Orthop Surg.* 2015;23(10):604-611.
5. Alaee F, Boehm S, Dobbs MB. A new approach to the treatment of congenital vertical talus. *J Child Orthop.* 2007;1(3):165-174.
6. Chang CH, Kumar SJ, Riddle EC, Glutting J. Macrodactyly of the foot. *J Bone Joint Surg Am.* 2002;84(7):1189-1194.
7. Zhang L.Y, Xiao B, Li Y. Two cases of macrodactyly of the foot: relevance in pediatric orthopedics. *J Pediatr Orthop B.* 2016; 25(2):142-147.
8. Sweetham R. Congenital curly toes: an investigation into the value of treatment. *Lancet.* 1958;2(7043):398-400.
9. Holmes LB, Nasri H, Hunt AT, Toufaily MH, Westage MN. Polydactyly, postaxial, type B. *Birth Defects Res.* 2018;110(2):134-141.
10. Katz K, Linder N. Postaxial type B polydactyly treated by excision in the neonatal nursery. *J Pediatr Orthop.* 2011;31(4):448-449.
11. Cohen BE, Nicholson CW. Bunionette deformity. *J Am Acad Orthop Surg.* 2007;15(5):300-307.
12. Chell J, Dhar S. Pediatric hallux valgus. *Foot Ankle Clin.* 2014;19(2):235-243.
13. Pfeiffer M, Kotz R, Ledl T, Hauser G, Sluga M. Prevalence of flat foot in preschool-aged children. *Pediatrics.* 2006;118(2):634-639.
14. Bouchard M, Mosca V. Flatfoot deformity in children and adolescents: surgical indications and management. *J Am Acad Orthop Surg.* 2014;22:623-632.
15. Skaggs D, Flynn J. *Foot problems in children.* In: *Staying Out of Trouble in Pediatric Orthopedics.* Philadelphia, PA: Lippincott Williams and Wilkins; 2006: 354-356.
16. Denning JR. Tarsal coalition in children. *Pediatr Ann.* 2016;45(4):e139-e143.
17. Mosca VS. The cavus foot. *J Pediatr Orthop.* 2001;21:423-424.
18. Coleman SS, Chesnut WJ. A simple test for hindfoot flexibility in the cavovarus foot. *Clin Orthop Relat Res.* 1977;123:60-62.
19. Ziebarth K, Krause F. Updates in pediatric cavovarus deformity. *Foot Ankle Clin.* 2019;24(2):205-217.
20. Lee C, Sucato DJ. Pediatric issues with cavovarus foot deformities. *Foot Ankle Clin.* 2008;13(2):199-219.

13

Leg Disorders

Ryan D. Muchow and Vishwas R. Talwalkar

Introduction to Leg Deformities

Children present with abnormal appearing lower extremities due to a variety of etiologies (**Table 13.1**) and at varied time points. Embryology and the uniqueness of the growth plate in children play significant roles in the development and management of pediatric lower leg deformity. Broad categories of limb deformity include congenital, metabolic/skeletal dysplasias, developmental, and acquired help group diagnoses based on etiology, timing of onset, and problem source, which allows for selection of the proper treatment. *Congenital* indicates an embryologic problem that results in aberrant anatomy present at birth; *metabolic disorders* can affect the bones and alter mineralization and ossification at different time points depending on the onset of the disorder; *skeletal dysplasias* represent mostly genetic issues that affect the growth plate; *developmental* refers to a problem of the growth plate or bone that is not initially present in a child's life and the deformity develops later, and *acquired* infers normal anatomy and alignment that becomes distorted secondary to an outside influence (eg, trauma or infection) on the growth plate.

Congenital Deformities of the Leg

Fibular Deficiency

Introduction

Fibular deficiency (or fibular hemimelia) is a lower extremity deformity marked most distinctly by the congenital absence of all or part of the fibula. This condition may be isolated or be a component of a family of congenital lower limb deficiency, which includes a spectrum of deformity that may encompass the femur, knee, tibia, ankle, and foot of the involved extremity. There is no known cause of fibular deficiency and there are no known genetic predispositions.

Table 13.1	The Causes of Lower Extremity Deformity Divided Into Four Broad Groups		
CONGENITAL	**METABOLIC/SKELETAL DYSPLASIA**	**DEVELOPMENTAL**	**ACQUIRED**
Fibular deficiency	Rickets	Blount disease	Cozen phenomenon
Tibial deficiency	Skeletal dysplasia	Congenital pseudarthrosis tibia/ anterolateral bowing	Partial growth arrest
	• Achondroplasia		
	• Diastrophic dysplasia		
	• Morquio syndrome		
	• Sanfilippo syndrome		
Posteromedial bowing			

Clinical Significance

The presentation and clinical impact of fibular deficiency is highly varied and dependent upon the degree of involvement of the leg and the presence and degree of other lower limb deformities at each anatomic site. The spectrum of anatomic involvement in addition to the fibula includes femoral shortening, tibial shortening, knee valgus, anterior cruciate ligament deficiency, tarsal coalition, and lateral foot ray absence. Based upon the Birch classification, there are two factors that most predict the functional outcome for patients with fibular deficiency: a preservable foot and limb length inequality.[1]

Physical Examination

Fibular hemimelia can typically be noted in an infant or small child given the associated congenital deformities. After gaining a general sense of the activity and age-appropriate function of the child, a focused physical examination of the lower extremities may reveal:[2]

Skin dimpling—Nonspecific and seen in various congenital deformities. Typically present over the tibia at the site of the bowing and/or knee in fibular deficiency (**Figure 13.1**).

Femoral shortening—In the supine position, the congenitally deficient femur will appear shorter when the hips and knees are flexed 90°. This is termed a positive Galeazzi sign (**Figure 13.2**). This can also be seen in patients with a congenitally dislocated hip. In the later instance, the femur is not shorter, the hip is dislocated posteriorly, and the femur appears shortened with this maneuver.

Limb-length discrepancy (LLD)—Because the bulk of children with fibular hemimelia have concurrent tibial shortening and some have femoral shortening, patients have reduced overall length of the involved limb (**Figure 13.3**).

Knee valgus, patella subluxation, and cruciate instability—Children with fibular hemimelia can have abnormalities at the knee. These include genu valgum (knock-knee deformity) as a result of lateral femoral condyle hypoplasia and the patella may subluxate laterally (**Figure 13.4**). Anterior and posterior knee instability is typically seen in older children as a result of cruciate deficiency (**Figure 13.5**).

Anterior bowing—Patients with fibular hemimelia will often have shortening of the tibia with angulation apex of deformity, which is predominately pointed anteriorly (**Figure 13.6**).

Ankle/hindfoot motion—In addition to the presence of hindfoot coalitions, patients can develop a "ball-and-socket" ankle. Therefore, inversion/eversion plus dorsiflexion/plantarflexion occurs through the ankle. Patients may display hypermobility or even instability at the ankle and have limited mobility of the midfoot.

Reduced lateral rays—In addition to bowing and shortening, the absence of rays from the lateral aspect of the foot is a hallmark of fibular deficiency (**Figure 13.7**).

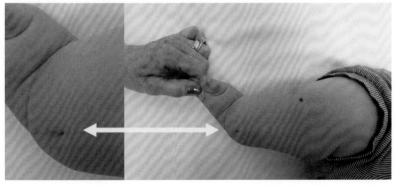

FIGURE 13.1 Skin dimpling can often be seen in congenital limb deformities such as in this patient with fibular hemimelia.

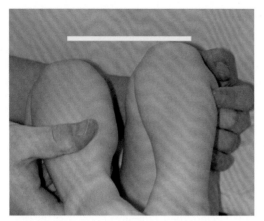

FIGURE 13.2 This child with congenital short femur has a positive Galeazzi sign with shortening of the right femur. This can also be seen in patients with a dislocated hip.

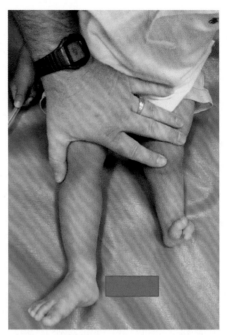

FIGURE 13.3 This child with fibular hemimelia has concurrent shortening of the femur, genu valgum, shortening of the tibia, and absent foot rays.

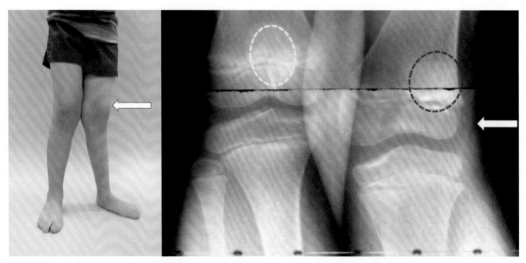

FIGURE 13.4 This child with congenital limb deficiency has multiple abnormalities of the left knee. This includes lateral femoral condyle hypoplasia (white arrow), patella (red circle) subluxation (not centered in the knee compared to normal patella [yellow circle]), as well as likely absence of the cruciate ligaments as hallmarked by the lack of tibial spine development.

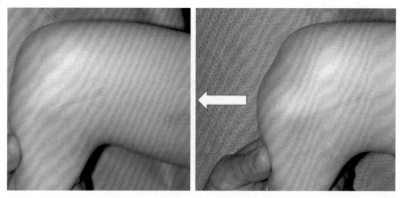

FIGURE 13.5 This child with congenital short femur has anterior instability of the knee joint due to congenital absence of the cruciate ligaments.

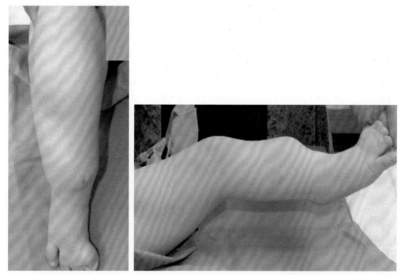

FIGURE 13.6 This child with fibular hemimelia has shortening of the tibia and an anterior and lateral bow of the tibia with an associate dimple at the apex of deformity.

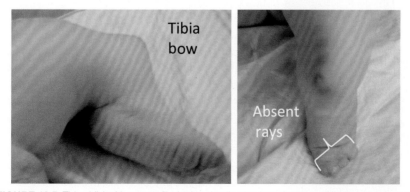

FIGURE 13.7 This child with severe fibular hemimelia also has absence of the rays of his foot.

Pitfalls in Diagnosis

In the milder forms of fibular deficiency, patients may evade early diagnosis. Having all five rays, minimal deformity, high functionality, and bilateralism could be factors that would result in a patient being diagnosed later in life. A progressive genu valgum or limb length inequality (in a mild, unilateral patient) revealing itself during the school-age years may be the first presenting sign (**Figure 13.8**).

Differential Diagnosis

- Congenital short femur and limb deficiency syndrome
- Tibial hemimelia
- Congenital foot deficiency
- Pes planovalgus (flatfoot)

Diagnostic Tests or Advanced Imaging

An anteroposterior (AP) radiograph of the lower extremities will provide ample information to confirm the diagnosis and aid in determining treatment based on the degree of involvement of the rest of the leg. One can compare femoral lengths, assess tibial deformity, and reveal the lateral ray deletions (**Figure 13.9**). Hindfoot coalition and the ball-and-socket ankle may be more easily detected on radiographs in the older child (**Figure 13.10**).

Treatment and When to Refer

This diagnosis is best treated by a pediatric orthopedic surgeon with specialty in limb deformities. The initial decision with a patient with fibular deficiency is dictated by the functionality of the foot—a nonfunctional, nonplantigrade foot typically requires amputation. Additional intervention is dictated by LLD, angular deformity, and knee stability.

Tibial Deficiency

Introduction

Tibial deficiency, or tibial hemimelia, is a lower extremity deformity that is defined by the partial or complete congenital absence of the tibia. It is much more uncommon than fibular hemimelia and while most cases are sporadic in cause, some forms of the disorder present in an autosomal dominant fashion. In contradistinction to fibular deficiency, most patients with tibial deficiency will have abnormalities of the upper extremity, hip, or spine.

Clinical Significance

The lower extremity deformity associated with tibial deficiency is significant, will affect the child's function, and typically requires surgical intervention. The key functional and treatment variable is the presence of an intact knee extensor mechanism to the tibia. If the proximal tibia is absent, there is no good attachment of the patella tendon to the lower limb.

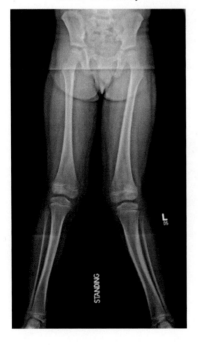

Symmetric fibular deficiency

FIGURE 13.8 This child has bilateral fibular hemimelia. There is asymmetric genu valgum of the left knee; however, limb lengths are fairly symmetric.

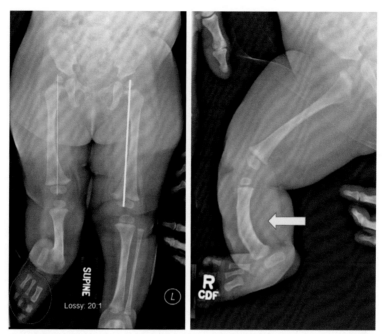

FIGURE 13.9 This child with congenital limb deficiency has a shortened right femur in comparison with the left, a shortened and bowed tibia consistent with fibular hemimelia, and an absence of toes of the affected foot.

Physical Examination

Given the involvement of other musculoskeletal systems in tibial deficiency, for example, upper extremity, spine, and hip, a thorough physical examination of the child is prudent. A focused lower extremity examination may reveal multiple lower limb anomalies (**Figure 13.11**)[3]:

Skin dimpling—Dimpling typically occurs at knee, ankle, or site of tibial involvement (**Figure 13.12**). In some cases, the dimpling may be the only sign of a shortened tibia.

Absence or duplication of medial (tibial) rays—Tibial deficiency often has severe polydactyly (**Figure 13.11**) with the more extensive duplication usually seen on the medial aspect of the foot (**Figure 13.13**).

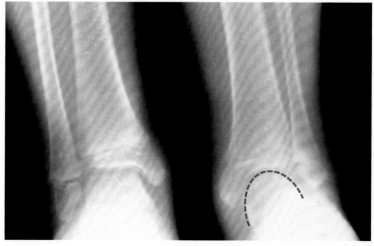

FIGURE 13.10 This child with left fibular hemimelia also has a ball-and-socket ankle as demonstrated by the spherical red line.

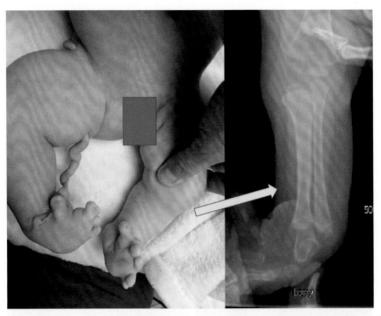

FIGURE 13.11 This child with multiple congenital deficiencies of the limbs demonstrates bilateral tibial hemimelia. There is multiple polydactyly and syndactylization of the feet in addition to clubfoot deformities. The left tibia is shortened in comparison to the fibula, consistent with tibia hemimelia.

Equinovarus foot—In patients with tibial hemimelia, the feet typically have an equinovarus position (**Figure 13.11**) or resemble clubfeet (**Figure 13.14**) (▶ **Video 13.1**).

Extensor mechanism—The ability to bear weight and/or perform knee extension is an important functional distinction (▶ **Video 13.2**).

In general, the proximal knee articulation may not be fully represented by the radiographs. In ▶ **Video 13.3**, we see that there is a much more articular stability during arthrography examination, which is represented in the radiographs in **Figure 13.13** (▶ **Video 13.3**).

Pitfalls in Diagnosis

Tibial deficiency is associated with involvement of the upper extremity, spine, and hip and with numerous inherited syndromes making the entire history and physical pertinent to the diagnosis. Further, assessing the function of the knee and the ability of the child to actively extend will aid the clinician in assigning a classification and guide treatment.

Differential Diagnosis

- Congenital short femur
- Fibular deficiency
- Clubfoot
- Polydactyly

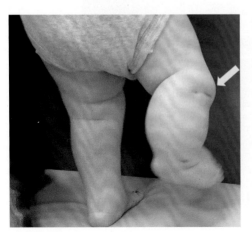

FIGURE 13.12 Similar to patients with fibular hemimelia, patients with congenital tibial abnormalities can also have skin dimpling at the site of deformity, such as this child with tibial hemimelia.

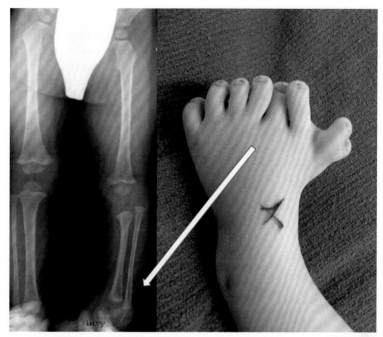

FIGURE 13.13 This child with tibial hemimelia has shortening of the tibia in comparison with the contralateral side, but also has extra digits along the medial aspect of his foot.

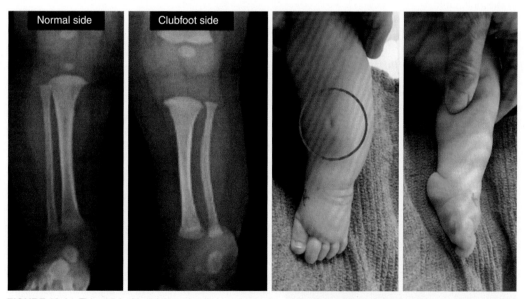

FIGURE 13.14 This child with tibial hemimelia has shortening of the tibia with comparison to the contralateral side. This side also has a clubfoot deformity, which has been partially corrected with casting. Please note the skin dimple on the pretibial surface of the affected side.

Diagnostic Tests or Advanced Imaging

AP lower extremity radiograph and two views of the tibia will allow thorough evaluation of bony structures of the patient's lower extremities to characterize any other deformities and properly classify the tibial deficiency. There are some reports of using MRI or ultrasound to determine the presence of a tibial anlage and the complete anatomy of the distal femur to gain an appreciation of the true function of the extensor mechanism when deciding between amputation types (**Figure 13.15**).

Treatment and When to Refer

Tibial deficiency is best treated by a pediatric orthopedic surgeon with access to prosthetic services given the vast majority of these patients require amputation of some variety. The child in **Figure 13.11** eventually underwent bilateral amputations and prosthetic fitting (**Figure 13.16**; ▶ **Video 13.4**).

Posteromedial Bowing

Introduction

Posteromedial bowing of the tibia is a deformity that is typically detected soon after birth. It can be associated with calcaneovalgus deformity of the foot and is quite dramatic in appearance, particularly in the newborn (**Figure 13.17**). The etiology of the deformity is unknown, but is thought to be a result of intrauterine packaging.

Clinical Significance

Repeated reassurance of the parents is often required. The calcaneal valgus deformity of the foot spontaneously corrects within the first 18 months while the posteromedial bowing of the tibia may take several years to straighten and this will result in a functional deficit in ankle plantar flexion until it fully straightens the posterior bow (**Figure 13.18**). Even though these deformities improve, the affected child may have a 3 to 4 cm discrepancy in tibial length. The limb length discrepancy may require treatment in the older child.[4]

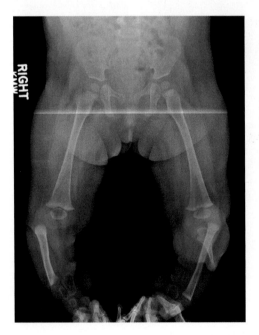

Physical Examination

A thorough newborn examination is necessary to look for any other deformities associated with intrauterine packaging (eg, metatarsus adductus, torticollis, dysplasia of the hip, and other limb deformities). The dorsum of the foot often is directly in contact with anterior shin and a medial dimple may be visible (**Figure 13.17**).

Pitfalls in Diagnosis

Recognition of this deformity in the proper clinical scenario is straightforward, but reassuring the family that it is often a self-limiting problem with a relatively

FIGURE 13.15 This child with bilateral tibial hemimelia will likely be a candidate for bilateral amputations due to the severe absence of the tibia, especially on the right side. Many of these patients will have an absent extensor mechanism as there is no place for the patella tendon to attach.

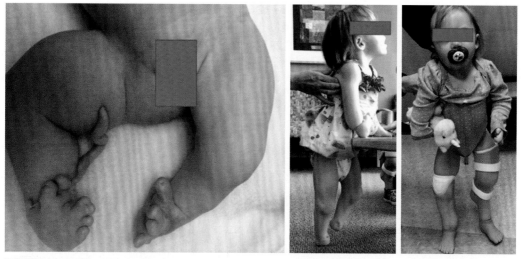

FIGURE 13.16 This child with bilateral congenital lower limb deformities underwent bilateral amputations and is now standing in appropriately positioned prostheses to accommodate her disparate limb lengths.

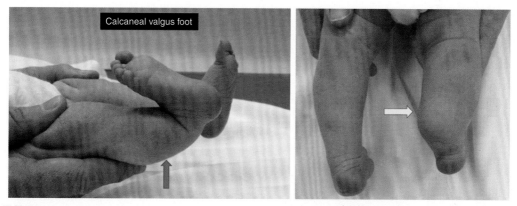

FIGURE 13.17 This newborn has a calcaneal valgus foot deformity in addition to posterior medial bowing of the tibia. Tibial deformity is noted by the blue and yellow arrows.

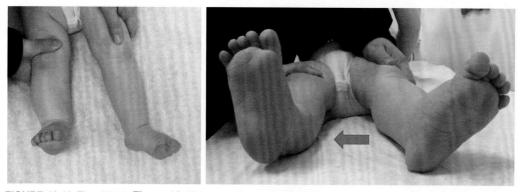

FIGURE 13.18 The child in **Figure 13.17** has grown and the foot deformity has corrected with a mild limb length discrepancy and some residual posterior bowing as noted by the blue arrow.

benign natural history can be more challenging. Often parents demand something should be done; so teaching the family how to stretch the anterior leg muscles and bracing of the foot and ankle may improve stability while the young child is learning to walk. This strategy can help parents feel like something is being done, but this is not always a necessary treatment for the child.

Differential Diagnosis

- Congenital vertical talus
- Anterolateral tibial bowing
- Tibial deficiency
- Fibular deficiency

Diagnostic Tests or Advanced Imaging

AP and lateral views of the lower extremity will reveal classic findings (**Figure 13.19**).

Treatment and When to Refer

Referral to a pediatric orthopedist within the first 4 weeks after birth is helpful to set parental expectations. Treatment of the residual leg length difference may range from observation to epiphysiodesis to limb lengthening that would be considered after the child is 10 to 12 years of age.

Leg Deformities as a Result of Metabolic Disorders and Skeletal Dysplasia

Rickets

Introduction

Rickets is a metabolic bone disease of either genetic or nutritional etiology that results in a failure of mineralization of cartilage and osteoid in the growing child. Affecting the growth plate primarily, the longitudinal growth is affected resulting in both decreased length and deformity. The strength of the long bones is also affected further contributing to the deformities visualized in the shaft of the bone.

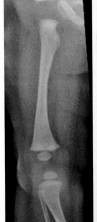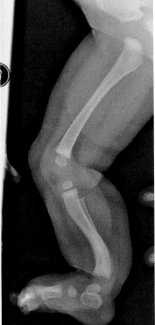

Clinical Significance

The clinical appearance of a patient with rickets depends on the age of onset and severity of the metabolic imbalance. Infants may experience some lethargy and muscle weakness contributing to delay in achieving developmental milestones. Classic bony manifestations of rickets include short stature, enlargement of the costochondral junctions ("the rachitic rosary"), pectus carinatum, delayed fontanelle closure in the skull ("hot cross buns"), dental defects, bowing of the extremities, and thickening of the ankles, knees, and wrists.

FIGURE 13.19 Radiographs of the child with posterior medial bowing of the tibia demonstrates a distal tibia bowing that is both medial and posterior.

Physical Examination

Lower extremity bowing—The direction of bowing, varus or valgus, correlates with the onset of disease and the typical physiologic limb alignment of the child at the time the disorder is manifested. As most forms of rickets are present at birth, that predicts for varus alignment. This is due to the fact that most babies are in varus, thus a congenital metabolic bone disease leads to progressive varus. Later presenting varieties of rickets, for example, renal osteodystrophy, may promote worsening valgus deformity (▶ **Video 13.5**). This is due to the fact that most children are in valgus after 3 years of age and if a metabolic insult occurs at that time, the bones will continue to progress into excessive valgus (**Figure 13.20**).

Pitfalls in Diagnosis

Once the clinical suspicion of rickets is made, identifying the type of rickets based on laboratory values can be challenging and is best managed by specialists in these disorders.

Differential Diagnosis

- Multiple varieties of rickets: nutritional, vitamin D-resistant, vitamin D-dependent, renal osteodystrophy
- Physiologic genu valgum or valgus
- Tibia vara
- Bony dysplasia

Diagnostic Tests or Advanced Imaging

A standing AP of the lower extremities will be able to highlight the varus deformity seen in congenital rickets and allow for diagnosis with classic appearances of widened physes and cupped metaphyses (**Figure 13.21**). Similar widened physis can be seen in late-onset rickets except for that the child is in valgus (**Figure 13.22**).

Laboratory testing is conducted to obtain blood levels of calcium, phosphate, creatinine, blood urea nitrogen, alkaline phosphatase, parathyroid hormone, 25-(OH) vitamin D, and 1, 25-(OH)$_2$ vitamin D. Urinalysis and other more specific testing will also be important. In general, it is wise to have metabolic bone specialists order the tests and manage the workup in order to avoid needless extra blood draws.

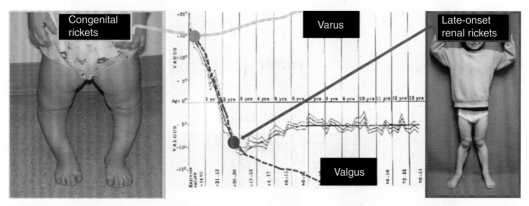

FIGURE 13.20 The graph in the middle demonstrates normal alignment of a growing child. When born, the normal child is in varus, or bowlegged, and with time, the child develops a knock-kneed, or valgus, positioning by the time he/she reaches 3 years of age. If a child is born with congenital rickets, his/her knee and leg will progress into more varus or bowlegged position. If a child develops rickets when he/she is already in a valgus position, his/her legs will continue on into a more knock-kneed appearance, such as this child with late-onset renal rickets.

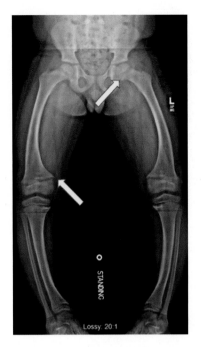

FIGURE 13.21 Radiographs of a child with early-onset rickets demonstrate widening of the growth plates and the hip, knee, and ankle. In addition, the shafts of the bones are bowed and the epiphyses are cupped.

Treatment and When to Refer

A tenet of rickets management is to ensure that the proper diagnosis is met and that the underlying metabolic disorder is maximally treated. Referral to a pediatric endocrinologist, pediatric nephrologist, or metabolic bone specialist is essential. Once the diagnosis is made, a referral to an orthopedic specialist can be beneficial for alignment management. Yet sometimes correction of the metabolic deformity can make a remarkable improvement in malalignment without surgical intervention (**Figure 13.23**).

Skeletal Dysplasia

Introduction

The appearance of individuals with skeletal dysplasia and the degree of disruption in musculoskeletal growth and function vary widely. Historically, these conditions have been classified by the appearance of the individual's facial features, limbs, and relative growth. More recently, the classification systems have been based on the location of genetic defects and/or the site of distorted function. Since the basis of this text is physical examination, the following descriptions will focus on the typical features and appearance of some common skeletal dysplasias.[5]

13-Year-old knee pain...creatinine 10

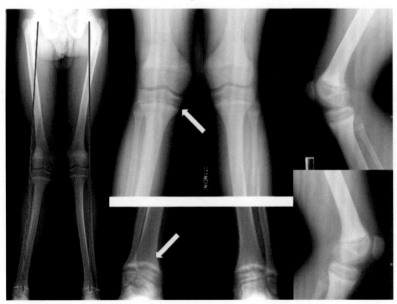

FIGURE 13.22 This 13-year-old boy presents to clinic with a knock-kneed appearance and knee pain. He has a remote history of obstructive ureters treated surgically but with no follow-up. He has late-onset renal rickets secondary to undiagnosed renal failure with widening of the growth plates and progressive valgus deformity.

1-Year-old with renal agenesis
on dialysis

7-Years after
renal transplant

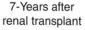

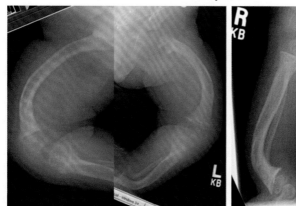

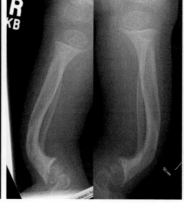

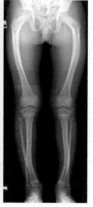

FIGURE 13.23 This one-year-old was born without kidneys and, as such, had severe metabolic bone disease. After a renal transplant, the child's skeleton straightened out to a great degree without any surgical intervention.

Clinical Significance

Accurate early identification of children with skeletal dysplasia is essential for appropriate timely treatment as well as counseling of families. Several dysplasias can impact growth and achievement of developmental milestones. Further, accurate diagnosis allows for initiation of treatment and avoidance of potentially dangerous activities such as contact sports in a child with upper cervical spine instability (Morquio syndrome or spinal epiphyseal dysplasia).

Physical Examination

Some people with skeletal dysplasia can be diagnosed immediately. Others remain a mystery until genetic testing is completed, or beyond. The pertinent examination features are:

Size—Is the child taller or shorter than average?

Head and face—Head circumference and skull shape as well as facial features (frontal bossing-achondroplasia) and ears (cauliflower ears-diastrophic dysplasia) can give clues to the type of dysplasia (**Figures 13.24** and **13.25**).

Ratios—Trunk to limbs ratio can be altered in disorders such as Marfan syndrome. Alterations in limb segments can be helpful in defining diagnosis. Mesomelic shortening implies shortening of the middle of the extremity, while rhizomelic implies shortening of the proximal portion of the limb. A classic example is achondroplasia (**Figure 13.24**).

Skin lesions—Hemangiomas can be seen in Klippel-Trenaunay-Weber syndrome; café-au-lait spots and neurofibromas are seen in neurofibromatosis.

FIGURE 13.24 This young boy with achondroplasia has classic rhizomelic shortening of the humerus as well as facial features such as frontal bossing.

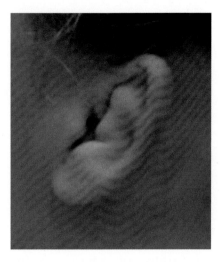

FIGURE 13.25 Cauliflower ears are classic phenotypic findings seen in patients with diastrophic dysplasia.

Chest deformities—Pectus carinatum and excavatum can be seen in Marfan syndrome.

Spinal deformities—Scoliosis and thoracolumbar kyphosis are seen in a variety of dysplasias such as mucopolysaccharidoses.

Limb deformities—Varus can be seen in a variety of dysplasias and includes achondroplasia (**Figure 13.26**) and valgus malalignment can be seen in different dysplasias such as pseudoachondroplasia and hypochondroplasia (**Figure 13.27**).

Hand and foot deformities—Short fingers and toes can be appreciated in diastrophic dysplasia (**Figure 13.28**) among others and long fingers and toes can be seen in Marfanoid patients (**Figure 13.29**).

Pitfalls in Diagnosis

The challenge with skeletal dysplasia is the significant overlap in clinical presentation with varied genetic etiology, as well as many dysplasias resemble metabolic bone diseases in appearance and radiographically. Additionally, individuals with the same diagnosis may have differences in disease severity. Identifying the correct diagnosis is important because of associations certain dysplasias have with other organ systems and upper cervical spine pathology.

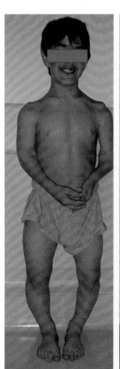

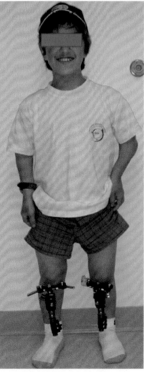

Differential Diagnosis

- Achondroplasia (**Figures 13.24** and **13.26**)
- Pseudoachondroplasia
- Hypochondroplasia
- Diastrophic dysplasia (**Figures 13.28** and **13.29**)
- Kniest dysplasia
- Multiple epiphyseal dysplasia
- Spondyloepiphyseal dysplasia
- Mucopolysaccharidoses = Hurler syndrome (**Figure 13.30**), Hunter syndrome, Sanfilippo syndrome (**Figure 13.31**), Morquio syndrome
- Chondrodysplasia punctata (**Figure 13.32**)
- Chondroectodermal dysplasia (Ellis-van Creveld syndrome)

FIGURE 13.26 This adolescent boy with bilateral genu valgum and achondroplasia underwent bilateral proximal tibial osteotomies for correction of his varus deformity.

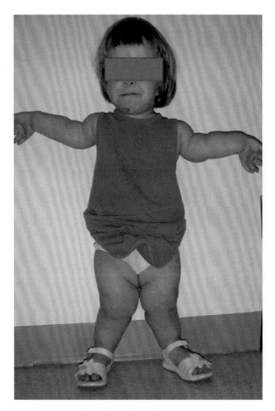

FIGURE 13.27 Valgus deformity of the lower extremities can be seen in many different skeletal dysplasias, including in this child with hypochondroplasia.

Diagnostic Tests or Advanced Imaging

Skeletal dysplasia should be considered in children with symmetric limb deformity and who have abnormal facies, spinal deformity, and who are less than the 10th percentile for height.

A good test to perform are X-rays of the entire skeleton known as a skeletal survey; images include the spine (especially cervical spine), lower and upper extremity, skull, hands, and feet.

Treatment and When to Refer

Establishing a diagnosis and outlining a plan of care for children with skeletal dysplasia often require multiple specialists. Early detection and referral to medical geneticists facilitates long-term planning and also allows patients to become involved in patient support groups for these relatively rare conditions. Simultaneous referral to pediatric orthopedics is appropriate.

⬤ *Developmental Causes of Limb Deformity*

Tibia Vara

Introduction

Idiopathic tibia vara, or Blount disease, is a deformity of the proximal tibia that presents in young children <4 years old (infantile form) and in the adolescent age group. Both types are seen most commonly in children who are overweight. Infantile tibia vara usually presents with excessive bowlegs from birth which worsens with time but is not initially painful. The late-onset variety usually becomes detectable in children older than 9 years of age with asymmetric genu varum and occasional

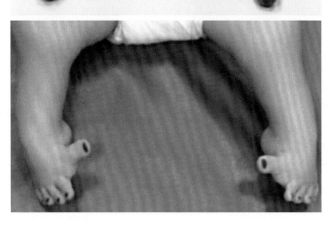

FIGURE 13.28 Children with diastrophic dysplasia will have shortened and widened fingers and classic findings of the Hitchhiker thumb.

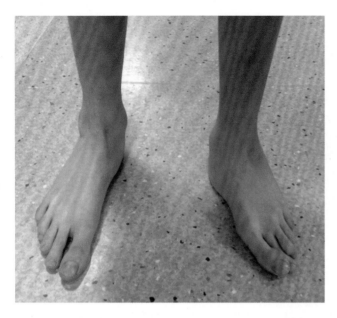

FIGURE 13.29 Patients with Marfan syndrome can have very long fingers and toes, such as this child with Marfan syndrome.

lateral knee pain. In both cases, the mechanical axis of the lower limb (the line of force from the hip to the ankle, which normally falls in the center of the knee) falls well medial to the knee (▶ **Video 13.6**).

Clinical Significance

Blount disease can lead to progressive deformity, disability, pain, and risk for arthritis at the knee as an adult. Early identification and treatment confers a greater chance of success for both infantile and adolescent forms of disease. The comorbidities associated with increased weight (diabetes and hypertension) may be of greater long-term clinical importance than their limb deformity and should not be ignored. Treatment of their limb deformities typically does not lead to resolution of their metabolic dysfunction.

Physical Examination

The child with infantile tibia vara deformity about the knee typically presents as an overweight child with bilateral disease that may be asymmetric with one side slightly worse than the other (**Figure 13.33**). Many are asymptomatic but some may complain of lateral-sided knee pain as the deformity worsens with time. The limb deformity is three-dimensional and internal tibial torsion is usually a component. Furthermore, there is often a lateral thrust of the knee while walking (▶ **Video 13.7**) that looks like the knee is partially giving way. Lateral ligamentous laxity may also be present.[6] Late-onset tibia vara is more often unilateral, and these patients have genu varum with some pain on ambulation but less likely to have a thrust in stance phase (**Figure 13.34**).

Pitfalls in Diagnosis

Discerning infantile tibia vara from physiologic bowing can be challenging in the younger child. Radiographs are usually not helpful in children less than 2 years of age. Radiographs in 3- and 4-year-old patients will likely show some changes of the proximal tibia (**Figure 13.33**). Standing radiographs of the late-onset group will usually be diagnostic for adolescent Blount disease (**Figure 13.34**).

Differential Diagnosis for Infantile Tibia Vara

- Physiologic bowing
- Physeal arrest
- Skeletal dysplasia such as focal fibrocartilaginous dysplasia (**Figure 13.35**)
- Metabolic bone disease (nutritional rickets)

Differential Diagnosis for Late-Onset Tibia Vara

- Growth arrest

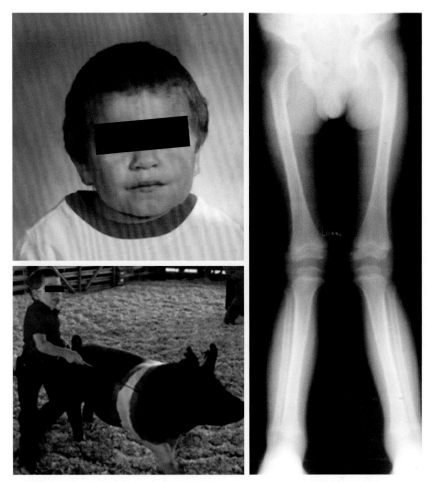

FIGURE 13.30 This young boy with Hurler syndrome has classic facial features. Skeletal manifestations include knock-kneed appearances and hip dysplasia. Thankfully, bone marrow transplants have reversed this otherwise fatal disease to allow a more normal life as seen in his 4-H picture.

Diagnostic Tests or Advanced Imaging

Standing AP radiograph of the lower extremities with the patellae pointing forward will identify the deformity, the location, and rule out other etiologies such as focal fibrocartilaginous dysplasia (**Figures 13.35**).

Treatment and When to Refer

Any ambulatory child with worsening varus alignment after the age of two should be referred to a pediatric orthopedist.

Anterolateral Bowing of the Tibia/Congenital Pseudarthrosis of the Tibia

Introduction

Anterolateral bowing of the tibia is the earliest manifestation of a continuum of tibial dysplasia that results in pseudarthrosis of the tibia. It can also affect the fibula with similar dysplastic bone that can lead to fracture and failure to heal. There is a significant association with neurofibromatosis Type 1 and fibrous dysplasia; however, the distinct pathophysiology remains elusive.[7]

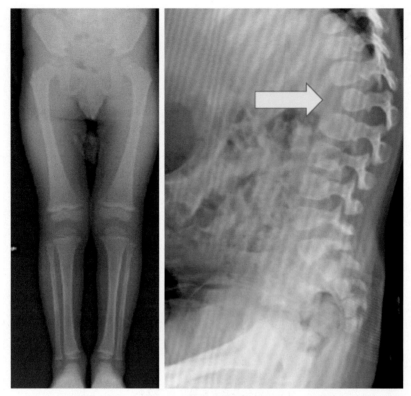

FIGURE 13.31 Many patients with mucopolysaccharidoses will have L1 or L2 vertebral body hypoplasia noted on the lateral X-ray. This boy with Sanfilippo syndrome has minimal skeletal deformity except for the skeletal hypoplasia in the spine.

Clinical Significance

Most patients are identified at birth or within their first year of life with deformity or a limp as the presenting signs.[8] Patients with anterolateral bowing of the tibia (**Figure 13.36**) typically proceed to develop fracture through the dysplastic bone (**Figure 13.37**) and the bone usually does not heal without surgical treatment and can lead to pseudarthrosis. Prior to fracture, a patient's function is typically limited due to progressive deformity and treatment involves bracing to prevent fracture.

Physical Examination

Anterolateral bowing of the tibia is almost universally unilateral where one will notice a shortened limb on the involved side, with a laterally positioned apex in the tibia and a medially positioned foot. There may be motion at the deformity if a true pseudarthrosis exists (▶ **Video 13.8**). It is important to look for skin manifestations of neurofibromatosis: café-au-lait spots, axillary and inguinal freckling, and subcutaneous neurofibromas.

Pitfalls in Diagnosis

The late-presenting tibia pseudarthroses are the mildest in severity and can be mistaken as a regular tibia fracture or a tibia stress fracture. Additionally, the practitioner should be aware of the association with neurofibromatosis and appropriately evaluate for this disorder.

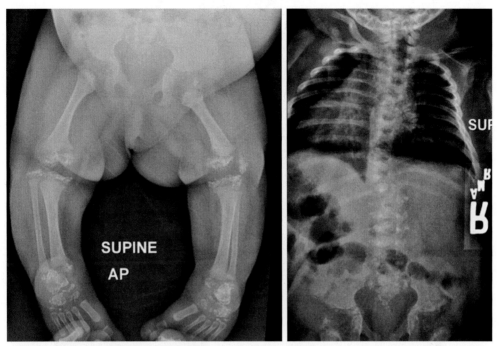

FIGURE 13.32 Children with chondrodysplasia punctata will have popcorn calcification throughout the skeleton, as seen in this affected child.

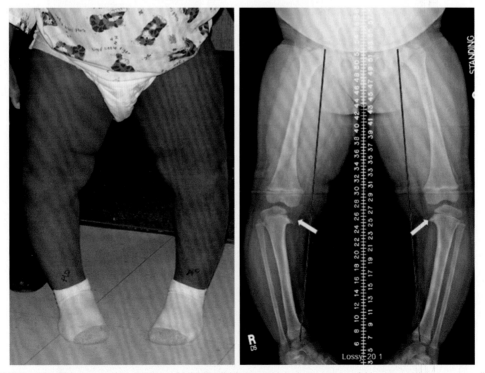

FIGURE 13.33 This young girl has bilateral infantile tibia vara, which demonstrates fairly symmetric varus as well as with deviation of the mechanical axis (medially displaced red lines) as well as changes in the proximal tibia (yellow arrows).

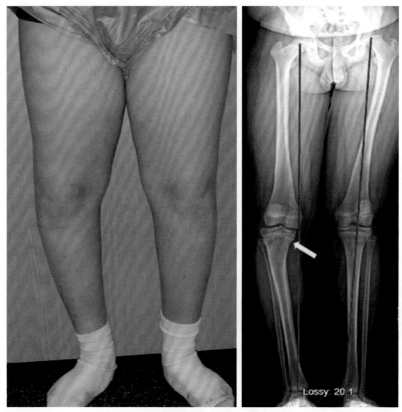

FIGURE 13.34 This boy with adolescent tibia vara has asymmetric varus with changes in the proximal tibia epiphyses, which are different from those found in infantile tibia vara.

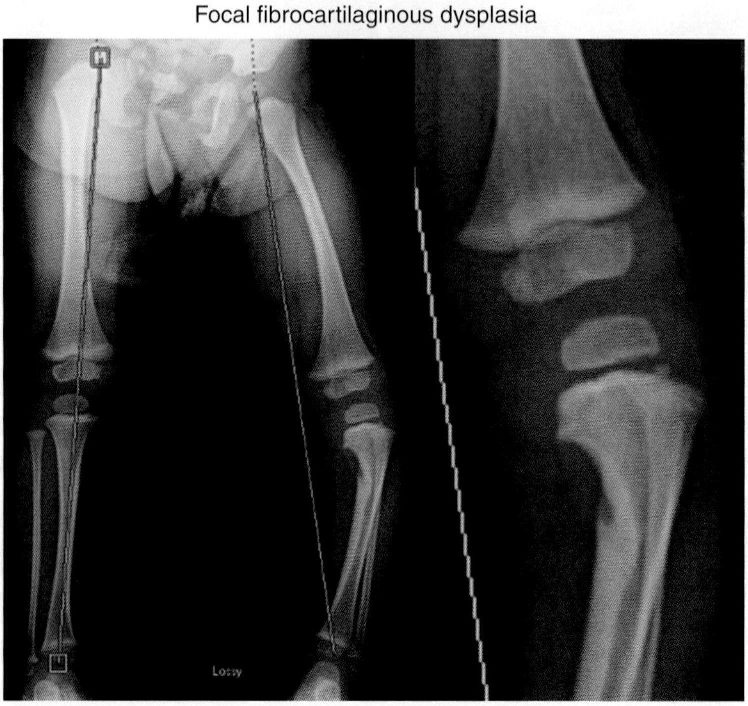

Focal fibrocartilaginous dysplasia

FIGURE 13.35 Focal fibrocartilaginous dysplasia can present with unilateral bowing at the knee, as seen in this child. On physical examination, this could be confused with persistent unilateral infantile tibia vara.

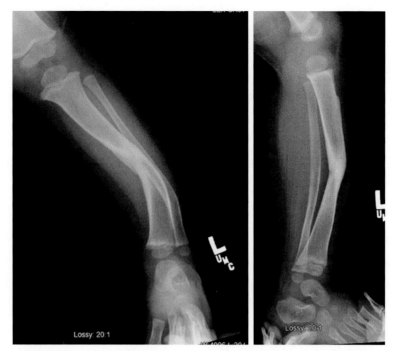

FIGURE 13.36 This child with anterior and lateral bowing of the tibia carries a diagnosis of neurofibromatosis and congenital pseudarthrosis of the tibia. This tibia has not broken yet, but sclerosis and dysplasia are present in the midtibial region.

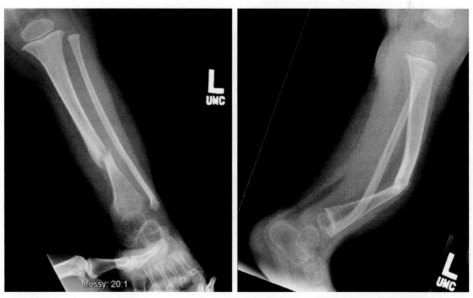

FIGURE 13.37 With time, the prior radiographs from this patient have progressed to the point of developing a fracture that does not heal.

Differential Diagnosis

- Tibia stress fracture
- Traumatic tibia fracture
- Anteromedial bowing

Diagnostic Tests or Advanced Imaging

Two views of the tibia should be appropriate to secure the diagnosis.

Treatment and When to Refer

Identification of pseudarthrosis of the tibia should prompt referral to a pediatric orthopedic surgeon as treatment will involve bracing and likely surgical treatment.

Acquired Causes of Limb Deformity

Cozen Phenomenon

Introduction

A fracture involving the proximal metaphysis of the tibia (**Figure 13.38**) is at risk for developing a growth phenomenon resulting in valgus of the proximal tibia (**Figure 13.39**). The underlying etiology for the valgus deformity is unclear and, as most cases resolve, it is unknown why normal growth is resumed and the deformity corrects itself.[9]

Clinical Significance

Following healing of the proximal tibial metaphyseal fracture, the proximal tibia grows in a valgus direction with the maximum deformity occurring around 1 year following the initial injury. Over time, the leg will straighten out in the majority of patients. The valgus knee is typically asymptomatic and rarely results in a functional deficit. It is helpful to counsel families at the initiation of treatment for the seemingly minor proximal tibial metaphyseal fracture of the possibility for the deformity and the need for recurrent visits.[10]

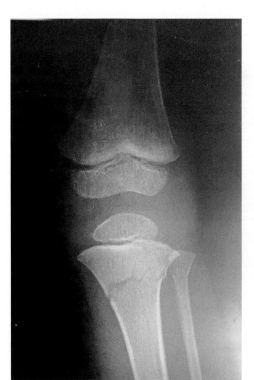

Physical Examination

The child is assumed to have normal anatomy and function given that the Cozen phenomenon occurs in a post-traumatic scenario without other genetic or metabolic variables affecting growth.

Lower extremity—The child will have a noticeable valgus deformity on inspection and gait with otherwise normal knee range-of-motion.

Pitfalls in Diagnosis

Recognizing the Cozen fracture and educating the family as to the possible valgus growth deformity are the most significant aspects to the care of these patients.

FIGURE 13.38 This child with a proximal tibia fracture is at risk for developing late-onset genu valgum due to abnormal asymmetric growth of the proximal tibia—Cozen phenomenon.

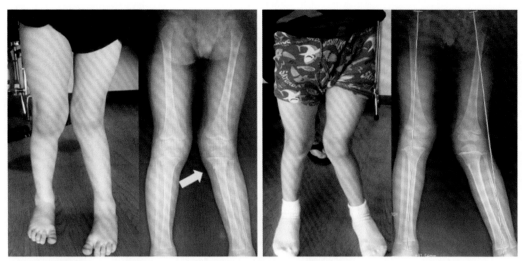

FIGURE 13.39 Over the year following the previous fracture, the child's limb has developed the Cozen phenomenon and progressed into excessive valgus.

Differential Diagnosis

- Post-traumatic partial growth arrest
- Postinfectious partial growth arrest

Diagnostic Tests or Advanced Imaging

AP radiograph of the lower extremities will identify the deformity, the location, and rule out other etiologies. AP and lateral views of the knee or tibia will identify fracture in the acute setting (**Figure 13.38**).

Treatment and When to Refer

Referral to a pediatric orthopedist is important to educate the family on natural history (usually benign) and treatment is indicated in the rare the patient that has extreme deformity that persists after 2 to 3 years. Treatment mostly involves observation and reassurance. If the deformity lasts longer than 3 years or there is a significant functional limitation, then growth plate stapling could be considered. This is preferable as corrective osteotomy may result in recurrence.

Partial Growth Arrest

Introduction

A partial growth arrest occurs when a previously normal and healthy physis experiences an insult, for example, trauma or infection, that results in partial cessation of growth. This growth arrest, or physeal bar, slows the growth plate in one spot while the remainder of the growth plate continues growing longitudinally resulting in an acquired limb deformity.

Clinical Significance

If a physeal bar has occurred, the deformity in the lower extremity will only get worse as the child grows. Therefore, close observation of a physeal injury is paramount (especially in children with significant growth potential) and early recognition is key to successful treatment.

Physical Examination

Lower extremity—The child will typically have a normal gait and normal examination of the involved joint. Identifying asymmetry in leg alignment and limb length is key to being suspicious of the diagnosis in the right historical setting (following infection or trauma).

Pitfalls in Diagnosis

Diligence in observation following an injury to a physis will help prevent significant deformity from a missed physeal bar. Clinical and radiographic evidence of normal physeal growth should be confirmed prior to discharging a patient from clinic after a physeal fracture or infection involving the physis. Sometimes the child needs to be followed for several years to ensure that growth is normal.

Differential Diagnosis

- Growth acceleration from inflammatory or neoplastic conditions
- Cozen phenomenon

Diagnostic Tests and Advanced Imaging

Plain radiographs of the involved joint plus standing lower extremity alignment films will both diagnose and determine the effect of the physeal injury. Advanced imaging in the form of CT or MRI is recommended to determine the extent of physeal involvement of the growth arrest (**Figure 13.40**).

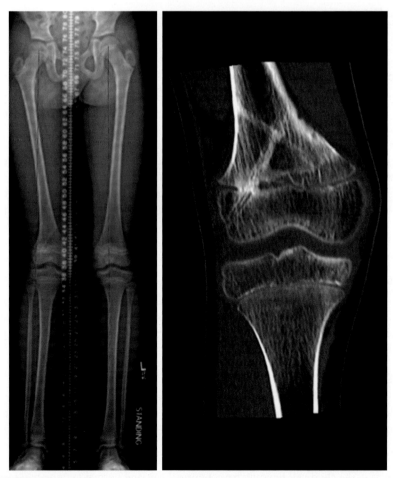

FIGURE 13.40 This child had suffered a distal femoral physeal fracture which was treated with closed reduction and pinning. A lateral growth arrest is present on CT scan, which accounts for the knock-kneed appearance of the limb due to asymmetric growth.

Treatment and When to Refer

As soon as a physeal bar is identified, the patient should be referred to a pediatric orthopedic specialist. Surgery will typically be indicated, and there is advantage to earlier treatment.

● Conclusion

The presence of a lower extremity deformity is able to be grouped into one of the four diagnostic categories: *congenital, metabolic/skeletal dysplasia, developmental,* and *acquired.* Knowledge of the disorders and a thorough history will assist the practitioner in placing patients in the diagnostic categories, while the physical examination should provide the final component to secure a diagnosis.

References

1. Birch JG, Lincoln TL, Mack PW, Birch CM. Congenital fibular deficiency: a review of thirty years' experience at one institution and a proposed classification system based on clinical deformity. *J Bone Joint Surg Am.* 2011;93(12):1144-1151.
2. Hamdy RC, Makhdom AM, Saran N, Birch J. Congenital fibular deficiency. *J Am Acad Orthop Surg.* 2014;22:246-255.
3. Jones D, Barnes J, Lloyd-Roberts GC. Congenital aplasia and dysplasia of the tibia with intact fibula: classification and management. *J Bone Joint Surg Br.* 1978;60:31-39.
4. Pappas AM. Congenital posteromedial bowing of the tibia and fibula. *J Pediatr Orthop.* 1984;4(5):525-531.
5. Warman ML, Cormier-Daire V, Hall C, et al. Nosology and classification of genetic skeletal disorders: 2010 revision. *Am J Med Genet A.* 2011;155A(5):943-968.
6. Blount WP. Tibia vara: osteochondrosis deformans tibia. *J Bone Joint Surg Am.* 1937;19A:1-10.
7. Andersen KS. Congenital pseudarthrosis of the leg. Late results. *J Bone Joint Surg Am.* 1976;58(5):657-662.
8. Roach JW, Shindell R, Green NE. Late-onset pseudarthrosis of the dysplastic tibia. *J Bone Joint Surg Am.* 1993;75(11):1593-1601.
9. Cozen L. Fracture of the proximal portion of the tibia in children followed by valgus deformity. *Surg Gynecol Obstet.* 1953;97(2):183-188.
10. Robert M, Khouri N, Carlioz H, Alain JL. Fractures of the proximal tibial metaphysis in children: review of a series of 25 cases. *J Pediatr Orthop.* 1987;7(4):444-449.

14

Knee Conditions

Eric W. Edmonds and Benton E. Heyworth

● *Introduction to Pediatric Knee Conditions*

In the realm of pediatric orthopedics and, in particular, pediatric sports medicine, the knee is by far the most commonly affected joint generating visits to caregivers of children and adolescents. Therefore, pediatric orthopedic specialists must have an intimate knowledge of knee anatomy, its function, and the physical examination maneuvers that allow for the diagnosis of pathologic conditions and injuries that affect the knee.

The most commonly seen musculoskeletal disorders affecting the knee of children can be traced to overuse phenomena, a discreet traumatic event, or an underlying congenital anomaly. Infectious, neoplastic, inflammatory, neurologic, genetic, and syndromic disorders will also affect the knee in childhood. However, the examination and diagnoses of these conditions are discussed in greater detail in previous chapters. The distinction between traumatic and isolated congenital knee issues will be discussed with an understanding that congenital issues can often lead to the traumatic issues via the level of activity that a child participates. One review article recently produced to highlight, "What's new in pediatric sports conditions of the knee" described tibial spine fractures, osteochondritis dissecans (OCD), and patella instability as the issues with the most recent publications.[1] However, the examination and diagnoses of these young patients would be incomplete without considering other sources of pathology, such as ligament injury, meniscus injury, and atraumatic knee pain associated with growth and the changing biomechanics of the lower limb.

The most common cause of knee pain in children is nontraumatic in nature.[2] In a Danish study that captured school-age children, the knee and ankle were the most common locations of pain, with the knee affecting over 15% of all children. The pain was found to be recurrent over the 3-year study, with pain lasting on average 8 weeks per episode and each child averaging 2.5 episodes per study year. Thus, familiarity with atraumatic overuse conditions is critical in evaluating a child's knee and development of a thoughtful differential diagnosis.

Perhaps the most studied conditions of adolescent knee in last 2 decades are ligament injury.[3] Injuries to the anterior cruciate ligament (ACL), classically the most studied condition in adult sports medicine, have now been appreciated as a condition primarily affecting the pediatric and adolescent populations and are the fear of most high school athletes. Studies have documented an increased rate of 150% over a recent 10-year period.[4] The posterior cruciate ligament (PCL) is also a debilitating injury that can affect young athletes, particularly in contact sports. Medial collateral ligament (MCL) and posterolateral corner (PLC) injuries get less literature-based attention but can be the bane of the treating provider if not promptly identified.[5]

Understanding that congenital and developmental risk factors can lead to traumatic knee injuries is underscored by the rising incidence of conditions, such as patellar instability, which can result from a multifactorial etiology that includes genu valgum, femoral anteversion, trochlear dysplasia, patellar dysplasia, and collagenous soft tissue makeup of the knee.[6,7] While the clinical history may clearly point to a diagnosis of patellar dislocation, the examination and diagnosis must include the evaluation of all of these etiologic factors in order to successfully manage the pathology and reduce the risk of recurrence.

The final topic to be discussed in this chapter is the childhood meniscus tear and the evaluation for discoid meniscus. If a clinically significant meniscus tear is identified, most authors will suggest surgical intervention, and the literature suggests that a much higher rate of successful repair can be obtained, compared with the adult population.[8] Therefore, identifying these injuries early is paramount to optimal treatment, and vigilance needs to be maintained in the evaluation of the pediatric knee.

● *Normal Knee Anatomy*

Ligaments

The ACL is a robust ligamentous structure composed of the anteromedial (AM) and posterolateral (PL) bundle. While more confluent than truly discreet substructures, the two bundles have been found to confer differing functional benefits. The AM bundle is tight in flexion and is the primary check against anterior translation of tibia on the femur, while the PL bundle is tight in extension[9] and is the primary constraint for rotation, thereby providing the rotational stability so essential to cutting and pivoting activities. For the average child, this stability is essential not only for sports but also for simple activities of daily life and free play. Of note, the collateral ligaments and capsule also contribute significantly to rotational stability. The MCL is composed of superficial and deep layers, with the superficial MCL proximal footprint lying just posterior to the medial femoral condyle (MFC) and the distal footprint lying 4-5 cm distal to the joint under the pes anserinus. The deep fibers have a distal footprint directly onto the edge of the tibial plateau near the meniscus. The MCL provides about 80% of valgus constraint at 25° of knee flexion.[10] The PLC is a complex of ligaments and tendons that provide stability to the lateral side of the knee[11] and some degree of rotational stability. The primary three constraints to stability include the lateral collateral ligament (LCL), the popliteus tendon, and the popliteofibular ligament. The PCL is approximately twice as strong and twice as thick as the normal ACL, and the tibial attachment is actually extra-articular in location.[12] Much like the ACL, it can be subdivided into two primary bundles, the anterolateral and posteromedial, with the former tight in flexion and the latter tight in extension. Structures about the knee joint can be seen in **Figure 14.1**.

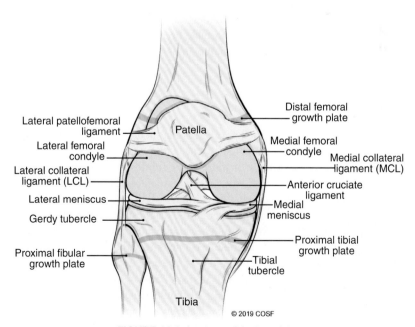

FIGURE 14.1 Anatomy of the knee joint.

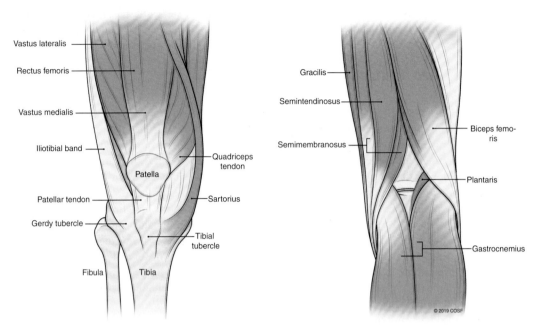

FIGURE 14.2 Muscles about the knee joint.

Muscles

Examining the muscles that affect knee function is important when considering sources of knee pain. The muscles whose tendons cross the knee joint can play a direct role in pain, such as the hamstrings, quadriceps, gastrocnemius, or popliteus. However, the muscles that reach the knee but do not cross the joint can also be a source of pain, such as plantaris, or the muscles that effect knee position during activity, such as the glutei and hip rotators, can have a role in knee pathology[13] (**Figure 14.2**).

It's important to remember that muscle weakness can mimic knee instability from ligamentous injury. The child whose knee buckles may feel unstable because the quadriceps muscle can reflexively stop contracting in the face of severe patella femoral pain.

● *Examination of the Knee*

Examination

Several overarching principles are critical to physical examination of the knee. While it may seem exhaustive to apply these principles to every patient with knee complaints, having a meticulous, consistent approach gives the examiner the best chance of appreciating subtle or rare findings and appreciating the complex interplay of different factors or underlying risk factors for different causes of knee pain. Such an approach will allow the examiner to developing a differential diagnosis without an excessive reliance upon advanced imaging, which should be a last step in the diagnostic process (**Table 14.1**).

The first principle for completing a thoughtful knee examination is that the nonpainful or unaffected knee should always be examined before the affected or painful knee. This will allow the examiner to better understand the patient's normal, baseline anatomy and knee function, as well as establish the patient's comfort level with basic examination techniques, such as palpation and range of motion. Children, much more than adults, may at least initially guard against performance of simple maneuvers or report discomfort with palpation of certain areas, even if not painful at rest or with activity. Such a comparative approach better allows for detection of true pathology and generally puts a young patient at greater ease with the process. Secondly, the examiner should always let the patient know what steps will be performed in the examination prior to

Table 14.1   A Stepwise Approach to the Physical Examination of the Knee

Step 1: Inspection

• Inspection is generally most effectively assessed with the patient in a standing position.

In the setting of an acute injury, supine inspection is performed.
Principles:

• For all steps in the examination, the examiner should inform the patient of how they will be examined.
• Always begin with contralateral limb if patient has unilateral symptoms.
• Examine the painful or injured part last.

Stepwise approach and points to document:

1. Standing alignment
   a. Frontal or coronal plane
      i. Neutral
      ii. Clinically significant varus versus valgus
   b. Sagittal plane
      i. Full extension versus flexion contracture
      ii. Full flexion versus extension contracture
2. Swelling
   a. None
   b. Soft tissue/extra-articular swelling
   c. Effusion/intra-articular fluid
   d. Posterior—popliteal fossa masses/swelling (possible Baker cyst)
3. Skin integrity
   a. Normal
   b. Bruising/ecchymosis
   c. Erythema/rash
4. Patellar position
   a. Neutral
   b. Lateralized
   c. Normal height
   d. Elevated … patella alta
   e. Lowered … patella baja
5. Localization of pain
   a. Patients should be instructed to point to the site of maximal discomfort (if simple provocative maneuver, such as a single leg hop, is needed to incite pain, precede with this step)
   b. Patients should be instructed to use one finger, without moving the finger
6. Gait
   a. Walking (see Chapter 4 on Gait)
   b. Running
   c. Single leg hop
      i. Normal/symmetric versus antalgic or buckling (*always* begin with contralateral limb if unilateral symptoms)

Step 2: Range of Motion Assessment
Principles:

• If any blocks to range of motion or asymmetries are appreciated, attempts should be made to assess the end point and whether they are rigid (boney/mechanical) versus soft (stiffness-based)
• Always recognize sources of "referred" pain to the knee from the hips (slipped capital femoral epiphysis or Perthes disease)

• *Stepwise approach and points to quantitate (degrees)*:

1. Hips
   a. Supine position … flexion/extension, abduction/adduction
   b. Prone position … internal/external rotation
      i. With hip extended, asymmetry in rotation detects underlying hip pathology.

(Continued)

Table 14.1	A Stepwise Approach to the Physical Examination of the Knee (Continued)

2. Ankles/feet
   a. Dorsiflexion/plantarflexion
   b. Inversion/eversion
3. Knees
   a. Extension
      i. Active (can the patient straighten to 0°?)
      ii. Passive (how much pain-free hyperextension can be achieved?)
   b. Flexion
      i. Active (can the patient pull the calf muscle against the posterior thigh?)
      ii. Passive (can the heel be made to touch the posterior thigh?)

Step 3: Effusion Test—The Fluid Wave Sign
Principles:

- Some of the most clinically significant and often missed diagnoses (such as a meniscus tear, anterior cruciate ligament (ACL) injury, osteochondritis dissecans (OCD), chondral injuries) have an associated effusion.
- Detection of this subtle sign is a critical step in a thoughtful knee assessment and may provide clear evidence of the need for magnetic resonance imaging (MRI).
- A lack of knee effusion provides reassurance for proceeding with other measures prior to pursuing an MRI.

Stepwise approach and points to document:

1. With the knee in full extension and the quadriceps muscle relaxed, the medial capsular fluid should be gently pushed/milked superior to the patella and across the suprapatellar pouch to the lateral side.
2. The lateral capsular fluid should then be pushed with a thumb at the lateral peripatellar soft spot in a medial direction.
3. The medial peripatellar soft spot should be observed carefully for the presence of a fluid wave, suggesting abnormal/excessive synovial fluid or hemarthrosis.
4. In patients with large effusions, it is impossible to confine the fluid to the lateral knee and to generate a fluid wave. The patella will float on the fluid and can be pushed down. The presence of ballotable patella is another sign of a knee effusion.

Step 4: Ligamentous Examination
Principles:

- If injury/symptoms are unilateral, always begin with contralateral limb to understand baseline status and normal features, given the spectrum of physiologic variability.
- Elimination of guarding is critical to the accuracy of these tests. Patients can be distracted with unrelated conversation or can be instructed to interlock their fingers and focus on pulling their hands apart; sometimes straining their upper body muscles will relax their lower body muscles.
- While among the most critical of ligamentous tests, the pivot shift maneuver should be reserved for the end of the ligamentous examination, so as not to create pain that may lead to greater guarding during the other attempted tests. At times, even slight guarding precludes an accurate/ unconfounded test.

Stepwise approach and tests to document:

1. Lachman test for ACL—With the knee flexed to 20°, stabilize the distal femur just above the patella with one hand and anteriorly translate the proximal tibia just below the patella with the other hand. Feel for distance traveled and whether the end point is firm and hard
   (normal implies the anterior cruciate is intact) or soft and indiscrete (possible ACL disruption).
2. Valgus stress test for medial collateral ligament—With one hand supporting the leg, the other hand should apply a medially directed force against the lateral aspect of the knee to assess laxity. This is done at full extension and in 30° of flexion.
3. Varus stress test for lateral collateral ligament—With one hand supporting the leg, the other hand should apply a laterally directed force against the medial aspect of the knee to assess laxity. This is done at full extension and in 30° of flexion.
4. Posterior sag—With the hip and knee flexed 90°, the amount of posterior displacement of the tibia is compared between the knees. Increased sag implies posterior cruciate ligament (PCL) deficiency.

Table 14.1	A Stepwise Approach to the Physical Examination of the Knee (Continued)

5. Drawer test—With the knee flexed 90°, the foot is stabilized by the examiner. The amount of anterior and posterior displacement is quantified. Increased displacement implies a cruciate injury.
6. Dial test—With the knee flexed (at 30° and 90°), increased external rotation of the tibia at the knee implies posterior/lateral injury of capsule, popliteus, and PCL.
7. Pivot shift test—With the knee fully extended and the tibia slightly internally rotated, the knee is gradually flexed to 15°-20°. Palpable reduction of the tibia as the knee is flexed implies an ACL-deficient knee.

Step 5: Meniscus Injury Tests
Principles:

- Several of the meniscal tests or signs, such as joint line tenderness and pain with hyperextension, are quite sensitive to meniscus injuries, particularly in the acute setting, but not necessarily very specific. In other words, other diagnoses, such as an ACL tear or severe bone bruise, may also be associated with positive joint line tenderness or positive pain with hyperextension.
- The overall number of meniscus signs, such as three out of five or four out of five, should be considered, especially as it relates to consideration toward the need for an MRI to definitely diagnose a patient's knee pain or knee injury.

Stepwise approach and tests to document:

1. Fluid wave sign for effusion (see above).
2. Pain with knee hyperextension—With one hand on the anterior aspect of the distal femur, above the level of the suprapatellar pouch, the other hand elevates the tibia from the ankle level, straightening the knee and passively applying slight hyperextension through the knee joint. A meniscus tear will often give pain on the affected side (medial or lateral) or may be described to be felt "in the back" of the knee, in part due to the posterior horn being the most commonly affected segment of the meniscus to sustain a tear/injury.
3. Pain with knee hyperflexion—With one hand on the anterior aspect of the distal tibia/ankle, the other hand supports the anterior aspect of the midthigh, effectively flexing the knee (and hip) and passively applying hyperflexion through the knee joint. Similar to the hyperextension maneuver, a meniscus tear will often give pain on the affected side (medial or lateral) or may be described to be felt "in the back" of the knee, in part due to the posterior horn being the most commonly affected segment of the meniscus to sustain a tear/injury. Most commonly, with a meniscus tear, there is pain with *both* hyperextension and hyperflexion, but occasionally one is positive while the other is negative.
4. Joint line tenderness—With the knee flexed to 70°-90°, the side of the thumb or the side of the index finger is placed along the medial or lateral aspect of the knee, respectively, to apply pressure to the several millimeter gap between the proximal tibial plateau and the femoral condyle. A meticulous, systematic examination will include separate assessments of the anterior horn (anteromedial/anterolateral), meniscal body (directly medial/lateral), *and* posterior horn (posteromedial/posterolateral).
5. McMurray test/maneuver—With the knee flexed to 70°-90° and with one hand supporting the knee, the other hand is used to rotate the tibia internally and externally while extending the knee toward 10°-30° of flexion. The tibial plateau is thereby loaded against the corresponding femoral condyle, squeezing the interposed meniscus which, in the face of a tear or contusion, will generate pain. The classic description of a positive test is one of palpable subluxation, or a palpable "pop," due to an unstable torn meniscus being felt by the examiner's thumb or index finger, which is placed over the joint line. However, more commonly today, people consider a positive McMurray test to be one of the knee pains generated by the maneuver. For clarity, the authors favor describing either a "pain and a palpable pop or snap with the McMurray test" or "pain, but no palpable pop or snap, with the McMurray test."

performing them. This tends to make patients more comfortable and establish an important level of trust in the encounter, which facilitates a meticulous examination. Thirdly, the hips and ankles should be examined for every patient reporting knee pain. This will help the examiner understand the patient's baseline level of flexibility and appreciate any underlying pathology in the adjacent joints that may be contributing to the patient's knee condition. Hip conditions not infrequently manifest themselves as nonspecific knee pain that is difficult to reproduce through palpation or provocative testing. This phenomenon is known as "referred pain," and in patients with hip conditions, this is due to the fact that obturator nerve innervates the hip capsule as well as the medial thigh and knee. Hip pathology, such as slipped femoral capital epiphysis or Perthes disease,

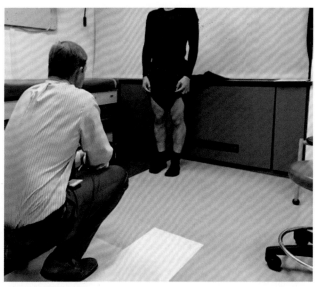

FIGURE 14.3 Inspection of the knee is often most effectively initiated from a squatted position several feet away from the standing patient. Appropriate exposure of the lower extremity should allow the examiner to visualize from the midthigh to the ankle, noting any asymmetry, swelling, and features of standing alignment.

may present with a complaint of knee pain or a slight limp, rather than with hip pain (see Chapter 16). Finally, a gait assessment should be performed on every patient that is able to do so (see Chapter 4). While acute injuries may preclude comfortable weight bearing, the walking and running gait should be assessed for all patients with atraumatic onset of knee pain. What is their foot progression angle? Do their patella point toward each other? Do they have an antalgic gait? Do they demonstrate circumduction?

When beginning the examination of the affected knee, the knee should be assessed first with direct visualization or inspection, often most effectively with the examiner squatting several feet away from a standing patient (**Figure 14.3**).

Is the skin intact? Is there an obvious effusion or hemarthrosis? Is it erythematous? Is the patella centered on the trochlea or is it dislocated (**Figure 14.4**)?

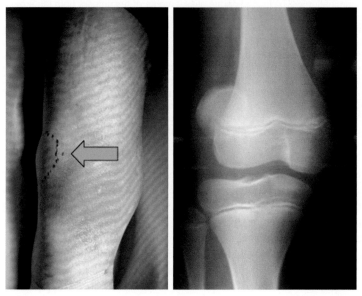

FIGURE 14.4 This figure demonstrates a laterally dislocated patella (outlined with a skin marker) (green arrow). Radiographic correlation is also provided.

Do their patella point toward each other? The standing coronal plane alignment should be assessed for the presence of genu valgum and genu varum. Next, having the child then point with one finger to the location of their greatest or most common site of pain is helpful in identifying the perceived location of pain. Do they localize the pain, or do they point at the entire anterior knee? Are there any masses on this knee of concern, compared with the contralateral knee?

Gentle palpation can then be performed to evaluate for masses or, more commonly, areas of tenderness. This is generally better done with the patient lying in the supine position on the examination table. The location of pain can be very telling, and the conditions that tend to generate pain at the various sites are listed here parenthetically. The locations that should always be palpated in a growing child include the inferior pole of the patella (Sinding-Larsen syndrome, patellar tendonitis), the superior pole of the patella (quadriceps tendonitis, midline superior, or bipartite patella, superolaterally), the tibial tubercle (Osgood-Schlatter syndrome), the medial joint line (medial meniscus tear), lateral joint line (lateral meniscus tear, discoid meniscus, or iliotibial [IT] band syndrome), anterior MFC (superomedial plicae or MFC OCD), anterior lateral femoral condyle (LFC OCD), medial patella and medial epicondyle (medial patellofemoral ligament, MPFL injury associated with patellar instability), pes anserinus (pes bursitis), and Gerdy tubercle (IT band syndrome). Specific sites can be further palpated as directed by the child, based on their understanding to the source of pain. Are there many sites that hurt, or is the pain localized?

One critical test for every child presenting with knee pain is assessment of a potential effusion, even with atraumatic onset of pain. The fluid wave test, performed with the knee in full extension, involves milking any fluid with one's fingers from the medial peripatellar space and suprapatellar pouch over to the lateral peripatellar region and then pushing, with the thumb, on the lateral peripatellar soft spot while inspecting the medial peripatellar soft spot. If there is even a trace effusion, the medial soft spot should show a discreet momentary outpouching, or a positive fluid wave sign, suggestive of an underlying effusion or hemarthrosis (▶ **Video 14.1**).

A pitfall exists when examining for an effusion in a very swollen knee. In this case it is impossible to milk all of the effusion to one side of the knee for the fluid wave test. In these cases, one can simply see if the patella is floating and can be pushed up and down. This is called a ballotable patella examination and can be accentuated by compressing the suprapatellar pouch and forcing the patella anterior (**Figure 14.5**; ▶ **Video 14.2**).

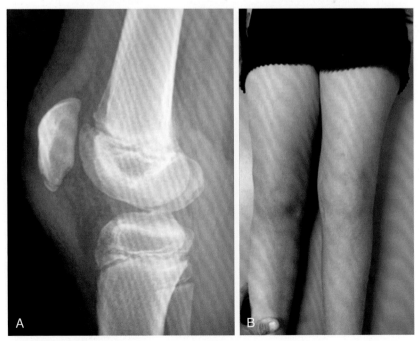

FIGURE 14.5 A, The x-ray above demonstrates a large knee effusion with the presence of a ballotable patella. B, On physical examination, the bony contour of the knee is lost.

Distinguishing soft tissue swelling and prepatellar bursitis (**Figure 14.6**) from an effusion is critical, and the latter is more concerning for causes of internal derangement, such as OCD or other cartilage disorders, Lyme arthritis of the knee, inflammatory joint disorders (**Figure 14.6**), meniscal tears, and ACL tears. In most cases, any effusion of unknown etiology should generate consideration of an MRI for further diagnostic workup.

The next step in every knee examination is a range of motion test. Ranging the knee in the supine position can be the most comfortable for an anxious patient. At this time, comparing the unaffected knee to the painful knee provides beneficial information, particularly for the recovery and changes over time. Because some children extend only to neutral, while others can even hyperextend 20°, lifting the heel off of the examination table while gently stabilizing the knee on the table is an important maneuver (**Figure 14.7**).

Is there a block to full extension? Is there a block to full flexion? This test should also be done actively, with the patient contracting the quadriceps muscle. Do they have a flexion contracture (**Figure 14.8**) or an extension lag (**Figure 14.9**)? In the former case, the knee cannot be straightened regardless of the position of the hip (extension or flexion) and cannot be manually straightened by the examiner. A child with extensor lag can be fully extended by an examiner but the patient cannot reach the same extent of extension usually as a result of quadriceps weakness.

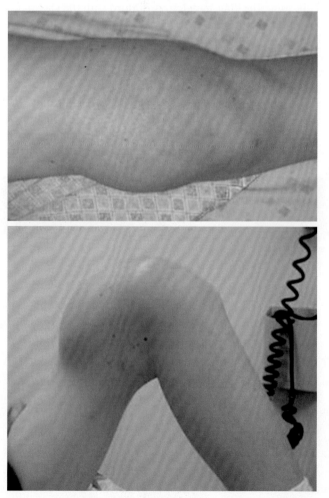

FIGURE 14.6 Photographs of a 14-year-old patient with severe intra-articular synovitis.

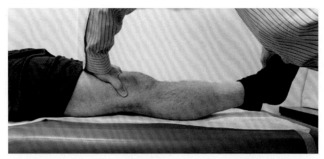

FIGURE 14.7 Hyperextension of the knee is demonstrated with the heel gently lifting off the examination table as the distal femur just above the knee is stabilized in extension. Quantifying a patient's normal hyperextension on the uninjured knee can help identify potential pathology, based on decreased or increased hyperextension on an injured knee or based on pain elicited during the maneuver.

A ligament examination can be performed next. When lateralization of the patella is associated with apprehension, or concern that the kneecap may dislocate, this is considered a positive patellar apprehension test (**Figure 14.10**).

The "moving patellar apprehension test," as described by Ahmad et al,[14] can also be done by slowly dropping the heel off the side of the bed with laterally directed pressure on the patella. Contraction of the quadriceps muscle to prevent any further flexion is considered a positive test and may be slightly more sensitive to patellar instability than the simpler version of the apprehension test in full extension. Next, the anterior drawer test, Lachman test (▶ **Video 14.3**), and pivot shift (▶ **Video 14.4**) test can be performed to assess ACL integrity. Assessment of the PCL is achieved with the posterior sag test and posterior drawer test (▶ **Video 14.5**).

Varus or valgus stress in full extension and 30° of flexion is critical if there is suspicion of potential injury to the collateral ligaments (**Figure 14.11**).

Finally, assessment of the dial test with the patient prone and the knee held by the examiner in both 30° and 90° of flexion checks the integrity of the PLC. When moving from assessment of the ligamentous structures to that of the meniscus, four cardinal signs of meniscus tears should be remembered: (1) effusion, (2) pain with hyperextension and/or hyperflexion, (3) joint line tenderness, and (4) positive McMurray testing. The McMurray test is performed by twisting the tibia, relative to the femoral condyles, while moving the knee from flexion to extension, and applying slight varus or valgus stress to

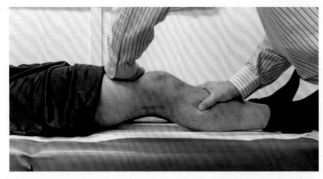

FIGURE 14.8 With a flexion contracture of the knee, the patient is unable to straighten the knee fully, with the joint seemingly forced into a fixed flexed position at terminal extension. However, most flexion contractures, which are common postoperatively, can be overcome with aggressive passive stretching exercises over time.

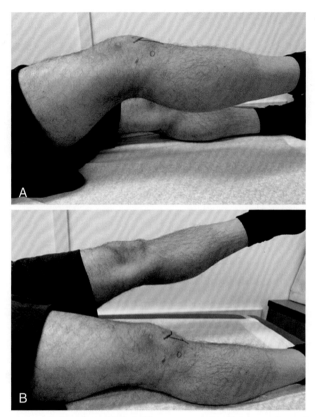

FIGURE 14.9 A knee extensor lag is seen with quadriceps muscle weakness and may be common in the early weeks following knee surgery or with an injury somewhere along the extensor mechanism. Here the patient is unable to achieve full extension of the knee with active hip flexion (A), as an attempted straight leg raise (SLR) is performed off the examination table. By contrast, a normal, proficient SLR can usually be performed on the uninjured or nonoperative, contralateral limb without an extension lag (B).

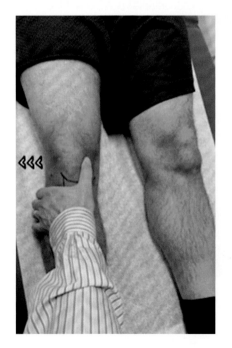

test the lateral or medial meniscus, respectively.[15] While the classic description of the test involved palpating a mechanical clicking or clunking at the joint line, as may be present with a lateral discoid meniscus, most people today consider pain with this provocative maneuver to be a "positive" McMurray test.

Next, an assessment of muscle flexibility is pertinent particularly when the history is atraumatic. The popliteal angle can be assessed with the patient supine on the bed. The hip is then flexed to 90°, pointing straight toward the ceiling. The knee is then held in space, while the ankle is pushed to make the knee straight (the whole limb pointing straight toward the ceiling) (**Figure 14.12**).

FIGURE 14.10 In the patellar apprehension test, the patient lies supine with the knee in extension as the examiner translates the patella laterally with their thumb. The test is considered positive is if the patient reports apprehension during passive displacement.

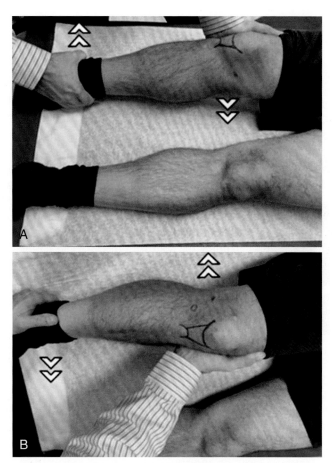

FIGURE 14.11 Testing of the collateral ligaments requires application of valgus and varus forces to a relaxed knee, both in full knee extension and with the knee flexed 20°. The valgus stress test stretches the medial collateral ligament as force is applied medially to the lateral aspect of the knee while the opposite hand stabilizes the leg at the ankle (A). The varus stretch test assesses the integrity of the lateral collateral ligament as force is applied laterally to the medial aspect of the knee while the opposite hand stabilizes the leg at the ankle (B). Either test is considered positive if there is an asymmetric end point with excessing gapping or less stability felt at the level of the joint.

An easy way to measure the result is starting with the knee bent to 90° and considering a completely straightened knee 180°. The achieved measurement is the recorded result. The examiner should not push, but just move the leg until tension is achieved, and the patient should not assist by flexing the quadriceps. The contralateral leg can be compared to identify the hamstring flexibility. The patient can then roll over into a prone position. Prone knee flexion can then be assessed with a "positive" Ely test, suggestive of tightness or a contracture to the rectus femoris, representing an inability to touch the posterior calf to reach the posterior thigh. Many quantify the severity of a positive Ely test by the number of clenched fists that could be placed between the heel and the posterior thigh (**Figure 14.13**).

Finally, an assessment of IT band flexibility can be achieved by performing an Ober test in the lateral decubitus position (with affected hip up), contralateral hip flexed to 90°, ipsilateral knee flexed to 90°, and allowing it to fall to the table. If the knee on the tested side does not reach the table, this is considered a "positive" Ober test, with IT band contracture representing a risk factor for IT band syndrome or bursitis (**Figure 14.14**).

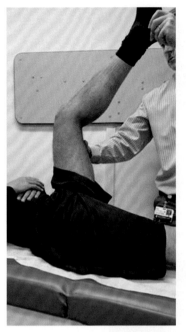

FIGURE 14.12 The popliteal angle is used to assess hamstring muscle tightness. While the patient is laying supine, the hip is passively flexed to 90° as the contralateral leg remains flat against the bed. The knee is then passively extended toward full extension by placing pressure on the posterior aspect of the ankle toward the ceiling until there is a firm resistance to movement or the patient reports discomfort or the inability to be extended further. A knee injury may confound the assessment of the normal flexibility of the knee or tightness of the hamstring secondary to knee pain.

Finally, quadriceps and hamstring muscle strength should be tested next. Is it normal? Does it cause discomfort? How does it compare to the contralateral side? A step-down test can be performed by having the child stand on a raised platform (such as an 8-in step stool) and lower themselves down on one leg, tapping the floor with their toe and raising back up to standing, almost like a single leg squat. Having an available hand out for support can be useful to keep your patient from falling. Does the ipsilateral hip move into adduction? Does the ipsilateral knee move into valgus? Can they raise back up to a standing position? Can they control the descent to the floor?

The above steps may not be applicable to every patient, due to discomfort, deformity, or disability. However, application of this systematic and comprehensive approach, individualized for the patient, based on their age and presentation, should optimize the diagnostic approach in the evaluation of pediatric and adolescent knee conditions. The below findings are designed to facilitate assessment of specific conditions that may be high on the differential diagnosis, based on the clinical history or physical examination.

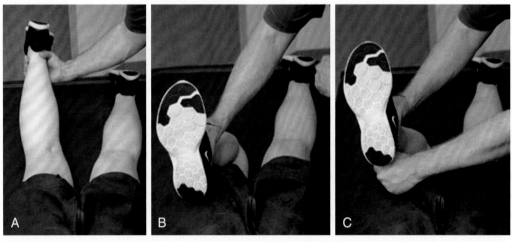

FIGURE 14.13 The Ely test is an assessment of tightness of the extensor mechanism, including the rectus femoris muscle-tendon unit. With the patient prone, the knee is passively flexed toward the posterior thigh (A). With maximum flexibility, the posterior heel is often able to touch the posterior thigh (B). Abnormal tightness, or a positive test, is seen when the heel cannot touch the posterior thigh (C) or the ipsilateral hip rises off of the table and can be quantified approximately by the number of fist widths between the heel and the posterior thigh.

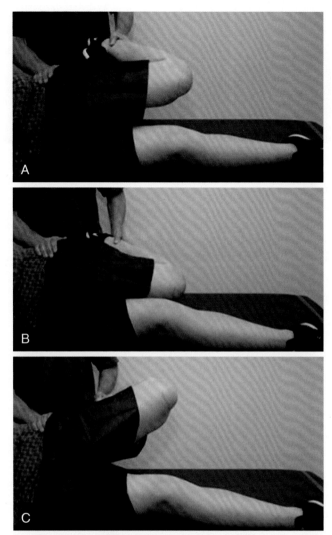

FIGURE 14.14 The Ober test assesses the flexibility or tightness of the iliotibial band (ITB). The patient lies in the lateral decubitus position. The hip is placed into slight abduction and extension while the knee is passively flexed (A). The patient is instructed to allow the knee to fall toward the table posterior to the contralateral, extended leg (B). In a positive test, there is limited adduction of the tested leg secondary to ITB tightness, preventing the knee from touching table (C). Both sides should be assessed to understand every patient's normal, baseline flexibility in this muscle-tendon unit.

Pertinent Findings in Common Knee Conditions

Congenital Knee Dislocation

Hyperextended or dislocated knees can be seen in the newborn nursery. In these cases, the infant's knee is difficult to flex. Hyperextended knees can be progressively flexed with serial casting, physical therapy, or bracing over a few weeks of treatment. Congenital knee dislocations may not respond to conservative methods and require surgical release (**Figures 14.15** and **14.16**).

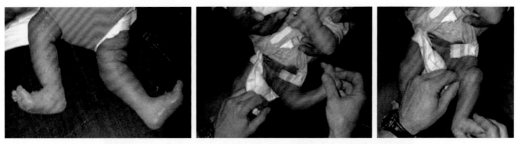

FIGURE 14.15 Physical examination of a child with congenital hyperextension of the knee.

Pitfalls in Diagnosis

One has to be cognizant that ipsilateral hip dislocation is common in children with congenital knee dislocation and ultrasound of the hip may be required to assess its location. Patients with knee dislocations may have systemic or syndromic disorders such as arthrogryposis or spinal dysraphism such as spina bifida. Examination of the back is important to rule out cutaneous signs of spinal dysraphism (hairy

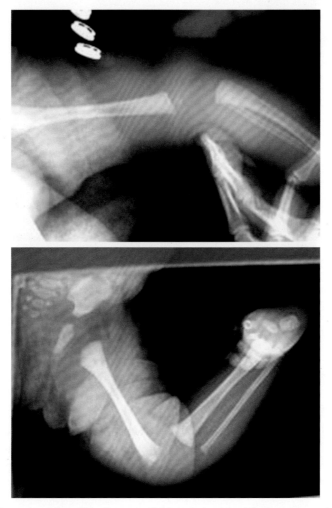

FIGURE 14.16 Radiographs of the child with congenital hyperextension of the knee shown in **Figures 14.15**. In the bottom panel the knee is significantly hyperextended. The top panel demonstrates that with manipulation the proximal tibia aligns with the femur axis.

patch, supragluteal cleft dimple, or lipoma), and detailed neurologic examination can gain insight into possible causes of muscle weakness (hamstring). Concurrent foot deformity is almost diagnostic for nonidiopathic causes of knee dislocation.

Diagnostic Tests or Advanced Imaging

Anteroposterior (AP) and lateral knee radiographs can infer whether the knee is simply hyperextended or if the tibia is dislocated anterior to the femur.

Treatment and When to Refer

Children should be referred to a pediatric orthopedist for evaluation and consideration of next best steps of treatment. Referral to pediatric geneticist or neurologist may be appropriate in the face of possible syndromes or paralytic muscle conditions.

Plica Syndrome

Plicae are synovial folds most commonly in the AM aspect of the knee. A plica is present in about 50% of the population and is thought to be a remnant of embryonic connective tissue that failed to fully resorb during development (**Figure 14.17**).

Luckily, most plicae are asymptomatic. Tenderness, particularly in conjunction with palpable snapping, is highly suggestive of an inflamed plica. Tenderness to palpation is over the superomedial area of the knee, adjacent to the patella, over the MFC, especially when the medial shelf plicae are palpable. As *symptomatic* plicae are relatively rare, it is a relative diagnosis of exclusion, such that all other examination findings tend to be normal. It can be difficult to ascribe anterior knee pain to a plica as a result of flexibility issues and pain or weakness with step-down testing. Many adolescents and preadolescents, the subpopulation most affected by the condition, can have similar signs and symptoms as a result of hip core weakness.

Osteochondritis Dissecans

OCD is a condition that develops in the joints, most often in the knee of children and adolescents. It occurs when a small segment of the bone dies and begins to separate from its surrounding region due to a lack of blood supply. The overlying cartilage may remain intact or the entire piece of necrotic bone and cartilage can displace (**Figure 14.18**).

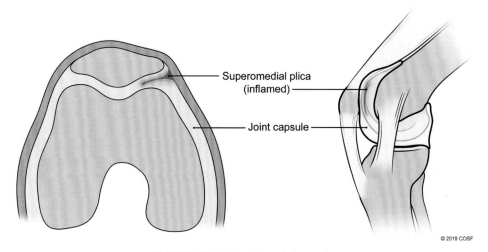

Superomedial plica (inflamed)

Joint capsule

© 2019 COSF

FIGURE 14.17 Rendering of a knee plica.

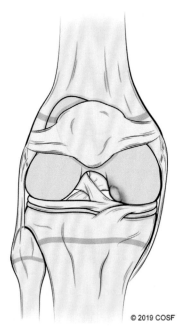

FIGURE 14.18 An illustration demonstrating a medial femoral condyle osteochondritis dissecans lesion.

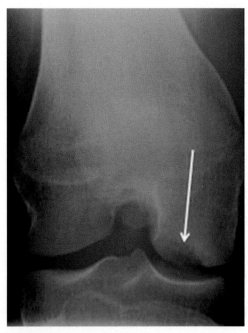

FIGURE 14.19 Osteochondritis dissecans lesions are found most commonly on the medial femoral condyle. On plain radiograph, cortical flattening or indistinct subchondral radiolucency (arrow) is best visualized on tunnel view.

Tenderness to palpation at the medial condyle itself (the AM area of the knee, sometimes just distal to a palpable plica) with or without an effusion may raise one's suspicion for a medial OCD lesion, which can be detected on a radiographic examination (**Figure 14.19**). While the lateral aspect of the MFC is the most common area of knee OCD, similar tenderness over the anterior lateral femoral condyle or trochlea may similarly suggest an OCD in these other, slightly less common areas.

Medial Meniscus Tear

Tenderness to palpation at the medial joint line is perhaps the most specific finding associated with this pathology (**Figure 14.20**), though MCL injuries (see below) may also yield this positive examination finding. Patients with medial meniscal tears will not have pain with valgus stress of the knee, whereby MCL injuries will.

Meniscus tears are associated with a hemarthrosis in 90% of cases, but only when seen in the acute setting. The McMurray test can also indicate a medial meniscus tear, particularly if mechanical symptoms are reproduced. If there is doubt concerning the origin of pain, and the child indicated that it was more anterior than posterior, then an Apley grind can be performed in the prone position. The knee is bent to 90°, and the foot is twisted back and forth with an axial load on the knee. This can elicit pain in the setting of an anterior horn tear. A bucket handle tear that is displaced will often result in an apparent flexion contracture, limiting full extension of the knee either passively or actively (**Figure 14.21**).

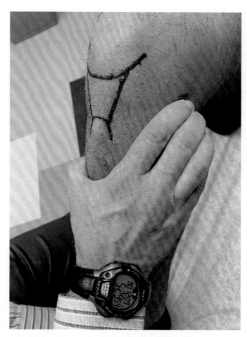

FIGURE 14.20 Palpation with the index finger of the medial joint line (which is likely to be positive with a medial meniscus tear, though other causes, such as a medial collateral ligament sprain, must be considered and ruled out).

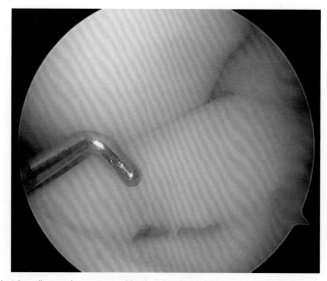

FIGURE 14.21 Bucket handle meniscus tear with visualization of the torn posterior horn and body of the medial meniscus displaced into the anterior aspect of the medial compartment and the intercondylar notch.

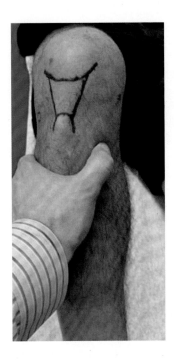

FIGURE 14.22 Palpation with the thumb of the pes anserine (a potential site of bursitis, which can cause anteromedial knee pain).

Pes Anserine Bursitis

Pes anserine bursitis is inflammation of the bursa located between the proximal tibia and the tendons of sartorius, gracilis, and semitendinosus on the medial side the knee. Tenderness to palpation over the anteroinferior aspect of the knee (**Figure 14.22**), or proximal medial tibial metaphyseal region, can indicate insertion pain of the hamstrings or a bursitis.

Often the slight soft tissue swelling or fluctuance of the bursitis can be palpated as well. All the ligament testing will be normal, but the hamstring muscles will often demonstrate relative inflexibility. The step-down test tends to be positive as well.

Symptomatic Bipartite Patella

Tenderness to palpation at the superolateral aspect of the patella, along the border of the patella itself, should raise suspicion for a symptomatic bipartite patella (**Figure 14.23**).

There may be a palpable prominence to the synchondrosis, but this is not consistently found. The quadriceps may demonstrate muscle tightness, and strength testing can elicit pain with active leg extension. Ligament testing and the remaining examination maneuvers are usually benign.

Discoid Lateral Meniscus and Lateral Meniscus Tears

Normal lateral menisci are C-shaped structures (**Figure 14.24A**), while a discoid meniscus is thicker than normal and often oval or disc shaped (**Figure 14.24B**).

People with discoid meniscus may go through their entire lives and never experience any problems. A discoid meniscus have few presenting examination findings, unless it is unstable in nature. These can be unstable posteriorly, anteriorly, or both. The instability can result in limitations in knee range of

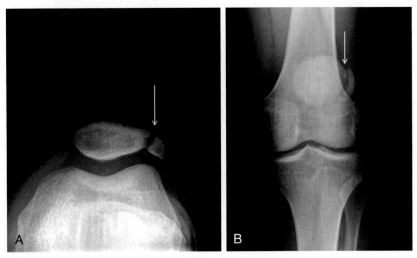

FIGURE 14.23 The separation between the patella and the unfused secondary ossification center of a bipartite patella is demonstrated (white arrow) on sunrise (A) and anteroposterior (B) views.

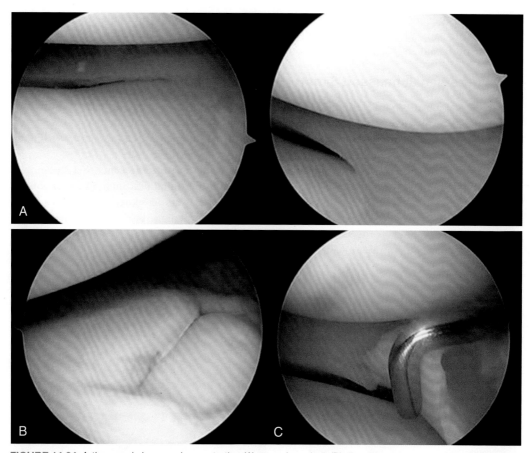

FIGURE 14.24 Arthroscopic images demonstrating (A) normal menisci, (B) discoid meniscus, and (C) meniscus tear (radial flap pattern at the posterior horn-meniscal body junction).

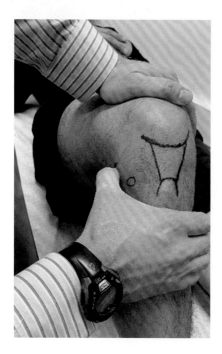

motion, or it can result in a near pathognomonic clunk of the knee with passive extension to flexion maneuver (▶ **Video 14.6**).

Discoid menisci are, however, more prone to injury and tearing than a normally shaped meniscus. Symptoms often begin during childhood. Much like traumatic tears in the medial meniscus, a torn lateral meniscus (discoid or not) will often be tender to palpation over the lateral joint line (**Figure 14.25**).

Just as in medial meniscal tears, a hemarthrosis or effusion is common in the acute setting of a tear. This can often be reproduced

FIGURE 14.25 Palpation with the thumb of the lateral joint line (which is likely to be positive with a lateral meniscus tear, though other causes, such as a lateral collateral ligament sprain or iliotibial band bursitis, must be considered and ruled out).

with active knee motion as well. A torn meniscus (**Figure 14.24C**) can also result in a limitation of motion, particularly a loss of extension in the setting of a bucket handle tear. A McMurray test can reproduce both pain and mechanical symptoms when the lateral meniscus is torn.

Sinding-Larsen Johansson Syndrome and Patellar Tendinitis

Sinding-Larsen Johansson (SLJ) disease is a possible cause of anterior knee pain in active children and adolescents. It is considered an overuse knee condition rather than a traumatic injury and is referred to as an apophysitis at the inferior pole of the patella where the patella tendon *originates* (**Figure 14.26**).

Tenderness to palpation at the inferior pole of the patella in preadolescents (8-12 years old) can be indicative of SLJ (**Figure 14.27**), while the same finding in adolescents (>12 years old) is more consistent with patella tendinitis, sometimes referred to as "jumper's knee" or "runner's knee."

The ligament testing and McMurray's will all usually be benign, but the muscle flexibility and strength can be poor, as this pathology often represents an issue related to the changing lower extremity biomechanics of the growing child. The step-down test can often be difficult to perform secondary to pain.

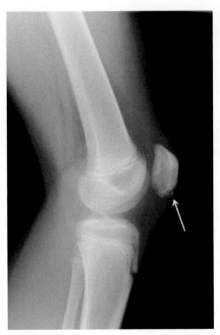

FIGURE 14.26 Lateral x-ray of the knee in a skeletally immature patient with Sinding-Larsen-Johansson syndrome (SLJS) shows a small ossification variant (arrow) on the inferior pole of the patella at the origin of the patellar tendon. While such bony findings are common in patients with SLJS and can be helpful in confirming a diagnosis, they are not definitively diagnostic, in that patients may have SLJS without such radiographic findings, and such radiographic findings may be present in patients without SLJS. Also, these findings must be differentiated from an acute avulsion injury or patellar sleeve fracture, based on history and physical examination.

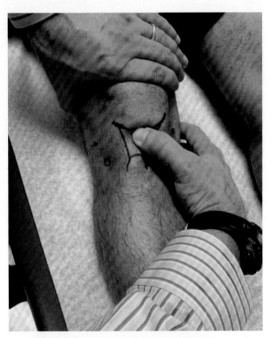

FIGURE 14.27 Tenderness associated with Sinding-Larsen-Johansson syndrome (usually in 8- to 12-year-old athletes) or patellar tendonitis (usually in older adolescents and adults) can be elicited with palpation along the inferior pole of the patella.

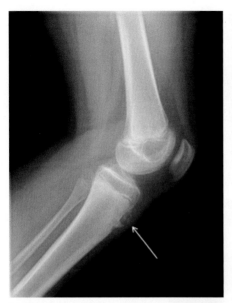

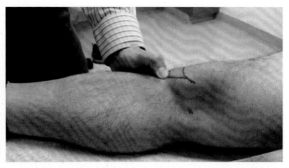

FIGURE 14.29 Examination of a patient with suspected Osgood-Schlatter disease should include palpation over the tibial tubercle, where tenderness can be elicited and a soft tissue or bony prominence may be appreciated upon inspection.

FIGURE 14.28 Osgood-Schlatter disease, also known as tibial tubercle apophysitis, can cause ossification variants and the appearance of fragmentation within or just proximal to the tibial tubercle (arrow) as seen in this lateral x-ray of a knee in a skeletally immature patient.

Osgood-Schlatter Syndrome and Patellar Tendon Ossicles

Osgood-Schlatter syndrome is another common cause of knee pain in growing adolescents. It is an inflammation (apophysitis) of the *insertion* of the patella tendon on the proximal tibia (**Figure 14.28**). With time, the repeated inflammation cycles can lead to development of the bone within the substance of the tendon and its insertion.

Tenderness to palpation over the tibial tubercle is nearly pathognomonic for Osgood-Schlatter syndrome in a growing child, usually seen in 12-16-year-olds (**Figure 14.29**).

They will have some combination of muscle tightness and weakness consistent, but an otherwise benign examination of the knee. The may occasionally have localized swelling caused by the inflammation of the still incompletely ossified apophysis. The step-down test can often be difficult to perform secondary to pain.

Anterior Cruciate Ligament Tear or Tibial Spine Avulsion

Disruption of the ACL complex is the most feared injury to the growing athlete. In children, the tendon may stretch before the ligament and the bony insertion is pulled off of the proximal tibia and is considered a tibial spine avulsion (**Figure 14.30**).

In older children and adolescents, the ACL may be disrupted within the substance of the ligament.

In either case, there is often a large hemarthrosis in the acute setting of an ACL tear. Tenderness to palpation at the lateral condyle is not uncommon due to the bone bruising incited by the traumatic event, but this is difficult to discern from the lateral joint line tenderness of an associated lateral meniscus tear. Patients will have a positive (asymmetric) Lachman test and anterior drawer test, which should be distinctly different from the contralateral knee. If there is an associated bucket handle meniscus tear that is displaced into the notch, then the ligament examination can be misleading

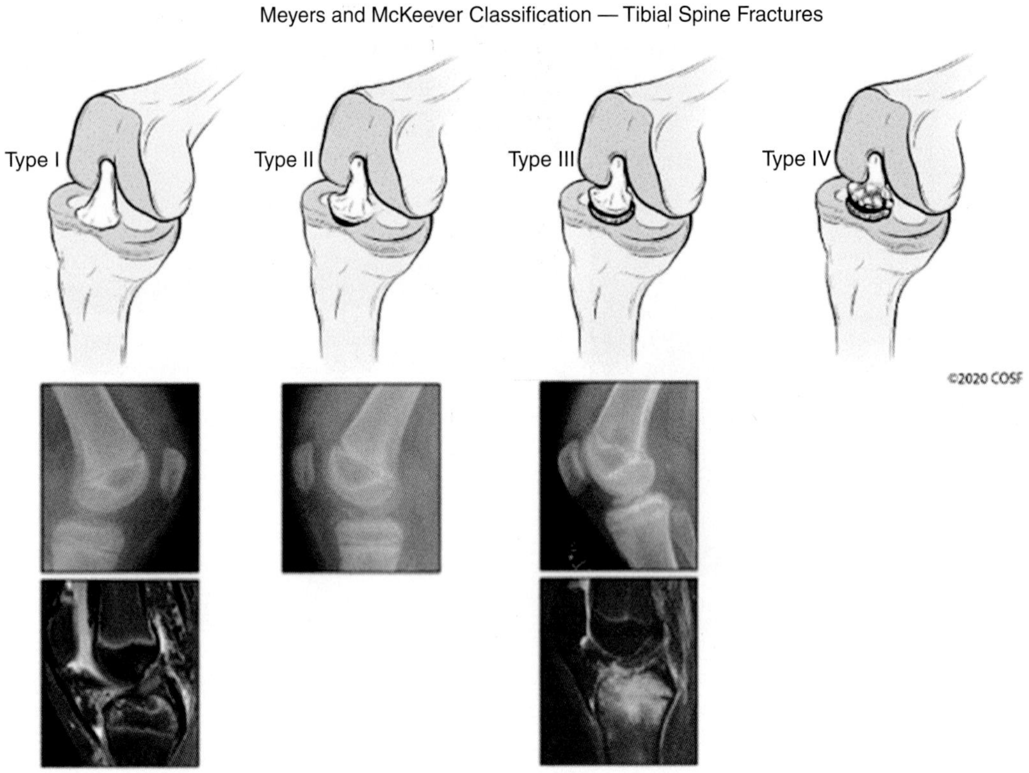

Meyers and McKeever Classification — Tibial Spine Fractures

©2020 COSF

FIGURE 14.30 The Meyers and McKeever Classification of Tibial Spine Fractures with corresponding imaging: Type 1: The fragment is elevated anteriorly, with minimal or no displacement. Type 2: The anterior edge of the fragment is hinged with an intact posterior edge. Type 3: The fragment is completely detached. Type 4: Comminution of the fragment.

and the Lachman and drawer testing can be negative (stable). If possible, then a pivot shift test should be performed, as this will be positive if testing is not precluded by muscle guarding. If findings are consistent for an ACL tear, then you must be sure to assess for associated collateral ligament injury and meniscus injury.

Posterior Cruciate Ligament

There is often a large hemarthrosis in the acute setting of a PCL tear. Tenderness to palpation is unlikely to find a specific area of pain in the setting of an isolated PCL, unless associated with a tibial avulsion. In that setting, posterior popliteal pain is possible. Patients will have a positive (asymmetric) posterior drawer test, which should be distinctly different from the contralateral knee. A positive posterior sag test is suggested by the anterior tibial plateau sitting posterior to the anterior aspect of the femoral condyles. If findings are consistent for a PCL tear, then you must be sure to assess for associated collateral ligament injury and/or meniscus injury.

Medial Collateral Ligament

There is sometimes, though rarely, a hemarthrosis in the acute setting of an MCL tear. In a delayed setting, there will often still be swelling over the medial knee. Tenderness to palpation may be present at the medial condyle, medial joint line, proximal medial tibia, or along substantial portions of the course of the MCL. Valgus stress testing will either elicit pain (unless presentation is delayed) or demonstrate laxity compared to the contralateral knee. The gait will often be antalgic. If findings are consistent for a MCL tear, then you must be sure to assess for associated ligament injury and meniscus injury.

A valgus force applied to the knee in a child with open growth plates can lead to a Salter-Harris fracture as opposed to an MCL tear. In both cases, pain with a valgus force will be present; yet in the case of a fracture, there will be tenderness located more proximally at the level of the growth plate. The growth plate is usually at a level at the midpoint of the patella and is the widest portion of the bone.

Lateral Collateral Ligament and Posterolateral Corner

Lateral collateral injuries are less common than MCL injuries. There is often a large hemarthrosis in the acute setting of a PLC complex tear. Tenderness to palpation at the lateral knee or the PL knee is common. There is often edema affecting the knee, even more so than finding the effusion. If findings are consistent for a PLC tear, then you must be sure to assess for associated cruciate ligament injury and meniscus injury. Varus stress testing of the knee can elicit instability if the LCL is involved. The dial test is good for discerning if the PLC injury is likely to be symptomatic in the long term regarding instability.

Patellar Instability

In the acute setting of a patella dislocation or subluxation, there will often be a hemarthrosis and there is tenderness at the location of MPFL disruption: along its course, at the medial patella, or on the medial epicondyle of the femur. Often they can have tenderness to palpation over the lateral femoral condyle where the patella strikes the condyle during the dislocation event (▶ **Video 14.7**).

The patient will have a positive apprehension test, and they will demonstrate laxity with lateralization compared to the contralateral knee. The gait analysis is important to identify underlying etiologies for the patella instability event, particularly femoral anteversion in the setting of external tibial torsion.

Pitfalls in Diagnosis of Knee Pathology

When it comes to knee pain and knee injuries, the pitfalls include not considering all of the different diagnosis. Patients and families want to "help you" make the diagnosis and may provide information that may have little importance. For instance, a 2-year history of knee pain that "might have followed a twisting knee event" and that "might have occurred" somewhere in that general time period is not an enough causation to confirm a traumatic etiology.

Key Points to Remember

1. Knee effusions can occur from trauma or inflammation such as Lyme disease, infection, or inflammatory conditions.
2. Vague medial-sided knee pain could be referred from the hip. One must perform a detailed assessment of hip rotation in the prone position. Any differences in rotational profile should dictate hip radiographic examination.
3. Bone and growth plates usually fail before ligaments tear in traumatized children.
4. Lots of different sites of knee pathology and pain can occur around the patella.
5. Symptomatic knee instability may not be ligament damage but may be reflexive muscle weakness from pain.
6. Asymptomatic knee crepitance/popping with motion may be normal.
7. When a knee radiograph "looks funny," consider a contralateral radiograph to assess what's normal.
8. Congenital knee conditions (discoid meniscus, cruciate aplasia, lateral femoral condyle hypoplasia) may not become symptomatic until later in life.

Diagnostic Tests or Advanced Imaging

Standard radiographs are always a good initial screening. In general, an AP and lateral image is required. A Merchant or Sunrise view can assess patella femoral congruity. A notch view can evaluate for OCD. Standing alignment films can assess limb lengths and determine alignment. AP and frog pelvis radiographs can evaluate for hip pathology. MRI studies are often ordered to confirm diagnosis suspected on physical examination.

Blood tests can be used to evaluate for inflammatory conditions. These include complete blood count, differential, sedimentation rate, and specific markers for inflammatory conditions.

Treatment and When to Refer

Children and adolescents should be referred when the diagnosis is uncertain and treatment strategies have yet to be clarified. Referral to pediatric orthopedist, pediatric sports medicine specialist, or nonoperative pediatric orthopedic provider is appropriate. Treatment is based upon diagnosis and can include activity modification, physical therapy, bracing, and occasionally surgical management.

References

1. Cruz A, Richmond C, Tompkins M, Heyer A, Shea K, Beck J. What's new in pediatric sports conditions of the knee. *J Pediatr Orthop*. 2018;38(2):e66-e72.
2. Fuglkjaer S, Hartvigsen J, Wedderkopp N, et al. Musculoskeletal extremity pain in Danish school children – How often and for how long? The CHAMPS study-DK. *BMC Musculoskelet Disord*. 2017;18(1):492.
3. Stanitski CL, Harvell JC, Fu F. Observations on acute knee hemarthrosis in children and adolescents. *J Pediatr Orthop*. 1993;13(4):506-510.
4. Shaw L, Finch CF. Trends in pediatric and adolescent anterior cruciate ligament injuries in Victoria, Australia 2005-2015. *Int J Environ Res Public Health*. 2017;14(6):599.
5. Kramer DE, Miller PE, Berrahou IK, Yen YM, Heyworth BE. Collateral ligament knee injuries in pediatric and adolescent athletes. *J Pediatr Orthop*. 2017.
6. Askenberger M, Janarv PM, Finnbogason T, Arendt EA. Morphology and anatomic patellar instability risk factors in first-time traumatic lateral patellar dislocations: a prospective magnetic resonance imaging study in skeletally immature children. *Am J Sports Med*. 2017;45(1):50-58.
7. Duppe K, Gustavsson N, Edmonds EW. Developmental morphology in childhood patellar instability: age-dependent differences on magnetic resonance imaging. *J Pediatr Orthop*. 2016;36(8):870-876.
8. Shieh A, Bastrom T, Roocroft J, Edmonds EW, Pennock AT. Meniscus tear patterns in relation to skeletal immaturity: children versus adolescents. *Am J Sports Med*. 2013;41(12):2779-2783.
9. Amis AA, Dawkins GP. Functional anatomy of the anterior cruciate ligament. Fibre bundle actions related to ligament replacements and injuries. *J Bone Joint Surg Br*. 1991;73(2):260-267.
10. Grood ES, Noyes FR, Butler DL, Suntay WJ. Ligamentous and capsular restraints preventing straight medial and lateral laxity in intact human cadaver knees. *J Bone Joint Surg Am*. 1981;63(8):1257-1269.
11. Gollehon DL, Torzilli PA, Warren RF. The role of the posterolateral and cruciate ligaments in the stability of the human knee. A biomechanical study. *J Bone Joint Surg Am*. 1987;69(2):233-242.
12. Lopes OV Jr, Ferretti M, Shen W, Ekdahl M, Smolinski P, Fu FH. Topography of the femoral attachment of the posterior cruciate ligament. *J Bone Joint Surg Am*. 2008;90(2):249-255.
13. Nascimento LR, Teixeira-Salmela LF, Souza RB, Resende RA. Hip and knee strengthening is more effective than knee strengthening alone for reducing pain and improving activity in individuals with patellofemoral pain: a systematic review with meta-analysis. *J Orthop Sports Phys Ther*. 2018;48(1):19-31.
14. Ahmad CS, McCarthy M, Gomez JA, Shubin Stein BE. The moving patellar apprehension test for lateral patellar instability. *Am J Sports Med*. 2009;37(4):791-796.
15. McMurray TP. The semilunar cartilages. *Br J Surg*. 1942;29:407-414.

Limb Alignment and Limb Length Discrepancies

Christopher A. Iobst and Raymond W. Liu

● Introduction to Pediatric Limb Deformity

Limb deformity is a frequent cause for evaluation in a young child. Parental concern regarding the appearance of the lower extremities is often encountered. This chapter focuses first on examining rotational deformities in the growing child, which are likely the most common reason for orthopedic referral. Next, coronal plane deformities, or deformities that are most apparent when viewed from the front or back, are reviewed. Finally, the evaluation and examination of limb length discrepancy (LLD) is discussed.

● Basic Normal Limb Development

Limb alignment in children changes naturally with development, particularly in the earlier years. Although these findings can be concerning to parents, many cases will spontaneously improve and only require reassurance. In other circumstances, such as substantial genu varum (bowlegs), more careful observation and treatment may be necessary.

Foot progression angle (FPA) is the angle between the long axis of the foot and the direction of gait (**Figure 15.1**). A slightly externally rotated FPA at maturity is normal, with only a small amount of change with development. An internally rotated FPA is often observed in younger children. In infants who have not begun to walk, the most common cause of in-toeing is metatarsus adductus. This can be confirmed by finding a curved lateral border to the foot on examination. In children who are noted to have in-toeing as they begin to walk (usually at 1 year of age), the most common cause is internal tibial torsion. In children older than 4 or 5 years of age, the most common cause of in-toeing is usually excessive femoral anteversion. Femoral anteversion is defined as an anterior rotation (in the transverse plane) of the proximal femur relative to the distal femur and knee. At birth, the average proximal femur is rotated 30° to 35° anteriorly, and with time, this decreases to 15° to 20° by skeletal maturity. Anteversion is a physical characteristic such as height; all humans have height, some are taller than others. Similarly, all normal humans have anteversion; yet some are born with a lot more anteversion (excessive) than the average values above. In these subjects, the neonatal external hip flexion contractures mask the effect of underlying femoral anteversion for the first years of life. However, as these external hip contractures gradually begin to disappear, the child with excessive femoral anteversion becomes more apparent. Neurological disorders can affect the ability of the femur to change its anteversion. For instance, patients with hemiplegia will have more internal rotation of the affected femur with persistent fetal anteversion which has not remodeled, presumably as a consequence of altered neuromuscular control.

When viewed from the front (coronal plane), children are generally born with genu varum or bowleggedness. This typically decreases until the age of 2 years when children begin to develop genu valgum. The valgus increases until around the age of 4 years and then gradually settles into its adult alignment of slight residual valgus by the age of 7 years.[1]

LLD is an inequality of the length of the extremities, most commonly referring to the lower extremities. It is common to see LLD in the general population, as the mean LLD has been found to be

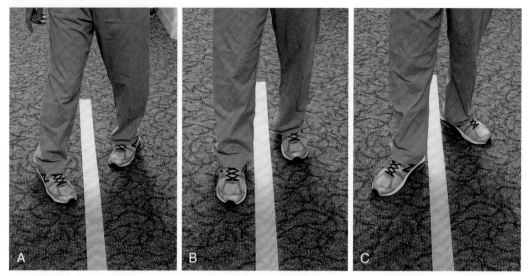

FIGURE 15.1 The foot progression angle (FPA) is the angle between the direction of gait and the direction of the foot. These images demonstrate (A) internal, (B) neutral, and (C) external FPA.

approximately 5 mm with a standard deviation of 4 mm.[2] In most cases, LLD increases proportionally with the child's overall limb growth. It is useful to know that boys reach half of their ultimate lower extremity lengths at 4 years of age, while girls do so at 3 years of age.[3] Thus, if one does diagnose LLD at these ages, it would be expected to double at skeletal maturity, while predictions at other ages can be quickly done with the multiplier method, where the discrepancy is factored by a multiplier based on the child's gender and age.[3]

In-toeing

Introduction

In-toeing is a common finding, particularly in growing children. The most common causes of in-toeing are metatarsus adductus, internal tibial torsion, and excessive femoral anteversion. Metatarsus adductus is a deformity at the level of the midfoot and is first diagnosed in newborns. Internal tibial torsion is an inward twisting of the tibia and is commonly diagnosed in children shortly after walking. Excessive femoral anteversion is an inward twisting of the femur and is commonly diagnosed after 4 to 5 years of age.

Clinical Significance and Natural History

In most cases, the diagnosis can be established by a careful physical examination, and the treatment is reassurance and observation as needed. Less commonly, children with significant metatarsus adductus can have foot pain or difficulty with shoe wear. Patients with internal tibial torsion and femoral anteversion can have difficulties with excessive tripping and/or persistent lower extremity pain with activities. By 10 years of age, most children will have reached their final adult rotational alignment. No substantial correction of rotation is expected to occur with growth after this age. In regard to the natural history of in-toeing, an osteological study found no association between femoral and tibial rotation and arthritis of the spine, hips, and knees, which provides reassurance to families concerned about in-toeing.[4] It is important to note that this study focused on a general population and thus should be used for reassurance in asymptomatic cases, rather than in cases with severe deformity, comorbidities such as cerebral palsy, or in children with significant symptoms.[4]

History and Physical Examination

The age at which the in-toeing was first noticed is an important component of the history. As noted above, in-toeing noticed in an infant suggests a foot origin, in-toeing with initial walking suggests tibial torsion, and later in-toeing is more likely secondary to excessive internal rotation in the femur. Prematurity and delayed onset of walking of 18 months or later should lead the clinician to suspect developmental delays such as that seen in mild cerebral palsy. Although asymmetric in-toeing is frequently reported by family members, the physical examination usually demonstrates symmetric rotation. In those cases, the asymmetry is simply due to the immature gait. If true asymmetry is noted, then neurologic conditions such as hemiplegia should be suspected. Changes in the in-toeing with growth are often noted by the family, and tripping while running is a common complaint of families. Pain is uncommonly reported in younger children, but knee pain may be reported in adolescents with excessive femoral anteversion.

Observational gait analysis is important for all of the clinical conditions in this chapter. Oftentimes, you will get a more natural gait pattern if you can observe the child before they reach the clinic room and before they become aware they are the center of attention. When performing a gait analysis, it is important the child is barefoot and the legs are fully exposed and you have a good distance (private hallway is ideal) from which to observe from the front and the side. This allows enough room for observing multiple gait cycles (▶ **Video 15.1**). During observational gait analysis, it is important to look at each aspect of the gait individually and then observing the gait as a whole package. It is critical to focus on each segment of the lower body individually (foot/ankle, knee, and hip) in both the frontal and sagittal planes. After assessing each level, the following questions should be pondered while watching the child walk: Is there any limping? Is there a full, smooth range of motion at each of the joints, or does the gait appear stiff at a particular level? Are there any compensatory maneuvers such as toe walking, vaulting, circumduction, or knee flexion? Is there any joint instability or thrust with gait? Are the legs straight or is there an associated angular deformity present? Is the FPA straight or rotated? For a more detailed description, please see Chapter 4 on Gait Analysis.

With in-toeing, the clinician will observe an internal FPA, in which the direction of the foot is rotated internally relative to the direction of the child's overall gait (**Figure 15.1**). Many children will self-correct their gait when observed. Asking a child to walk fast or run is usually enough of a distraction to get them to revert to their baseline gait pattern. It is also very useful to observe the child when he/she is first walking into the clinic and not aware that he/she is being observed.

The key portion of the physical examination involves a series of maneuvers in the prone position called the "*rotational profile*." Femoral rotation, tibial torsion, and foot alignment of each limb are assessed in the rotational profile. The foot can be examined for metatarsus adductus by determining that the lateral border of the foot is not straight but convex. The degree of deformity can be assessed with the heel bisector line which is an imaginary line drawn that bisects the heel, and the physician observes which toe this line passes through (**Figure 15.2**). In a normal foot, the heel bisector line passes between the second and third toes, while in a foot with metatarsus adductus the line is lateral to this. If the foot has metatarsus adductus, it is appropriate to determine if the adductus is flexible or fixed by trying to correct the position of the foot. If the foot can be corrected to a normal position where the lateral border of the foot is straight, observation is generally the only treatment necessary.

Internal tibia torsion is most commonly assessed by measuring the thigh foot angle in the prone position with the knee flexed to 90°. The angle between the thigh and the axis of the foot represents the thigh foot angle (▶ **Video 15.2**). Generally, this is between neutral and 10° externally rotated. It is important to allow the foot to naturally dorsiflex to neutral. The clinician should be careful to avoid accidently manipulating the foot into a rotated position which leads to an inaccurate thigh foot angle. If the clinician is unsure about the true proper movement of the foot, or if there is foot deformity, then the thigh malleolar axis can be utilized. In this measurement, a line perpendicular to a line passing between the medial and lateral malleoli is used as the second line to compare to the axis of the thigh (**Figure 15.3**). Thigh malleolar axis is approximately 20° greater than thigh foot angle, and so the normal range is approximately 20° to 30° externally rotated.

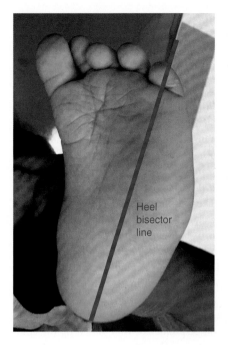

FIGURE 15.2 The heel bisector line is the intersection between a line bisecting the hindfoot and the toes. Normally, this line should pass through the webspace between the second and third toes. In this child with metatarsus adductus, the line is more lateral, intersecting the webspace between the fourth and fifth toes.

Children with excessive femoral anteversion may be able to substantially internally rotate their feet in stance (**Figure 15.4**). Children with excessive femoral anteversion can be easily placed into a W-sitting position due to their increased hip internal rotation (**Figure 15.5**).

In general, each child will have about 90° of total hip rotation; excessive femoral anteversion is assessed by comparing internal and external rotation of the hip with the hip in extension. In the case of a very nervous toddler, internal rotation can be assessed with the knees bent over the side of the table while the child is lying on their back next to their parent. For less anxious children, hip motion is best assessed with the child in a prone position, keeping the pelvis level on the examination table. Hip internal rotation is measured with the feet rotated away from each other, while hip external rotation is measured with the feet rotated toward each other, flexing the knees such that the tibia tends to cross (▶ **Video 15.3**). It is important that the knees are kept together, particularly in external hip rotation. Allowing the knees to separate from each other will result in measuring a falsely higher external rotation angle. Generally, a child with 75° of hip internal rotation and significantly less external rotation (15°) is defined as having excessive femoral anteversion. However, any substantial mismatch with more internal than external rotation could contribute to a negative FPA and in-toeing.

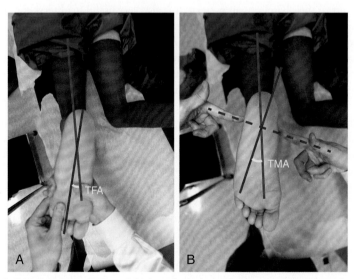

FIGURE 15.3 Both thigh foot angle (TFA) and thigh malleolar axis (TMA) can be used to evaluate tibial torsion. In both cases, the child is prone and the knee is flexed 90°. The blue line represents the axis of the thigh. A, For TFA, the foot is dorsiflexed to neutral and the red lines represents the foot axis. The TFA is the angle (yellow) between the thigh and foot. B, For TMA, a line connecting the medial and lateral malleoli is determined (dotted red line). The TMA is the angle (yellow) between a line orthogonal to this (solid red line) and the thigh axis.

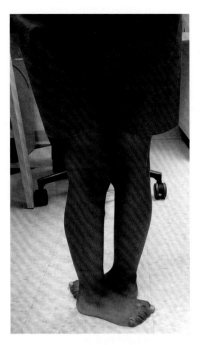

FIGURE 15.4 This child with excessive femoral anteversion can substantially internally rotate both hips and bring the feet nearly 180° to each other.

Pitfalls in Diagnosis

In diagnosing metatarsus adductus, it is important to be sure that the child does not have a clubfoot, as metatarsus adductus is one of the components of a clubfoot. If the child has good dorsiflexion range of motion in the ankle, then the diagnosis of clubfoot is unlikely. It is important to make sure the foot is angulated in the inward direction, as a foot in the opposite direction would likely be a calcaneovalgus foot in an infant.

Internal tibial torsion can be difficult to diagnose in a child with foot deformity. As described above, in concomitant cases of foot deformity, it is preferable to use thigh malleolar axis. Because proper dorsiflexion of the foot can be difficult to position, it is reasonable to check thigh malleolar axis whenever examining thigh foot angle and evaluating the child more carefully if the thigh malleolar axis is not 20° more externally rotated than the thigh foot angle as expected. Internal tibial torsion can also masquerade as genu varum, or the two conditions can occur in tandem. See below including a description of the "cover-up test" to differentiate between the two.

Excessive femoral anteversion is generally fairly straightforward to diagnose by comparing hip internal rotation with hip external rotation. The main pitfall is that in patients with excessive femoral anteversion, concurrent internal or external tibial torsion can be overlooked. With combined femoral anteversion and internal tibial torsion, the child can have a large negative FPA. With combined femoral anteversion and external tibial torsion, the two deformities compensate for each other with a fairly neutral FPA. However, this combination (also known as miserable malalignment) tends to place more stress on the patellofemoral joint, and knee pain can occur, particularly in older children in the adolescent age range.

Differential Diagnosis

Subtle cerebral palsy can present with asymmetric in-toeing. Although parents may notice more in-toeing on one side than the other in children with routine femoral anteversion or internal tibial torsion, it is important to be sure that the child does not have spastic hemiplegia. In cerebral palsy, the child generally exhibits increased tone when the extremities are manipulated for examination. Also, irregularities when walking in the hallway can be helpful

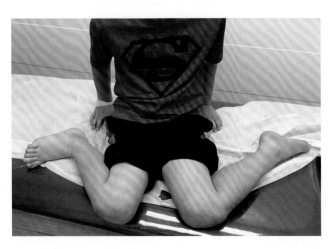

FIGURE 15.5 It is common for children with excessive femoral anteversion to sit in a W-position, with the hips internally rotated. This sitting position should be discouraged, as it is thought to prevent proper remodeling of the femur with growth.

and particularly obvious with the child running, which can produce posturing of the upper extremity (see Chapter 4 on Gait Analysis).

Diagnostic Tests or Advanced Imaging

Rotational deformities are mostly diagnosed and managed without imaging. Femoral anteversion and tibia torsion are not readily apparent on plain radiographs, although subtle signs such as apparent coxa valga (a neck shaft angle greater than 145 degrees) can be seen with excessive femoral anteversion. In metatarsus adductus, an anteroposterior (AP) view of the foot will confirm and quantify the adductus deformity, although this is not necessary for diagnosis.

Advanced imaging such as computed tomography (CT) and magnetic resonance imaging (MRI) can be used to quantify the magnitude of femoral anteversion and tibia torsion. However, this is generally unnecessary for diagnostic purposes and is mainly considered as a presurgical test.

Treatment

In most cases, the causes of in-toeing can be treated with observation. Metatarsus adductus generally improves with observation. Metatarsus adductus that cannot correct past neutral can be treated with serial casting. On occasion, surgery is recommended to correct the foot if the deformity has persisted into childhood and is symptomatic.

Since many parents are frustrated by their child's gait and assume that there must be something wrong, they can be dissatisfied with the answer from the physician that no treatment is necessary. It is controversial whether it is wise to advice against W-sitting. On one hand, there are no data to suggest it makes a difference, and most parents are wise to pick their battles carefully. Others may advocate this approach as a way to placate families who feel that they must do something and will provide the parents with something to monitor their child and often appease their need to have something done (**Figure 15.5**). Bracing has not been shown to be effective and is not used for these conditions. Excessive femoral anteversion and external tibial torsion are also largely treated with observation. In older children with persistent symptoms of the above miserable malalignment, physical therapy might be utilized to help the child strengthen and compensate for the deformity. Surgical reconstruction for patella femoral pain as a result of "miserable malalignment" can be recommended for children with persistent deformity and/or persistent pain recalcitrant to normal conservative measures.

When to Refer

As noted above, most children with in-toeing can be treated with reassurance to the parents that it should improve spontaneously. Some families may be unsatisfied with observation as the only form of treatment because older family members may have worn braces or special shoes for similar conditions in the past. A child with metatarsus adductus that is not correctable to a neutral position or a walking child having difficulties with shoe wear or foot pain should be referred. Internal tibia torsion or excessive femoral anteversion with persistent symptoms, such as excessive falling or pain that limits activity, should also be referred. For children with substantial residual rotation after the age of 8 years, a referral to a pediatric orthopedic surgeon is reasonable to educate families and to discuss treatment options.

● Out-toeing

Introduction

Out-toeing is less common than in-toeing, particularly at younger ages. It is normal to have a slightly externally rotated FPA by adulthood. Out-toeing in infants generally originates from an external hip rotation contracture due to intrauterine positioning, which generally starts to improve by 18 months of age as they learn to walk. Out-toeing in walking children commonly originates from external tibial torsion or in children with excessively flat feet.

Clinical Significance and Natural History

Most cases of out-toeing can simply be observed. External rotation hip contractures generally resolve on their own as the child continues to walk. External tibial torsion tends to persist but is generally asymptomatic. Sometimes children will report pain, generally in the later juvenile or adolescent age ranges, with pain from external tibial torsion potentially affecting the knee, shin, ankle, or foot. An osteological study did not find any association between external tibial torsion and arthritis of the spine, hips, or knees.[5]

History and Physical Examination

Children who have just begun to walk and have out-toeing generally have external hip rotation contractures. Children who have been out-toeing since walking age are more likely to have external tibial torsion. One should particularly suspect other etiologies with unilateral out-toeing, as physiologic out-toeing is commonly bilateral with external tibial torsion. It is useful to determine if there is any history of breech delivery, increasing suspicion for potential hip dysplasia. On the other hand, children who begin to out-toe in the juvenile and early adolescent age ranges may have other pathologies such as Legg-Calve-Perthes disease or slipped capital femoral epiphysis (SCFE).

As with in-toeing, it is important to perform observational gait analysis as described above (▶ **Video 15.4**). Children with out-toeing will have an external FPA (**Figure 15.1**). External rotation contracture of the hip generally occurs in infants and young toddlers and can be examined in the supine position, with substantially more external hip rotation than internal hip rotation (▶ **Video 15.5**). External tibial torsion can be diagnosed based on the thigh foot angle, as described above (▶ **Video 15.2**). Again, it is useful to concurrently assess the thigh malleolar axis (**Figure 15.3**) to avoid being deceived by the foot position. This is particularly important in the case of flatfoot, where midfoot collapse and an abduction deformity of the midfoot can lead to the false diagnosis of external tibial torsion.

Pitfalls in Diagnosis

An externally rotated gait can occur as a compensation pattern for knee pain, knee stiffness, ankle pain, ankle stiffness, or drop foot (inability to actively dorsiflex the ankle). It is important to bring the knees and ankles through a full range of motion and note any pain with this movement. A drop foot should be noticeable on observation of gait, as the foot will strike the floor awkwardly and often with a noticeable sound. Knee or ankle pain or stiffness can present with an antalgic gait, where the child is trying to decrease the amount of time on the affected lower extremity. A child with an externally rotated gait, loss of internal rotation, and new-onset knee pain over the age of 8 years should be evaluated with an AP and frog pelvis radiograph for a possible SCFE.

Differential Diagnosis

An externally rotated gait is common after a lower extremity injury. This almost always improves as the child recovers. Observation of gait in the hallway, including running motion, is very helpful. Increased tone on examination should alert the clinician for possible cerebral palsy. It is important to rule out other hip pathologies with out-toeing. In children with limited hip internal rotation, one should rule out Legg-Calve-Perthes disease if the child is of age 4 years or older and SCFE if the child is approaching puberty.

Flatfoot can present as an out-toeing gait. In children with flat feet and a tight Achilles tendon, the foot cannot fully dorsiflex through the ankle. Consequently, the foot bends through the ligamentously lax midfoot causing a combination of dorsiflexion and abduction of the midfoot (▶ **Video 15.6**), which appears as out-toeing.

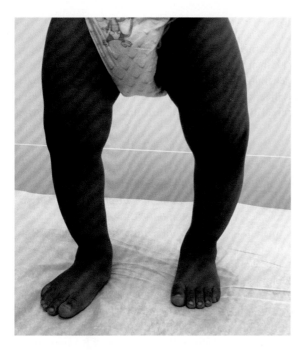

FIGURE 15.6 Toddler standing with bilateral genu varum. Note the curve is symmetric in both limbs and is a long sweeping curve without any acute deformity in the femur or tibia.

Diagnostic Tests or Advanced Imaging

Infants and toddlers with suspected external rotation contracture of the hip and children with external tibial torsion do not require imaging. Imaging, if obtained, is generally unremarkable. In children of age 4 years and older with limited internal rotation of the hip, a standing AP pelvis and supine frog lateral pelvis radiograph should be obtained to look for hip pathology such as Legg-Calve-Perthes disease or in preadolescents, SCFE. Although CT and MRI can be used to quantify the magnitude of external tibial torsion, this is rarely done and generally only necessary for surgical planning.

Treatment

External rotation contracture of the hips resolves and external tibial torsion can also be treated with careful observation. Bracing has not been shown to be effective for out-toeing. In older children with persistent symptoms, physical therapy might be utilized to help the child improve flexibility and strength. Surgical options are recommended for children with persistent deformity and persistent pain recalcitrant to normal conservative measures. Children may note improved function as well as improved pain after correction.

When to Refer

External rotation contracture of the hip generally does not require referral. However, external tibial torsion with significant pain that limits activity should be referred. External rotation with new-onset hip or knee pain can indicate an SCFE or Legg-Calve-Perthes disease and demands immediate referral to a pediatric orthopedic surgeon. Limping (even if painless) combined with an externally rotated gait should also merit referral to a pediatric orthopedic surgeon.

● Genu Varum

Introduction

Bowlegs, also known as genu varum (knee deviated away from the midline), is a Latin term, which translates to the knees bent outward. Bowing is natural in children until the age of 18 to 24 months (**Figure 15.6**). This physiologic bowing is often a result of some deformity in both the femur and tibia and is usually symmetric. Asymmetric bowing or persistent bowing after 3 years of age is not normal and warrants further investigation (**Figure 15.7**).

Clinical Significance/Natural History

Genu varum in the adult population results in asymmetrical loading of the medial portion of the knee joint and can begin to cause knee pain and in severe cases can develop arthritic joint disease

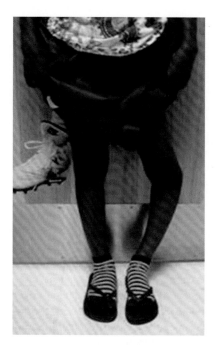

FIGURE 15.7 Standing view with asymmetric bowing of the left lower extremity. Note there is an acute deformity that can be identified in the left proximal tibia.

in the knee as the patient ages. Thankfully, the vast majority of infants and early toddlers with varus deformity have physiologic bowing which resolves by 4 years of age. In the minority of children with bowlegs, their deformity is secondary to metabolic bone disease, skeletal dysplasia, or Blount disease. These children may have persistent varus into adulthood with a natural history described above (**Figure 15.8**).

History and Physical Examination

It is common for parents to bring their child to the physician with concerns about the shape of the legs and the gait pattern, especially between the ages of 12 and 24 months. The clinician must be able to differentiate between normal physiologic bowing and abnormal bowing (examples include dysplasia, rachitic conditions, Blount disease). The key questions to ask are when the bowing was first noticed and whether it is getting better or worse over time. A toddler whose height is greater than the 25th percentile is unlikely to have skeletal dysplasia, while a toddler who is obese could be at risk for infantile Blount disease especially if the child was an early walker (9-10 months). It is also important to discover whether there was any previous trauma or infection to the lower extremities and whether any prior treatment was attempted. Finally, a family history of bowing requiring treatment and a diet history (looking for vitamin D or calcium deficiency) should be ascertained.

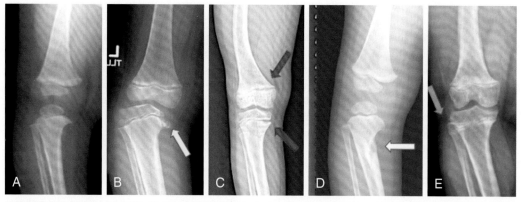

FIGURE 15.8 Varus panel: Five images of different types of varus deformity around the knee. A, Patient with physiologic bowing. Notice that the appearance of the physis in the distal femoral and proximal tibial is normal. B, Patient with Blount disease. Notice the irregularity of the medial proximal tibial physis characteristic of this condition (yellow arrow). C, Patient with hypophosphatemic rickets. Notice the irregularity and widening of the physis in both the distal femur and the proximal tibia (red arrows). D, Patient with focal fibrocartilaginous dysplasia. Notice the well-circumscribed lesion in the proximal tibia at the junction of the metaphysis and diaphysis (white arrow). In this condition, the physis is normal in the distal femur and proximal tibia. E, Patient with achondroplasia. The varus in these patients is related to relative overgrowth of the fibula compared with the tibia (orange arrow).

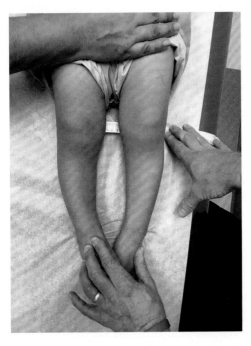

FIGURE 15.9 The intercondylar distance is measured by placing the limbs in full extension with the patient in the supine position. The patella should point directly anterior in each limb, and the medial malleoli should be gently touching. The distance between the medial femoral condyles can be measured with a ruler or with the clinician's fingers.

The physical examination should begin with calculation of the child's body mass index. Obese children have a propensity to develop pathologic bowing. Observational gait analysis is performed; internal tibial torsion may coexist with the bowing of the limbs. An internally rotated tibia can accentuate the appearance of the genu varum by causing the knees to point outward in order to keep the feet straight while walking. This external rotation of the knee makes even normal alignment appear more bowlegged (apparent genu varum). A lateral thrust may be noted with gait indicating laxity of the lateral collateral ligament (▶ **Video 15.7**). This occurs when the knee abruptly shifts into a varus position (fibular head and upper tibia shift laterally) during the stance phase of ambulation. While examining the patient standing, the stature and posture may raise suspicion for an underlying diagnosis, such as rickets or skeletal dysplasia.

Assessment of each leg's alignment in the frontal and sagittal planes with the patient in the standing and supine positions should be performed. While the patient is standing with both knees fully extended and the feet flat on the floor, the examiner can look at the posterior sacral dimples or the level of the iliac crests to determine if there is any leg length discrepancy. The examiner should determine whether there is symmetry of the lower extremities (unilateral or bilateral). If deformity is present, the clinician should isolate where it is located (eg, in the femur or tibia or both). The clinician should differentiate whether the bowing appears as a gentle curve or as a more pronounced curve in one portion of the limb (**Figures 15.6** and **15.7**). The intercondylar distance can be measured with the patient standing and supine (**Figure 15.9**). This represents the distance between the medial femoral condyles when the ankles are just touching each other. A graphical chart produced by Heath and Staheli provides the normal range for the intercondylar distance by age.[4] The level of the fibular head should be determined. Normally, the top of the fibular head sits below the joint line. Relative overgrowth of the fibular head closer to the joint line can be seen in skeletal dysplasias, tibial hemimelia, and Blount disease. A rotational profile with the patient in the prone position can assess femoral rotation, the thigh foot angle, and the thigh malleolar axis. The integrity of the collateral ligaments should be tested with varus and valgus stress of the knee in extension and in 30° of flexion.

Pitfalls in Diagnosis

In many instances, the physician is trying to distinguish physiologic bowing from pathologic bowing. Physiologic bowing tends to be symmetric in both the limbs, with a long sweeping curve. Pathologic bowing tends to be more acute in appearance and is usually focused in the proximal tibia. Tibial torsion can also make bowing look worse than it really is. The cover-up test can be helpful in discerning whether the bowleggedness in gait is due to actual bowing or if it is a compensation for internal tibial torsion (**Figure 15.10**). A toddler with internal tibial torsion will often externally rotate their legs when they walk. This may be due to concurrent hip external rotation contractures or the child may actively externally rotate so their feet do not collide. Regardless of the reason, when walking with the feet turned out the proximal tibia will appear bowed even though the child does not have genu varum. This is where the cover-up test can help. In this test, the examiner should place the child supine on the examination table with both legs fully extended and the patella pointing straight anteriorly. Covering the feet and lower portion of the tibia will give a more accurate account of the amount of varus at the knee by removing the contribution from torsion from the examiner's sight. The prone examination of the thigh foot angle is the best way to quantify how much torsion is present.

When in doubt, serial examinations every few months are still the most effective way to discern pathologic from physiologic bowing. Clinical photographs of the child standing are an effective way to monitor the progress of limb alignment without using an x-ray. If bowing is progressively getting worse instead of better or if the bowing has not resolved by the age of 2½ years, then a referral to a pediatric orthopedist for radiographs is warranted.

Differential Diagnosis

While physiologic bowing and Blount disease are the most common causes of bowing in a toddler, the clinician should be cognizant of several other potential causes of genu varum. Metabolic bone disease (renal osteodystrophy, dietary vitamin D deficiency, hypophosphatemic rickets), focal fibrocartilaginous

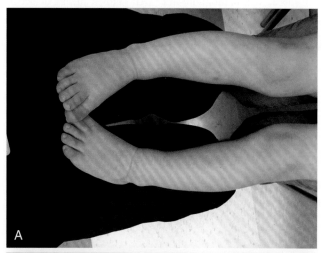

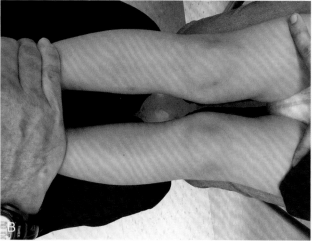

dysplasia of the tibia, posttraumatic or postinfectious deformity of the femur or tibia, and skeletal dysplasia (metaphyseal chondrodysplasia, mucopolysaccharidoses, achondroplasia) are other potential sources of bowing. The history, physical examination, and radiographs are usually sufficient to distinguish most of these diagnoses from one another.

Diagnostic Tests or Advanced Imaging

A standing hip to ankle bilateral lower extremity film is the most effective method to analyze the alignment (**Figure 15.11**). Dedicated standing AP and lateral films of the tibia and/or

FIGURE 15.10 A and B, The cover-up test is used to differentiate deformity caused by genu varum from deformity caused by internal tibial torsion. Place the child supine and fully extend both knees with the patella pointing straight up (A). Then cover the distal 1/2-1/3 of the tibia with your hand to isolate the deformity at the knees. B, If there is true genu varum, the bowing will be noticeable at the level of the knees. If the knees look straight, then the apparent bowing is due to the internal tibial torsion.

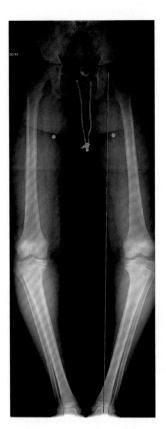

FIGURE 15.11 An example of a standing full-length bilateral lower extremity radiograph. Note this patient has bilateral genu varum. The mechanical axis (red line) is drawn on the left leg from the center of the hip to the center of the ankle. The line passes medial to the center of the knee indicating varus is present.

femur can then be ordered if deformity is identified on the long leg film. Radiographs in those younger than 2 years are generally not very helpful unless there is clear asymmetry between the two limbs. Radiographs should be ordered when (1) the child is older than 2 years with progressively worsening varus deformity, (2) the varus deformity is unilateral or asymmetric, (3) the site of bowing is acute rather than a gentle curve, and (4) the clinical findings suggest possibility of a pathologic condition (short stature, fibular overgrowth, history of trauma or infection, etc.).

Radiographic abnormalities in the periphyseal area will be present in many etiologies. Blount disease will show irregularities in the posteromedial proximal tibial physis. If the varus is caused by physeal injury from trauma, infection, or neoplasm, characteristic radiographic findings will be apparent. The radiographic feature of focal fibrocartilaginous dysplasia is a pathognomonic, well-defined lucent defect in the medial cortex of the proximal tibia. Skeletal dysplasias typically demonstrate abnormal epiphyseal or metaphyseal regions in multiple bones. Metabolic bone disease is characterized by widening of the physes. If metabolic bone disease is suspected, additional laboratory work may be necessary to pinpoint the diagnosis.

Treatment

The treatment for physiologic bowing is observation, education, and reassurance. Most children will grow out of the varus by the age of 2 years, and any concomitant internal tibial torsion should continue to gradually improve during the preschool years. Special shoes, braces, or therapy is not necessary for physiologic bowing. Serial examination with clinical photographs every few months is the most reliable method to monitor a young child with bowing.

When to Refer

Bowing that persists past the age of 2 years or documented worsening of bowing over several visits should be evaluated by a pediatric orthopedist. Any child with asymmetric bowing or acute bowing of the limb, a child with a lateral thrust with gait, if the measured intercondylar distance is more than two standard deviations from the mean based on the Heath and Staheli chart, then the clinician should refer to a pediatric orthopedist.

● Genu Valgum

Introduction

Genu valgum (knee deviated toward the midline of the body), also known as knock-knees, describes a patient's standing lower extremity alignment where the knees are close together and the ankles are spread apart (**Figure 15.12**). Between approximately 2 and 8 years of age, symmetric genu valgum is the expected alignment and is known as physiologic genu valgum. The lower extremities settle into their adult alignment pattern of approximately 7° of valgus by 7 years of age. Understanding this pattern of development helps the clinician distinguish between normal physiologic alignment and abnormal alignment.

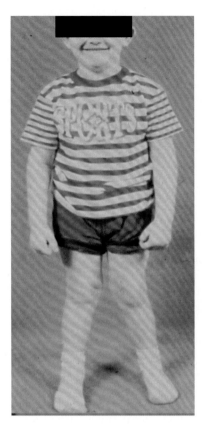

FIGURE 15.12 Standing photograph of a patient with bilateral symmetric genu valgum. Genu valgum is normal in children from 2 to 7 years of age.

Clinical Significance/Natural History

Adult patients with genu valgum may complain of knee pain and easy fatigability when walking long distances. Many patients will comment that their knees rub together when they walk and running appears awkward. In genu valgum, the patella may subluxate laterally due to increased stress through the quadriceps extensor mechanism. This patellar subluxation can cause knee pain, wearing of the patellofemoral articular cartilage, and eventually can progress to complete patellar dislocation in severe genu valgum. Long-standing genu valgum can also cause degenerative knee joint disease by asymmetrically overloading the lateral compartment during weight bearing.

History and Physical Examination

The history should determine when the valgus was first noticed and whether or not it is getting worse with time. The clinician should also find out if there is any associated pain or impairment of function. If the valgus is asymmetric, common etiologies such as trauma or infection should be investigated (**Figure 15.13**). A family history may discover other family members with a similar valgus appearance. Short stature can indicate the presence of a skeletal dysplasia. If there is a history of swollen, erythematous, and warm valgus knees, a rheumatologic process may be the cause. Increased circulation around the knee can cause tibial overgrowth relative to the fibula. Patients with renal disease can have progressive valgus as a result of renal osteodystrophy.

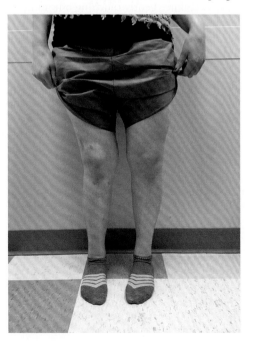

Observational gait analysis is performed to detect thrust with stance phase which indicates that collateral ligament instability exists (▶ **Video 15.8**). Some patients compensate for genu valgum by walking with an in-toeing gait. This maneuver shifts the foot medially, which helps the center of gravity to fall in the center of the foot. The patient's stature and posture may reveal an underlying diagnosis, such as rickets or skeletal dysplasia. There should be symmetry to the alignment of each lower extremity. The leg lengths should be assessed with the patient standing. The iliac crest heights and the posterior sacral dimples are good leg length landmarks. Leg alignment should be assessed in the frontal and sagittal (viewed from the side) planes with the patient in the standing and supine positions. This will allow the clinician to evaluate if there is unilateral or bilateral deformities,

FIGURE 15.13 This patient has asymmetric genu valgum. The left lower extremity is straight and the right lower extremity has a knock-kneed appearance.

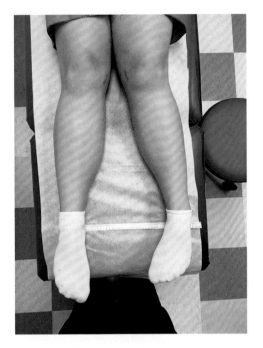

FIGURE 15.14 The intermalleolar distance can be used to quantify the amount of genu valgum. With both lower extremities fully extended and the kneecaps pointing straight anteriorly, the medial femoral condyles should be brought together until they are just touching. The distance between the ankles can then be measured with a ruler or with the clinician's fingers.

gauge the symmetry of the lower extremities, and pinpoint the location of a deformity (eg, in the femur or tibia). The foot should be evaluated in a full weight bearing position to look for pronation, forefoot abduction, and hindfoot valgus.

The hip, knee, and ankle joint range of motion must be examined. Collateral ligament instability can cause or exacerbate genu valgum. The collateral ligament stability of the knee should be examined with varus and valgus stress in full extension and in 30° of flexion. The iliotibial band may be tight in patients with genu valgum and should be evaluated using the Ober test (▶ **Video 15.9**). Any pediatric patient presenting with concerns regarding the knee must have a thorough hip examination. As described above, the rotational profile should be checked in the prone position to judge the shape of the foot, the thigh foot angle, and the amount of internal/external rotation of the hip. Patellar instability or maltracking during flexion/extension of the knee may become evident with progressive valgus deformity of the knee. The intermalleolar distance provides an objective measurement of the amount of genu valgum (**Figure 15.14**). Placing the child supine on the examination table and extending the knees allows this distance to be measured. The lower extremities are rotated until each patella points straight to the ceiling. With the medial femoral condyles of each knee gently touching one another, the space between the medial malleolus of each ankle can be measured with a tape measure. A normal intermalleolar distance should measure less than 8 to 10 cm. As a reference, Heath and Staheli have produced a graphical chart that provides the normal ranges of the intermalleolar distance for each age.[4] Alternatively, in children between 2 and 8 years of age, placing the examiner's hand between the medial malleoli and counting the number of fingerbreadths needed to span the distance can quickly measure the intermalleolar distance. Normally, the separation between the malleoli should be no more than two to four adult-sized fingerbreadths. The parents can be shown how to do this test at home to monitor the alignment.

Pitfalls in Diagnosis

A knock-kneed appearance without true genu valgum (apparent genu valgum) can occur in several clinical scenarios. The overall body morphology should be noted as obesity leads to "knock thighs." In this case, the genu valgum appearance is a result of the thigh soft tissue bulk that forces the lower extremities apart. Standing full-length AP radiographs in these children are usually normal. Losing weight solves this issue. Another valgus appearing situation is a child with pes planus valgus foot (flatfoot) deformities. The severe pronation of the foot forces the knee into a valgus position in order to keep the foot flat on the floor. Finally, children with excessive femoral anteversion can appear valgus due to the inward rotation of the knee during stance phase (anatomic knee flexion visualized out of plane).

Differential Diagnosis

The most common cause of symmetric excessive genu valgum is idiopathic or unresolved physiologic valgus. Radiographically there is no obvious abnormality to the femoral condyles or the physes of the distal femur and proximal tibia. In contrast, radiographic abnormalities can be seen in renal osteodystrophy and skeletal dysplasia in those who present with symmetric genu valgum. These patients have characteristic history and physical examination findings that guide the diagnosis. Asymmetric genu valgum can result from injury to the lateral portion of the distal femoral or proximal tibial physis from trauma or infection. Asymmetric growth following a proximal tibial metaphyseal fracture (Cozen phenomenon) can create genu valgum. Asymmetric genu valgum can also occur from congenital limb deficiency such as fibular hemimelia or congenital short femur; these children usually have other issues such as shortening or foot deformity which makes the diagnosis obvious (**Figure 15.15**).

Diagnostic Tests or Advanced Imaging

If substantial genu valgum (greater than 10°) is present on examination, or if there appears to be asymmetry between the two limbs, then radiographs are recommended. Documented worsening valgus on serial examinations should also be evaluated radiographically. A standing full-length AP radiograph of the lower extremities is the best screening examination (**Figure 15.16**). True genu valgum will have lateral deviation of the mechanical axis from the center of the knee. Typically, advanced imaging with CT or MRI is not necessary. Laboratory work is not generally necessary in the evaluation of genu valgum unless there is a concern for undiagnosed renal osteodystrophy.

Treatment

The decision to treat genu valgum depends on the age of the patient, the etiology, and the magnitude of the deformity. Children are expected to have symmetric knock-knees between 2 and 8 years of age; parents of children this age can be reassured that treatment is usually not necessary. Asymmetric angulation

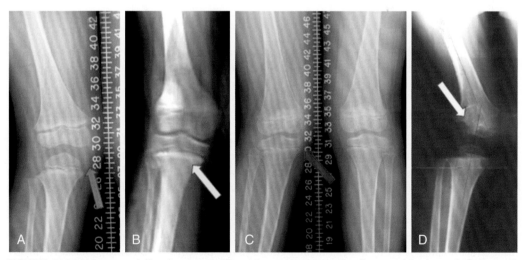

FIGURE 15.15 Valgus panel: Four images of different types of valgus deformity around the knee. A, Patient with physiologic valgus. Despite the angular deformity at the knee, the appearance of the physis in the proximal tibia is normal (orange arrow). B, Patient with renal osteodystrophy. Notice the abnormally widened physis in the proximal tibia characteristic of this condition (yellow arrow). C, Patient with Cozen phenomenon. The appearance of the physis in the affected right proximal tibia is normal (red arrow) and symmetric with the unaffected left leg. The deformity is located in the right tibial metaphysis. D, Patient with skeletal dysplasia (pseudo achondroplasia). There is marked irregularity to the physis and epiphysis of the distal femur (white arrow).

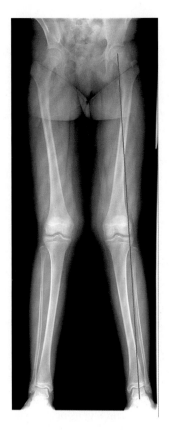

FIGURE 15.16 An example of a standing full-length bilateral lower extremity radiograph in a patient with genu valgum. The mechanical axis (red line) is drawn on the left leg from the center of the hip to the center of the ankle. The line passes lateral to the center of the knee indicating valgus is present.

between the two extremities or severe angulation interfering with function, however, requires further investigation even when occurring in the appropriate age groups.

For mild deformity in a child with more than 3 years of growth remaining, observation with serial standing full-length radiographs every 6 to 12 months is preferred. If the mechanical axis deviation remains mild or is improving over time, then no treatment is necessary. However, if there is evidence of gradually worsening genu valgum in those older than 8 years, then referral to a pediatric orthopedic surgeon is warranted. For patients with apparent genu valgum (knock thighs) caused by obesity, guided weight loss can be curative. Bracing does not correct real genu valgum, if flatfoot deformities are contributing to the valgus, medial arch supports can be helpful in alleviating any knee pain.

When to Refer

Children that present with progressive genu valgum out of the expected age range (greater than two standard deviations from the mean based on Heath and Staheli) have asymmetric genu valgum or who have abnormal screening radiographs should see a pediatric orthopedic surgeon.

● Leg Length Discrepancy

Introduction

LLD is a common presenting concern for pediatric patients and their families (**Figure 15.17**). Studies have shown that approximately 70% of the population has up to 1 cm of discrepancy. Despite its prevalence, however, most LLDs do not require any treatment.

Clinical Significance/Natural History

LLD can be categorized as either congenital or developmental. Congenital LLD represent etiologies arising from abnormal embryological development of the limb, such as congenital femoral deficiency, tibial, or fibular longitudinal deficiency. Developmental LLD occurs after birth and results from some insult or pathological process to a previously normal physis. Examples of a developmental LLD include trauma, infection, or neoplastic invasion of the physis. LLDs can also be classified as static or progressive. A fractured femoral shaft that heals with 2 cm of shortening is an example of a static discrepancy. A progressive LLD describes a situation in which a physis is not functioning properly from either a congenital or a developmental etiology, and the LLD is constantly increasing in size with time.

There does not seem to be any clear evidence that back pain, hip pain, or knee pain will develop in individuals with an LLD measuring less than 1.5 to 2 cm at maturity. Untreated leg length discrepancies greater than 2 cm may be a contributing factor for low-back pain, hip pain, or knee pain later in life if left untreated.

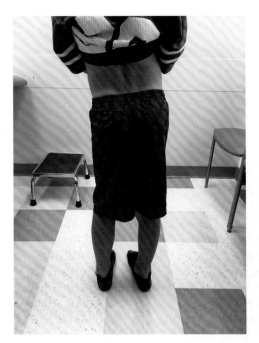

FIGURE 15.17 Photograph of a patient standing with a leg length discrepancy (right lower extremity is longer than the left). Note the asymmetric posterior sacral dimples just above the tilted waistband.

History and Physical Examination

A series of seven questions should uncover most of the information necessary to make an adequate assessment. (1) When did you discover the LLD? Significant LLDs are usually discovered early in life; a teenage patient with a minimal LLD is unlikely to be significant at growth cessation. (2) Do you notice the discrepancy? They may describe compensatory gait changes that have developed to accommodate the discrepancy such as toe walking on the short side or circumduction of the long leg. If they do not notice any difference in the leg lengths or gait, then the current LLD is probably not significant. (3) Has the discrepancy been changing over time? Significant discrepancies will slowly increase in size each year. (4) Is there any history of fracture or infection involving the bones in the lower extremities? (5) Has the family noticed any associated deformity or asymmetry to lower limbs? (6) Is there any family history of LLD? Some common causes of LLD such as skeletal dysplasias can be hereditary. (7) Has there been any treatment in the past?

Observational gait analysis is performed prior to more static testing (▶ **Video 15.10**).

A visual inspection of the patient is performed in a standing position: Are the knee heights symmetric? Are the limbs symmetric in girth? Is there obvious asymmetric angular deformity? Are the shoulder heights equal? Is there a mild scoliosis? Are the iliac crests at the same level? In thin patients, the posterior sacral dimples can be seen and used as a guide. If they are not in the same level, then a pelvic obliquity exists. Premeasured lifts of various sizes can be placed under the short side to balance the pelvis and thus approximate the size of the discrepancy (▶ **Video 15.11**).

Patients with an LLD can have a compensatory curve of the lumbar spine that must be differentiated from true scoliosis. To properly examine the spine for scoliosis, the leg lengths must be equalized with blocks put under the short limb to create a level pelvis. In this position, any abnormal findings from Adam forward bending test should be attributed to the spine and not an LLD. A second method is to examine the spine with the patient in an upright sitting position (▶ **Video 15.12**). In the sitting position, the shoulder heights can be assessed and Adam forward bending test can be performed.

The examination continues on the examination table with both legs fully extended (**Figure 15.18**). One can measure the supine leg lengths with a tape measure from the anterior superior iliac spine to medial malleolus. This can be difficult in patients with hip and knee contractures and can be unreliable secondary to obesity. A visual inspection of the skin should be performed looking for any cutaneous lesions. Café au lait spots are a hallmark of neurofibromatosis. Hemangiomas or other vascular abnormalities may indicate an underlying vascular etiology of the LLD such as Klippel-Trenaunay-Weber syndrome (**Figure 15.19**). The symmetry of the patient should be assessed. Hemihypertrophy patients have a spectrum of presentation. Mild cases may only have slight differences in calf and thigh circumference and a small LLD. As cases increase in severity, the entire one half of the body can be involved with asymmetry in the foot size, the arm length, the hand size, the chest size, and the face.

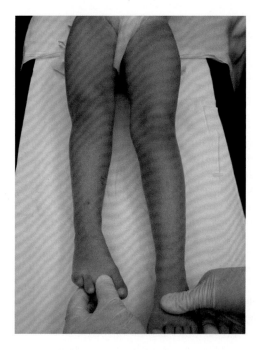

FIGURE 15.18 Supine examination of the leg lengths with both hips and knees fully extended. The medial malleolus is a good landmark to visualize the lengths of each limb relative to one another. This patient also has asymmetric knee heights.

It is important to differentiate structural LLD where the bones are of different length from functional or apparent LLD. In these instances, the bones are of equal length, but joint contractures (foot equinus, knee flexion, or hip flexion contractures) can create the appearance of an LLD (▶ **Video 15.13**). Similarly, hip adduction contractures can make the limb functionally short while hip abduction contractures can cause the limb to appear long. The hip abductor flexibility can be assessed using the Ober test (▶ **Video 15.9**). The patient should lie on one side with both knees pulled up to the chest. The hip of the uppermost limb is then extended with the knee kept in flexion. By extending the hip, the knee of the upper limb should be clear of the other inferior limb. The upper limb can then be lowered toward the examination table to allow the flexed knee to attempt to touch the table. The test is then repeated on the opposite side. Asymmetry in flexibility between the two sides indicates the presence of an abduction contracture.

A Galeazzi test (flexing both hips and knees to 90°) with the hips in neutral abduction and adduction alignment will demonstrate the length of the femoral segment (hip to knee) of each limb (▶ **Video 15.14**). Always remember that a patient with a dislocated hip will have a functional discrepancy with a short limb gait and a positive Galeazzi test. These patients have normal lengths of their femurs but are functionally short due to proximal migration of the dislocated hip. A reverse Galeazzi test can be performed in the prone position with the hips extended to neutral and the knees flexed to 90° (▶ **Video 15.15**). The difference in the resting position of the plantar surface of the foot represents the difference in limb length from the knee to the bottom of the foot.

The range of motion of the knee should be tested. A knee flexion contracture will make the limb appear shortened (▶ **Video 15.16**). Hamstring tightness can be evaluated in the supine position by flexing the hip and knee to 90° and then extending the knee until resistance. The angle between the maximally extended leg and an imaginary vertical line

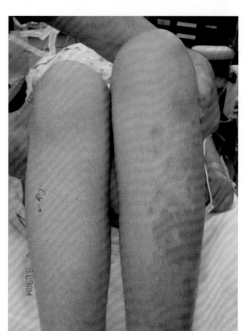

FIGURE 15.19 A patient with a vascular malformation on the side of the longer limb. A thorough skin examination to look for café au lait spots, hemangiomas, or other skin abnormalities will help to determine the underlying etiology of the limb length discrepancy. The girth of the limbs should also be compared.

perpendicular to the table is the popliteal angle. The stability of the knee ligaments should be tested. Many of the congenital limb deficiencies have an absent or incompetent anterior cruciate ligament (▶ **Video 15.17**).

An equinus contracture will cause the limb to look longer. The ankle should be maximally dorsiflexed with the knee in extension and the foot inverted and then again with the knee flexed (▶ **Video 15.18**). A foot that can be dorsiflexed with the knee flexed indicates a tight gastrocnemius muscle alone, if the foot cannot be dorsiflexed with the knee in 90° indicates a gastrocnemius and soleus contracture.

The foot should be inspected. Fewer than five complete rays may indicate longitudinal deficiency of the fibula or postaxial limb deficiency. The presence of a clubfoot or evidence of previous clubfoot treatment may provide the etiology of the discrepancy. Subtalar and midfoot motion should be tested. Patients with longitudinal deficiency of the fibula or postaxial limb deficiency may have a fused subtalar joint or tarsal coalitions.

Pitfalls in Diagnosis

Deformities of the spine, such as scoliosis, can cause obliquity of the pelvis that mimics LLD. Examination of the spine in the upright sitting position can help distinguish true spinal deformity from compensatory spinal curvature due to an LLD. If there is any doubt, upright thoracolumbar spine radiographs can be obtained with blocks under the short limb to balance the pelvis. In infants or toddlers, a missed unilateral hip dislocation can present as an LLD. Asymmetric hip abduction with the hips flexed to 90° on supine examination will help to make this diagnosis. Radiographs can be used to verify the dislocation, if necessary. Finally, joint contractures can cause a functional LLD. A hip flexion or adduction contracture can cause the limb to appear short, while a hip abduction contracture can cause the limb to look long. Knee flexion contractures shorten the limb and plantar flexion (equinus) contractures of the ankle will lengthen the limb. Testing for full range of motion at each joint in both lower extremities will allow the clinician to assess for functional or apparent LLD.

Differential Diagnosis

Mild LLD can have congenital or developmental causes such as tibial bowing (posteromedial or anterolateral) or clubfoot. Large, progressive LLDs can result from long bone deficiencies (femoral, tibial or fibula deficiency). Other causes of LLD, such as injury to the physis from trauma, infection, or neoplasm, are also progressive, but the LLD does not start until after the inciting incident. Other common causes of LLD such as Blount disease, Perthes disease, vascular malformations, and multiple hereditary exostoses will have characteristic findings on physical examination or radiographs. Conditions such as Russell-Silver or Ollier disease are also known to have LLD. Neuromuscular diseases can have both structural and functional LLD, and a careful examination is necessary to differentiate the contribution of each to the overall LLD. If hemihypertrophy is suspected, the patient should be referred for appropriate screening, including regular abdominal ultrasounds to monitor for Wilms tumor, adrenal carcinoma, and hepatoblastoma.

Diagnostic Tests or Advanced Imaging

Clinical examination should be sufficient to diagnose most clinically relevant LLD. If there is any question, then a standing full-length radiograph of the lower extremities from the pelvis to the foot is the most effective radiograph (**Figure 15.20**). This radiograph can quantitate the discrepancy and allows visual examination of the entire skeleton and includes important information such as foot height or the presence of diaphyseal deformity. Assessment of length can be made with a scanogram (**Figure 15.21**), but this film requires the patient to be still (difficult in toddlers) and does not include all of the skeleton.

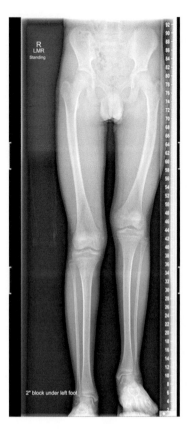

FIGURE 15.20 Standing anteroposterior bilateral lower extremity radiograph. Note there are blocks placed under the left foot to level the pelvis. The technician has notated the size of the blocks on the radiograph. There is a ruler next to the patient which can be used for calibration of measurements, if necessary.

Treatment

A shoe lift is an excellent way to manage many LLDs. A 1-cm lift can be accommodated inside a shoe before the foot no longer fits comfortably in the shoe. Adding a lift to the bottom of the shoe can accommodate the remainder, keeping in mind that many patients actually feel more comfortable with a lift that leaves the limb a little short. Lifts greater than 5 cm become heavy and tend to be unstable for the patient to walk on. Patients with projected discrepancies greater than 2 cm may be a candidate for surgical interventions.

When to Refer

Infants or toddlers with progressive, congenital causes of LLD should be referred to a pediatric orthopedic surgeon due to the progressive nature of these conditions. Similarly, any patient with functional limitations or pain due to LLD should be referred.

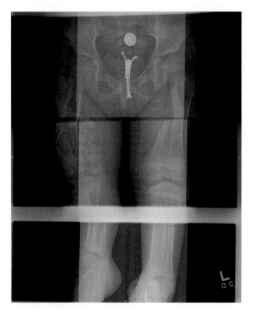

FIGURE 15.21 An example of a scanogram radiograph used to measure leg lengths. This radiograph may be used if it is not possible to obtain a full standing lower extremity radiograph. There are several disadvantages of the scanogram compared to the standing lower extremity radiograph. The scanogram is not a weight-bearing film and does not include foot height in the measurements. It also omits the diaphyseal portions of the femur and tibia making deformity analysis impossible. Finally, if the patient moves during the process of obtaining the three separate images, then the measurements will not be accurate.

● *Conclusion*

Children with pediatric limb deformity are a relatively common finding. Mainly, causes such as excessive femoral anteversion, tibial torsion, physiologic bowing, genu valgum, and mild LLD can be treated with simple observation and reassurance. Children with more severe deformity, deformity that does not properly correct with growth and development, or deformity that is causing symptoms in the child can benefit from an orthopedic referral and potential treatment.

References

1. Salenius P, Vankka E. The development of the tibiofemoral angle in children. *J Bone Joint Surg Am.* 1975;57(2):259-261.
2. Liu RW, Streit JJ, Weinberg DS, et al. No relationship between mild limb length discrepancy and spine, hip or knee degenerative disease in a large cadaveric collection. *Orthop Traumatol Surg Res.* 2018;104:603-607.
3. Paley D, Bhave A, Herzenberg JE, Bowen JR. Multiplier method for predicting limb-length discrepancy. *J Bone Joint Surg Am.* 2000;82-A(10):1432-1446.
4. Heath CH, Staheli LT. Normal limits of knee angle in white children – Genu varum and genu valgum. *J Pediatr Orthop.* 1993;13:259-262.
5. Weinberg DS, Park PJ, Morris WZ, Liu RW. Femoral version and tibial torsion are not associated with hip or knee arthritis in a large osteological collection. *J Pediatr Orthop.* 2017;37:e120-e128.

Hip Disorders

Matthew D. Milewski and Pablo Castañeda

● Introduction

Many different conditions can affect the hip of the growing child; some occur in childhood and some can be detected at birth with findings specific for developmental dysplasia of the hip (DDH) or congenital hip deficiencies. Examples of hip problems in older children include developmental pathology (Perthes disease), neurologic manifestations (eg, hip contractures for cerebral palsy), inflammatory (infection), and neoplastic conditions. Adolescents can present with pain and lack of hip function as a result of late sequela from DDH or Perthes. The older child and adolescent can have pain and decreased function from slipped capital femoral epiphysis (SCFE) or from trauma and overuse injuries. The physical examination of the hip is crucial for any child presenting with low back, hip, or knee pain. The major innervating nerves for the hip originate in the lumbosacral region that can make it difficult to distinguish between primary hip pain and radicular lumbar pain, especially in older children. It is also crucial to examine the hip in patients presenting with a limp, leg length discrepancy, or rotational abnormality such as in-toeing or out-toeing.

● Anatomy

The hip joint is a ball and socket synovial joint designed to allow polyaxial motion while transferring load between the upper and lower body. The acetabular rim is lined by a special fibrocartilage called the labrum that adds depth and stability to the femoral acetabular joint; when this is torn, patients can complain of pain and popping. The articular surfaces are covered by hyaline cartilage that dissipates shear and compressive forces during load-bearing and hip motion.

The hip joint's wide range of motion is second only to that of the glenohumeral joint and is enabled by the large number of muscle groups that surround the hip. The flexor muscles include the psoas, rectus femoris, pectineus, and sartorius muscle. The gluteus maximus and hamstring muscle groups allow for hip extension. The major abductor muscles such as the gluteus medius and minimus, the piriformis obturator externus and internist and quadratus femoris muscles insert around the greater trochanter. Major muscles that adduct the hip include the gracillis, adductors longus, brevis, and magnus.

There are several important growth centers in the pelvis including the triradiate cartilage that separate the ilium, ischium, and pubis bones, and this cartilage is responsible for deepening of the socket with growth. There are multiple sites of tendon and muscle attachments that originate from (or insert on) apophyseal growth centers; these areas can be subject to chronic tension and develop symptoms of tendonitis. These sites of muscle attachments can also be subject to acute severe muscle strain, and avulsion fractures can also occur (**Figures 16.1-16.3**). Potential sites of apophyseal injury in the hip region include the ischium (hamstring origin), anterior superior iliac spine (sartorius origin), anterior inferior iliac spine (rectus femoris origin), iliac crest (external oblique origin), lesser trochanter (psoas tendon insertion), and greater trochanter (gluteus medius insertion). The apophysis of the superior iliac spine is the last to fuse and is susceptible to injury up to 25 years old.

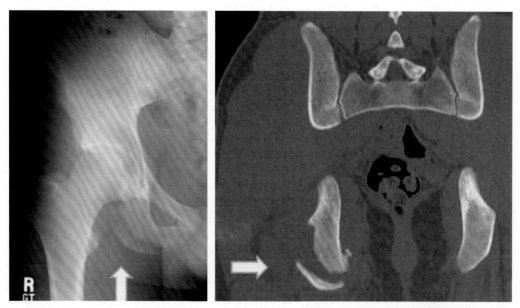

FIGURE 16.1 This soccer player has an avulsion of his ischial tuberosity as a result of powerful hamstring contraction during sprinting.

● *History*

Infection, inflammatory autoimmune disorders, and benign or malignant tumors can present at any age and should be considered in the differential diagnosis for hip pain or hip dysfunction; yet age can narrow the differential diagnosis and can direct the history. Perinatal, family, and birth history are important for infants who may be at higher risk for DDH. Most children have a 1/1000 chance of developing a dislocated hip. Yet other factors can increase this incidence; a firstborn female born breech into a family with a positive family history has a 1/100 chance of hip dislocation. Interestingly, infants and toddlers

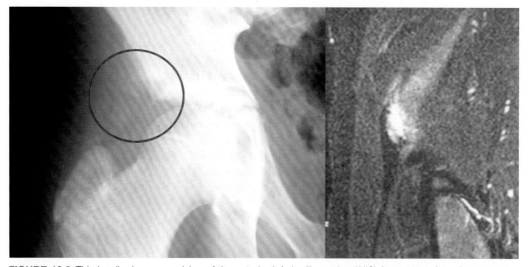

FIGURE 16.2 This hurdler has an avulsion of the anterior inferior iliac spine (AIIS) from rectus femoris contraction noted on x-ray and confirmed with MRI.

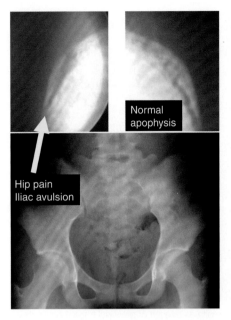

Normal apophysis

Hip pain Iliac avulsion

FIGURE 16.3 This wrestler developed acute right iliac crest pain during a match and has an iliac apophysis fracture that is noted when the pelvis x-ray is magnified.

with congenital hip dislocation rarely if ever complain of hip pain. In prepubescent children, history should focus on decreases in function, pain, and presence of a limp. A comprehensive review of systems (ROS) will be important and should include a history of trauma, determining the presence of fever and other systemic symptoms. Adolescent patients with hip pain should be asked about antecedent trauma or inciting activity, factors that increase or decrease pain, mechanism of injury, and time of onset questions. Other questions should document altered functions such as the ease of getting in and out of the car, putting on shoes, running, walking, and going up and down stairs. SCFE, apophyseal avulsion fractures should be considered for those adolescents with acute onset of a painful limp. In the more skeletally mature, hip pain can be the result of residual hip deformity (from old trauma, DDH, Perthes disease, or SCFE), musculotendinous strain, ligamentous sprain, contusion, or even bursitis. Degenerative osteoarthritis can occur from residual deformity but is uncommon in the childhood and early adolescent population.

Key Point

Location of the pain is important because the layperson may localize "hip pain" to basic anatomical regions that may not be a sign of true hip joint pathology. Although the anterior hip and groin pain is suggestive of hip joint pathology, other common locations of "hip pain" may not be. This includes the anterior thigh (femur pathology), the posterior aspect of the hip and buttock (referred pain from the spine or SI joint), and the lateral aspect hip (trochanteric pain or abductor muscle weakness).

Ability to Walk and Observational Gait Analysis

In children of walking age, special attention should be paid to the ambulatory status and the quality of their gait. Pain and a limp do not necessarily always coexist; for example, children with Perthes will often limp without complaining of pain. On the other hand, a refusal to bear weight in a child who was walking previously should raise the concern for a traumatic or septic origin. It can be difficult to determine the precise location of pain, and younger children may just hold the hip in a position of comfort in flexion and external rotation (the hip joint has more room for swelling when it is flexed and externally rotated). Older patients commonly express their pain localized to one of three anatomical regions: the anterior hip and groin, the posterior hip and buttock, and the lateral hip. It should also be noted that pain along the medial aspect of the distal thigh and knee can be referred pain from hip pathology.

The examination of the hip begins as the child walks to the examination room and can be further observed in shorts in the clinic hallway. It is best to examine the child's gait from in front and behind the patient. It can also be useful to ascertain whether they are able to jog or do light running. Having the child perform toe walking, heel walking, and repetitive single leg hopping is also useful to ascertain whether a gross functional or strength limitation is present. (Please see Chapter 4 on Observational Gait Analysis.)

Patients who have pain in one of their limbs will have decreased time in stance relative to swing phase; they try to get off of the painful limb as soon as possible and transfer weight to the nonaffected side. This is termed *an antalgic gait* and can be due to pathology anywhere in the limb; yet a hip source is suspected when other alterations are noted. For instance, hip pathology should be suspected in the antalgic child (decreased stance phase) with a Trendelenburg gait. By shifting the body over the affected side (Trendelenburg gait), the child decreases the force (and pain) across the affected hip. Similarly, if an adolescent has an antalgic gait with a positive foot progression angle (because their hip is externally rotated), hip pathology such as a SCFE should be considered.

Stance assessment is also useful to determine if there is a limb length discrepancy as noted with asymmetry in the height of the iliac crest, or buttocks. It should be followed by a Trendelenburg test, which is a single leg stance whereby the gluteus medius of the limb in stance is tested while the contralateral limb is taken off the ground. After examination of gait, consideration should always include cursory examination of the lumbar spine, knee, and ankle bilaterally, as pathology in these areas could impact hip function. These examinations will be covered in other chapters.

General Physical Examination of the Hip

In this chapter, we will present a general approach for examination of the hip regardless of suspected pathology and will follow with consideration of examination specific for common pathology.

General hip examination is ideally performed in a systematic manner.

1. *Assessment of Leg and Hip Asymmetry* is crucial to measure and is done with the patient in the standing (if able) and supine position. In the supine position, limb atrophy can signal a longstanding hip problem. Palpation of the muscles can identify masses. In the standing position, pelvic height asymmetry can also be used to detect a limb length discrepancy. Yet remember that hip pathology can present as a functional limb length discrepancy even though the lengths of the femur or tibia may be equal. For instance, a patient with a severe hip flexion contracture will be functionally shorter on that side. In addition, pelvic obliquity can be a result of asymmetric hip joint contracture (see below) and can also present with a functional discrepancy in length. Pelvic obliquity in the standing position can also be a result of rigid spine conditions such as lumbosacral scoliosis.

2. *Palpation for Tenderness and Ecchymosis* can signal traumatic injuries. Avulsions fractures around the pelvis are common in adolescent athletes and manifest as bruising and or tenderness to palpation along the anterior pelvic brim (for ASIS or AIIS avulsions) (**Figure 16.4A** and **B**), posteriorly along the ischial tuberosity in the gluteal fold (for ischial/hamstring avulsions) along with less commonly about the proximal femur (for greater or lesser trochanteric avulsions) (**Figure 16.4C**; ▶ **Video 16.1**).

3. *Detection of Hip Joint Effusion*, as opposed to other joints; a hip effusion cannot be directly palpated but can be suspected based on the presence of hip that lies in a flexed, abducted, and externally rotated position (**Figure 16.5**).

   It is in this position that accommodates the most intra-articular volume. If the leg is held in a flexed and adducted position, the examiner should be alert to the possibility of iliopsoas irritation or infection such as with a psoas abscess.

4. *Documentation of Hip Motion* is important to refine the potential differential diagnosis for hip pathology.

Key Point

When moving the hip through the different arcs of motion, it is critical that the examiner keeps his/her hand on the pelvis to detect the movement of the pelvis once the limits of motion are reached. As an example, one could easily record spurious increased hip flexion by not appreciating the pelvis rolling back once femoral acetabular impingement is reached. Similarly, without having a hand on the pelvis one would be challenged to know when thigh abduction from the hip is maximized and which point the pelvis would begin shifting as the thigh is further abducted.

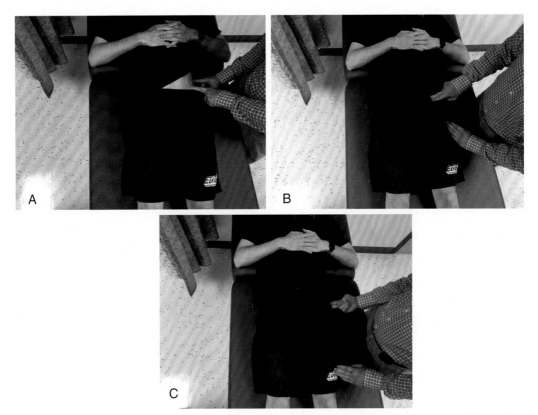

FIGURE 16.4 A, An athlete who avulses his anterior superior iliac spine (ASIS) as a result of severe sartorius contracture would have pain and tenderness at the examiner's left finger. His right finger is on the iliac crest. B, A hurdler with an avulsion of the anterior inferior iliac spine (AIIS) as a result of his extreme contraction of his rectus femoris will have pain in the anterior groin with palpation and with attempted hip flexion. C, A child with greater trochanter avulsion will have severe pain over his trochanter (examiner's right hand) and will likely not be able to walk well.

Measuring the hip range of motion has consistently been shown to be highly reliable and can be useful in identifying pathology. Hip flexion, abduction, and adduction are usually assessed in the supine position (**Figures 16.6-16.8**).

Hip extension and internal and external rotation are best assessed in the prone position (**Figures 16.9-16.11**).

Assessing pain during range of motion can be helpful in identifying inflammatory conditions, in general a hip with pathology will have limited abduction and internal rotation. Pelvic obliquity and a functional limb length discrepancy can be noted in patients with a unilateral adduction contracture. It is further important to record the range of motion at each visit and compare it with prior past measurements; there are many conditions that manifest increasing disease severity through decreasing abduction over time. For example, a child with Perthes disease and worsening loss of motion may have progressive extrusion of the hip.

Key Point

Unilateral decrease of internal rotation on the affected side is a specific finding pointing to the hip joint as a source of pathology.

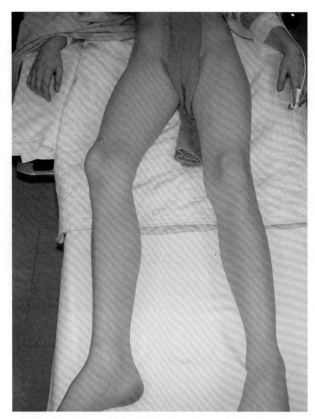

FIGURE 16.5 This boy with a left septic hip lays with his hip abducted, flexed, and externally rotated. The large collection of fluid within the hip is best accommodated in this position.

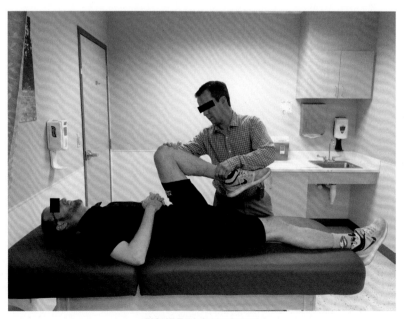

FIGURE 16.6 Hip flexion.

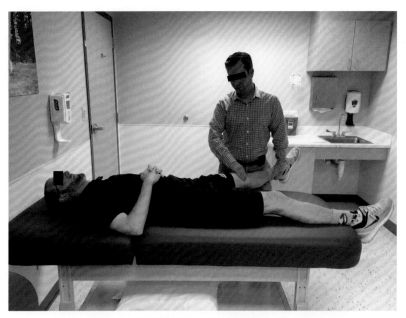

FIGURE 16.7 Hip abduction.

The degree of femoral anteversion can also be estimated on physical exam using the technique described by Ruwe and Deluca[1] by palpating the greater trochanter in the prone position and the maximum lateral trochanteric prominence was related to the degree of internal rotation of the hip (**Figure 16.12**).

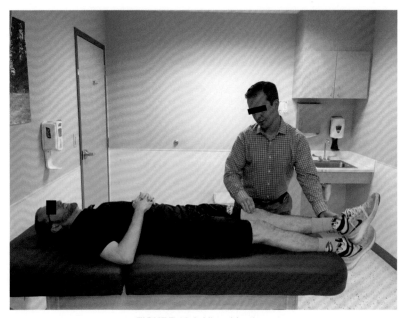

FIGURE 16.8 Hip adduction.

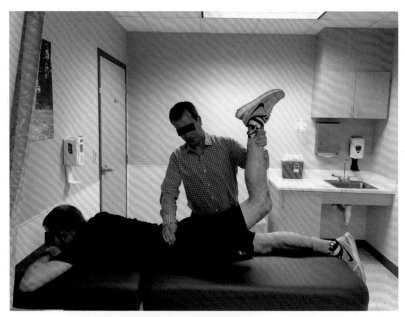

FIGURE 16.9 Hip extension.

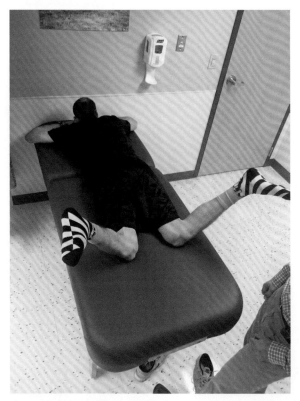

FIGURE 16.10 Hip internal rotation is best documented in the prone (hip extended) position. Any decrease in the hip internal rotation is a sign of hip pathology.

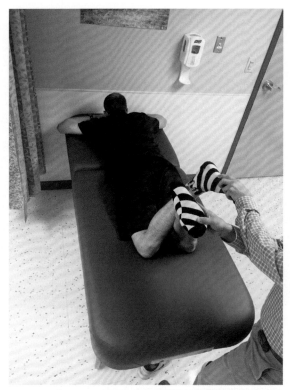

FIGURE 16.11 Hip external rotation. In general, children will have a total of 90° of hip rotation in the prone position. If there is a 60° of internal rotation, one should expect 30° of external rotation.

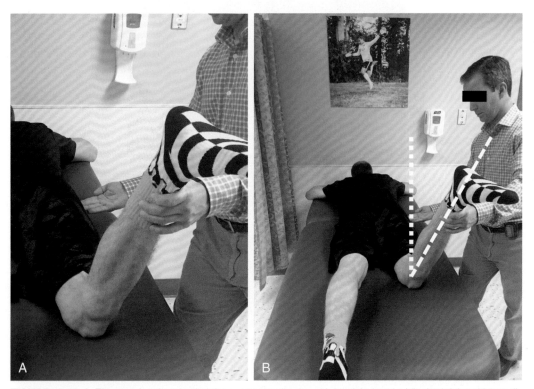

FIGURE 16.12 A, The examiner is palpating the greater trochanter with his right hand while the left hand internally rotates the hip. The point at which the greater trochanter is maximal is measured from vertical, and this angle is considered an estimate of femoral anteversion.

5. *Strength Testing* is done in both the supine and the prone position. Standard 5-point manual muscle strength testing should be done for flexion, extension, adduction, abduction, and internal and external rotation. Assessment of the hip muscle strength has been shown to be reliable, but appears to be less helpful in identifying specific tendinous pathological conditions. For instance, pain is nonspecific especially when it comes from the gluteus minimus or medius. Posterior pain when performing a squat can be useful in identifying gluteus medius pathology. Special tests that should be considered in this young population include the Trendelenburg test to assess for hip abduction weakness or altered hip mechanics as a result of hip varus or trochanteric overgrowth. The child should be asked to stand on a single leg for about 30 seconds without leaning to one side. The pelvis should be observed from behind to see if it dips to the opposite side (positive test) or elevates (negative test) (**Figure 16.13**). Again, a positive test is indicated if the pelvis drops toward the unsupported side during a single-leg stance. In children, a useful way of doing this is by having them balance by putting their hands on the examiner's hands and determining if there is a subtle difference in the amount of force needed to maintain balance (▶ **Video 16.2**).

6. *Specific Tests.*

   a. The FABER (Flexion, Abduction, External Rotation) test is crucial for the comprehensive examination of the hip test (**Figure 16.14**). This test assesses both the hip joint along with sacroiliac pain or irritation. The leg to be tested is flexed at the knee with the thigh abducted and externally rotated such that the foot is placed across the front of the contralateral knee. The examiner will then place additional pressure on the ipsilateral knee to bring the hip into further abduction. Pain elicited on the ipsilateral hip anteriorly is suggestive of hip pathology. Pain elicited on the contralateral side posteriorly is suggestive of sacroiliac joint pathology.

   b. The Thomas test is useful for assessing hip flexor tightness or contracture. The cooperative patient can lie supine and hold the contralateral/uninvolved knee to their chest, while allowing the ipsilateral/involved leg to lie flat. The knee is held to the torso to help flatten out lumbar lordosis and stabilize the pelvis. If the iliopsoas is tight or the hip joint is contracted, the ipsilateral/involved leg will be unable to fully extend at the hip and this would be a positive Thomas test. It is usually done with the patient supine. In patients with a knee contracture, it will be impossible for the

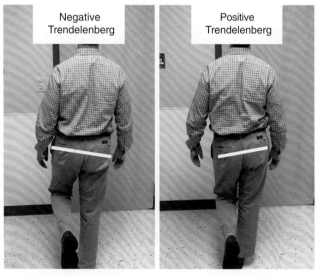

FIGURE 16.13 The Trendelenburg test for gluteus medius function. If the patient has normal right gluteus medius function, the pelvis elevates on the left when standing on his right leg. If the right gluteus medius is weak or if there is altered hip mechanics, the left hip will dip while standing on his right leg.

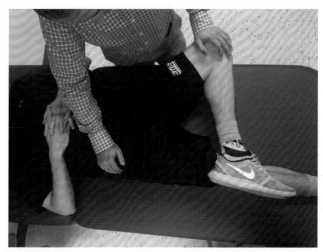

FIGURE 16.14 FABER test. With the left leg placed in a "Figure-4" position (**F**lexion, hip **AB**bduction, and **E**xternal **R**otation) over the right thigh; the examiner stabilizes the right pelvis while the left knee is pressed down. Left groin pain implies left hip pathology. Right buttock pain implies right SI joint pathology.

limb to lay flat thus the Thomas test should be done with the contracted leg and foot off the bed (**Figure 16.15**). Alternatively, the hip contracture can be documented moving from a standing position to a supine position in ambulatory patients (▶ **Video 16.3**).

c. Ober test is an important part of both the hip and knee examination. It helps quantify iliotibial band tightness and symptoms (▶ **Video 16.4**). The child should lie on the contralateral side with both the hip and knee flexed to 90°. The examiner should then stabilize the pelvis with one hand to keep it perpendicular to the exam table. The other hand should then slightly extend the hip, fully abduct the ipsilateral hip and allow the leg/knee to adduct until it cannot adduct further (**Figure 16.16**). A positive test is usually indicated by less adduction compared with the contralateral side, pain with passive adduction in this position, or bilateral decreased ability to adduct to at least neutral adduction/abduction.

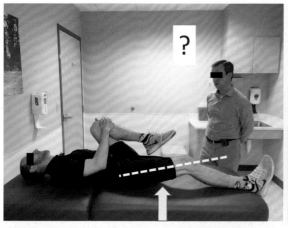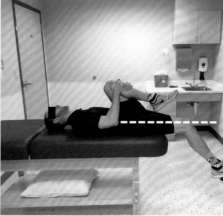

FIGURE 16.15 The Thomas test. The patient holds his left knee maximally flexed, which stabilizes his pelvis. The right hip lays flexed (white line) and implies that the patient has a right hip contracture (yellow arrow). The examiner wonders if the inability to get the knee flat is due to primary hip contracture or a stiff knee, which prevents it from laying flat. In the second panel, the leg is allowed off of the table and thus removes any knee flexor contribution. In this case, the hip is neutral and thus the patient has no hip contracture.

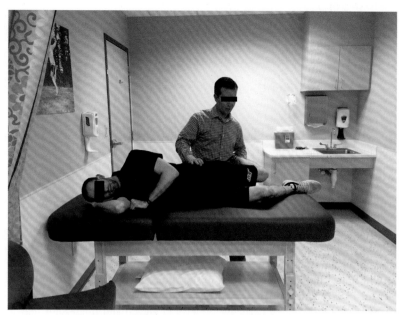

FIGURE 16.16 Ober test.

⬤ *Pathology-Specific Examination*

Developmental Dysplasia of the Hip

Dysplasia of the hip can be used to describe any radiographic abnormality of the femoral head or acetabulum; dislocation is a term used to describe the situation where the femoral head is completely displaced from the hip socket and subluxated hips are partially displaced. Dislocated hips and subluxated hips are all considered dysplastic; yet not all dysplastic hips have displacement as described earlier. DDH is a term that is used for children whose hips are displaced or unstable at birth. Examination of the newborn hip is critical to detect these conditions. In newborns and infants, the most important pathology to rule out is DDH, which is present in 1 in 1000 children and is 10× greater in firstborn females who are born breech to a family with a history of DDH.

During the examination of infants, the baby should be comfortable, warm, and in a relatively quiet environment; a dark room can also keep the baby calm and many clinicians advocate for some form of soothing low-volume background music. The test should be postponed if the baby is crying and fussy. The Ortolani and Barlow maneuvers are performed to detect hip instability in the newborn, and these are performed with the baby laying on a firm surface with the hips flexed 90° (**Figure 16.17**).

The Ortolani test essentially reduces a dislocated hip by abducting the flexed hip and lifting the femoral head into the acetabulum with upward pressure on the greater trochanter with the examiner's fingers. When a palpable clunk is appreciated, this is considered a test of reduction of a dislocated hip (▶ **Video 16.5**).

On the contrary, the Barlow test detects hip laxity with the potential for dislocation; hip displacement is provoked by adducting the flexed hip with downward and lateral pressure on the knee. With a positive Barlow test, the examiner can feel the head of the femur sliding out of the acetabulum; once the pressure is released and the femur is abducted, the examiner may feel the hip slide/pop back into place. It should be noted that lesser degrees of instability can be difficult to detect; in fact, there must be at least 9 mm of displacement of the femoral head from the acetabulum to be clinically detectable even in experienced hands.

Key Point

A newborn with a fixed hip dislocation will be Ortolani and Barlow negative; in this situation, the hip is not unstable, and it is fixed outside of the socket. As the infant ages, the examination is marked by "adaptive changes" in the hip examination.

Limited hip abduction is the most important adaptive change seen in older infants and toddlers with a dislocated hip. With the hip flexed to 90°, the affected hip will lack about 20° to 30° of abduction, and the adductor longus tendon will appear tight in the groin of the affected hip (**Figure 16.18**). The femur will also appear short (▶ **Video 16.6**).

One must always remember that children with bilaterally dislocated hips will have a symmetric lack of hip abduction that can be hard to detect. The use of Klisic line is an important tool to confirm hip dislocation and is very helpful in patients with bilaterally dislocated hips. A line drawn from the greater trochanter to the ASIS will lie proximal to the umbilicus in a normal hip but will be inferior to the umbilicus when the hip is dislocated (**Figure 16.19**).

Asymmetry in limb length can be the first observation pointing toward a unilaterally dislocated hip in the older infant (▶ **Video 16.7**). The femur itself is not shorter, the appearance is owed to the proximal displacement of the femoral head. Asymmetry of gluteal and thigh folds may also be noted, but these can be nonspecific findings. On a firm table, the examiner can provocatively flex the hips and knees and by holding the heels together (Galeazzi test), can observe the height of the knees to determine if there is a real or apparent limb length discrepancy (**Figure 16.18**). Usually, there will be no detectable asymmetry in children with bilaterally dislocated hips (**Figure 16.20**).

Yet the careful clinician can suspect this with a toddler who stands with a fore-shortened thigh and a lordotic waddling gait (**Figure 16.21**).

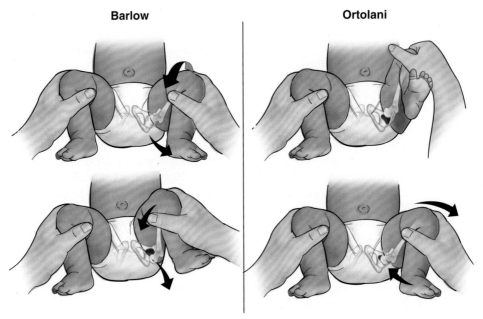

Barlow   **Ortolani**

FIGURE 16.17 Barlow test is demonstrated here with adduction and posteriorly directed force on the femur will allow the unstable hip to dislocate posteriorly. Ortolani test is also demonstrated here with abduction and anteriorly directed force allowing the dislocated hip to reduce.

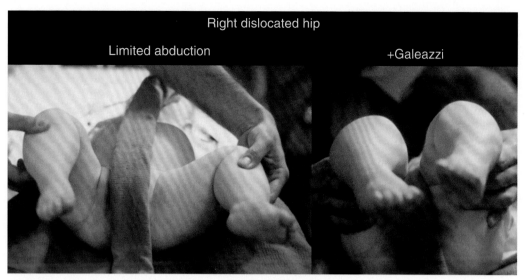

FIGURE 16.18 Examination of the infant with a right dislocated hip shows "adaptive changes." These include limited abduction on exam along with asymmetric relative knee height consistent with a positive Galeazzi test.

Diagnostic Testing and When to Refer

1. Ultrasound is a test that can be ordered to screen for hip dysplasia and, in general, is indicated in infants with risk factors for hip dysplasia. It requires no sedation and involves no radiation. In those patients with a normal examination, but who have risk factors (positive family history or breech presentation), pediatricians and primary care providers are well advised to wait until the infant is 6 weeks old as ultrasound before this can have false-positive findings for acetabular dysplasia. Ultrasound can be ordered to confirm hip instability or the patient can be referred to a pediatric

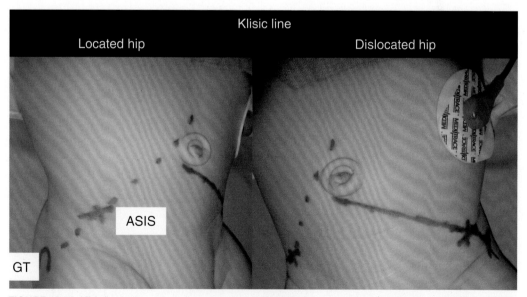

FIGURE 16.19 Klisic line is drawn from the greater trochanter (GT) to the anterior superior iliac spine (ASIS) and should normally project proximally to the umbilicus. In the hip that is dislocated, the line will project inferior to the umbilicus.

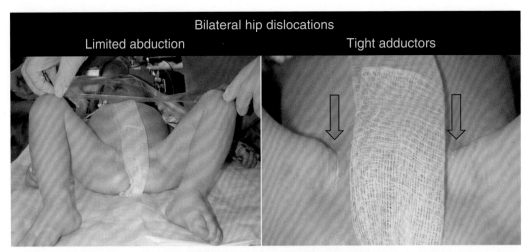

FIGURE 16.20 This child with bilaterally dislocated hips has symmetric abduction, which is limited to about 25° on each side. The experienced clinician will note the tight hip adductors (blue arrows). The use of Klisic line here is helpful.

orthopedist for evaluation. More than 4 mm of displacement on a sonographic equivalent of the Barlow test is considered relevant and can be detected on ultrasound-enhanced physical exam.

2. Office-based ultrasound of the hip is simple, reliable, effective, and easy method for trained pediatric orthopedists to assess the hip.

Ultrasound-enhanced physical exam of the infant's hip can be performed in three steps:

a. The first is to determine the location of the femoral head in relation to the acetabulum, the transducer should first be held parallel to the shaft of the femur at the height of the greater trochanter. By identifying the femoral head and its position in relation to the triradiate cartilage the hip can be determined to be either located or dislocated.

b. The second step is evaluating stability, displacement can be evaluated by reproducing the Barlow maneuver and taking the hip through adduction with posterior and lateral pressure applied while maintaining the transducer on the joint. More than 4 mm of displacement of the femoral head from the acetabulum is considered abnormal and should be treated. A normal hip under stress will not have any separation between the femoral head and the acetabulum after the age of 4 weeks. Hips can thus be considered to be either stable or unstable with this test.

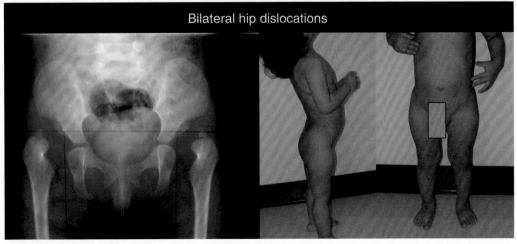

FIGURE 16.21 This girl with bilateral hip dislocations has lordosis of her lumbar spine that accommodates the bilaterally dislocated hips. She will walk with a waddling gait.

c. The third step in the ultrasonographic exam of the hip is to determine the shape, and this is determined by turning the transducer 90° on its axis, producing a so-called coronal image. This allows evaluation of the shape of the femoral head that should be round, and the bony acetabulum should cover at least 50% of the femoral head and the angle between the ilium and the bony roof should be at least 60°; this is the so-called alpha angle. The soft tissues can also be evaluated, and the angle between the ilium and the cartilaginous roof is the so-called β angle that should be at the most 55° (▶ **Video 16.8**).

3. Radiographs should be obtained in any infant or toddler with adaptive physical examination findings. An AP and frog pelvis films should be ordered in any infant or toddler with suspected hip dislocation. Radiographs are not of benefit in infants with Ortolani or Barlow positive hips. In these cases, a radiograph with the hip located will be reassuring but does not characterize the true instability present. Any child with radiographic dysplasia or displacement needs to be referred to a pediatric orthopedist as soon as possible.

Perthes Disease

Perthes disease will present in children (males > females) between 3 years and up to 11 or 12 years of age; the typical age of presentation is from 4 to 8 years. In general, there will be an insidious onset of a limp with or without pain. A 6-year-old boy who presents with an antalgic limp with a positive foot progression angle and who has no pain is a not an uncommon presentation. Past medical history is obtained to determine exposure to steroids, neonatal sepsis, or previous trauma that can lead to radiographic appearance consistent with avascular necrosis. The parents should be queried for any family history of clotting disorders such as sickle cell or thalassemia. Other important history is to determine a family history of skeletal dysplasia (multiple epiphyseal dysplasia). A comprehensive ROS is important to rule out constitutional symptoms that can signal systemic disorders (leukemia, hypothyroidism, sickle cell trait, infection, etc.) that can also lead to avascular necrosis.

The child with early Perthes disease will have an antalgic gait with a positive foot progression angle. There may be a decreased hip range of motion in gait. Concern for Perthes disease should be raised in those individuals with a decrease of internal rotation in the prone position (**Figure 16.22**). Patients will also have a decrease in hip abduction in the supine position and a child in the acute stages of Perthes may have a spasm of the adductor muscles.

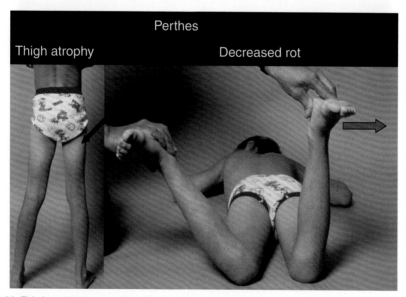

FIGURE 16.22 This boy with longstanding Perthes disease has thigh atrophy (black arrow). Prone examination of the child with Perthes will reveal decreased internal rotation (red arrow).

The physical examination findings for Perthes vary as the disease evolves. In the early fragmentation stages, the child will present as above. Yet in the healed stage, the patient will have a much less irritable hip and may have a remarkably similar hip range of motion despite an oval or oblong-shaped femoral head. As time progresses, these now-adolescent patients may have findings consistent with femoral acetabular impingement (see below).

Diagnostic Testing and When to Refer

1. Radiographs should be ordered in all patients with possible Perthes disease and an AP and frog pelvis x-ray is the test of choice. In the initial stage, the child may have a slightly smaller ossific nucleus while the joint space may seem wider. As time progresses, the femoral epiphysis will demonstrate radiographic fragmentation.
2. Hematologic evaluation. Bilateral Perthes disease is rare but does occur, the caveat is that if apparent Perthes disease is bilateral, and both hips are in the same stages of progression (fragmentation or reossification); one should consider a systemic cause of avascular necrosis mentioned earlier (**Figure 16.23**).

In those cases, blood should be sent for basic metabolic panel, complete blood count with differential and thyroid-stimulating hormone; should those be normal, referral to a pediatric geneticist may be appropriate to evaluate for skeletal dysplasia (**Figure 16.24**).

1. If a patient is suspected of having Perthes disease despite normal-appearing radiographs, one could get a repeat radiograph in 4 months looking for early fragmentation. Alternatively, it may be best to order an MRI in patients with an obviously irritable hip, but other more significant diagnoses (infection, neoplasia) are higher in the differential diagnosis (**Figure 16.25**).

Any child with suspected Perthes disease should be referred to a pediatric orthopedist.

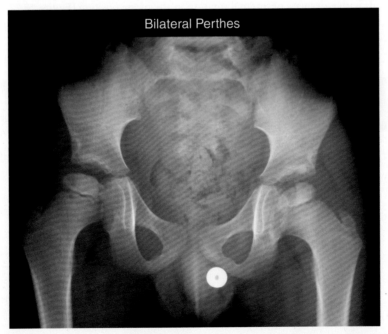

FIGURE 16.23 Anteroposterior radiograph reveals bilateral femoral epiphyseal changes consistent with Perthes disease. Note that each side is in a different stage of the disease course. A child with suspected bilateral Perthes disease based upon radiographs that show similarly appearing hips is always a concern for a systemic disorder.

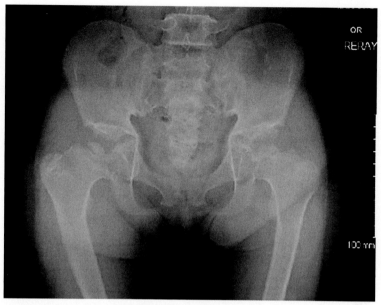

FIGURE 16.24 This child has abnormally developing hips that are symmetric radiographically. Due to her short stature, she was referred to a geneticist who diagnosed multiple epiphyseal dysplasia.

Slipped Capital Femoral Epiphysis

Slipped capital femoral epiphysis is typically encountered in older children and adolescents who are overweight. Pediatric orthopedists classify these hips as "stable" if they can walk with or without crutches (**Figure 16.26**).

"Unstable" hips are those patients in severe pain who cannot ambulate even with aids (**Figure 16.27**). Those with gradual slipping (stable slip) may present with achy groin pain, vague knee pain with or without a limp. Alternatively, some patients may have severe sudden slipping (unstable slip) that presents with acute pain that is similar to that which one would encounter with a fracture. These patients will be unable to walk even with crutches. Those with unstable slips have a higher rate of complications.

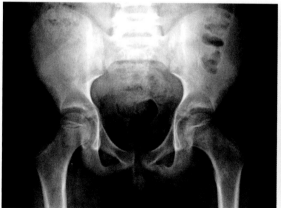
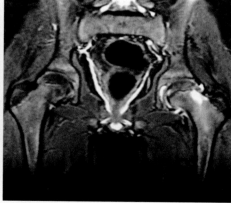

FIGURE 16.25 This 8-year-old boy with an irritable left hip was suspected of having Perthes disease and was confirmed on MRI.

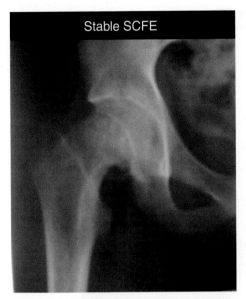

FIGURE 16.26 Anteroposterior radiograph of the right hip in a patient with a stable slipped capital femoral epiphysis (SCFE). This child is likely able to walk even though his antalgic gait may demonstrate external rotation of the foot.

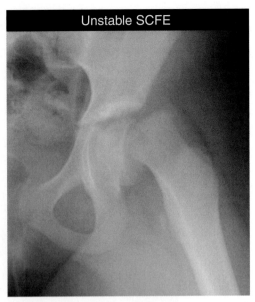

FIGURE 16.27 Anteroposterior radiograph of the left hip in a patient with an unstable slipped capital femoral epiphysis (SCFE). In contrast this child will be unable to walk as a result of severe pain. Unstable hips present with severe pain similar to fracture symptoms.

The past medical history should be obtained to rule out endocrinopathy, history of renal disease, or other metabolic bone diseases that can lead to weakness of the growth plate and slipping of the epiphysis. These patients are considered to have "atypical slips." Atypical slips should be suspected in patients who are younger than 9 years old or older than 16. Patients with normal BMI between 9 and 16 could also have an underlying pathology (**Figure 16.28**).

General physical examination is always important for those adolescents suspected of having an atypical SCFE (**Figures 16.29-16.31**).

The orthopedic examination of the patient with a stable slip will have an antalgic limp with a positive foot progression angle. In the supine position, the limb will be slightly abducted and lay in external rotation. In the prone position, there will be a decrease in the internal rotation of 20° to 40°. Special attention should be paid to the adolescent patient presenting with obligate external rotation (Drennan sign), with hip flexion, as this is often pathognomonic for a slipped capital femoral epiphysis or SCFE (**Figure 16.32**; ▶ **Video 16.9**).

Key Point

Any child or adolescent with vague, nonreproducible knee pain must have a detailed hip exam performed looking for a loss of internal rotation in the prone position, or have an AP and lateral hip radiograph performed.

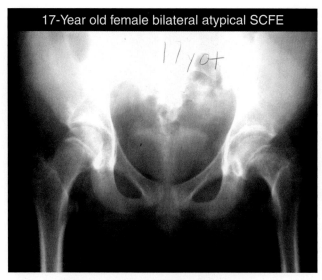

FIGURE 16.28 This 17-year-old girl has bilateral slipped capital femoral epiphysis (SCFE). She is 17 years old with open growth plates, which is "atypical" (most girls' growth plates close at 14). Thus, she is suspected of having a metabolic condition until proven otherwise.

Diagnostic Testing and When to Refer

1. Radiographs should be ordered in all patients with possible SCFE and an AP and frog pelvis x-ray is the test of choice for stable slips. Frog pelvis radiographs will be too painful in the unstable SCFE, thus a true lateral of the hip is ordered. One should note posterior and inferior displacement of the epiphysis.
2. If a patient is suspected of having a SCFE disease despite normal-appearing radiographs, it may be best to order an MRI in patients. Patients with a "pre-slip" can have edema of the metaphysis of the femoral neck.

Any child with suspected SCFE should be referred to a pediatric orthopedist.

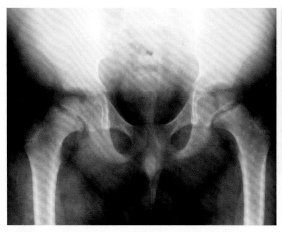
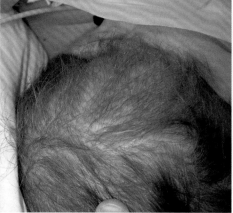

FIGURE 16.29 This 14-year-old boy has bilateral slipped capital femoral epiphysis (SCFE) with open triradiate cartilages, which is unusual. His relative skeletal immaturity demanded a physical examination that revealed an enlarged thyroid and coarse hair loss consistent with his undiagnosed hyperthyroidism.

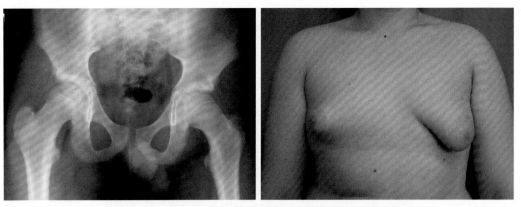

FIGURE 16.30 While this 15-year-old boy's left stable slipped capital femoral epiphysis (SCFE) on radiographs appears typical, his asymmetric gynecomastia is not and indicated an endocrine evaluation for an abnormality in pituitary function.

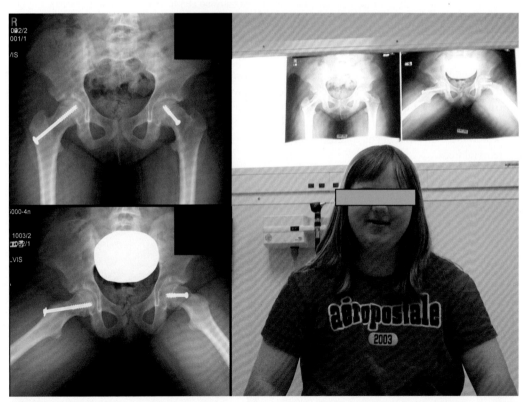

FIGURE 16.31 Children with Down syndrome with slipped capital femoral epiphysis (SCFE) should always be evaluated for thyroid hormone deficiency (atypical SCFE) and like all atypical slips; consideration for treatment of both the symptomatic and nonsymptomatic hip.

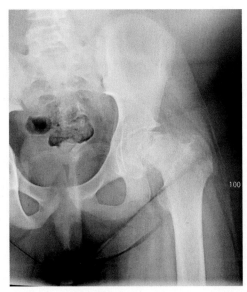

FIGURE 16.32 This 14-year-old girl with severe stable slipped capital femoral epiphysis (SCFE) will lay on the examination table with an external foot rotation. She will have a positive Drennan sign (▶ **Video 16.9**).

Hip Pathology in the Young Athlete

In the young or adolescent athlete with hip pain, a few additional physical examination tests are important. Certainly, extra attention should be paid to the traumatically injured athlete in regards to palpation for possible pelvic avulsion fractures. Developmental changes in the young growing athletic hip including proximal femoral and acetabular morphologic changes can lead to femoroacetabular impingement (FAI). As the name describes, with hip flexion there is abnormal contact between the femoral neck and the edge of the fibrocartilage of the bony acetabulum that can lead to pain and possibly lead to eventual degenerative arthrosis of the hip (**Figure 16.33**).

There are several key examinations to help evaluate for FAI.

1. The flexion adduction internal rotation (FADIR) test involves the examiner bringing the young athlete's affected side flexed hip and knee into adduction and internal rotation and pain with this maneuver are considered a positive test (**Figure 16.34**).
2. Another important test is the Scour test, which is similar to the FADIR test except it adds posteriorly applied pressure to the adducted femur by the examiner in the first part of the examination. The test is repeated in the abduction. A positive test is a reproduction of the patient's pain in adduction.
3. A third similar test is called Third test.[2] The first part of this test is the FADIR test. The second part is compression by the examiner of the femur into the acetabular socket similar to the Scour test. The third part is the distraction of the joint (ie, opposite pressure of the compression). Here, a positive test is pain with the FADIR and compression portion of the exam but the relief of the symptoms with distraction. It may have some additional sensitivity and specificity for hip labral pathology. Multiple examinations are important for the examination of the young athlete with suspected FAI and labral pathology (**Figure 16.35**; ▶ **Video 16.10**).

In addition to iliotibial band symptoms, there are other extra-articular causes of hip and groin pain in the young athlete. Iliopsoas tendonitis can cause snapping hip, and this can be tested by examining the patient supine and then bringing the hip from the flexed and externally rotated position into an extended and internally rotated position (**Figure 16.36**).

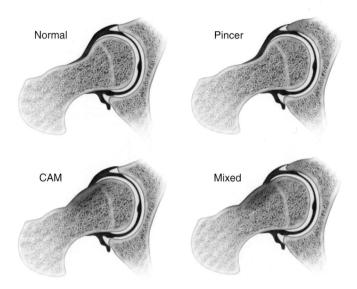

FIGURE 16.33 FAI can result from excessive anterior coverage of the hip by the labrum and bone of the hip and is termed "pincer impingement." When there is an anterior bump on the femoral neck or decreased offset, there can be "cam impingement" with hip flexion. In some instances, both mechanisms are possible.

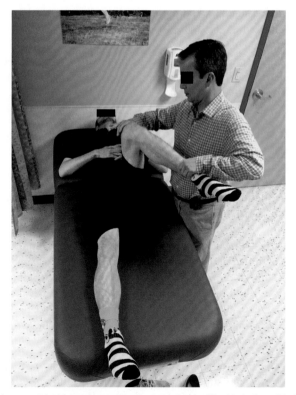

FIGURE 16.34 The impingement test is performed to document pain. The hip is flexed to 90° and if pain is reproduced with adduction and internal rotation; impingement is suspected.

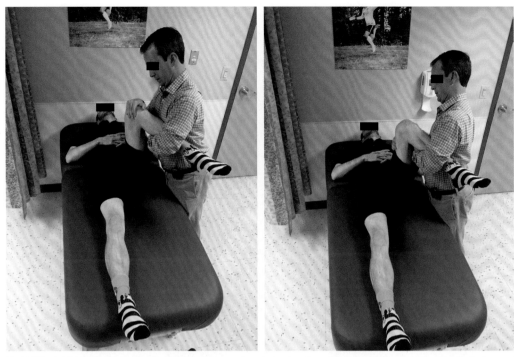

FIGURE 16.35 Third test. In the first panel, the examiner is forcing the adducted hip posteriorly with hip flexion and extension, which should generate pain in the afflicted hip. In the second panel, the examiner is lifting the femur anteriorly and relief of pain is specific for hip pathology.

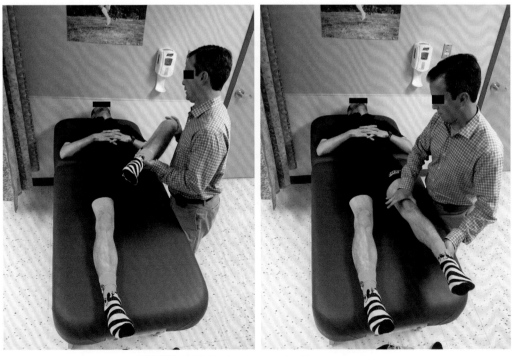

FIGURE 16.36 Testing for snapping iliopsoas tendon.

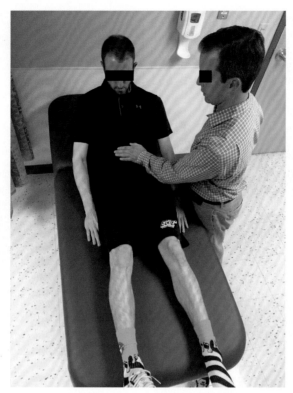

FIGURE 16.37 The resisted sit-up test can help discern hip pathology from a sports hernia.

Pain or snapping constitutes a positive test. Also, many young athletes with groin pain may be suffering from a sports hernia. A resisted sit-up test can help distinguish this entity from intra-articular hip pathology. Again, the patient is supine. The young athlete should be asked to do a sit-up with their knees extended. This should be repeated with the examiner providing gentle counter pressure at the abdomen. Pain in the groin with this maneuver can be consistent with a sports hernia and requires further evaluation (**Figure 16.37**; ▶ **Video 16.11**).

Diagnostic Testing and When to Refer

1. Radiographs should be ordered in all patients with possible FAI and an AP and frog pelvis x-ray is the best test to screen for other pathology. Any patient with undiagnosed hip pain and popping should be referred to a specialist in pediatric hip pathology before ordering advanced imaging. Today's specialists have protocols for advanced imaging that are not examined in routine MRI exams obtained at centers not focused on this patient population.

References

1. Ruwe PA, Gage JR, Ozonoff MB, DeLuca PA. Clinical determination of femoral anteversion. A comparison with established techniques. *J Bone Joint Surg Am.* 1992;74(6):820-830.
2. Myrick KM, Nissen CW. Third test: diagnosing hip labral tears with a new physical examination technique. *J Nurse Practioners.* 2013;9:501-505.

Chest and Shoulder Deformity

Dennis E. Kramer and Derek M. Kelly

● Basic Bony Anatomy, Development and Function

The pediatric shoulder girdle changes dramatically from the embryological period to adulthood, and each bone (scapula, clavicle, and humerus) has certain characteristics which are clinically relevant (**Figure 17.1**).

The scapula develops from embryological cartilage that migrates distally from the cervical spine to take its final position along the posterior chest wall during the first trimester. This has clinical importance as an undescended scapula (Sprengel deformity) may have residual tissue (fibrous, cartilaginous, or bone) that connects the scapula to the cervical spine.[1]

The clavicle connects the sternum to the shoulder girdle and the shaft of the clavicle primarily by intramembranous ossification, a process whereby the bone develops directly from mesenchymal tissue rather than going through endochondral ossification.[2] Defects in this embryological process can result in clavicular pathology such as congenital pseudarthrosis of the clavicle or even complete absence seen in cleidocranial dysplasia. The ends of the clavicle develop and grow by means of endochondral ossification, and the medial clavicular physis typically is the last one in the body to close sometime during the middle 20s. Consequently, sternoclavicular injuries in children are primarily growth plate fractures and rarely dislocations. The lateral clavicle articulates with the acromion process of the scapula through

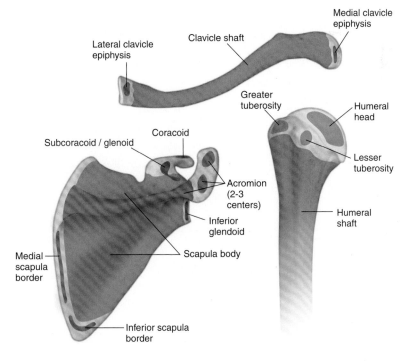

FIGURE 17.1 Shoulder physes and apophyses: location and name of each.

a capsular and ligamentous structure called the acromioclavicular (AC) joint. Sprains and dislocations to this joint can occur in children, but, similar to the medial clavicle, the lateral clavicle of the growing skeleton is much more prone to fractures than ligamentous injuries.

The proximal humerus develops from three primary ossification centers: the greater and lesser tuberosities and the humeral head. These three coalesce and eventually fuse with the humeral shaft. Greater than 80% of the growth of the humerus comes from the shoulder and thus a great deal of remodeling can be expected in fractures in this area that are displaced. This also means, however, that damage to the proximal humeral physis that leads to early cessation of growth can result in noticeable limb length inequalities.

The primary functions of the shoulder girdle are to help position the hand in space and transfer weight from the upper extremity to the torso. To accomplish these tasks, the shoulder has a large number of muscular attachments to accomplish weight transfer and to produce a wide variety of possible motions (**Figure 17.2**). The motions of the shoulder are made up of a complex interplay between

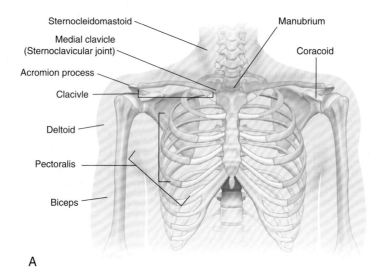

A

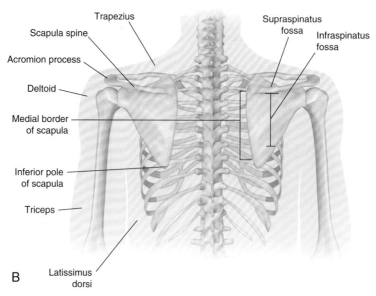

B

FIGURE 17.2 Boney anatomy of the pediatric shoulder region.

scapulothoracic and glenohumeral motions. While scapulothoracic motion is important to full shoulder function, most shoulder motion comes from the glenohumeral joint. The glenohumeral joint is largely unconstrained, moving through a large arc of motion within the glenoid. This makes the shoulder prone to conditions of instability, but it also means that large deformities of the proximal humerus can exist with little impact on overall shoulder function.

● General Physical Examination

Bony Anatomy/Surface Landmarks

Figure 17.3 shows the surface landmarks of the shoulder girdle in a pediatric patient along with the corresponding bony structures. During the physical examination, close attention should be paid to asymmetries. These are particularly noticeable at the sternoclavicular joint, acromion, AC joint, inferior pole of the scapula, and scapular spine. Swelling, bruising, or tenderness to palpation near these bony landmarks can indicate trauma or infection. Suspected bony trauma should be palpated very carefully to avoid a painful experience for the pediatric patient.

Shoulder Range of Motion

The glenohumeral joint is a ball-and-socket joint in which the ball is the head of the humerus and the socket is the glenoid which is directly attached to the scapula or shoulder blade. The glenohumeral joint is designed to allow the greatest arc of motion of any joint in the human body. Shoulder range of motion is a combination of glenohumeral and scapulothoracic motion. Maximal range of shoulder motion typically occurs through combined glenohumeral and scapulothoracic motion in a 2:1 ratio.[3] When necessary, true glenohumeral motion can be differentiated from combined glenohumeral/scapulothoracic motion in any range of motion test by stabilizing the scapula to prevent scapulothoracic range of motion (**Figure 17.4**).

The shoulder physical examination should always be performed bilaterally to provide comparison. Range of motion can be evaluated with the patient supine or upright. If active range of motion is limited, passive range of motion and/or isolated glenohumeral motion should also be assessed.

Forward flexion of the shoulder is assessed by asking the patient to stand straight and with elbows extended and forearms supinated, to raise arms vertically to maximal height above the head (forward and perpendicular to the plane of the body) (**Figure 17.5**). The zero starting position is with the arm at the side of the body. The amount of forward elevation is referenced off the plane of the body in the sagittal plane. Conversely, shoulder extension involves backward motion of the arm in the sagittal plane, referenced off the body. Typical normal forward elevation is 150° to 180°.

Shoulder abduction is measured in the horizontal plane of the body by raising the arm away from the medial side of the body to maximal height above the head (**Figure 17.5**). Normal shoulder abduction is typically 150° to 180° and involves both glenohumeral and scapulothoracic motion with a 2:1 ratio. Shoulder adduction is more difficult to measure because the body blocks movement toward its medial plane. Shoulder adduction can be assessed by having the patient forward flex the arm to 90° and then bring the arm toward the medial plane of the body with the elbow either extended or flexed.

Shoulder internal/external rotation can be measured with the patient supine and the arm abducted to 90° and the elbow flexed to 90°. In this position, the examiner can stabilize the scapula by placing his or her palm over the patient's shoulder and applying mild pressure to its anterior aspect to isolate true glenohumeral rotation. Internal and external rotations are then assessed by rotation of the forearm cephalad (external rotation) or caudad (internal rotation) with the forearm perpendicular to the floor (0°) considered as the starting position (**Figure 17.6**).

Shoulder internal and external rotation can also be measured with the patient standing and the arm at the side of the body with the elbow flexed 90°. In this position, external rotation is measured

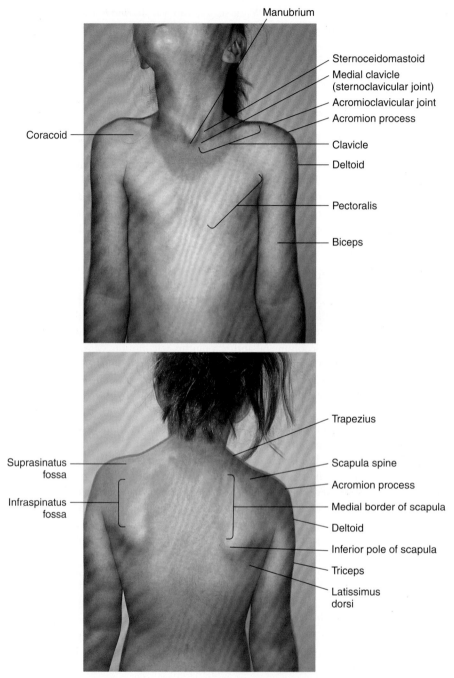

FIGURE 17.3 Bony and muscular landmarks of the chest and shoulder. AC, acromioclavicular; SC, sternoclavicular.

by rotation of the forearm away from the body and referenced off the zero position of the forearm perpendicular to the body. Internal rotation is more difficult to assess with this technique because the chest wall blocks motion and is typically assessed by having the patient reach behind his or her back and determining the highest vertebral level the patient can reach with his or her thumb (**Figure 17.7**).

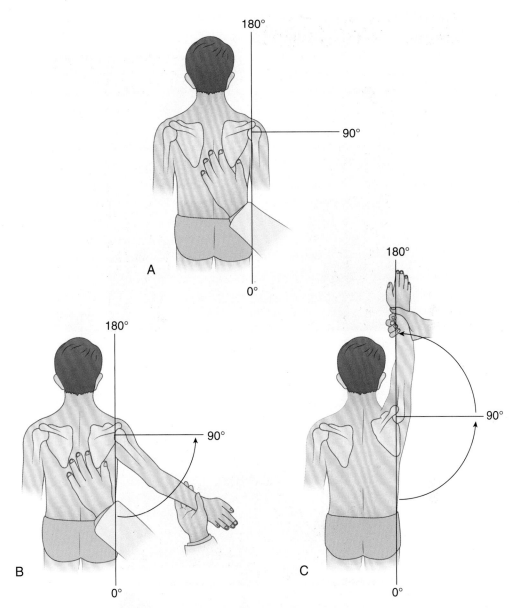

FIGURE 17.4 Total shoulder abduction is about 180 degrees and is the sum of motion at the glenohumeral joint and scapulothoracic motion. The examiner can isolate glenohumeral motion by first stabilizing the scapula with her left hand (A). The examiner can record glenohumeral motion by abducting the arm with her right hand until the scapula starts to move on the thorax (B). The contribution to total abduction via scapulothoracic motion is realized by releasing the scapula (C) and documenting total abduction.

Scapulothoracic motion, or motion between the anterior scapula and the posterior chest wall, can be assessed for dyskinesis by comparison to the other side. The patient is asked to do 10 wall push-ups and 10 full shoulder abduction exercises. The examiner looks for evidence of abnormal scapulothoracic motion (dyskinesis) present as a "hitch" or jump in an otherwise smooth motion pattern. Motion and position should be examined both in the ascending phase and in the descending phase of the arm. Dyskinesis will be noted more frequently in the descending phase of arm movement.

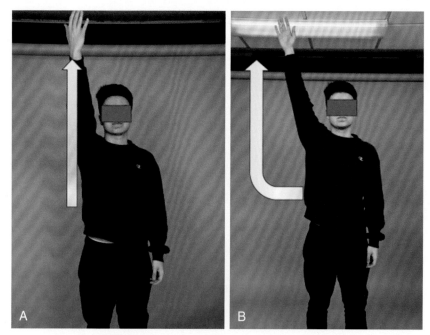

FIGURE 17.5 (A) Forward flexion and (B) abduction.

Internal rotation

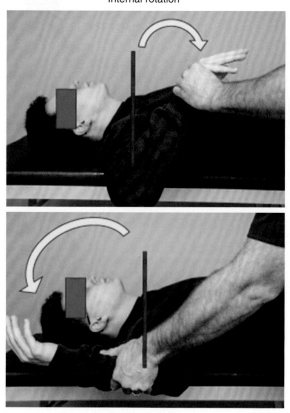

External rotation

FIGURE 17.6 Internal and external shoulder motion measured in the supine position.

Internal rotation

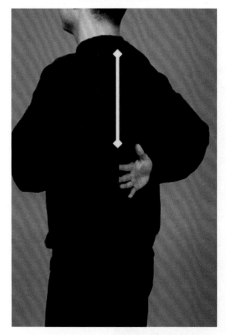

Shoulder Muscle Testing (▶ Video 17.1)

Shoulder muscle testing is done bilaterally to assess for weakness in specific shoulder muscles. Muscle strength typically is recorded on a 0 to 5 scale: 0: no palpable muscle contraction; 1: muscle flicker; 2: muscle contracture producing full joint movement with gravity eliminated; 3: full joint movement against gravity only (no resistance); 4: near-normal muscle strength; and 5: normal strength. A grade of 4 allows the examiner to subjectively grade strength as 4+ (near-normal/slight weakness) or 4− (profoundly weak but able to contract against resistance greater than gravity).

The rotator cuff is a group of four muscles that surround the shoulder like the cuff of a shirt. Two rotator cuff muscles—the more anterior supraspinatus and more posterior infraspinatus—lie on top. The subscapularis is positioned in front of the shoulder, and the teres minor lies in the back of the shoulder. The rotator cuff muscles all form tendons that attach to the head of the humerus. The top supraspinatus and infraspinatus work to bring the arm above the head and are most important in overhead sports.

Surrounding the rotator cuff muscles is the deltoid muscle. The deltoid muscle originates at the clavicle and acromion and attaches to the lateral humerus, surrounding and enveloping the rotator cuff anteriorly, posteriorly, and laterally. The deltoid muscle is tested with the arm adducted to the side and the elbow flexed to 90°. The patient is asked to forward flex (anterior deltoid), abduct (middle deltoid), and extend (posterior deltoid) the arm against resistance.[3] The biceps muscle forms two cordlike tendons that lie in the anterior shoulder region and help to flex the elbow and supinate the forearm. The biceps strength is best assessed with the arm adducted (at the side) and the elbow flexed to 90°. The patient is asked to flex the elbow or supinate the forearm against resistance.

The supraspinatus typically is assessed by the "full can" and "empty can" tests. These tests are done with the shoulder forward flexed to 90° in the plane of the scapula (30° of adduction). The examiner asks the patient to forward flex (push upward toward the ceiling) with the thumb up (full can) and thumb down (empty can) while the examiner attempts to push the arm downward. The patient's strength is assessed in comparison to the other side (**Figure 17.8**). The full can test specifically evaluates the anterior supraspinatus, while the empty can evaluates the posterior supraspinatus.

The infraspinatus is assessed by having the patient externally rotate the humerus from neutral with the elbow flexed and the arm in varying degrees of abduction (30°, 60°, and 90°) (**Figure 17.9**).

Subscapularis strength is best assessed by the "belly press" and "lift-off" tests. For the belly press test, the patient is asked to place his or her palms on the abdomen with the elbows parallel to the coronal plane of the body. The patient then forcibly pushes the elbows anteriorly. Subscapularis weakness is suggested by wrist flexion or dropping of the elbow behind the body during this maneuver (**Figure 17.10**). The "lift-off" test asks the patient to place the back of the hand on the lumbar spine and then lift the hand away from the back (internal rotation) (**Figure 17.10**). Inability to do this indicates subscapularis weakness or insufficiency.

Full can anterior supraspinatus

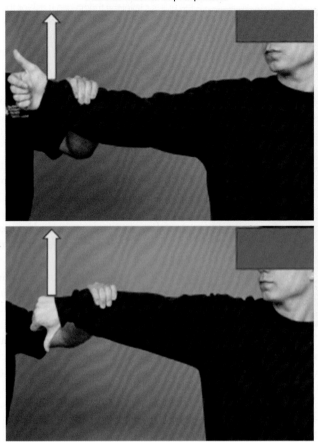

Empty can posterior supraspinatus

FIGURE 17.8 Testing the strength of the different insertions of the supraspinatus muscle. Resistance is compared to the other side.

Infraspinatus strength testing

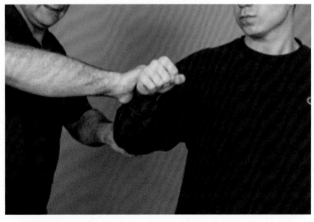

FIGURE 17.9 Testing the strength of the infraspinatus muscle.

Subscapularis: belly press test   Lift-off test

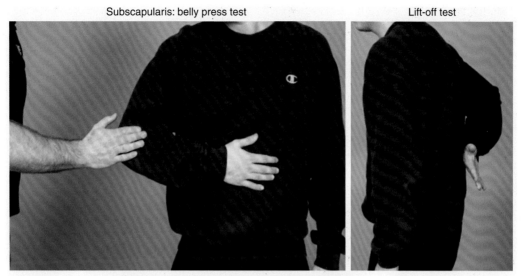

FIGURE 17.10 Testing the strength of the subscapular muscle.

Periscapular muscle strength can be difficult to quantify. A good provocative maneuver to evaluate scapular muscle strength is to have the patient do an isometric "pinch" of the scapulae in retraction. Scapular muscle weakness can be noted as a burning pain in less than 15 seconds. Normally, the scapula can be held in this position for 15 to 20 seconds without pain or muscle weakness.

● Radiographic Studies

Plain Radiographic Imaging

As with all radiographic examinations, two orthogonal views are ideal to avoid missing important findings. The glenohumeral anteroposterior (AP) radiograph will characterize basic shoulder anatomy and pathology and is oriented 5° to 10° from a straight AP of the chest to account for the obliquity of the scapula. The orthogonal view can be a scapular Y view or an axillary view, and these can document shoulder dislocations (usually anterior) as well as scapular body or glenoid fractures. A number of special views can help in the diagnosis of a wide variety of conditions, but a complete list of these views is beyond the scope of this text. A list of common additional views and their potential indications is provided in **Table 17.1**.

Table 17.1	Specialized Radiographic Views of the Shoulder
VIEWS	**INDICATIONS**
Scapular anteroposterior (AP) and lateral	Scapular trauma or deformity or suspected neoplasia
Cross-body lateral or transthoracic lateral	Trauma when shoulder range of motion is limited by pain
Shoulder internal and external rotation	Visualization of the entire humeral head. Hill-Sachs lesions or tuberosity fractures
Shoulder apical oblique (Garth) view	Bankart or Hill-Sachs lesions
Bicipital groove (Fisk) view	Pathology of the intertubercular groove
Shoulder outlet (Neer) view	Coracoacromial arch deformity or impingement
Stryker notch view	Glenohumeral articulation, humeral head defects
Clavicular AP and AP cephalad	Acromioclavicular joint trauma or degeneration, clavicular trauma or deformity
Sternoclavicular AP, lateral, and serendipity views	Sternoclavicular trauma or deformity

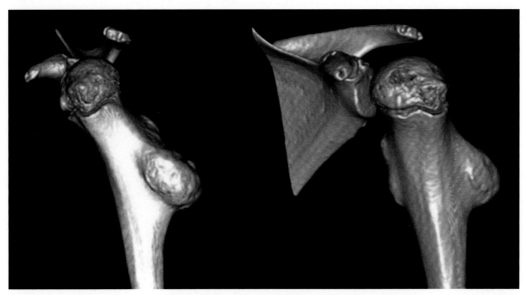

FIGURE 17.11 Three-dimensional computed tomography reconstruction of a 10-year-old female patient with a large posterior humeral osteochondroma. This test is not needed for diagnosis but for surgical planning purposes and is best ordered at the discretion of the surgeon.

Computed Tomography Scan Imaging

Computed tomography (CT) of the shoulder region can be used to further define bony anatomy, particularly when additional information in the axial plane is needed, such as in trauma, congenital deformity, or neoplasia. However, the CT should not be the first imaging test ordered due to increased exposure of the patient to ionizing radiation (**Figure 17.11**).

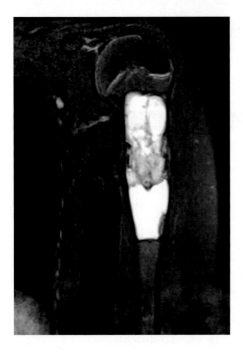

Magnetic Resonance Imaging

Magnetic resonance imaging (MRI) can be used when information is needed about the soft tissues of the shoulder region such as the rotator cuff, glenohumeral joint capsule, labrum, AC joint, pectoralis, and deltoid. In some cases, MRI of the glenohumeral joint can be enhanced with arthrography (injection of MRI contrast material into the joint before the MRI) to accentuate injuries to the labrum and surrounding structures. MRI should not be ordered in hopes that an abnormal finding might explain vague pain; rather, MRI of the shoulder is most helpful to confirm a diagnosis already suggested by history and physical examination (**Figure 17.12**).

FIGURE 17.12 Magnetic resonance imaging scan of pediatric shoulder showing a large unicameral bone cyst in the proximal humeral metaphysis.

● *Disorders of the Clavicle*

Congenital Pseudarthrosis of Clavicle

Introduction

Congenital pseudarthrosis of the clavicle most commonly affects the right clavicle, except in cases of sinus inversus or dextrocardia, when the left clavicle is at risk. A suggested etiology of the pseudarthrosis is pressure of the nearby subclavian artery during embryological development.[4] Females are more commonly affected than males. Unlike congenital pseudarthrosis of the tibia, congenital pseudarthrosis of the clavicle is unrelated to neurofibromatosis and, unlike cleidocranial dysplasia, there does not seem to be a direct genetic link.

Clinical Significance and Natural History

The bone does not heal without intervention; yet the condition is only rarely painful and may bother some children after activities involving the upper extremity.[5]

History and Physical Examination

Examination of a newborn reveals a painless prominence over the midshaft of the clavicle (**Figure 17.13**). As the child ages, the cosmetic deformity can become more pronounced, with a subcutaneous bony spike and a drooping shoulder girdle.

Diagnostic Tests or Advanced Imaging

Radiographs will demonstrate a dysplastic clavicle with defect in the midportion of the clavicle. A CT scan may be required to gain an accurate assessment of fragment size prior to consideration of surgical repair.

Treatment

Treatment includes stabilization and bone grafting of the area if the cosmetic or functional complaints warrant surgical treatment[6] (**Figure 17.14**).

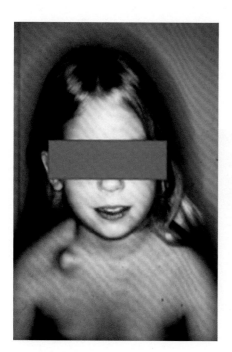

When to Refer

Referral to a pediatric orthopedist is indicated to confirm the diagnosis and discuss treatment options.

Cleidocranial Dysplasia

Introduction

Cleidocranial dysplasia or dysostosis is a genetic defect in the *CBFA1* gene whose gene product functions as a regulator of osteoblast differentiation and as an osteoblast transcription factor. The trait is transmitted by autosomal dominant inheritance.[7] One of the characteristic clinical features of cleidocranial dysplasia is hypoplasia or complete absence of the clavicles.[8]

Clinical Significance and Natural History

While the clavicular defect is perhaps the most pronounced physical finding of cleidocranial dysplasia, the genetic defect also results in abnormal bony development

FIGURE 17.13 This 5-year-old girl has a painless right clavicle pseudarthrosis.

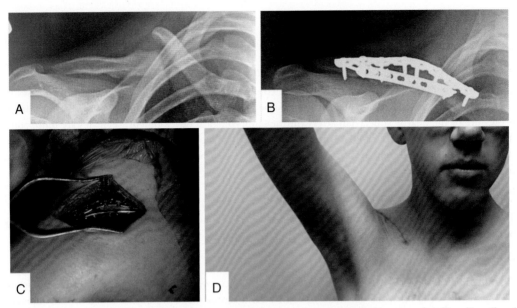

FIGURE 17.14 A, This 15-year-old boy has pseudarthrosis of the right clavicle that is uncomfortable with golf and other overhead activities. B and C, Open reduction and repair with iliac crest bone graft is performed. D, After surgery he is asymptomatic.

in the bones that undergo intramembranous ossification such as the pelvis. The pelvis demonstrates characteristically small iliac wings and widened pubic symphysis and sacroiliac joints. Children with this disease also have abnormal development of the cranium and facial bones, resulting in a wide skull and small face.

History and Physical Examination

Often patients can directly appose their shoulders in front of their chests (**Figure 17.15**; ▶ **Video 17.2**).

Diagnostic Tests or Advanced Imaging

Hip and spine imaging are also warranted because scoliosis and coxa vara are not uncommon.[9]

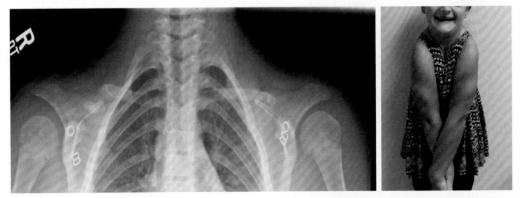

FIGURE 17.15 This 8-year-old girl with cleidocranial dysostosis has hypoplastic clavicles and can bring her shoulders together.

Treatment

Treatment is not needed for the clavicle; the hips may require treatment depending on the severity of dysplasia if it exists.

When to Refer

Genetics referral should be considered for children diagnosed with cleidocranial dysplasia.

Poland Syndrome

Introduction

Patients with Poland syndrome are missing the pectoralis minor muscle and the sternal head of the pectoralis major muscle. They also have at least one of a possible number of hand and finger deformities, including brachydactyly, hypoplasia, and syndactyly. Disruption of the arterial supply of the subclavian artery during the first trimester is one proposed mechanism for Poland syndrome.[10] Poland syndrome most commonly affects the right side, but it can affect either and rarely is bilateral.

Clinical Significance and Natural History

Function of the affected shoulder rarely is affected dramatically—shoulder ROM and strength typically are similar to the normal side—but the cosmetic deformity prompts many patients to seek plastic surgery solutions, including pectoralis silicone implants for both men and women and breast augmentation for women.

History and Physical Examination

Physical examination findings include a flattened chest wall and altered appearance of the anterior axillary fold (**Figure 17.16**). Patients with Poland syndrome may also have absent or hypoplastic ribs and shortened ipsilateral upper extremities.

When to Refer

There is not much that an orthopedist can do to improve the natural history of the absent muscles, but referral may be required to optimize hand function.

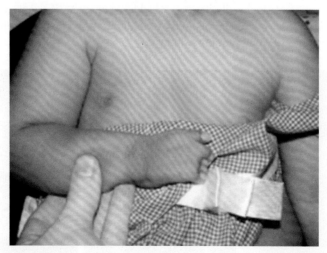

FIGURE 17.16 This child with Poland syndrome has absent right pectoralis muscle with complex deformity of the hand.

● *Disorders of the Scapula*

Sprengel Deformity

Introduction

Sprengel deformity results from premature arrest of the caudal migration of the scapula from the cervical spine that occurs during the first trimester. Severity of the deformity depends on how far the scapula descends relative to the normal position. In severe cases, an omovertebral connection (defined as fibrous or osseous connection) can be found between the superior-medial pole of the scapula and the cervical spine.

Clinical Significance and Natural History

Sprengel deformity has both functional and cosmetic consequences. A blunted shoulder and an altered neck line are common cosmetic concerns for the more severely affected. From a functional standpoint, the primary limitation is shoulder abduction. The scapula is rotated so that the glenoid faces caudally; the scapular musculature often is hypoplastic and weak, further limiting scapulothoracic abduction motion.

History and Physical Examination

Physical examination reveals asymmetric neck lines, asymmetry in the position of the two scapulae, and varying degrees of limitation in shoulder abduction on the affected side (**Figure 17.17**).

Pitfalls in Diagnosis

Milder deformities often are mistaken for scoliosis because of the asymmetry about the thorax and the apparent elevation of one shoulder. In addition, one should recognize that other organ systems begin to develop in the first trimester and may also have been affected. Children with Sprengel deformity and congenital spine deformities can have renal and cardiac abnormalities.

Diagnostic Tests or Advanced Imaging

Plain radiographs can reveal the elevation of the scapula and occasionally the omovertebral bone. CT scan may be needed to further characterize this. Spine radiographs should be obtained to fully evaluate for congenital spine deformity which can often be seen.

Treatment

Treatment rarely is indicated for mild deformity, but surgical correction can be offered to patients with severe cosmetic concerns or functionally limiting shoulder abduction. The surgery involves release of the medial periscapular muscles of origin followed by mobilization and caudalization of the scapula and reattachment of the muscles (Woodward procedure[11]).

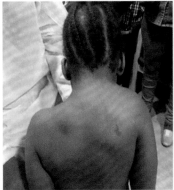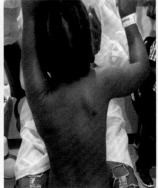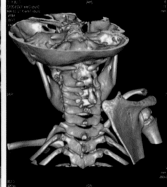

FIGURE 17.17 This 6-year-old girl has a clinically elevated right shoulder blade that has limited shoulder abduction. Computed tomography scan confirms elevated scapula and some congenital abnormalities in the cervical spine.

When to Refer

Patients should be referred to an orthopedist to evaluate the scapula position and its limits on function and to help screen for other associated problems.

Scapular Winging

Introduction

Scapular winging should be thought of as a symptom of a disease rather than the disease itself, much like a fever which is a physical finding of a large number of possible conditions. Winging is simply abnormal protrusion of the medial border of the scapula either during rest or during range of motion (**Figure 17.18; ▶ Video 17.3**).

Clinical Significance and Natural History

Ultimately the natural history is more dependent on the cause of the scapular winging. Those with poor scapular control can have limited active shoulder abduction and a sense of decreased power with push-off.

History and Physical Examination

While some conditions, such as Sprengel deformity or subscapular osteochondroma, might result in winging at rest, other conditions produce winging only during certain motions or actions. To elicit winging, the patient may either attempt a press-up from the prone position on the examination table or a push-off from the wall. Scapular winging also may appear during attempted shoulder abduction or forward elevation, when weakness of scapular stabilizers would be more pronounced.

Pitfalls in Diagnosis

Multiple conditions can affect the appearance and position of the scapula and include cleidocranial dysplasia and Sprengel deformity mentioned above. Causes of prominence or winging include subscapular osteochondroma (**Figure 17.19**). The serratus anterior muscle serves to maintain close opposition between the scapula and the chest wall during scapular motion, thereby improving the

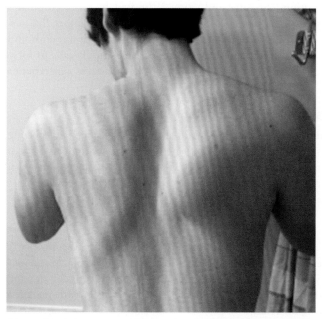

FIGURE 17.18 This adolescent male has asymmetric scapular winging that becomes obvious with a wall push-off.

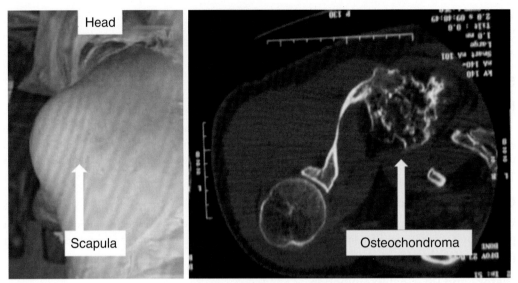

FIGURE 17.19 This patient has a prominent scapula as a result of large osteochondroma off the medial border of the scapula.

efficiency of scapulothoracic function. Dysfunction of this muscle leads to winging. Long thoracic nerve palsy (trauma or overuse) leads to serratus anterior muscle weakness (more common in adults). In children and adolescents, winging of the scapula is more likely due to muscular dystrophy.

Facioscapulohumeral dystrophy is one of the more uncommon forms of muscular dystrophy, but the true prevalence is not well known because many with the condition have milder symptoms and may not present for treatment. The inheritance pattern is autosomal dominant. Symptoms usually begin before the age of 20. Facial muscle weakness develops first (**Figure 17.20**), but the most significantly involved muscles are the levator scapulae, rhomboids, and trapezius (**Figure 17.21**). On physical examination, shoulder abduction is limited by weak scapular stabilizers while the deltoid remains strong (▶ **Video 17.4**). It is important to remember that, even though muscular dystrophies are systemic disorders, the degree of weakness and dysfunction in the shoulder may be asymmetric. When shoulder abduction is attempted, the scapula fails to forward flex and instead protrudes, elevates, and rotates inward (▶ **Video 17.4**). Patients can experience fatigue and pain about the shoulder.

Diagnostic Tests or Advanced Imaging

Radiographs and advanced imaging are of limited utility unless one is suspecting a mass effect that is leading to scapula asymmetry (**Figure 17.19**). When muscular dystrophy is suspected, laboratory testing usually reveals a normal creatinine kinase level. Genetic testing usually is diagnostic, but when genetic testing is equivocal and facioscapulohumeral dystrophy is still suspected, a biopsy can be obtained from the supraspinatus muscle.

Treatment

Treatment depends on the diagnosis, but, regardless of the etiology, therapy plays a large role. Scapular stabilization exercises can be used to maximize shoulder function and help replace some of the functions of deficient muscles. Surgical treatment is indicated when the cosmetic or functional deficit cannot be overcome with therapy alone. Scapulothoracic fusion can help with weakness and improve upper extremity function (**Figure 17.22**).

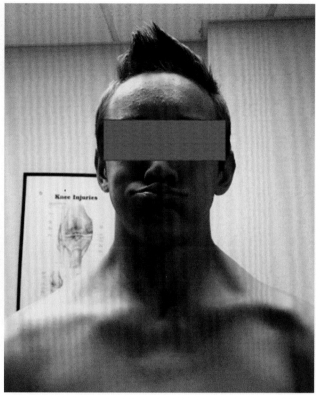

FIGURE 17.20 This boy with facioscapulohumeral muscular dystrophy has difficulty smiling and pursing his lips.

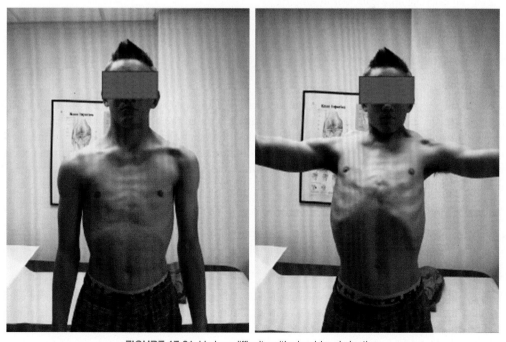

FIGURE 17.21 He has difficulty with shoulder abduction.

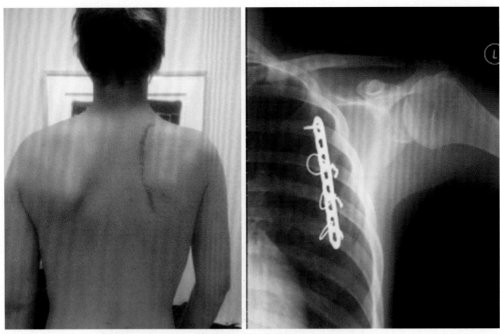

FIGURE 17.22 This 18-year-old boy has undergone scapulothoracic fusion that increased his function by stabilizing his scapula.

When to Refer

Referral to a pediatric orthopedist is certainly appropriate to confirm diagnosis, and pediatric neurology consult can help diagnose muscular dystrophy.

● *Disorders of the Proximal Humerus and Glenohumeral Joint*

Little League Shoulder

Introduction

Little League shoulder is a stress injury to the proximal humeral physis caused by repetitive micro-trauma. It occurs most often in male overhead throwers between the ages of 12 and 14 years. In these athletes, a strong rotational torque across the proximal humeral physis is produced by an imbalance between the rotator cuff muscles (which attach proximal) and the pectoralis major, deltoid, and triceps muscles (which attach distal). Poor throwing mechanics and an excessive number of pitches can predispose to this condition.[12,13]

Clinical Significance and Natural History

Considered an overuse injury, symptoms usually respond to appropriate rest and training to improve mechanics. Because of the remodeling potential of the proximal humerus, growth disturbances are rare.

History and Physical Examination

Patients with Little League shoulder typically present with anterolateral shoulder pain and loss of velocity following an increase in their throwing regimen. Physical examination findings are subtle, with the diagnosis typically made by clinical signs. Some athletes may have weakness with resisted shoulder abduction and internal rotation.

Diagnostic Tests or Advanced Imaging

Bilateral AP radiographs in internal and external rotation may demonstrate proximal humeral physeal widening or irregularity with metaphyseal demineralization, which is best seen in comparison to the contralateral shoulder (**Figure 17.23**).

Treatment

Treatment typically includes an initial period of rest from pitching (2-3 months), followed by rehabilitation and a gradual return to throwing. Developing proper throwing mechanics; limiting the number of pitches; and educating coaches, players, and parents are all crucial in the prevention of Little League shoulder.

Shoulder Instability

Introduction

The glenohumeral joint allows the greatest arc of motion of any joint and is the most commonly dislocated joint in adolescents.[14,15] The bony anatomy of the glenohumeral joint has been described as a "golf ball on a tee" configuration in which the humeral head (golf ball) has tremendous flexibility with limited bony restraints from the glenoid (tee). Stability is achieved through a combination of static (ligamentous) and dynamic (muscular) forces. The dynamic stabilizers (rotator cuff muscles) function during the midrange of motion to compress the humeral head against the relatively flat glenoid.[16] The static stabilizers include the glenohumeral ligaments, capsule, and labrum and function at the end range of motion to limit abnormal humeral head translation. These static stabilizers typically are injured in glenohumeral dislocations. Injury to static and dynamic restraints can impair shoulder function in a young athlete.[14,15,17]

By definition, "shoulder instability" includes acute dislocation typically from athletic endeavors. One of the most common acute traumatic shoulder injuries in athletes is a glenohumeral dislocation.[18] Anterior glenohumeral joint dislocations typically are traumatic injuries, and patients present holding the affected arm in abduction and external rotation with the humeral head palpable anteriorly (**Figure 17.24**). The typical mechanism of dislocation is a forced external rotation moment on the abducted arm. Patients with a history of shoulder dislocation may develop symptomatic anterior instability, but some

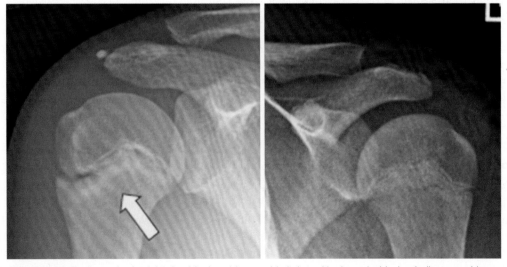

FIGURE 17.23 Radiograph of a right shoulder in a 14-year-old pitcher with physeal widening (yellow arrow) in comparison to the nondominant left shoulder.

AP view

Axillary view

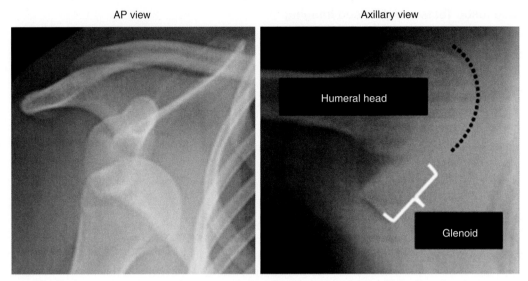

FIGURE 17.24 Radiographs of an athlete with an anterior dislocated humeral head. The axillary view demonstrates the humerus anterior to the glenoid. AP, anteroposterior.

patients with joint laxity can have instability in multiple planes without a history of trauma, and this atraumatic form of instability is called multidirectional instability (MDI). In this chapter, we consider three different clinical scenarios: (1) acute shoulder dislocation, (2) recurrent posttraumatic anterior instability, and (3) atraumatic MDI.

Clinical Significance and Natural History

Acute first-time shoulder dislocations are generally treated conservatively with a period of sling immobilization (1-3 weeks) followed by a course of physical therapy focusing on periscapular and rotator cuff strengthening exercises. Return to contact sports generally is not allowed until a full shoulder range of motion and a full return of strength have been achieved.

High rates of recurrent instability (50%-100%) have been reported after first-time dislocations in patients younger than 20 years of age, leading to some controversy regarding operative versus nonoperative management in adolescents with first-time shoulder dislocations.[19,20] Early referral to a shoulder surgeon may be beneficial.[19,21]

MDI is characterized by symptoms of subluxation in more than one direction (anterior, posterior, or inferior) in the absence of a major traumatic event.[22] MDI typically affects overhead athletes who participate in sports that require repetitive shoulder abduction and external rotation such as swimming (butterfly stroke) and gymnastics. Underlying glenohumeral laxity coupled with repetitive microtrauma can lead to painful MDI. Evaluation for hyperlaxity syndromes such as Ehlers-Danlos may be necessary.

History and Physical Examination

Posttraumatic Anterior Instability

The physical examination for recurrent posttraumatic anterior instability begins with visual inspection of the front and back of the shoulder focusing on scapular position and muscle atrophy. Active and passive range of motion can be assessed with the expectation that the injured shoulder will lack active abduction/external rotation, which stresses the injured anterior capsule. A thorough neurovascular examination should then be completed. Finally, evaluation of the individual rotator cuff muscles for weakness is necessary.

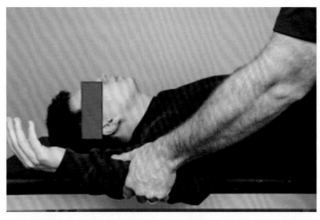

FIGURE 17.25 A positive apprehension test exists when this athlete's shoulder is externally rotated and he feels as if his shoulder will become unstable.

A few provocative maneuvers can assist with diagnosis, and affected patients often have a positive "*apprehension* test" and "*relocation* test."[23] These tests are reserved for assessing shoulder stability after rehabilitation of an acute glenohumeral dislocation, typically at least 6 weeks after injury. The *apprehension* test is done by having the patient lie supine and place the shoulder in 90° of abduction and gradually externally rotating the arm to 90° of external rotation (**Figure 17.25**). In this position, if the patient has symptoms of glenohumeral instability, the test is positive. It is important to note that this test is positive if it causes apprehension; pain alone is a less reliable finding.

The *relocation* test follows the apprehension test and evaluates relief of the sensation of instability in the above position when a posteriorly directed force is placed on the glenohumeral joint (**Figure 17.26**). Once again, the patient is positioned supine with the shoulder in 90° of abduction and progressively rotated to 90° of external rotation. When the patient begins to feel nervous, the examiner applies a posteriorly directed force to the humeral head. This maneuver stabilizes the humerus, and the test is considered positive if apprehension is relieved.

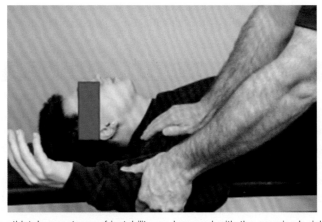

FIGURE 17.26 If the athlete's symptoms of instability are lessened with the examiner's right hand stabilizing his shoulder, this is considered a positive relocation test.

Multidirectional Instability

The physical examination for MDI is critical to help determine the direction(s) of glenohumeral instability that most typically replicate the patient's symptoms (**Table 17.2**). It is important to document generalized ligamentous laxity, which includes skin hypermobility tests as well as a Beighton score assessment.[24]

The *load and shift* test can be used to assess the amount of AP translation of the humeral head against the glenoid. In this test, the patient is positioned supine or upright and the examiner grasps the patient's arm with one hand and proximal humerus with the other hand (**Figure 17.27**). The examiner then centers the humeral head into the glenoid fossa before placing an anteriorly or posteriorly directed force on the humeral head to sublux the humerus out of the glenoid. The examiner then assesses for the amount of laxity[25]:

Grade 0: minimal displacement
Grade 1: humeral head reaches glenoid rim
Grade 2: humeral head dislocates over rim but spontaneously reduces
Grade 3: humeral head dislocates and does not spontaneously reduce

The *jerk test* can be used to assess posterior instability. In this test, the patient is supine and the arm is forward flexed to 90° and internally rotated 90° with the elbow flexed. The examiner grasps the elbow while stabilizing the scapula, axially loads the humeral head onto the glenoid, and then horizontally adducts the arm across the body while placing a posteriorly directed force to the humerus[26] (**Figure 17.28**). The examiner feels for posterior subluxation of the humerus out of the glenoid. The arm is then abducted while the examiner allows the humeral head to reduce back into the glenoid, feeling for a clunk or jerk as this occurs. Once again, it is important to note that the test is positive only if it reproduces symptoms of instability.

The *sulcus* sign can also be used to assess for inferior instability.[27] In this test the patient is either standing or seated with the arm at the side while the examiner stabilizes the shoulder and applies an inferiorly directed force on the elbow. The test is done with the shoulder in both neutral and 30° of external rotation. Excessive downward displacement of the humeral head that does not improve with external rotation suggests MDI of the shoulder or deficiency of the rotator interval.[26] If the test is positive, a sulcus appears in the subacromial region as the humeral head translates in the inferior direction. The sulcus sign is graded by the amount of inferior translation: grade I: <1 cm; grade II: 1–2 cm; and grade III: >2 cm.

Pitfalls in Diagnosis

The physical examination for shoulder instability in a pediatric patient can be challenging. Most importantly, it requires a relaxed patient to prevent guarding, which can interfere with the examination. While many tests for laxity of the shoulder have been described, it is important to note that any physical test

Table 17.2	Assessment Criteria for the Beighton Score (Maximal Score of 9)	
MANEUVER	**POSITIVE FINDING**	**SCORING**
Passive dorsiflexion of fifth metacarpophalangeal joint	≥90°	1 point per side
Passive hyperextension of the elbow	≥10°	1 point per side
Passive hyperextension of the knee	≥10°	1 point per side
Passive apposition of the thumb to flexor side of forearm	Entire thumb is in contact with flexor side of the forearm	1 point per side
Forward flexion of the trunk	Palms in contact with ground	1 point

Modified from Beighton P, Solomon L, Soskolne CL. Articular mobility in an African population. *Ann Rheum Dis*. 1973;32:413-418.

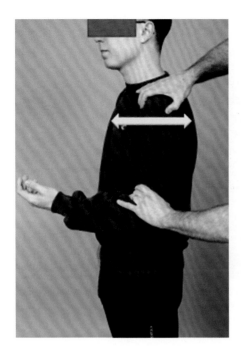

FIGURE 17.27 In the load and shift test, the examiner documents the degree of anterior and posterior displacement that can be produced.

for laxity in the shoulder should *reproduce* the patient's symptoms of instability to be considered positive. This distinction helps differentiate physiologic *laxity* from pathologic *instability.*[28] Comparison to the contralateral shoulder should always be done. Normal physiologic laxity tends to decrease with age, as the passive stabilizers tighten, but can be increased in patients with glenohumeral instability.[29] Laxity should not be confused with instability, particularly in young patients.

Diagnostic Tests or Advanced Imaging

Patients with acute shoulder dislocation require radiographs to confirm that the shoulder is dislocated with or without fracture. Axillary view radiographs will help make the diagnosis by depicting the location of the humeral head in relation to the glenoid (**Figure 17.22**).

Patients with a history of trauma and recurrent anterior instability also require radiographs to rule out old fractures (Hill-Sachs depression). An MRI arthrogram can be obtained by the treating orthopaedist to evaluate for injury to the static restraints. The most common injury pattern in anterior shoulder dislocations is a tear of the anterior-inferior labrum off the glenoid (Bankart tear) at the attachment point of the anterior band of the inferior glenohumeral ligament, along with a humeral head compression injury (Hill-Sachs depression) (**Figure 17.29**).

In MDI, radiographs and MRI images typically are normal except for a patulous glenohumeral joint.

Treatment

Surgical stabilization may be appropriate for patients with recurrent posttraumatic anterior instability for which conservative treatment fails. Nonoperative management is the primary treatment for MDI. A comprehensive physical therapy program focusing on postural work and rotator cuff and

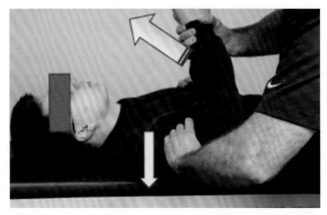

FIGURE 17.28 The jerk test is performed to detect posterior instability. First, the examiner adducts the arm across the chest (blue arrow) and then tries to translate the humeral head posteriorly (yellow arrow).

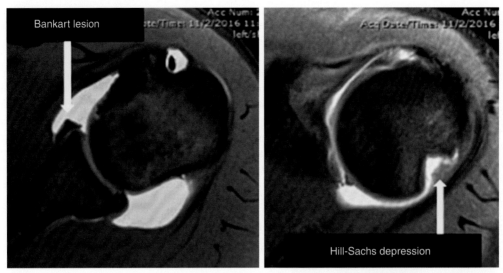

FIGURE 17.29 A magnetic resonance imaging arthrogram is obtained to document anatomic abnormalities in an athlete with anterior instability. The detached labrum (Bankart lesion) is noted. The Hill-Sachs depression occurred at the time of the dislocation when the anterior glenoid impacted the posterior humeral head.

periscapular strengthening can be beneficial. Surgery is indicated for patients with symptoms of MDI that affect activities of daily living and in whom at least 6 months of rehabilitation have failed to relieve symptoms.

When to Refer

All patients with a history of shoulder instability merit referral to a pediatric sports medicine specialist.

Internal Impingement (Swimmer's Shoulder)

Introduction

Shoulder pain without instability in an overhead athlete often comes from internal impingement caused by a combination of scapular protraction, muscle imbalance, and capsular contracture. This causes a posterior-superior shift in the glenohumeral rotation point, which leads to internal impingement of the greater tuberosity on the posterior-superior labrum and undersurface of the infraspinatus during abduction and external rotation mechanisms (such as throwing or swimming).

Clinical Significance and Natural History

Patients present with anterolateral shoulder pain with overhead activities. Physical examination often finds rotator cuff weakness, scapular protraction, and limited passive internal rotation, which signifies a tight posterior capsule. Typically, there also is some micro-anterior instability as evidenced by excessive external rotation of the shoulder.

History and Physical Examination

The physical examination for internal impingement generally focuses on identifying glenohumeral internal rotation deficits (*GIRD*) and evaluating for tears of the superior labrum. To determine if the patient has GIRD, the examiner should quantify passive internal and external rotation of the symptomatic and asymptomatic shoulders as previously described. The total arc of motion for each shoulder is the sum of internal and external rotation. It is normal for the patient's dominant shoulder to have increased external rotation and decreased internal rotation compared to the other

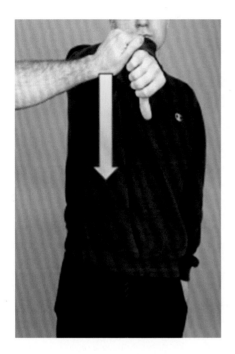

FIGURE 17.30 Pain with resisted downward force is indicative of impingement syndrome.

side. GIRD is defined as loss of more than 25° of internal rotation in the affected arm because this amount seems to predispose patients to SLAP tears.[30] In addition, a total arc of motion loss of more than 10° on the affected side may be a significant physical examination finding that is indicative of posterior capsular contracture on the affected side, which predisposes the patient to internal impingement.

The *O'Brien active compression test* is useful for evaluating the superior labrum for tears. In this test the patient is asked to place the shoulder in 90° of forward flexion and 10 degrees of adduction past neutral with the elbow fully extended. In this position the patient is asked to resist a downward force placed on the hand (**Figure 17.30**). The test is repeated with thumbs up (shoulder external rotation) and thumbs down (shoulder internal rotation). A positive result is obtained when the maneuver causes pain in the thumbs-down position only.

Diagnostic Tests or Advanced Imaging

Plain radiographs are indicated if the patient's pain is not typical for impingement. MRI may be normal or demonstrate posterior capsular contracture, superior labral tears (SLAP tears), or fraying of the undersurface of the infraspinatus.

Treatment

Initial treatment for internal impingement consists of physical therapy for posterior capsular stretching, scapular stabilization, and rotator cuff strengthening. Persistent symptoms often are due to labral tears, which are indications for operative management.

When to Refer

Patients with signs of persistent shoulder pain and/or impingement merit referral to a pediatric sports medicine specialist.

References

1. Matsuoka T, Ahlberg PE, Kessaris N, et al. Neural crest origins of the neck and shoulder. *Nature*. 2005;436:347-355.
2. Gardner E. The embryology of the clavicle. *Clin Orthop Relat Res.* 1968;58:9-16.
3. Montgomery S, Suri M. Physical examination of the shoulder: the basics and specific tests. In: Cohen SB, eds. *Musculoskeletal Examination of the Shoulder: Making the Complex Simple.* Thorofare, NJ: Slack Inc; 2011.
4. Lloyd-Roberts GC, Apley AG, Owen R. Reflections upon the aetiology of congenital pseudarthrosis of the clavicle. With a note on cranio-cleido dysostosis. *J Bone Joint Surg Br.* 1975;57:24-29.
5. Shalom A, Khermosh O, Wientroub S. The natural history of congenital pseudarthrosis of the clavicle. *J Bone Joint Surg Br.* 1994;76:846-847.
6. Schnall SB, King JD, Marrero G. Congenital pseudarthosis of the clavicle: a review of the literature and surgical results of six cases. *J Pediatr Orthop.* 1988;8:316-321.

7. Lee B, Thirunavukkarasu K, Zhou L, et al. Missense mutations abolishing DNA binding of the osteoblast-specific transcription factor OSF2/CBFA1 in cleidocranial dysplasia. *Nat Genet.* 1997;16:307-310.

8. Chung SM, Nissenbaum MM. Congenital and developmental defects of the shoulder. *Orthop Clin North Am.* 1975;6:381-392.

9. Richie MF, Johnston CE III. Management of developmental coxa vara in cleidocranial dysostosis. *Orthopedics.* 1989;12:1001-1004.

10. Bavinck JN, Weaver DD. Subclavian artery supply disruption sequence: hypothesis of a vascular etiology for Poland, Klipped-Feil, and Möbius anomalies. *Am J Med Genet.* 1986;23:903-918.

11. Woodward JW. Congenital elevation of the scapula: correction by release and transplantation of muscle origins. A preliminary report. *J Bone Joint Surg Am.* 1961;43:219-228.

12. Keeley DW, Hackett T, Keirns M, et al. A biomechanical analysis of youth pitching mechanics. *J Pediatr Orthop.* 2008;28:452-459.

13. Sabick MB, Kim YK, Torry MR, et al. Biomechanics of the shoulder in youth baseball pitchers: implications for development of proximal humerus epiphysiolysis and humeral retroversion. *Am J Sports Med.* 2005;33:1716-1722.

14. Chen FS, Diaz VA, Loebenberg M, et al. Shoulder and elbow Injuries in the skeletally immature athlete. *J Am Acad Orthop Surg.* 2005;13:172-185.

15. Kocher MS, Waters PM, Micheli LJ. Upper extremity injuries in the paediatric athlete. *Sports Med.* 2000;30:117-135.

16. Levine WN, Flatow EL. The pathophysiology of shoulder instability. *Am J Sports Med.* 2000;28:910-917.

17. LU B, Kelkar R, Flatow EL, et al. Glenohumeral stability. *Clin Orthop Relat Res.* 1996;330:13-30.

18. Culpepper MI, Niemann KMW. High school football injuries in Birmingham, Alabama. *South Med J.* 1983;76:873-875.

19. Jakobsen BW, Johannsen HV, Suder P, et al. Primary repair versus conservative treatment of first-time traumatic anterior dislocation of the shoulder: a randomized study with 10-year follow-up. *Arthroscopy.* 2007;23:118-123.

20. Handoll HH, Almaiyah MA, Rangan A. Surgical versus non-surgical treatment for acute anterior shoulder dislocation. *Cochrane Database Syst Rev.* 2004(1):CD004325.

21. Robinson CM, Jenkins PJ, White TO, et al. Primary arthroscopic stabilization for a first-time anterior dislocation of the shoulder. *J Bone Joint Surg Am.* 2008;90:708-721.

22. Paxinos A, Walton J, Tzannes A, et al. Advances in the management of traumatic anterior and atraumatic multidirectional shoulder instability. *Sports Med.* 2001;31:819-828.

23. Walton J, Paxinos A, Tzannes A, et al. The unstable shoulder in the adolescent athlete. *Am J Sports Med.* 2002;30:758-767.

24. Smits-Engelsman B, Klerks M, Kirby A. Beighton score: a valid measure for generalized hypermobility in children. *J Pediatr.* 2011;158(1):119-123.

25. Tzannes A, Murrell GA. Clinical examination of the unstable shoulder. *Sports Med.* 2002;32:447-457.

26. Lizzio VA, Meta F, Fidai M, et al. Clinical evaluation and physical exam findings in patients with anterior shoulder instability. *Curr Rev Musculoskelet Med.* 2017;10:434-441.

27. Neer CS III, Foster CR. Inferior capsular shift for involuntary inferior and multidirectional instability of the shoulder: a preliminary report.1980. *J Bone Joint Surg Am.* 2001;83:1586.

28. Mora MV, Ruiz-Ibán MA, Heredia JD, et al. Physical exam and evaluation of the unstable shoulder. *Open Orthop J.* 2017;11:946-956.

29. Beighton P, Horan F. Orthopaedic aspects of the Ehlers-Danlos syndrome. *J Bone Joint Surg Br.* 1969;51:444-453.

30. Burkhart SS, Morgan CD, Kibler WB. The disabled throwing shoulder. Spectrum of pathology. Part I: pathoanatomy and biomechanics. *Arthroscopy.* 2003;19:404-420.

Pediatric Elbow and Forearm Conditions

Joshua M. Abzug, Danielle A. Hogarth, and Dan A. Zlotolow

Introduction

Outside of the hand, the elbow is the most critical joint for the function of the upper limb. Therefore, preservation and restoration of stability and motion, in that order, are the highest priorities when treating elbow and forearm pathology. Forearm axial stability is also important, particularly as it affects the elbow and the wrist. Any pathology of the elbow or the forearm that affects the relative lengths of the radius and ulna can lead to dysfunction, deformity, and/or pain at the wrist. Likewise, some of the muscles of the forearm cross both the elbow and the wrist, and all of the muscles that originate in the forearm cross the wrist, except for the pronator quadratus. Primary and secondary muscle/tendon dysfunction can also affect the wrist. Any examination of the elbow and forearm must also at least consider potential pathology at the wrist as well. Common pathologies that afflict the pediatric elbow and forearm include congenital, traumatic, neurologic, neoplastic, sport-related, and other various conditions.

Congenital differences are present at birth but are occasionally not diagnosed until later in life. For example, radial head dislocations and radioulnar synostoses are often diagnosed after 5 years old, when limitations of forearm motion become limiting for recreational activities. Other congenital differences are immediately apparent at birth, such as congenital amputations, but much to the surprise of the parents commonly are not diagnosed in utero. This presents a difficult time for the family."[1,2]

Traumatic injuries to the elbow and forearm are very common in children and include fractures, dislocations, and soft tissue injuries. Because a child's ligaments are typically stronger than their bones, avulsion injuries are common. Plastic deformation can likewise pose diagnostic and treatment challenges. The pediatric elbow in young children is also particularly problematic diagnostically because of its large cartilaginous component, even past mid-childhood. Monteggia fracture-dislocations are often missed because of the combination of plastic deformation of the ulna and incomplete ossification of the capitellum. Likewise, medial condyle and epicondylar fractures are commonly missed or underappreciated because of the lack of ossification of the trochlea.

Pediatric tumors of bone in the elbow and forearm are most commonly benign lesions. Osteocartilaginous tumors can be seen inside the bone (enchondroma), on the surface of a bone (sessile osteochondroma), or growing out from the bone (pedunculated osteochondroma). Soft tissue tumors are most commonly hematologic in origin. Malignant neoplasms are rare but do occur, so an appropriate index of suspicion is warranted.

Neurologic disorders that affect the elbow and forearm can be local affecting the peripheral nervous system, such as cubital tunnel syndrome, or more proximal, such as cerebral palsy, which affects the central nervous system. Proximal neurologic disorders, such as a brachial plexus injury, that involve the elbow and forearm are typically more difficult to treat because they often comprise a larger scope of injury. Children with cerebral palsy can not only develop contractures of their elbow and forearm but also can exhibit athetoid movements or poor volitional muscle control.

Lastly, as sports participation and intensity have increased in the pediatric population, so have the prevalence and severity of sports-related injuries. The elbow of the growing child is particularly susceptible to overuse injuries from repetitive valgus overload, as seen in pitching and upper-limb weight-bearing sports. Typically, it is the most competitive and hardworking junior athletes who place themselves at the highest risk.

● General Physical Examination

Any examination of the elbow and forearm should include the shoulder, wrist, and hand. Although specific tests will be covered under specific diagnoses, the general upper limb examination detailed below should routinely be performed on all patients when possible. Children who are unable to follow commands may be lured to instead follow objects placed just out of reach. Stickers placed on the palm or back of the hand can also be used to induce supination or pronation, respectively.

Observation

All physical examinations should initially begin with observation of the child, looking for normal growth and development, deformities, skin lesions, and use of the limb in the office. For the majority of diagnoses, the contralateral limb can be utilized as a "normal" comparison, but this is certainly not true for all diagnoses. For an acute complaint, the skin should be assessed for swelling, tissue loss, ecchymosis, deformity, abrasions, etc. The carrying angle, an angle that defines the alignment of the limb at the elbow, can be observed and compared between sides. This angle is formed between the long axis of the humerus and the long axis of the forearm and is typically 11° to 14° of valgus in children (**Figure 18.1**). Overhead throwers will commonly have a greater carrying angle due to the repetitive valgus stresses placed on the elbow during the sports activities. Cubitus varus or "gunstock" deformity is commonly the result of a malunion about the elbow (**Figures 18.2** and **18.3**).

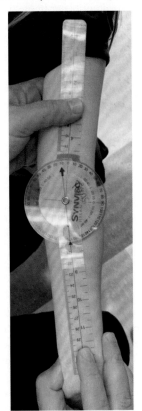

Topographical Inspection by Palpation

The next component of the physical examination should include palpation of anatomic landmarks. It is always optimal to begin away from the symptomatic area and progress toward it to gain trust with the child as well as to minimize any unnecessary discomfort during the examination. The bony landmarks about the elbow should be palpated purposefully to aid the practitioner during the examination. One should not just "grab" the elbow with a whole hand to determine tenderness. Rather, the structures about the elbow should be palpated utilizing 1 to 2 fingers so that the practitioner can differentiate the true areas of tenderness. The areas that should be palpated in particular include the supracondylar region, the lateral aspect of the joint and capitellum, the medial epicondyle, the radial neck, and the olecranon. One should also palpate the lateral "soft spot" to assess for fullness that may indicate a joint effusion. Palpation of the forearm should include assessing for any areas of tenderness, fullness, and/or abnormal bony anatomy (▶ **Video 18.1**).

FIGURE 18.1 Clinical photograph of a 5-year-old child with 12° of valgus measured between the long axis of the humerus and the long axis of the forearm. (Courtesy of Joshua M. Abzug, MD.)

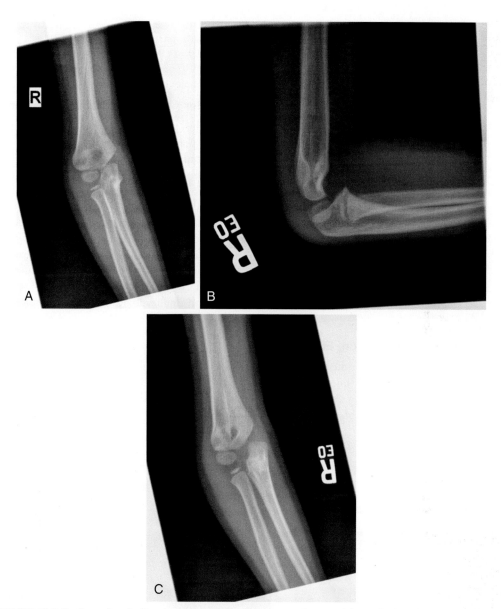

FIGURE 18.2 Radiographs of a 5-year-old child with cubitus varus after sustaining a displaced supracondylar fracture healed in malroation and in varus deformity. A, Anteroposterior view. B, Lateral view. C, Oblique view. (Courtesy of Joshua M. Abzug, MD.)

Range of Motion

Active and passive range of motion should be assessed in all children. The normal range of motion about the elbow is approximately 140° of flexion and 0° to −10° of hyperextension. A goniometer should be utilized during the examination to obtain true values. Normal forearm supination is approximately 85° and pronation is approximately 60° to 70°. Careful assessment must be performed to assess for true forearm rotation as opposed to pseudorotation that is occurring through the carpus when the examiner rotates the forearm by the hand (**Figure 18.4**). Therefore, the examiner should assess forearm pronation-supination by rotation at the distal 1/3 of the forearm as opposed to holding at the hand (▶ **Video 18.2**).

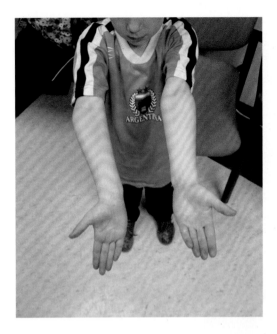

FIGURE 18.3 Clinical photograph of a 5-year old child with cubitus varus on the right. Carrying angle is 25° of varus, whereas the normal left side has a carrying angle of 8° of valgus. (Courtesy of Joshua M. Abzug, MD.)

Shoulder Abduction, Elbow Extension

With the patient either sitting or supine, instruct the patient to reach as high as they can away from the body. This tests both shoulder abduction and elbow extension. If the patient is unable to abduct the shoulder, elbow extension will have to be tested independently by the examiner holding the shoulder in abduction and asking the patient to reach as high as they can. If the patient is unable to extend the elbow, they may be reluctant to abduct the shoulder, so as to not hit themselves in the face or on the head with their hand when their elbow collapses.

Shoulder External Rotation, Elbow Flexion

Instruct the patient to reach for the back of their neck. This assessed shoulder external rotation and also tests elbow flexion at the same time. If the patient is unable to externally rotate the shoulder, test elbow flexion independently by asking the patient to reach for their mouth. If the patient is unable to abduct the shoulder, test for external rotation with the elbows at the side.

Pseudorotation

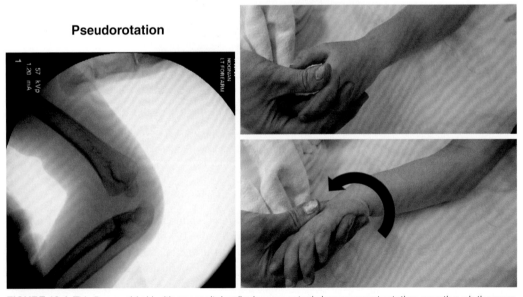

FIGURE 18.4 This 5-year-old girl with congenital radioulnar synostosis has apparent rotation even though the proximal forearm is fused. This motion occurs at the wrist and not the forearm.

Elbow Flexion, Forearm Rotation

With the elbows at the side and flexed approximately 90°, instruct the patient to turn the palms up and down. Forearm motion is assessed by looking and feeling for the relative positions of the radius and ulna, not the position of the hand, as the wrist itself can produce up to 60° of pronation and supination.[3]

Wrist Flexion and Extension, Radial and Ulnar Deviation

Test passive extension by instructing the patient to place the palms together with the fingers pointing to the ceiling and raise their elbows up while keeping the hands down. Test passive flexion by instructing the patient to place the back of the hands together with the fingers pointing to the floor and lower their elbows while keeping the hands up. Active extension is tested with the forearm in pronation, and active flexion is tested with the forearm in supination. Radial and ulnar deviation require a hands-on approach from the examiner to assess passive movement. The wrist should be moved into radial, and then ulnar deviation. Pain with ulnar deviation should be noted as a sign of ulnocarpal impaction.

Overall Stability

Following the assessment of a range of motion, one can assess the stability of the elbow, although this examination is quite limited in an awake child due to co-contraction of muscles, pain, and fear. The lateral ligamentous structures can be assessed by applying a varus force while internal rotation is applied to the elbow, with the elbow flexed about 30°. In contrast, the medial ligamentous structures can be assessed by applying a valgus force with external rotation to the elbow, with the elbow flexed about 30°. One can attempt to perform the posterolateral pivot shift test to assess the lateral ligamentous complex by applying a valgus and axial load to the elbow while flexing the elbow with the forearm in supination and arm overhead. A positive test implies posterolateral subluxation when there is a clunk with greater than 40° of flexion (▶ **Video 18.3**).

Neurovascular Examination

A neurovascular examination should also be performed on all patients. This includes a motor and sensory assessment of the peripheral nerves throughout the upper extremity (▶ **Video 18.4**). Although the examination needs to be focused depending on the complaints, the major peripheral nerves including the median, ulnar, and radial nerves should be assessed in all patients. In younger patients, this may be difficult but certain maneuvers can be helpful. For example, one can utilize the tenodesis effect to assess for tendon continuity following a forearm laceration. Alternatively, the forearm musculature can be squeezed in a young child, and the hand can be observed for digital flexion. Knowledge of tendon congruity can aid in differentiating a tendon injury from a nerve injury.

When evaluating potential sensory injuries, normative data in the pediatric population have been established for Semmes-Weinstein monofilament testing, as well as moving and static two-point discrimination.[4] Threshold testing utilizing a monofilament can be performed uniformly in children as young as 5 years of age and density testing utilizing two-point discrimination can be performed in children as young as 7 years old.[4] An examiner can also assess for sensibility in the younger child utilizing the wrinkle test, where the hand is placed in cold water for 5 minutes and wrinkling of the skin occurs in the digits that have intact neurological input. Parts of the hand that do not wrinkle are likely denervated.

The vascular assessment of the limb begins with the observation of the color of the skin. Additionally, the temperature of the digits should be noted, and capillary refill testing can be performed. One should then palpate the radial and ulnar pulses and compare the strength of the palpation with the contralateral limb. The hands should be pink and warm (**Figure 18.5**).

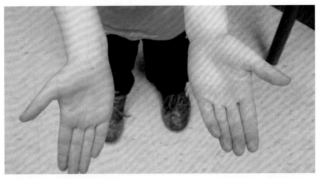

FIGURE 18.5 Clinical photograph of a bilateral vascular assessment of the hands demonstrating adequate pink coloration. (Courtesy of Joshua M. Abzug, MD.)

Congenital Differences

Coronoid Insufficiency

Introduction

Coronoid insufficiency is rare and presents typically in early adolescence with either recurrent or chronic elbow dislocation. Because of the late presentation, and because elbow trauma is ubiquitous in children, differentiating a congenital from a posttraumatic coronoid insufficiency is nearly impossible, but may have some relevance in management.

History and Physical Examination

On examination, the elbow becomes unstable axially with increasing extension. Once reduced, there is no varus or valgus instability.

Differential Diagnosis

Heterotopic ossification is a sign that the etiology may be traumatic in origin and not congenital insufficiency. Pain is typically not a factor in congenital insufficiency but is often seen with posttraumatic deficiencies.

Diagnostic Tests or Advanced Imaging

A global assessment of the elbow bony anatomy is important and may require either an arthrogram or a magnetic resonance imaging (MRI) in addition to palpation and range of motion assessment. If the elbow is completely ossified, a CT scan with 3D reconstruction is preferred. The coronoid is either small or absent while the remainder of the elbow is typically unaffected.

Treatment

There is no current treatment for elbow instability due to coronoid insufficiency. For patients who are unable to function with their instability, an elbow fusion is the only current option. Theoretical procedures such as using the ipsilateral or contralateral olecranon tip to replace the coronoid have not been sufficiently proven in this patient population.[5,6]

Radial Head Dislocation

Introduction

Differentiating between posttraumatic and congenital radial head dislocations is often a matter of conjecture, as birth trauma can result in a radial head dislocation.[7] It is our belief that the vast majority of "congenital" radial head dislocations are missed Monteggia fracture-dislocations or nursemaid's elbows, either from birth trauma or early childhood trauma. However, bilateral radial head dislocations are more likely to truly be a congenital condition in nature.

History and Physical Examination

Children often present in late childhood when restricted forearm motion is functionally limiting or when the child or parents notice a "mass" on the posterolateral aspect of the elbow. Other symptoms such as a limitation of elbow flexion can be seen if the radial head is anteriorly dislocated. Lateral dislocations are typically the most benign, as the position of the radial head does not interfere with elbow motion but does promote valgus instabiity. Medial dislocations present with gross valgus instability and limited elbow flexion.

Differential Diagnosis

One possible differentiator of congenital as opposed to traumatic radial head dislocations may be the development of the capitellum. A normal convex capitellum suggests that there was a radial head to contour against at least at some point in development (**Figure 18.6**). We consider all radial head dislocations with a normal capitellum to be of traumatic origin. Likewise, all patients with an irregularly angled ulna are managed as missed Monteggia fracture-dislocations (**Figure 18.7**).

Diagnostic Tests or Advanced Imaging

Plain radiographs are typically sufficient to obtain the diagnosis. A CT scan and/or MRI can be obtained if one thinks the dislocation is traumatic in origin, such as a missed Monteggia fracture-dislocation, and preoperative assessment is being considered.

Treatment

The keys to treating radial head dislocations are to determine (1) the cause of the dislocation, (2) the timing of the dislocation, (3) if it is reducible, and (4) if the radial head/capitellar anatomy would allow/sustain a reduction. Congenital radial head dislocations have so far proven difficult if not impossible to reduce. However, neonatal Monteggia injuries are amenable to relocation, particularly with the use of three-dimensional modeling techniques.[7] Restoring the bony anatomy is the most important component, with annular ligament reconstruction often not required. Reducible/dislocatable joints can be stabilized with an annular ligament reconstruction. Our annular ligament reconstruction transfers the distal biceps tendon to the medial origin footprint of the annular ligament, with half of the tendon left in continuity and the other half passed over the radial head, under the PIN, and docked into the footprint of the lateral annular ligament origin.

Congenital

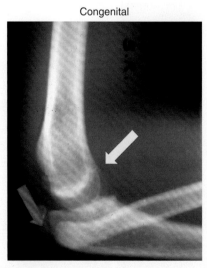

FIGURE 18.6 This adolescent male has likely congenital dislocation as his mother has similar radiographs. The capitellum is hypoplastic (yellow arrow) and the proximal radius is elongated and the radial head lacks the normal concave appearance (red arrow).

Posttraumatic

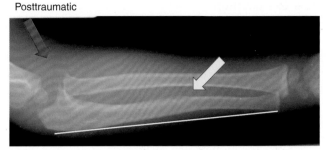

FIGURE 18.7 This child with an anterior dislocation radial head (red arrow) is likely a missed Monteggia as evidenced by anterior ulna bow that is normally straight (white line) and with evidence of old fracture (yellow arrow).

Radioulnar Synostosis

Introduction

Radioulnar synostosis is a rare, congenital condition where parts of the radius and ulna fail to separate. This congenital condition limits forearm rotation, so limitations are functionally relevant.

History and Physical Examination

Typically, the presentation is delayed until late childhood when the child is attempting to catch a ball. Children with extreme rotational positions (beyond 30° of supination or 60° of pronation) will present earlier. Parents will often assert that the loss of motion is new and in many instances provide photographic mis-evidence of such. The child will have no motion at the forearm, but typically will demonstrate hyperrotation at the radiocarpal joint, even up to 60° of both pronation and supination.[8]

Diagnostic Tests or Advanced Imaging

Plain radiographs are pathognomonic (**Figure 18.8**), and there is nothing else in the differential.

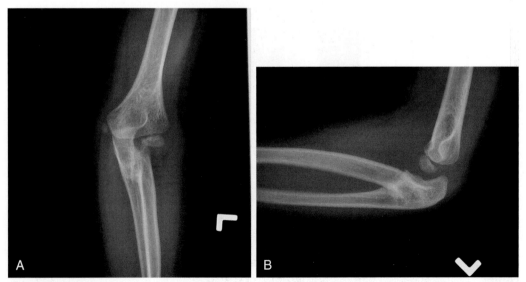

FIGURE 18.8 Radiograph of elbow demonstrating proximal radioulnar synostosis. A, Anteroposterior view and (B) lateral view. (Courtesy of Joshua M. Abzug, MD.)

Treatment

Attempts to restore forearm motion have proven fruitless in the vast majority of cases. Surgical treatment is reserved for patients in too much supination or pronation to accomplish daily activities. A transverse osteotomy is performed at the synostosis site, with resection of a 1-cm wafer of bone to limit soft tissue tension after rotation (▶ **Video 18.5**).

Transverse Deficiencies

Introduction

Congenital transverse deficiencies are very commonly misdiagnosed as resulting from amnionic bands. Although amniotic bands are a cause of congenital amputation, more common causes such as symbrachydactyly are not well known to frontline providers (**Figure 18.9**). Transverse deficiencies most often are due to a failure of formation or differentiation, rather than from intrauterine amputation. Loss of the apical ectodermal ridge (AER) results in hypodactyly or cleft hand, loss of mesoderm results in symbrachydactyly with or without Poland syndrome, and loss of the zone of polarizing activity (ZPA) results in ulnar deficiency with or without thumb dysplasia.

History and Physical Examination

When constriction banding does occur, evidence of bands in the ipsilateral limb or other parts of the body are pathognomonic (**Figure 18.10**). With cleft hand, imaging is unnecessary to make the diagnosis. Radiographs are only rarely used for preoperative planning.

Differential Diagnosis

There are many causes of transverse deficiencies, including symbrachydactyly (loss of mesoderm), hypodactyly (loss of AER), ulnar deficiency (loss of ZPA), amnionic bands, and intrauterine compartment syndrome.

Diagnostic Tests or Advanced Imaging

There are no diagnostic tests to perform.

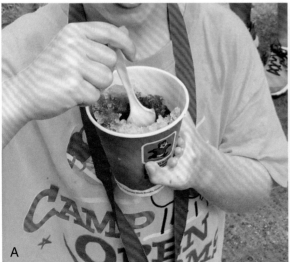
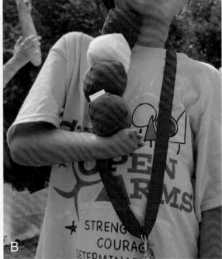

FIGURE 18.9 Clinical photographs of children with symbrachydactyly. A, Type 2 symbrachydactyly with the ability to grasp using the thumb and small finger. B, Type 4 symbrachydactyly without prehensile function. (Courtesy of Joshua M. Abzug, MD.)

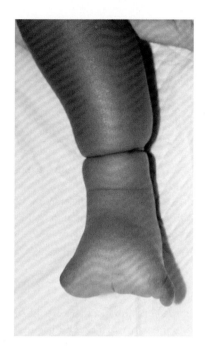

FIGURE 18.10 This child with amputations has a pathognomonic constriction band.

Treatment

Most children require no treatment for their transverse deficiencies and can manage fine with the occasional adaptive device such as a bicycle modification or swim fin. However, as prosthetics improve, there may be a role for targeted muscle reinnervation and osseointegration in older children.

Ulnar Deficiencies

Introduction

Although ulnar deficiencies can present as a transverse deficiency, more commonly children show a predilection for ulnar sided limb deficiency. Thumbs can be dysplastic in many patients.[9]

History and Physical Examination

All four limbs and the spine can be involved. Lower extremity deformities include proximal focal femoral deficiency and fibular hemimelia. Children should also be screened for congenital spinal abnormalities and scoliosis. We routinely obtain a one-time spine screening radiograph on presentation. Genetic evaluation rarely turns up anything with the exception of ulnar-mammary syndrome.

Differential Diagnosis

Monodactylous symbrachydactyly or cleft hand cleft feet can look like a monodactylous ulnar deficiency. Symbrachydactyly with one digit can be differentiated by the presence of an ulna and ulnar sided carpal structures. Cleft hand cleft feet can easily be differentiated by the presence of the small finger in the monodactylous type.

Treatment

Surgical options are highly specific to the particular deficiency of each individual child. Common options include pollicization for children with deficient thumbs, thumb reconstruction for children with duplicated thumbs, and syndactyly releases. Optimizing function often requires creativity and the development of novel techniques.

Radial Deficiencies

Introduction

The factors that lead to radial deficiencies are poorly understood. Associated cardiac, hematologic, and/or other organ system abnormalities are the norm. Holt-Oram syndrome is autosomal dominant and presents with cardiac septal defects and variable phenotypes of radial hypoplasia. Fanconi anemia is pancytopenia that results in complete bone marrow destruction at approximately 7 years old and can be found alongside any other cause of the radial deficiency. Treatment of the hematopoietic collapse is through a bone marrow transplant. Failure to find a matching donor in time results in the death of the child. Any child with a radial deficiency should, therefore, be screened for Fanconi anemia by obtaining a chromosomal challenge test, to maximize the time to search for a donor. Very few institutions perform the test, and insurance companies may initially deny coverage and therefore vigilance is necessary. Thrombocytopenia and absent radius syndrome has a pathognomonic phenotype with absent radii and broad, flat thumbs. Platelet counts can vary dramatically from patient to patient but tend to improve with age. Diamond Blackfan syndrome is a more rare condition but also has associated cardiac and hematologic disorders, with anemia as the most common presentation. Inheritance is most often autosomal dominant.

History and Physical Examination

The examination is mostly observational in the young child. The practitioner should assess the global shoulder and elbow motion by having the child reach up above their head and to their mouth, belly, and back. To assess hand function, hand the child a variety of different sized and shaped objects.

Differential Diagnosis

Amniotic bands can lead to amputation of the thumb but are rarely single bands. Usually, there is evidence of another banding on the same limb or elsewhere. Structures proximal to the amputation are preserved, unlike radial deficiency.

Diagnostic Tests or Advanced Imaging

Diagnostic tests for associated conditions are required for any child with preaxial deformity. This includes triphalangeal thumb, thumb polydactyly, thumb hypoplasia, and radial deficiencies. Referral to a hematologist and a geneticist is a reasonable approach to insure the workup is appropriate. This usually includes renal ultrasound, echocardiogram, a spine radiograph, and chromosomal challenge testing (for Fanconi anemia). In patients with thumbs but absent radii, a CBC is required primarily to assess platelet count.

Treatment

Patients without elbow flexion beyond 90° are not candidates for centralization or radialization-type procedures because they require radial deviation of their wrist to reach their mouth. If the child uses the thumb as a thumb, they are not candidates for pollicization. If the child uses the index finger for pinch and grasp and ignores the thumb, reconstruction of the neglected thumb is not advisable. If the child uses an ulnar sided grasp pattern and ignores the thumb and the index finger, neither thumb reconstruction nor pollicization are indicated.

If there is a thumb, joint stability guides treatment. No reconstruction is possible with an unstable basal joint at the thumb. If only the MP joint is unstable, an MP arthrodesis or chondrodesis should be included in the reconstructive plan. When considering thumb reconstruction or index finger pollicization, assess both intrinsic and extrinsic muscles acting on the thumb. If the size of the thumb is less than that of the small finger, ablation of the thumb and index finger pollicization is preferred over thumb reconstruction (**Figure 18.11**).

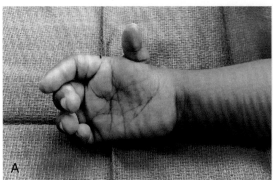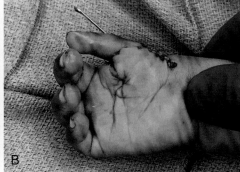

FIGURE 18.11 Clinical photograph of a Type IIIB hypoplastic thumb (A) preoperative and (B) status post index finger pollicization. Note the unstable thumb carpometacarpal joint preoperatively. (Courtesy of Joshua M. Abzug, MD.)

Arthrogryposis

Introduction

A condition with many names (arthrogryposis, arthrogryposis multiplex congenita, congenital contractures), many diagnostic codes, and over 300 causative conditions, arthrogryposis is a descriptive diagnosis that incorporates any condition that results in multiple joint contractures at birth. The most common cause of congenital contractures is amyoplasia, an idiopathic disorder characterized by hypoplasia or aplasia of skeletal muscle and occasionally the diaphragm. Although rare, absence or severe hypoplasia of the abdominal musculature can result in gastroschisis. Other causes include spinal muscular atrophy (SMA), Emery-Dreyfus muscular dystrophy (MD), and over 12 distinct inheritable disorders known jointly as the distal arthrogryposes.

History and Physical Exam

Despite a lack of muscle development, tendons can be robust and restrictive of joint motion. The flexor carpi ulnaris tendon attaches the pisiform to the volar forearm fascia leading to the typical wrist flexion and ulnar deviation contracture that is present. This tendon can be palpated quite easily because there is no surrounding muscle to obscure it. Most commonly, children with amyoplasia present with nearly symmetrical internally rotated and adducted shoulders, extended elbows (without elbow flexion creases) (**Figure 18.12**), flexed wrists, and stiff fingers with the MP joints in a neutral position. Finger proximal interphalangeal joint flexion contractures (camptodactyly) and atypical clasped thumbs are typical. In neonates, the posture is often confused with a bilateral brachial plexus (Erb) palsy, which is even more rare.

Children with SMA or MD, or other neuromuscular diseases tend to have progressive contractures and muscle loss. Children with amyoplasia and distal arthrogryposis tend to improve with age. The distal arthrogryposes are a set of distinct conditions with characteristic phenotypes and genotypes. The shoulders and elbows are relatively spared while the hands are most affected, hence the name "distal" arthrogryposis.

Differential Diagnosis

The most common misdiagnosis is bilateral brachial plexus birth injury (BPBI). Differentiating the two diagnoses is simple: children with BPBI will have normal passive joint motion up to 3 months old. After that age, children with BPBI will have a predictable pattern of contractures, primarily at the shoulder, specific to the number of roots involved.

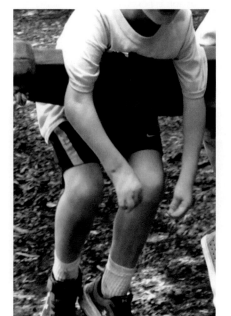

Diagnostic Tests or Advanced Imaging

We do not recommend any testing for these children but referral to a neurologist or geneticist may be indicated in children with a progressive decrease in function.

Treatment

Children with amyoplasia and distal arthrogryposis tend to improve with age. Children with elbow extension contractures that limit hand to mouth functions can be dramatically helped by performing an elbow release and triceps lengthening.[10] Best results are seen in children under 2 years, with most patients gaining the ability to feed themselves (**Figure 18.13**).[10] Shoulder internal rotation contractures can create the appearance of forearm pronation and should be corrected with an external

FIGURE 18.12 Clinical photograph of a child with amyoplasia. Note the lack of elbow flexion creases. (Courtesy of Joshua M. Abzug, MD.)

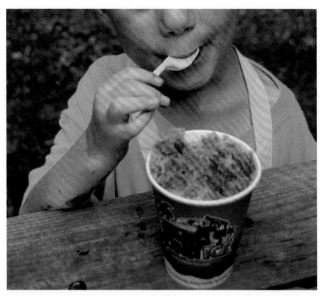

FIGURE 18.13 Clinical photograph of a child with amyoplasia. Note the child using the table to assist with passive elbow motion to permit bringing the hand to the mouth for feeding. (Courtesy of Joshua M. Abzug, MD.)

rotation humeral osteotomy before addressing the forearm (▶ **Video 18.6**). If the forearm is in excessive pronation or supination for the patient's functional needs, our preferred technique is the creation of a one-bone forearm, as rotational osteotomies of the radius, ulna, or both often regress.

● *Traumatic Injuries*

Introduction

Traumatic injuries about the child's elbow and forearm are extremely common from activities including falls from playground equipment, trampolines, and sporting activities, among others.

History and Physical Exam

When examining the child's upper limb following a traumatic injury, it is extremely important to observe, assess, and then palpate.[11] Following this algorithm will limit the child's pain and anxiety while allowing the practitioner to develop a relationship with the child before causing any pain. The initial observation should focus on the color of the extremity to assess the vascular status, the presence or absence of any lacerations or wounds, the presence or absence of substantial swelling or ecchymosis, and the child's active motion of the involved extremity. Subsequently, one can assess the neurovascular status of the extremity by palpating the radial/ulnar pulses, assessing capillary refill. One can assess the neurologic status of the extremity, typically by having the child perform movements of the digits (ie, flexion of the thumb IP joint to assess the median and anterior interosseous nerves, extension of the digits at the MP joints to assess the radial and posterior interosseous nerves, and crossing the fingers to assess the ulnar nerve). Lastly, the practitioner should palpate the upper extremity, starting at sites away from the likely injured area and working toward it.

Palpation of the child's forearm is fairly straightforward; however, when palpating a child's injured elbow, the examiner needs to have a focused exam and not just "grab" the child's elbow with a whole hand. Rather, the practitioner should utilize one or two fingers to palpate specific areas of the child's elbow as noted above. Tenderness to palpation in the supracondylar region is associated with supracondylar humerus fractures, tenderness on the lateral aspect of the elbow at the level of the joint is associated with lateral condyle fractures, tenderness to palpation on the lateral aspect of the elbow at the level of the radial neck is associated with radial head and neck fractures, tenderness to palpation on the medial aspect of the elbow proximal to the joint line is associated with medial epicondyle fractures, and tenderness to palpation posteriorly is associated with olecranon fractures. While concomitant injuries can occur, as well as more rare pediatric and adolescent elbow fractures, the aforementioned ones are the most common.

Lacerations from an open fracture or from a traumatic object must be assessed for tendon and nerve involvement. This requires a thorough assessment of the structures distal to the laceration, including a motor and sensory neurologic exam. The tenodesis effect and/or squeezing a child's forearm musculature can confirm the integrity of the forearm musculature and tendons. Sensory testing utilizing light touch in a child old enough to cooperate with the exam can indicate damage to a major peripheral nerve, including nerves that are only sensory in nature, such as the medial and lateral antebrachial cutaneous nerves.

Children may also present after a traumatic forearm or elbow injury that was not initially treated or treated by another provider. It is possible that a fracture healed in poor alignment, can lead to cubitus varus (more common) or cubitus valgus. This is assessed by looking at the carrying angle of the child's extremity (as described earlier) and comparing it to the contralateral side. Individuals with longstanding cubitus varus may develop posterolateral rotatory instability, due to the laxity that develops over time to the lateral ligamentous structures.[12] This is best assessed for utilizing the pivot shift test; however, this test is difficult to obtain a positive result when the patient is awake and is better performed in a patient that is under anesthesia. Patients with longstanding cubitus valgus may develop tardy ulnar nerve palsy due to the prolonged stretch on the ulnar nerve. Assessment of ulnar nerve function distal to the elbow can aid in this diagnosis. If a child presents late following an injury with an abnormal neurovascular exam, it is important to look for any scars from lacerations/wounds that may be present. Ideally, in all late presenting cases, the practitioner can review the initial injury radiographs to determine what the initial injury was and the subsequent treatment.

Tumors of the Elbow and Forearm

Introduction

Patients with tumors about the elbow and forearm typically present with concern regarding a noticeable "bump" (**Figure 18.14**). When seeing these patients, the practitioner should always begin the thought

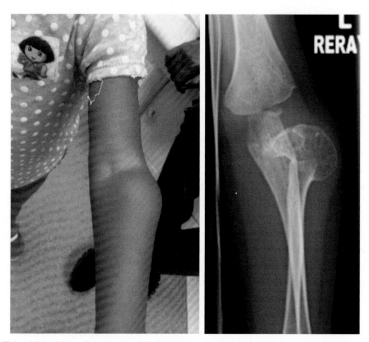

FIGURE 18.14 This child with undiagnosed multiple hereditary osteochondromatosis presents with a painful and swollen elbow with limited forearm range of motion.

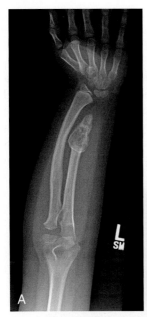

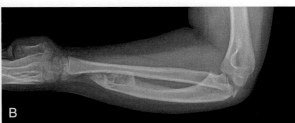

FIGURE 18.15 Radiographs of a benign ulnar osteochondroma in an 8-year-old girl causing limited pronation. Note the radial bowing. (Courtesy of Joshua M. Abzug, MD.)

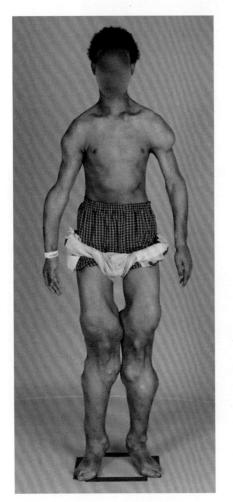

FIGURE 18.16 Clinical photograph of a child with multiple hereditary exostoses involving bilateral upper and lower extremities. (Courtesy of Shriners Hospital for Children, Philadelphia, PA.)

process with a wide differential diagnosis, as many non-tumor conditions can present with a "bump." Some examples may include an infectious process, a radial head dislocation, and a malunion of a fracture.

An osteochondroma is a benign bone tumor that grows adjacent to the physes and is contiguous with the medullary canal. The "bump" is firm and nonmobile. Tenderness to palpation may or may not be present. In some instances, the tumor has obliterated the physis, leading to bowing of the bone. This most commonly occurs about the distal ulna, causing the forearm to be bowed. Typically, a plain radiograph can confirm the diagnosis (**Figure 18.15**). Patients can have multiple hereditary exostoses, also known as multiple osteochondromatosis, which is a rare autosomal dominant condition (**Figure 18.16**). Patients with this condition may present with multiple bumps; cosmetic deformities of the forearms; pain due to impingement of nearby tendons, nerves and blood vessels, or pathologic fractures. Besides addressing the acute issue, the practitioner must monitor these children for the malignant transformation of a tumor, which has been reported in up to 5% of patients.[13]

A bone cyst such as a unicameral bone cysts or aneurysmal bone cyst (ABC) commonly presents in the second decade of life with the patient complaining of localized pain and swelling or following a pathologic fracture. Plain radiographs will show the cyst, which is a lytic metaphyseal lesion with an "eggshell" sclerotic border (**Figure 18.17**). An MRI can differentiate between these tumors by showing internal septations, often containing fluid-fluid levels, which is diagnostic of an ABC (**Figure 18.18**).

Ollier disease, multiple enchondromatosis, is a rare condition that has multiple enchondromas present, typically affecting one side of the body and can affect the growth and development of the arm (**Figure 18.19**). Maffucci syndrome is a rare, congenital enchondromatosis in which the patients also have multiple hemangiomas. Patients may present with painless or painful swelling of the elbow or forearm or a limb length discrepancy. The radiographic appearance of Ollier disease and Maffucci syndrome is the same except that one can see multiple phleboliths present in the Maffucci syndrome radiographs. These tumors should be observed over time as 30% of patients will ultimately develop a malignant neoplasm.

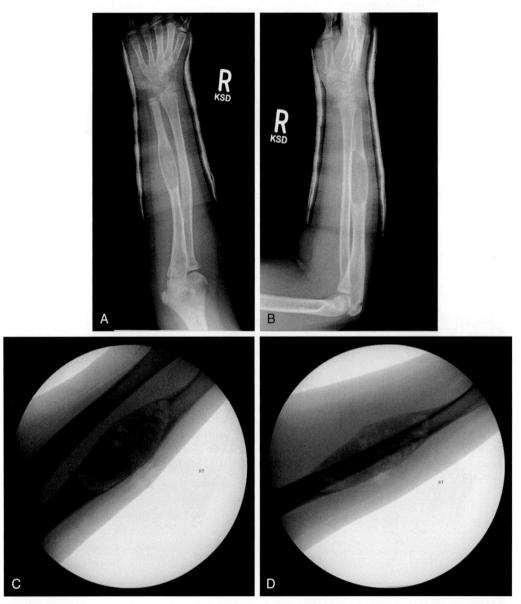

FIGURE 18.17 Unicameral bone cyst of ulna diaphysis. A, Anteroposterior and (B) lateral views. Postoperative X-rays after curettage and filling with bone graft substitute (C and D). (Courtesy of Joshua M. Abzug, MD.)

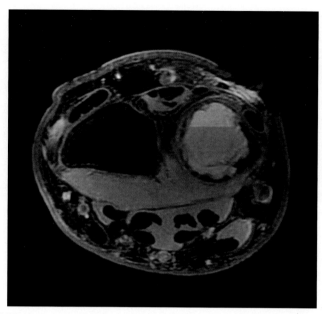

FIGURE 18.18 Axial MRI of an aneurysmal bone cyst in the distal ulna. Note the fluid-fluid level. (Courtesy of Joshua M. Abzug, MD.)

Hemangiomas of infancy are vascular tumors that present within the first month of life and subsequently go through various phases, including rapid growth and proliferation, followed by a slow involution phase and then ending with resolution. Superficial hemangiomas appear lobulated as a bright red papule, nodule, or plaque, whereas deeper lesions have a blue- or skin-colored appearance. As the vast majority of lesions undergo complete resolution, observation is the mainstay of treatment.

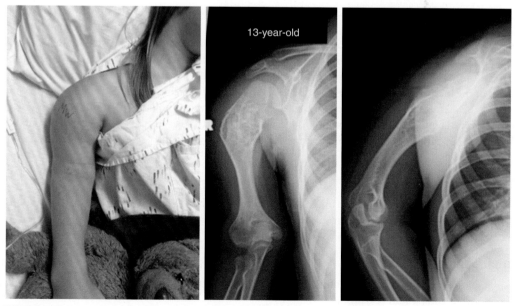

FIGURE 18.19 This adolescent with a shortened humerus is a result of a proximal growth arrest and deformity from Ollier disease.

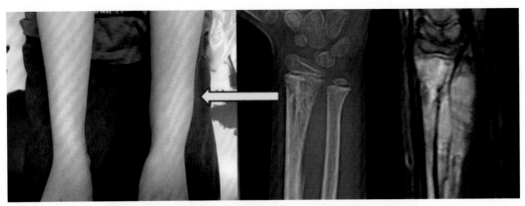

FIGURE 18.20 This 7-year-old boy presents with a painful wrist mass, and MRI and plain films suggest a malignant process, Ewing sarcoma was later confirmed on biopsy.

Although most tumors are benign, one should always keep malignant Ewing sarcoma and osteosarcoma in the differential diagnosis of painful mass with ominous bony destruction with or without soft tissue mass (**Figure 18.20**).

Neurologic Disorders

Cubital Tunnel/Ulnar Nerve Subluxation

Introduction

Compression neuropathies affecting the upper extremity are much rarer in children as compared to adults.

History and Physical Exam

The most common compressive neuropathy affecting the elbow and forearm region is cubital tunnel syndrome. Patients typically present with the instability of the ulnar nerve with elbow range of motion that leads to complaints of pain and/or numbness and tingling about the elbow and/or the ring and small fingers. The physical examination should include a Tinel's test about the cubital tunnel and a cubital tunnel compression test. Tinel's test is performed by having the practitioner tap on the ulnar nerve at the level of the cubital tunnel to elicit the subjective complaints. A cubital tunnel compression test can be performed by having the patient hyperflex the elbow and hold the position for 1 minute, in an attempt to reproduce their symptoms. The examiner should also assess the ulnar nerve for instability by having the patient flex and extend the elbow while palpating for the nerve to subluxate during this motion.

Differential Diagnosis

Any lesion along the course of the ulnar nerve proximal to the elbow can lead to similar symptoms. For example, a tumor in the lower trunk of the brachial plexus or thoracic outlet syndrome can lead to patients complaining of pain/numbness in the ulnar digits.

Treatment

Surgical intervention, including an ulnar nerve decompression and transposition, is effective at resolving symptoms of cubital tunnel syndrome.

Pronator Syndrome/Radial Tunnel Syndrome

Introduction

Other less common compression neuropathies affecting the elbow and forearm include radial tunnel syndrome and pronator syndrome. Pronator syndrome involves compression of the median nerve in the forearm, typically beneath the lacertus fibrosis, within the pronator teres muscle, or under the arch of the flexor digitorum superficialis muscle. It can also occur about the elbow if there is a supracondylar process present, as the nerve can be compressed beneath the ligament of Struthers. Depending on the location of the compression, the symptoms will occur with differing movements. Radial tunnel syndrome is due to compression of the radial nerve within the radial tunnel. This is a syndrome that only causes pain and is elicited on examination by noting tenderness to palpation distal to the lateral epicondyle along the course of the radial nerve. Additional testing can assess for pain with resisted supination and/or pain with resisted long finger extension.

Differential Diagnosis

Any compression of the median or radial nerve proximal to the forearm/elbow region can lead to similar findings and therefore the patient needs to be assessed beginning from their cervical spine and working distal.

Treatment

A diagnostic injection into the radial tunnel can produce pain relief while confirming the diagnosis (**Table 18.1**).

Spinal Cord Injury/Myelitis

Introduction

Injuries to the spinal cord can be due to trauma, autoimmune disorders, ischemia, and viral injury. The etiology often determines the pattern of injury. There are a multitude of traumatic spinal cord injuries, from central cord to complete injuries to Brown-Sequard. Virally mediated injuries have recently gained media attention as polio-like Acute Flaccid Myelitis (AFM) increases in incidence worldwide. In AFM, the virus attacks the muscle and the anterior horn cells, while excluding injury to the afferent and sympathetic cells and tracks.

Transverse myelitis (TM) can be differentiated from AFM by the presence of spasticity in the lower extremities and sensory loss in the upper and lower extremities. The neural injury in TM also tends to be contiguous, whereas AFM is patchy with some predilection for loss of shoulder function.

History and Physical Exam

Traumatic spinal cord injuries have a clear history of trauma. Patients with TM typically report a febrile illness a couple of weeks before the onset of weakness. AFM differs from TM in that, although it is also associated with a febrile illness, the neurologic injury occurs within a few days of onset of the illness.

Table 18.1	Compression of Pronator Syndrome and Respective Movements
LOCATION	**MOVEMENT TO ELICIT SYMPTOMS**
Between supracondylar process and ligament of Struthers	Flexion of elbow against resistance
Beneath lacertus fibrosis	Active flexion of elbow with forearm in pronation
Within pronator teres muscle	Resisted pronation during wrist flexion
Under arch of flexor digitorum superficialis muscle	Resisted flexion of long finger superficialis

At the heart of any upper extremity neurologic exam in children are the Active Movement Scale (AMS) (**Table 18.2**) and the British Research Council Manual Muscle Testing. In children over 7 years, sensory testing with 2-point discrimination and Semmes-Weinstein filaments are reliable.[4] Reflexes are hyperactive in upper motor neuron injuries.

Treatment

Surgical options include the full armamentarium of nerve injury procedures. Within 12 months of injury, and perhaps up to 18 months in AFM, nerve transfers are the mainstay of treatment. Beyond that, tendon and free muscle transfers are the only options.

Brachial Plexus Injury

Introduction

Traumatic brachial plexus injuries are uncommon in the pediatric population, but birth injuries occur with an incidence of 1 to 3 per 1000 live births.[14] Narakas classification is a useful grading scale for plexus injuries, with grades (1) upper plexus injuries, (2) extended upper plexus injuries, (3) global injuries, and (4) global injuries with Horner syndrome.[15] Grade 1 injuries involve weakness or paralysis in the C5-C6 distribution. The result of the deltoid and biceps involvement limits shoulder abduction and external rotation as well as elbow flexion and forearm supination. Grade 2 injuries affect the C5-C7 distribution and therefore present with the same weaknesses as Grade 1 but with the addition of limited shoulder internal rotation as well as difficulties with wrist and digit extension. Grade 3 injuries affect the entire brachial plexus (C5-T1) and therefore present as weakness or paralysis of the entire upper extremity. Grade 4 injuries have the same presentation as Grade 3 injuries but have the addition of Horner syndrome, a facial neural deficit that can present as a drooped eyelid and/or constricted pupils.

The roots can be stretched distal to the dorsal root ganglia to a point of demyelination (neuropraxia), axonal rupture without disruption of the epineurium (axonotmesis), and complete nerve ruptures (neurotmesis). Alternatively, preganglionic injuries (avulsions) disconnect the roots from the spinal cord.

History and Physical Exam

The AMS is valid throughout childhood and can be obtained even in newborns just by observing their movements. The Mallet examination (which characterizes upper extremity strength and function) is only possible after about 3 years old (**Figure 18.21**). In children with brachial plexus injuries, the children will have a muscle imbalance that can lead the shoulder to become dysplastic and tight as early as 3 months old. An ultrasound is useful as a screening test for shoulder dysplasia in children up to 1 year old,[16] but does not visualize the glenoid as well as an MRI.

Table 18.2	Active Movement Scale
SCORE	**DESCRIPTION OF MOVEMENT**
0	No contraction
1	Contraction without movement
2	Less than 50% joint motion with gravity minimized
3	More than 50% joint motion with gravity minimized
4	Full motion with gravity minimized
5	Less than 50% joint motion against gravity
6	More than 50% joint motion against gravity
7	Full motion against gravity minimized

Upper Extremity Brachial Plexus Clinic Form

Patient's Age: _____ Visit Type: ___ Routine follow up ___ Post-op follow up (___ months)

History of Condition: _____

PROM: ER (scapula stabilized, shoulder add) _____   IR (scapula stabilized, shoulder add) _____

   Scapulo-Humeral Abduction Contracture: _____   Elbow Extension: _____

Active Movement Scale (AMS)

		Gravity Eliminated	Score
Shoulder Abduction	_____		
Shoulder Adduction	_____	**Gravity Eliminated**	**Score**
Shoulder Flexion	_____	No contraction	0
Shoulder External Rotation	_____	Contraction, no motion	1
Shoulder Internal Rotation	_____	<50% motion	2
Elbow Flexion	_____	>50% motion	3
Elbow Extension	_____	Full Motion	4
Forearm Supination	_____	**Against Gravity**	
Forearm Pronation	_____	<50% motion	5
Wrist Flexion	_____	>50% motion	6
Wrist Extension	_____	Full Motion	7
Finger Flexion	_____		
Finger Extension	_____		
Thumb Flexion	_____		
Thumb Extension	_____		
Total	_____		

Toronto Score

Elbow Flexion	(0-2)	_____
Elbow Extension	(0-2)	_____
Wrist Extension	(0-2)	_____
Finger Extension	(0-2)	_____
Thumb Extension	(0-2)	_____
	Total	_____

Table for Scoring Toronto
(all movement scored against gravity)

	Grade	Weight
No Joint Mov't	0	0.0
Flicker	0+	0.3
<50%ROM	1-	0.6
=50%	1	1.0
>50% ROM	1+	1.3
Good but not full	2-	1.6
Full ROM	2	2.0

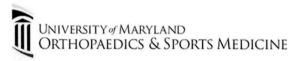

Modified Mallet classification
(grade I = no function, Grade V = normal function)

	Grade I	Grade II	Grade III	Grade IV	Grade V
Global abduction	Not testable	No function	<30°	30° to 90°	>90°	Normal
Global external rotation	Not testable	No function	<0°	0° to 20°	>20°	Normal
Hand to neck	Not testable	No function	Not possible	Difficult	Easy	Normal
Hand on spine	Not testable	No function	Not possible	S1	T12	Normal
Hand to mouth	Not testable	No function	Marked trumpet sign	Partial trumpet sign	<40° of abduction	Normal
Internal rotation	Not testable	No function	Cannot touch	Can touch with wrist flexion	Palm on belly, no wrist flexion	

UNIVERSITY *of* MARYLAND
ORTHOPAEDICS & SPORTS MEDICINE

FIGURE 18.21 Clinical documentation form for a brachial plexus birth palsy evaluation including the Modified Mallet Classification schematic. (Courtesy of Joshua M. Abzug, MD.)

Treatment

Early management focuses on maintaining passive shoulder external rotation and includes stretching exercises, splinting, and botulinum toxin injections. Global injuries that do not recover lower trunk function by 3 months of age should undergo a plexus exploration and nerve grafting with nerve transfers as needed. Upper and extended upper injuries can wait until 5 to 6 months old for a plexus exploration is warranted. In these groups, the lack of elbow flexion beyond 90° (AMS of 6) by 6 months old is a rough indication for exploration and nerve grafting and nerve transfers. This decision can be influenced by other factors such as C7 recovery, wrist extension, and active shoulder motion that also play a role in decision-making.

Nerve grafting is performed with sural nerve autograft. The results of allograft nerve and conduits are currently under investigation. Common nerve transfers include spinal accessory to suprascapular, radial to axillary, ulnar to biceps, and median to brachialis. Other nerve donors that surgeons should be able to transfer before undertaking any plexus reconstruction include intercostals, long thoracic, and medial pectoral. Contralateral C7 transfers have shown great promise but require specialized training before they can be attempted.

Spasticity/Cerebral Palsy

Introduction

Cerebral palsy is the physical manifestation of a static brain injury; although the original insult does not change, the challenge for the patient is that the manifestations can evolve with time. Muscle spasticity can affect limb movement and control, muscle contractures can develop and lead to altered motion, and this can eventually result in joint contracture or bony deformity. Although most pediatric orthopedists have been well trained to focus on the effects of the spine and lower extremity (walking), similar considerations are needed to improve upper extremity function.

History and Physical Exam

Progressive neurologic deficits should be referred to a neurologist for diagnosis, as CP is static and nonprogressive. Spasticity can increase as the child grows, typically peaking around 12 years. The physical examination should test passive and voluntary active motion of each joint. Classic upper extremity pathology in spasticity include various degrees of spasticity or contracture at each level. Some patients can have dynamic involuntary shoulder abduction, and elbow flexion contractures are common, with some patients having no active elbow extension. The forearm is often in pronation despite a spastic biceps tendon, due to spasticity in the pronator teres (PT) and pronator quadratus that overwhelms the supination power of the biceps and instead takes up some excursion of the biceps to further worsen the flexion contracture of the elbow. The wrist is usually flexed and ulnarly deviated with various degrees of finger flexion, the thumb can be adducted and flexed within the palm.

Treatment

Similar to the lower extremity, the bulk of treatment for upper extremity involves physical therapy, stretching, botulinum toxin injection, and splinting. The surgical treatment for children with no volitional control of their elbow or forearm is to release the joints as required to make it easier for their caretaker to dress and bathe the child. For the child with active elbow motion both in flexion and extension, lengthening of the brachialis, with or without the brachioradialis and the biceps, can be very helpful to augment elbow extension. Pronator rerouting does not biomechanically create a supinator, as routing around the radius still leaves the PT on the same side of the axis of rotation. It does, however, weaken the pronator. Other muscle releases and transfers are useful to improve the appearance and function of the hand.

● Overuse Injuries

Sports-related injuries about the elbow and forearm are quite common in the pediatric and adolescent populations. Although these may include fractures, they more commonly include overuse injuries about the elbow. These injuries are most commonly seen in athletes that do overhead throwing (**Figure 18.22**), play racquet sports, or weight-bear on the upper extremities, such as gymnasts and cheerleaders. Common overuse diagnoses include Little League elbow and lateral epicondylitis.

Little League Elbow

Introduction

Overuse injuries are commonly seen in overhead throwing athletes, such as baseball players. Little League elbow is a condition that occurs most commonly in pitchers who place excessive valgus stress on their elbows (**Figure 18.23**).

History and Physical Examination

Patients often present complaining of medial sided elbow pain and/or a decrease in the velocity of their throws. The history of the thrower must be obtained, specifically asking about pitch counts and pitch types. Little League has published guidelines for pitchers based on age, regarding optimal pitch numbers and types per given day, as well as minimum rest periods. A pitcher/parent unfamiliar with pitch counts and type restrictions is a "red flag" for the practitioner and likely correlates with the patient having an overuse injury. Examination of a child with suspected Little League elbow should

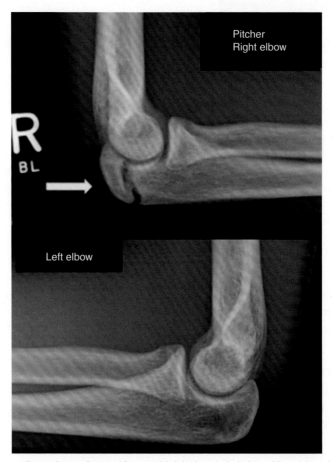

FIGURE 18.22 These radiographs are from a 16-year-old right-handed pitcher with activity-related pain at his olecranon. Radiographs of his contralateral elbow reveal that his olecranon physis is closed. This pattern is consistent with traction apophysitis from overuse.

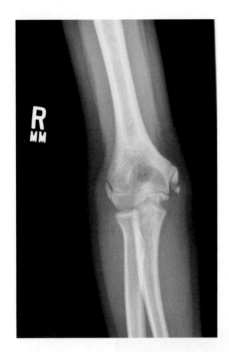

FIGURE 18.23 Radiograph of an 11-year-old male with a medial epicondyle avulsion fracture sustained after pitching during baseball. Note the physeal widening of the medial epicondyle physis. (Courtesy of Joshua M. Abzug, MD.)

include an assessment of shoulder motion, looking for excessive external rotation and limited internal rotation, termed glenohumeral internal rotational deficit. Elbow range of motion, both active and passive, should also be assessed. Patients commonly have tenderness to palpation about the medial epicondyle region.

Differential Diagnosis

It is important to note whether a pitcher that felt a "pop" on the medial aspect of their elbow may have sustained a medial epicondyle avulsion fracture and/or an injury to the ulnar collateral ligament (UCL).

Diagnostic Tests and Advanced Imaging

Although physical examination is typically all that is needed to make the diagnosis of Little League elbow, plain radiographs are often obtained to rule out fractures of the medial epicondyle and osteochondritis dissecans (OCD) lesions.

Treatment

The recommended course of treatment is dictated by the severity of the injury and the presence of associated injuries. Early recognition of Little League elbow with complaints of pain only during activity has been shown to resolve with cessation of activity, use of ice, and prescription of anti-inflammatory medications. Patients complaining of persistent pain, even during rest, are suggested to adhere to regular anti-inflammatory utilization, elbow immobilization in a brace or cast, and adherence to a throwing specific physical therapy regimen. For cases with an associated medial epicondyle fracture and/or UCL injury, surgical treatment is warranted for fixation and/or repair, respectively, followed by therapy rehabilitation for a gradual return to sport.

Elbow Osteochondritis Dissecans

Introduction

The valgus stress placed on the elbow during throwing and seen when an athlete weight-bears on their upper extremities, may lead to compressive forces and microtrauma about the radiocapitellar joint. This microtrauma, along with the tenuous blood supply to this region, is thought to be the etiology of OCD of the capitellum.

History and Physical Examination

Patients with this diagnosis commonly present complaining of pain on the lateral aspect of the elbow, decreased throwing velocity, a lack of full elbow extension, and popping/catching if a loose body or cartilage flap is present. The examination should include an assessment of active and passive elbow range of motion. The maximum flexion of the elbow exposes the capitellum on the posterior-lateral aspect of the elbow to permit palpation of this region. Tenderness at this location is very consistent with an OCD lesion. Although the examiner takes the elbow through a range of motion, he/she should place their thumb and index finger on either side of the elbow at the level of the joint to assess for the presence of crepitus, locking, or popping, which typically occurs when a loose body is present. The examiner can also apply axial loading of the forearm against the capitellum, while rotating the forearm, to determine if this causes pain.

Differential Diagnosis

One can experience popping of the elbow secondary to a plica, a snapping triceps, or ulnar nerve sub-luxation. Additional causes of pain on the lateral aspect of the elbow include lateral epicondylitis, radial tunnel syndrome, and fractures.

Diagnostic Tests and Advanced Imaging

Standard elbow radiographs (AP and lateral views) should be obtained if a loose body is suspected (**Figure 18.24**). MRI is recommended to identify the location of the lesion, as well as to determine if a loose body is present (**Figure 18.25**).

Treatment

OCD that is stable and does not have an associated loose body can be treated with rest and subsequent reevaluation of the lesion to ensure it has resolved. Persistence of the OCD despite prolonged rest warrants surgical intervention. Elbow arthroscopy to debride the lesion and remove any loose bodies is the mainstay of treatment. Depending on lesion size, stability, location, etc., microfracture or osseocartilaginous transplant may be performed in an attempt to "heal" the OCD lesion following the debridement.

Lateral Epicondylitis

Introduction

Some sports, such as racquet sports, may place additional stress on the lateral aspect of the elbow leading to lateral epicondylitis (tennis elbow) and/or apophysitis. Patients may, therefore, experience pain about the lateral epicondyle or just distal to it.

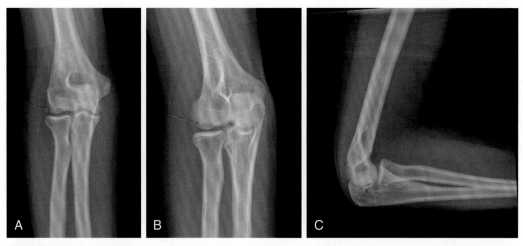

FIGURE 18.24 Radiographs of an elbow osteochondritis dissecans (OCD) in a 13-year-old female volleyball player. Note the lucency in the capitellum. A, Anteroposterior view, (B) oblique view, and (C) lateral view. (Courtesy of Joshua M. Abzug, MD.)

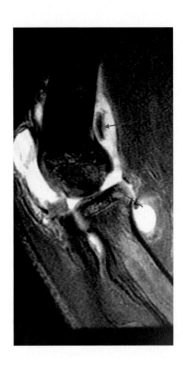

FIGURE 18.25 Lateral view of an elbow MRI of an osteochondritis dissecans (OCD) lesion of the capitellum (bottom arrow) and loose body entrapped in the joint space (top arrow). (Courtesy of Joshua M. Abzug, MD.)

History and Physical Examination

Physical examination should consist of an assessment of elbow range of motion. Patients commonly have tenderness to palpation about the lateral epicondyle or just distal to it. The examiner can also assess for inflammation in this region by resisting wrist extension, which reproduces the pain about the lateral epicondyle. Of note, medial apophysitis can be assessed for utilizing resisted wrist flexion to assess for pain about the medial epicondyle.

Differential Diagnosis

The differential diagnosis for lateral epicondylitis includes radial tunnel syndrome, fractures, and OCD lesions.

Diagnostic Tests and Advanced Imaging

Physical examination is often adequate to diagnose lateral epicondylitis; however, plain radiographs are often obtained to rule out an OCD lesion.

Treatment

Lateral epicondylitis is treated with rest from the inciting activity, anti-inflammatory medication, and physical/occupational therapy. Surgical intervention is typically not necessary in the pediatric and adolescent populations.

● Conclusion

There is a wide variety of diagnoses that occur in the child's elbow and forearm region that range from congenital differences to traumatic injuries. Knowledge of the development of the upper extremity as well as the normal anatomy will aid the examiner in correctly diagnosing the condition. Observation alone is always a critical part of any evaluation, followed by palpation and assessment of range of motion. Radiographs and advanced imaging are really utilized as confirmatory adjuncts to a good physical examination.

References

1. Bradbury ET, Hewison J. Early parental adjustment to visible congenital disfigurement. *Child Care Health Dev.* 1994;20(4):251-266.
2. Bristor MW. The birth of a handicapped child: a wholistic model for grieving. *Fam Relat.* 1984;33:25-32.
3. Morrey BF, Askew LJ, Chao EY. A biomechanical study of normal functional elbow motion. *J Bone Joint Surg Am.* 1981;63(6):872-877.
4. Dua K, Lancaster TP, Abzug JM. Age-dependent reliability of Semmes-Weinstein and 2-point discrimination tests in children. *J Pediatr Orthop.* 2019;39:98-103.
5. Alolabi B, Gray A, Ferreira LM, Johnson JA, Athwal GS, King GJ. Reconstruction of the coronoid process using the tip of the ipsilateral olecranon. *J Bone Joint Surg Am.* 2014;96(7):590-596.
6. Wegmann K, Knowles NK, Lalone EE, et al. The shape match of the olecranon tip for reconstruction of the coronoid process: influence of side and osteotomy angle. *J Shoulder Elbow Surg.* 2019;28(4):e117-e124.
7. Smith WR, Kozin SH, Zlotolow DA. Delayed treatment of a neonatal type-I Monteggia fracture-dislocation: a case report. *J Pediatr Orthop B.* 2018;27(2):142-146.

8. Tsai J. Congenital radioulnar synostosis. *Radiol Case Rep.* 2017;12(3):552-554.

9. Goldfarb CA. Congenital hand differences. *J Hand Surg Am.* 2009;34(7):1351-1356.

10. Richards C, Ramirez R, Kozin SH, Zlotolow DA. The effects of age on the outcomes of elbow release in arthrogryposis. *J Hand Surg Am.* 2019;44:898.e1-898.e6.

11. Edmond T, Laps A, Case AL, O'Hara N, Abzug JM. Normal ranges of upper extremity length, circumference, and rate of growth in the pediatric population. *Hand (N Y).* 2019. doi:10.1177/1558944718824706.

12. O'Driscoll SW, Spinner RJ, McKee MD, et al. Tardy posterolateral rotatory instability of the elbow due to cubitus varus. *J Bone Joint Surg Am.* 2001;83(9):1358-1369.

13. Murphey MD, Choi JJ, Kransdorf MJ, Flemming DJ, Gannon FH. Imaging of osteochondroma: variants and complications with radiologic-pathologic correlation. *Radiographics.* 2000;20(5):1407-1434.

14. Abzug JM, Mehlman CT, Ying J. Assessment of current epidemiological and risk factors surrounding brachial plexus birth palsy. *J Hand Surg Am.* 2018;1(1):e1-e10.

15. Al-Qattan MM, El-Sayed AA, Al-Zahrani AY, et al. Narakas classification of obstetric brachial plexus palsy revisited. *J Hand Surg Eur.* 2009;34(6):788-791.

16. Donohue KW, Little KJ, Gaughan JP, Kozin SH, Norton BD, Zlotolow DA. Comparison of ultrasound and MRI for the diagnosis of glenohumeral dysplasia in brachial plexus birth palsy. *J Bone Joint Surg Am.* 2017;99(2):123-132.

Hand and Wrist Problems

Roger Cornwall

● Introduction

The hand and wrist are the most frequently injured parts of a child's body,[1] and the hand is the second most common anatomic location for congenital anomalies.[2] Several features of the problems that occur in the hand and wrist make the physical examination a critical part of this evaluation. First, because of the development of the skeletal structures from cartilage to bone during childhood, injuries or abnormalities may not be readily apparent on conventional radiographs. Second, soft tissue injuries and disorders are quite common in the hand and frequently do not involve radiographic abnormalities that can aid in the diagnosis. Finally, decisions regarding treatment for many injuries and disorders are often based on physical examination findings rather than any other diagnostic testing.

The physical examination of the pediatric hand and wrist can be challenging. The regional anatomy is complex, and localization of pain and other symptoms can be challenging for young children to describe. Furthermore, several specific tests require patient participation in tasks that may be difficult to comprehend by a young child or painful to perform in an acutely injured hand. Therefore, it is quite helpful to have an armamentarium of passive tests and clinical signs that can be used to elucidate physical examination findings without relying on patient participation. This chapter will highlight such pearls, as it describes the physical examination of common traumatic and atraumatic conditions in the pediatric and adolescent hand and wrist.

● The Injured Wrist

Fractures at the distal end of the forearm are among the most common fractures in humans at any age.[3] The mechanism is typically a fall on an outstretched hand with resulting axial load on the hyperextended wrist. Occasionally, the load will occur on a flexed wrist, such as when gripping the handlebars of a bicycle. Additionally, twisting injuries to the forearm can produce fractures or soft tissue injuries. Many different types of fractures and injuries can result from these mechanisms, and the physical examination is a critical step in making the diagnosis and determining treatment.

Distal Radius Fractures

Incomplete fractures can occur as the malleable nature of pediatric bone can allow deformation of the cortex without complete fracture. Such fractures, referred to as buckle fractures, tend to be stable and can be successfully treated with symptomatic support only.[4] Despite this, careful evaluation is necessary to rule out severe injuries that require more definitive care.

Swelling and deformity may not be present, thus observation of the child is quite helpful. Does the child use the hand for bimanual tasks or when trying to climb onto the examination table? A wrist that is not painful at rest may become painful when force is applied to it, so the child will display a willingness to use the hand up to a certain amount of force. It is not uncommon for the child to present several days after the fracture when pain has persisted longer than the caregivers would have expected from a minor injury. Visual inspection can reveal deformity, even if the fracture is incomplete. When a child falls on an outstretched hand, if the wrist is extended during the injury, the wrist may appear extended. However, the volar apex of even substantial extension deformity (15°-20°) can be hidden by the abundant volar soft tissue around the wrist. Conversely, even subtle flexion of the bone may be readily apparent, as the dorsal apex of the deformity is not well hidden by the scant soft tissue coverage dorsally. Soft tissue injury is rare in the setting of a distal radius buckle fracture, but a thorough examination of the skin in the hand and upper extremity should be performed to rule out associated wounds from the fall.

Tenderness to palpation may only be present on the buckled side of the bone: dorsal in extended fractures and volar in flexed fractures. Circumferential tenderness should prompt concern for a physeal fracture of the distal radius. This injury requires proper orthopedic immobilization and follow-up rather than purely symptomatic treatment. In addition, tenderness should be assessed throughout the extremity, as distal radius buckle fractures can coexist with more proximal fractures, such as a supracondylar humerus fracture.

Complete fractures of the distal radius that do not involve the physis are also common and usually have greater degrees of swelling and deformity. Additionally, the child will be more reluctant to use the hand than in the case of an incomplete fracture. Complete distal radius fractures also commonly involve the distal ulna as well, so tenderness at the ulna is frequently present. In addition, wrist pain with rotation of the forearm is common, given the typical involvement of both forearm bones. A thorough soft tissue examination is important to rule out open fractures.

When a distal radius fracture is suspected, it is important to obtain an anteroposterior and lateral radiograph centered at the wrist. Radiographic images are generated from a single point source of radiation that spreads out as a cone shape through the tissue onto the film. Bone at the center of the film is accurately characterized by the perpendicular radiation; bone at the periphery is distorted by the oblique radiation. Sometimes forearm radiographs (which are focused on the forearm) must be obtained to locate the fracture, especially in young children who cannot locate the pain. However, a radiograph that is not centered at the level of the injury will not fully characterize the amount of displacement. As a result, angulation of a distal radius fracture may be underappreciated on radiographs of the entire forearm.

Key Point: It is important that the joints proximal and distal to a fracture are examined and radiographed as injuries at these areas are common and could be overlooked by the more displaced injury. Regardless, radiographic identification of any complete fracture of the distal radius and/or ulna requires orthopedic referral for further evaluation and definitive management.

Distal Radius Physeal Fractures

The physis of the distal radius is frequently injured, and displaced fractures have a 5% risk of causing a growth disturbance and potentially require corrective surgery.[5] Prompt identification of significantly displaced physeal injury is important to optimize outcome. Delay of reduction beyond 7 days can increase the risk of subsequent growth arrest, so prompt referral is of paramount importance.

A variable amount of swelling, visible volar ecchymosis, and deformity may indicate significant displacement of the physeal fracture. Less displaced fractures may not be initially swollen, and circumferential tenderness around the physis is the key physical examination finding especially in nondisplaced fractures with normal radiographs. Lister tubercle is a helpful landmark to locate the distal radius physis dorsally (**Figure 19.1**). Radiographs should be obtained in any child with tenderness around the growth plate. Referral to an orthopedic specialist is necessary even if the radiographs are normal.

Growth plate injuries at the radius may be a result of a high energy mechanism and thus vigilance is needed to detect other problems. Significant displacement can lead to open fracture of the radius or distal ulna and thus antibiotics and surgical treatment are needed to prevent infection. Any pinhole lesions that are adjacent to fracture are considered open until proven otherwise. A distal radius physeal fracture with substantial dorsal displacement can stretch or compress the median nerve as it enters the carpal tunnel; a compromised nerve should prompt emergent reduction of the fracture. Affected median nerves can have decreased sensation in the volar aspect of the thumb, index, middle, and radial side of the ring finger, as well as the radial aspect of the palm. While some of the intrinsic hand muscles

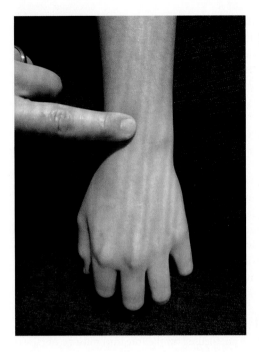

FIGURE 19.1 Depiction of the location of tenderness in a distal radius physeal fracture. Lister tubercle serves as a helpful landmark for the physis.

can be affected by median nerve injury, detection of abnormal sensation is more reliable. As with any wrist injury, the remainder of the upper limb should be examined for tenderness and ipsilateral injury.

Scaphoid Fractures

The scaphoid is the most commonly fractured carpal bone. Injuries typically occur in adolescents, with a peak incidence of 15 years,[6] and are quite rare in children under 10 years of age. Several complications can arise after fractures of the scaphoid; thus, proper alignment and healing are essential for long-term function of the wrist. To complicate matters, occult fractures may not be detected by radiographs for several weeks after the injury. Even when the diagnosis is made properly, proximal fractures rarely heal without surgery. More distal fractures heal in >90% of cases, but the average time to heal in this location is 9 weeks.[6] Finally, fractures of the scaphoid in adolescents frequently present as established nonunions where surgery and prolonged immobilization are required to achieve healing.

Any mechanism capable of causing a distal radius fracture can also cause a scaphoid fracture, so a scaphoid fracture should be on the differential diagnosis in such injuries. Swelling is rarely present and associated subcutaneous soft tissue injury is rare. The classic hallmark is tenderness in the anatomic snuffbox (**Figure 19.2**). It is important to differentiate between snuffbox tenderness and distal radius tenderness, because scaphoid and distal radius fractures can coexist. Have the patient actively extend the thumb to make the extensor pollicis longus and extensor pollicis brevis tendons prominent; the snuffbox sits in the hollow between these two tendons. Two additional pearls are helpful in differentiating between snuffbox and physeal tenderness. First, ask the patient which site is more tender. A scaphoid fracture is suspected if the snuffbox is more tender than the distal radius. Second, ask the patient "if you had to put a ball point pen dot on the spot that your wrist hurts the most, where would you put that dot?" Patients with scaphoid fractures typically point to the radial side of their wrist, whereas patients with distal radius fractures point to the dorsal side of their wrist.

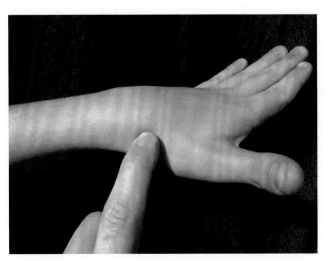

FIGURE 19.2 Depiction of the location of anatomic snuffbox tenderness in the setting of a scaphoid fracture. The snuffbox can be localized by asking the patient to actively extend the thumb, accentuating the extensor pollicis longus and brevis tendons that form the snuffbox.

These fractures typically are also tender at the distal pole of the scaphoid, which is palpable as a prominence at the radial side of the wrist flexion crease. Finally, scaphoid fractures typically cause radial-sided wrist pain with passive radial deviation of the wrist. **The presence of these three findings (snuffbox tenderness, scaphoid tubercle tenderness, and radial-sided wrist pain with passive radial deviation of the wrist) should raise concern for the provisional diagnosis of a scaphoid fracture until proven otherwise.**

Plain radiographs including a posteroanterior (PA), lateral wrist, and scaphoid view (PA radiograph in ulnar deviation) should be obtained. The latter view allows better identification of a fracture as ulnar deviation extends the scaphoid into view. Yet a fracture should still be suspected if the exam is positive and the radiographs are negative. At this point, the wrist can be immobilized with repeat radiographs obtained at weekly or bi-weekly intervals. However, only 85% of initially occult fractures have positive radiographs within 5 weeks of injury. Alternatively, magnetic resonance imaging (MRI) can be obtained, which will identify fractures within 24 hours of injury with high sensitivity.

Once the diagnosis of a scaphoid fracture is made, referral to an orthopedist is required and treatment may consist of cast immobilization until healed or surgery based upon location, the displacement, and the chronicity.

Triangular Fibrocartilage Complex Injuries

The triangular fibrocartilage complex (TFCC) cushions the articulation between the ulna and the carpus, and it stabilizes the articulation between the radius and the ulna via dorsal and volar radioulnar ligaments that originate from the base of the ulnar styloid and insert onto the dorsal and volar rim of the distal radius. Most injuries of the TFCC follow an acute injury[7] such as a hyper-twisting injury to the forearm, a fall or excessively forceful lifting. Additionally, TFCC tears can coexist with displaced distal radius fractures, especially when such fractures include a fracture of the ulnar styloid. Sometimes, a discrete injury is not known, and symptoms from a TFFC tear can appear insidiously.

Typically, patients with TFCC tears can very precisely localize pain on the ulnar side of the wrist, most focally in the soft spot just distal to the distal ulna (the ulnar fovea, **Figure 19.3**). Additionally, ulnar-sided wrist pain with active and/or passive forearm supination is quite specific for TFCC injuries. Other provocative test findings include ulnar-sided pain with gripping or with dorsal/volar translation of the distal radioulnar joint (DRUJ).[8]

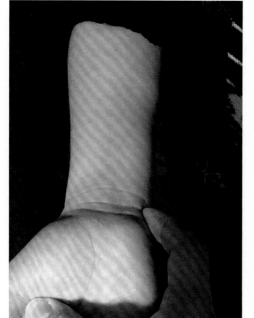

Radiographs of the wrist should be obtained to rule out injuries that can mimic or coexist with a TFCC tear, such as an ulnar styloid fracture or dorsal avulsion fracture from the triquetrum. MRI has relatively poor accuracy for diagnosing TFCC tears. Arthroscopic surgical evaluation of the TFCC is the only method for making a definitive diagnosis in the rare patient who does not heal with immobilization in a long arm cast (to prevent forearm rotation) and subsequent therapy.

Carpal Ligament Injuries

Injuries of the ligaments connecting the carpal bones are uncommon in children, although they can occur in adolescents from high-energy hyperextension

FIGURE 19.3 Depiction of the location of tenderness in the setting of a triangular fibrocartilage injury. Note that pain in this location is also made worse with active and/or passive supination.

injury. Two versions require specific mention as they can cause substantial loss of function: scapholunate interosseous ligament (SLIL) disruption and perilunate dislocation.[9]

The SLIL is a U-shaped array of fibers that connects the scaphoid and the lunate along their dorsal (primary stabilizer), proximal, and volar edges. Complete tearing of these fibers can cause separation of the scaphoid and lunate with progressive collapse of the carpus and subsequent arthritis. Two key physical exam features help to identify this injury and differentiate it from distal radius fractures and scaphoid fractures. First, patients will localize tenderness just distal to the distal radius. Second, the Watson test can elicit pain specific to SLIL injuries (▶ **Video 19.1**). In this test, pressure is placed with the thumb volarly on the distal pole of the scaphoid, and the wrist is passively radially deviated. This combination of forces applies stress to the SLIL. If the dorsal fibers of the SLIL are injured, the maneuver will cause dorsal wrist pain, even though no direct pressure is applied dorsally. If the SLIL is completely torn, the maneuver can subluxate the scaphoid and cause a painful clunk when pressure is relieved, akin to the Ortolani and Barlow maneuvers for hip dysplasia. Plain static radiographs are notoriously difficult to utilize in the pediatric wrist suspected of having a scapholunate ligament disruption.[1,10] Therefore, any clinical suspicion for an SLIL injury should prompt referral to a specialist for further evaluation.

Perilunate dislocations are severe ligamentous injuries to the wrist, typically occurring in adolescents from a high-energy injury involving wrist hyperextension. The short radiolunate ligament, which connects the volar rim of the radius to the volar pole of the lunate, is among the strongest ligaments in the wrist. Therefore, when the wrist is forcefully hyperextended, this ligament keeps the lunate secured against the radius while the remainder of the carpal bones dislocate dorsally around it. In the most severe case, the lunate is pushed volarly out of the radiocarpal joint where it can apply substantial pressure to the median nerve in the carpal tunnel. Unfortunately, due to the normally complex and overlapping anatomy of the carpal bones, these injuries can be missed initially on plain radiographs.

Adolescents with perilunate dislocations have pronounced swelling with limited and painful motion. Median nerve function may not be normal because of stretch of the nerve from the dislocation or pressure on the nerve from a displaced lunate. Proper early identification is important, because emergent reduction is required to relieve pressure on surrounding structures, especially the median nerve. Definitive treatment requires surgical stabilization of the carpus and repair or reconstruction of the torn intercarpal ligaments, along with release of the carpal tunnel when indicated. However, because of the severe nature of this injury, persistent stiffness and dysfunction can often follow appropriate treatment.

● The Injured Hand

Hand injuries are extremely common in children and adolescents.[1] Many hand injuries can heal reliably with minimal treatment and good outcomes, but several types of fractures and injuries can cause serious and permanent problems if not properly recognized or treated. The physical examination is critical in identifying these injuries, in some cases even radiographs are inconclusive. This section will describe the more common, and the particularly problematic, types of injuries in the hand and digits, focusing on the utility of the physical examination to identify and assess problematic injuries.

Metacarpal Fractures, Dislocations, and Ligament Injuries

The evaluation of the injured metacarpal region of the hand begins with a careful history, as the mechanism of injury can be helpful in assessing the risk of associated severe soft tissue problems.[11] Finger and metacarpal fractures commonly occur by axial loading, such as in a fall on a closed fist or in a punching injury. The boxer's fracture, or fracture of the small finger metacarpal neck, is one of the more common fractures (**Figure 19.4**). These injuries can include lacerations of the skin overlying the metacarpal head, damaging the extensor tendon and penetrating the metacarpophalangeal (MCP) joint. If the object punched is an opponent's tooth, oral bacteria can contaminate the MCP joint and lead to septic arthritis. Any full thickness skin injury over the metacarpal heads warrants radiographs to rule out an underlying open fracture. Ruling out joint penetration requires insufflation of the joint with sterile saline to

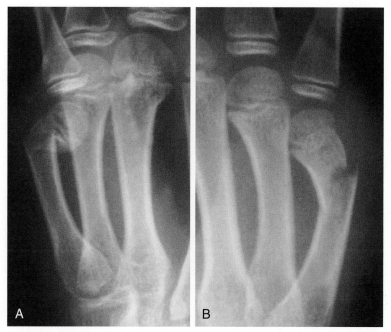

FIGURE 19.4 A, A true boxer's fracture of the metacarpal neck of the fifth ray. B, This fracture is more in the diaphysis and should not be considered a boxer's fracture.

(Waters PM, Skaggs DL, Flynn JM, Rockwood CA. Rockwood and Wilkins Fractures in Children. Philadelphia, PA: Wolters Kluwer; 2020.)

check for egress from the wound, a procedure best done in an emergency department by a qualified specialist. Ruling out extensor tendon injury can be difficult, as the tendon will retract proximal to the wound when the MCP joint is extended. Direct visualization of the tendon through the wound is typically required, again with proper anesthesia and sterile technique.

In young children, crush injuries to the metacarpal region, such as in a gate or industrial door, can cause multiple metacarpal fractures with severe associated soft tissue swelling. Such swelling can progress to compartment syndrome of the hand. The dorsal skin of the hand is very loose and dorsal swelling can be quite dramatic even without a compartment syndrome. However, the palmar skin is firmly anchored to the metacarpals with vertical fibrous septae, so substantial pressure is required to elevate the skin of the palm into a convex shape. **Therefore, swelling with a convex palm should raise suspicion for actual or impending compartment syndrome (Figure 19.5).** If a compartment syndrome is suspected or the child is at risk for developing one, referral to a specialist and inpatient admission may be warranted to allow close observation, as swelling can peak in the first 24 to 48 hours after injury. Immediate surgical compartment release, within 6 hours of the compartment syndrome, is required to prevent tissue necrosis and permanent dysfunction.

Beyond examining for associated soft tissue injuries, careful examination for rotational malalignment is critical, especially in the finger metacarpals. Only physical examination will reliably identify the rotational displacement as fractures may appear to be nondisplaced on radiographs. Flexion of the MCP joints will reveal overlapping of fingers when a severe rotational deformity is present (**Figure 19.6**). Comparing to the opposite hand is helpful to identify less significant malalignment seen as subtle convergence or divergence of fingers. In the young and/or apprehensive child, finger flexion can be achieved by passive extension of the wrist that generates tension in the finger flexor tendons. Pronating the forearm during this maneuver will add the force of gravity to the effect of tenodesis flexing the fingers, requiring the patient to actively extend the fingers to resist finger flexion.

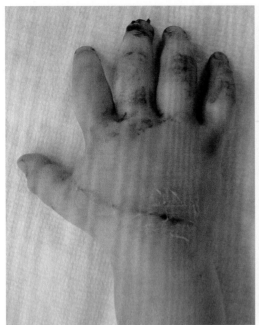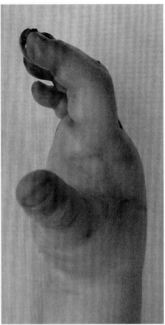

FIGURE 19.5 Swelling associated with compartment syndrome in the hand from a crush injury resulting in multiple metacarpal fractures in a 3-year-old child. Note the convexity of the palm.

Fractures at the base of the metacarpals can be associated with injuries of the carpometacarpal (CMC) joints. These dislocations or joint malalignments can be difficult to identify on plain radiographs because of the overlapping metacarpals and the arch of the carpus. On physical examination, dorsal prominence of the metacarpal bases can be seen and/or palpated. In the thumb, CMC dislocation can cause a swan neck deformity due to the compensatory hyperextension of the MCP joint. Any deformity noted in the region of the CMC joints should warrant additional imaging such as computed tomography to aid in treatment planning.

MCP dislocation is nearly always a dorsal dislocation. Physical examination for this injury is critical as it can be missed on radiographs. Because of the swelling that rapidly occurs dorsally, the injury may not be associated with obvious deformity other than resting hypertension of the digit (**Figure 19.7**). Palpation in the palm may identify a prominent metacarpal head, and even tented, puckered, or ischemic overlying skin. A neurologic examination is critical, as the dislocation can cause injury to the digital nerves stretched over the volarly

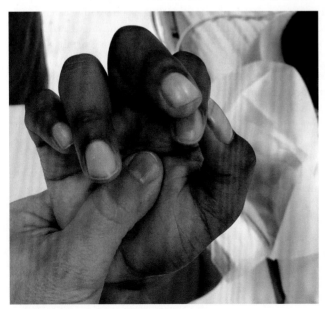

FIGURE 19.6 Rotational deformity resulting from a displaced middle finger metacarpal fracture. Note the overlapping of the middle and index fingers.

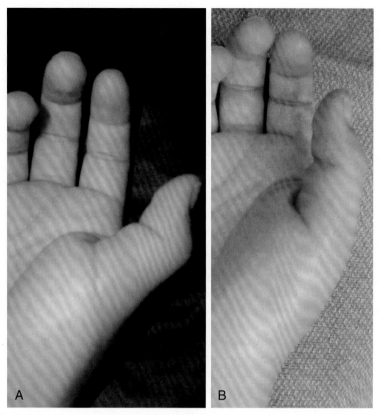

FIGURE 19.7 Typical clinical appearance of a thumb metacarpophalangeal joint dorsal dislocation. Note the subtle hyperextension deformity of the metacarpophalangeal joint (A) corrected after reduction (B).

prominent metacarpal head. Prompt reduction is required, emergently if neurologic compromise or skin ischemia is present; up to 50% of dislocations will require surgical reduction.

MCP ligament injuries of the thumb are also diagnosed clinically. Knowing the direction of displacement of the thumb can help to determine the injured structure. A pure hyperextension injury causes a volar plate rupture with volar tenderness and swelling throughout the thenar eminence. A radial deviation injury typically injures the ulnar collateral ligament, which tends to avulse from the insertion at the base of the proximal phalanx. The joint will be tender ulnarly and swelling will be present in the first web space. Passive radial deviation of the thumb in 30° of flexion will produce ulnar-sided pain and may reveal instability of the thumb when compared to the contralateral side. With sufficient displacement, the adductor aponeurosis may be interposed and the ulnar collateral ligament may be palpable beneath the skin in the first web space, the so-called Stener lesion. In adolescents, similar injuries may be seen as displaced, intra-articular avulsion fractures from the base of the proximal phalanx by the ulnar collateral ligament. Therefore, radiographs of injured thumb MCP joints are always warranted.

A hyperflexion or ulnar deviation injury of the thumb typically injures the radial collateral ligament, which typically avulses from the origin on the metacarpal head. Tenderness and focal swelling will be present at the dorsoradial aspect of the metacarpal head, and radial-sided pain will be reproduced with passive flexion and/or ulnar deviation. Fortunately, most thumb MCP ligament injuries are incomplete and can heal reliably with conservative management; operative treatment is reserved for a Stener lesion, substantial laxity, displaced fractures, or a failed conservative treatment.

The most important finger MCP collateral ligament is the radial collateral ligament of the index finger that resists force applied during pinch. **Since the collateral ligaments of the finger MCP joints** are lax in extension but taut in flexion, stability should be assessed by flexing the MCP joint maximally and applying deviation stress (▶ **Video 19.2**). Treatment of finger collateral ligament injuries typically involves protected early motion, as stiffness tends to be a more troublesome outcome than persistent instability, in contrast to the thumb MCP joint. Regardless of the ligament injured and the digit involved, radiographs should always be obtained, as intra-articular fractures at the origin or insertion of the collateral ligaments are typically more common than isolated ligament injuries in children and adolescents.

Phalanx Fractures, Dislocations, and Ligament Injuries

Phalanx fractures are among the most common injuries in children[12] and can cause permanent dysfunction if treatment is not appropriate and timely. All too often, patients with finger injuries will be brought for medical attention after several weeks when the "jammed" digit does not improve. Radiographs should be obtained if any deformity is present or delayed-onset ecchymosis (2-3 days later) occurs. Radiographs should be isolated to each injured finger with separate lateral radiographs of each finger, as overlapping fingers will hide subtle injuries.

Physical examination is important to supplement the findings of the radiographs; for instance, rotational deformity can be ascertained by physical examination as described previously (**Figure 19.8**). Additionally, coronal malalignment of a phalanx fracture may be more apparent on physical examination than on radiographs. Remodeling does occur in some phalangeal malunions when the deformity occurs in the plane of adjacent joint motion and if near the physis at the proximal end of the phalanges. Fractures at the distal end of the phalanges do not reliably remodel and tend to impede interphalangeal (IP) joint motion. To complicate matters, many periarticular fractures in the phalanges are unstable once reduced, so surgical stabilization techniques such as pin fixation are often required. Such surgeries are easier, safer, and more successful within the first 2 weeks of injury, so a strategy of waiting for several weeks to see if swelling will subside or motion will improve is fraught with peril.

A Seymour fracture is a physeal or periphyseal fracture of the distal phalanx with avulsion of the proximal end of the nail and the torn nailbed interposed in the fracture[13,14] (**Figure 19.9**). This injury constitutes an open fracture, with a risk of infection, growth arrest, and nail deformity if not immediately recognized and treated appropriately. There is often bleeding around the cuticle and there is

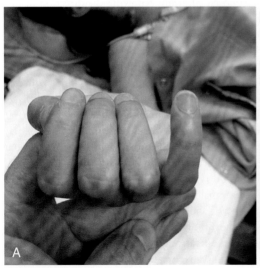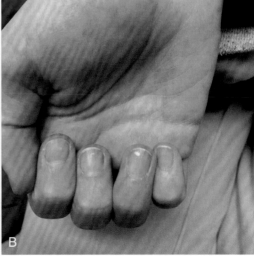

FIGURE 19.8 Rotational deformity resulting from a small finger proximal phalanx fracture (A) and ring finger middle phalanx fracture (B).

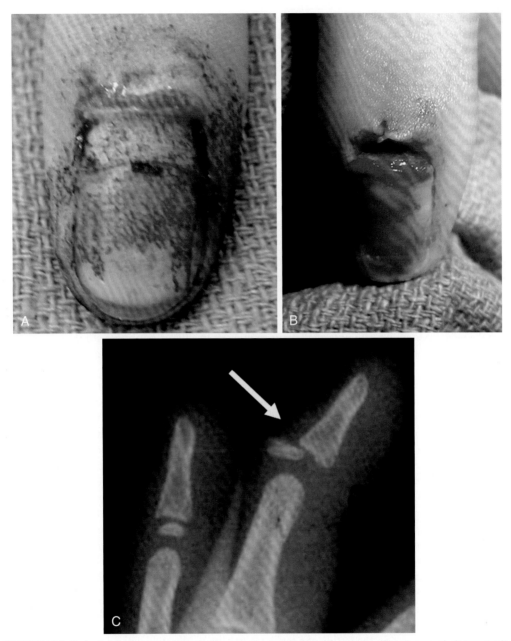

FIGURE 19.9 Typical clinical appearance of a Seymour fracture before (A) and after (B) nail removal, demonstrating the open physeal injury. Radiographic appearance of Seymour fracture (arrow) (C).

typically no subungual hematoma, since the blood that would have collected under the nail came out when the nail was avulsed. The only way to rule out an open Seymour fracture is to obtain adequate radiographs, including an isolated lateral of the injured digit, and to remove the nail to examine the nailbed. Irrigation and debridement of the fracture can prevent infection, which can occur within days if the injury pattern is missed. Infection, once allowed to form, almost universally causes a growth arrest of the distal phalanx, which in a young child can cause visible deformity. Therefore, any avulsed fingernail should be evaluated with radiographs before an attempt is made to simply reduce the nail.

Nailbed injuries can also occur with a fracture of the tuft of the distal phalanx.[15] The presence of a hematoma under an anatomically aligned nail with aligned skin does not warrant nail removal. Trephination of a subungual hematoma can be performed, but appropriate antibiotics should be given to prevent infection. Any displacement of the nail itself or of the fingertip skin suggests the presence of a displaced nailbed laceration that needs repair. Nailbed repair should be done by qualified individuals. Many complications of improperly repaired nailbeds can occur, some leading to permanent deformity.

Hand Soft Tissue Injuries

Closed tendon injuries can occur from an axial load, including a mallet finger, or rupture of the terminal extensor tendon. Conversely, traction on an actively flexing finger can cause a rupture of the flexor digitorum profundus tendon, or jersey finger. Tendon and nerve injuries in the setting of penetrating trauma usually require surgical repair. Diagnosis depends on understanding the mechanism of injury and an appropriate physical examination. Lacerations with a knife can involve lacerations of deep structures in line with the blade. Lacerations with broken glass involve more widespread damage to structures even distant from the skin injury. Lacerations from dog bites tend to involve substantial soft tissue damage from the shaking by the dog, while cat bites tend to deeply penetrate and inoculate deep compartments such as joints and flexor tendon sheaths.

Observation of the resting posture of the hand is the first step in evaluating for tendon disruption. With the wrist in extension, all joints of all digits should rest in a flexed position, with the most flexion in the small finger and the least in the index finger. The thumb should rest flexed at the MCP and IP joints.

The use of the tenodesis test to provide tension on the flexor and extensor tendons is very helpful for children who cannot follow directions. Passively extending the wrist should cause flexion of all digits, as does squeezing the volar compartment of the mid forearm. If any joint of any digit rests in an extended position with the wrist extended, discontinuity of the tendon that flexes that joint should be suspected (**Figure 19.10**). Similarly, passive wrist flexion should produce digit extension. One must consider the possibility of an extensor tendon injury if any joint droops during an attempt to extend the digit against gravity, or when the examiner passively flexes the wrist to extend the fingers. The extensor tendons to the middle, ring, and small fingers are interconnected over the metacarpals, so an injury to any of these tendons may only produce a slight extensor lag or droop at the MCP joint (**Figure 19.11**).

If the patient is able to comply with instructions, ask the patient to activate each tendon individually against resistance. Absence of joint motion with muscle activation implies complete tendon rupture, whereas pain with resisted activation implies partial tendon injury (or underlying associated bone injury—radiographs should be obtained). If a patient is unable to move any joint distal to a penetrating injury, a tendon or nerve injury should be assumed until proven otherwise.

Nerve injury should be specifically ruled out in the setting of penetrating trauma. It is important to remember that young children do not complain of numbness. However, a child will not use a numb part of the hand. For instance, in the setting of a median nerve injury, the child will nearly instantly develop grasp patterns using the small and ring fingers, avoiding the use of the thumb, index, and middle fingers (**Figure 19.12**). Second, wrinkling of the skin in water depends on intact sensory nerve function; after a laceration to a digital nerve, that nerve's side of the fingertip will not wrinkle, whereas the intact side will (**Figure 19.13**). Finally, the skin of a numb finger will be dry at rest with abnormal moisture and sweat pattern. Similar tricks exist for discerning motor nerve function. For instance, if children are asked to cross their fingers (which tests finger adduction—ulnar nerve motor function) and they cannot do so actively, they will reach over with their opposite hand to do so passively. A sticker placed on the small fingertip will promote thumb opposition to the small finger. A sticker placed on the thumbnail or fingernail will promote thumb or finger extension. A sticker placed on the hypothenar eminence will promote supination.

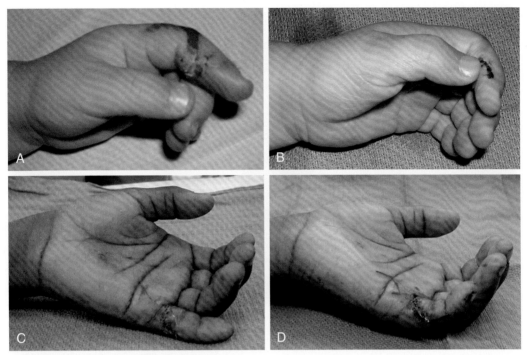

FIGURE 19.10 Altered cascade of finger flexion from flexor tendon injuries. Index finger with resting extended posture of the distal interphalangeal joint indicating flexor digitorum profundus injury (A), with flexion restored after tendon repair (B). Small finger with resting extended posture of proximal and distal interphalangeal joints indicating laceration of the flexor digitorum profundus and superficialis tendons (C), with restored flexion after repair (D).

Overall, the rarity of tendon and nerve injuries in the child's hand can lead to failure to include these injuries on the differential diagnosis of hand complaints. When in any doubt, immediate referral to a hand specialist is advisable. Tendon and nerve repairs achieve optimal outcomes if performed acutely, and delay of repairs beyond 2 weeks from injury frequently requires secondary salvage procedures.

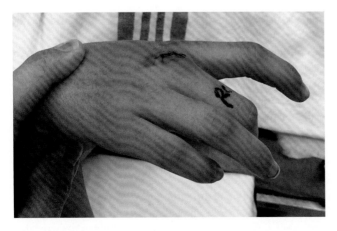

FIGURE 19.11 Extensor lag resulting from extensor digitorum communis tendon laceration in the middle finger. Note the persistent flexion despite using passive wrist flexion to induce finger extension through tenodesis.

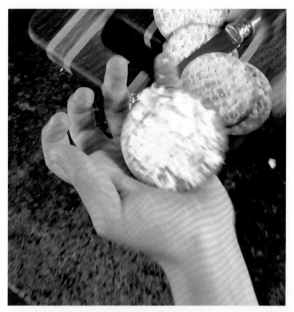

FIGURE 19.12 Altered prehension pattern following median nerve injury. Note the avoidance of the radial side of the hand due to numbness in the median nerve distribution.

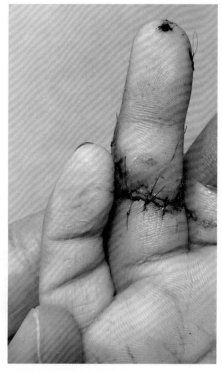

FIGURE 19.13 Lack of wrinkling in the ring finger tip (compared to the small finger tip) due to digital nerve laceration in the ring finger. Also note the resting extended posture of the ring finger distal interphalangeal joint due to laceration of the flexor digitorum profundus tendon.

● The Deformed Wrist

Deformity of the wrist can be noted at birth in association with congenital anomalies or appear later due to atypical development or growth. Eliciting a good history, including during pregnancy and peripartum, is helpful in understanding the cause of deformity. The physical examination is important to help understand how the child is functioning and what compensatory mechanisms are in place for functional tasks. Radiographs are essential for understanding the pathology leading to deformity and will guide the clinician toward optimal treatment for these conditions. Most patients with an acquired or congenital deformity of the wrist should be evaluated by a qualified pediatric orthopedic or upper extremity specialist, so that a correct diagnosis can be made, along with the prescription of an appropriate treatment plan and ordering of ancillary tests to evaluate for potentially morbid coexisting pathology.

Post-Traumatic Deformity

The most common deformities of the wrist result from previous trauma, and any history of injury (even minor) and treatment should be obtained, along with injury radiographs. Post-traumatic deformity can be due to malunion or physeal arrest of the distal radius or distal ulna. Children have a great remodeling potential at the distal radius and ulna, but this decreases closer to skeletal maturity and persistent deformity is possible despite initial remodeling. Although physeal arrest in the distal radius has a low incidence (1%-7%) following physeal fracture,[5] patients should be screened for at least 3 to 6 months following injury to ensure that normal growth has returned.

For most patients with post-traumatic wrist deformity, the main complaint is likely to be deformity and bony prominence. Sagittal plane deformity may be hidden in extension and more prominent in flexion as noted in the wrist fracture section above. Loss of motion of the wrist (flexion/extension) and forearm rotation are commonly reported with deformity of the distal radius. If present, the exact location of pain is helpful in determining the pathology present, as ulnar abutment will cause pain centrally in the wrist due to edema within the lunate, while TFCC injuries or DRUJ instability will lead to ulnar-sided wrist pain.

On examination, the entire arc of motion of the wrist should be assessed, including forearm pronation and supination and wrist flexion, extension, radial and ulnar deviation. Any patient that has volar DRUJ instability[16,17] in supination most likely has an apex volar malunion of the radius (▶ **Video 19.3**). Additionally, loss of radial inclination of the wrist leads to prominence of the ulnar head, and excessive sagittal plane deformity of the distal radius can lead to an alteration of wrist range of motion and adaptive carpal instability patterns.[18] Maximum power grip is obtained between neutral and 15° of wrist extension and between neutral and 15° of ulnar deviation[19] and loss of radial inclination or increasing volar tilt can lead to weakness of wrist and hand function.

Standard AP and lateral radiographs of the wrist are important in the setting of deformity, as they most often will illuminate the diagnosis. Distal radius physeal arrest may lead to angular deformity or ulnar positive variance (radius is short compared to the ulna) and possible ulnar impaction into the carpus. An MRI is useful to help determine how much physeal arrest is present and can guide treatment for osteotomy or physeal bar excision in the younger patient. CT is valuable for patients with deformity and pain from intra-articular malunions of the distal radius or DRUJ. In patients with central and ulnar wrist pain, an MRI can help to determine if a TFCC injury is present versus ulnar impaction. Treatment of these conditions requires referral to a pediatric orthopedic or hand surgery specialist.

Congenital Deformity

Congenital deformity of the wrist is typically apparent at birth[2] and a detailed history is helpful for assessing these deformities. Radiographic evaluation of the elbow, forearm, wrist, and hand is imperative for patients with congenital deformity, as the entire limb must be evaluated prior to initiating treatment. Careful examination of the entire upper extremity is vitally important for a thorough understanding of the patient's condition and its impact on function.

In a patient with radial longitudinal deficiency (**Figure 19.14**), his or her wrist will have good function in flexion and radial deviation, but often have limited wrist extension. In patients with an absent radius, the ulnar length can be up to 60% shorter than the unaffected ulna. This length discrepancy (as defined by a percentage of the unaffected side) remains stable during growth, but the absolute length difference will continue to expand until skeletal maturity. Functional testing in patients with congenital wrist deformity should be performed, with various tests used in the literature.[20] Some of these patients will additionally have limited elbow flexion, such that their wrist flexion and radial deviation allow for them to reach their head to their mouth with the affected extremity. Correction of the wrist by centralization, without assessing their loss of elbow flexion, will place the wrist and hand away from their head and mouth and decrease functional use of the arm. Additionally, patients with severe radial longitudinal deficiency can have hypoplasia of the glenohumeral joint and musculature, which consequently

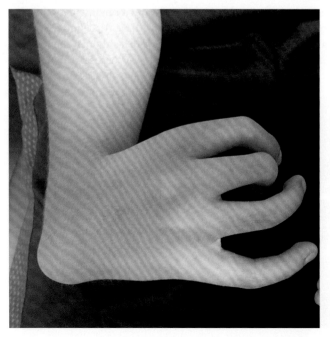

FIGURE 19.14 Radially deviated wrist posture in an adolescent with untreated severe radial longitudinal deficiency (absence of radius). Also note the absence of the thumb.

limits the overall use of the entire upper limb. Thumb hypoplasia and web space deficiency are frequently seen in patients with radial longitudinal deficiency. Conversely, patients with the much less common ulnar longitudinal deficiency can have hypoplasia of the ulnar digits.[21] Patients with ulnar longitudinal deficiency may have a radiohumeral synostosis, which can be malrotated up to 180°, or an unstable, hypoplastic elbow with limited function. The passive and active motion of the wrist in flexion/extension and pronation/supination should be evaluated, as well as hand function, especially of the thumb and index fingers.

Congenital radioulnar synostosis is commonly diagnosed around age 3 to 5 in children who have difficulty with supination tasks such as hygiene and sports. Although forearm rotation is completely absent, patients develop compensatory pronation and supination through the carpus, which may fool the examiner (▶ **Video 19.4**).

In patients with congenital wrist deformity, further testing is required to evaluate for potentially morbid associated conditions. Radial longitudinal deficiency is associated with Holt-Oram syndrome (congenital heart defects and conduction deficits), thrombocytopenia absent radius syndrome (completely absent radius with thrombocytopenia at birth), Fanconi anemia (disorders of bone marrow, including agenesis of red and white blood cells between 5 and 10 years of age, as well as increased risk of acute myeloid leukemia), VACTERL association (vertebral anomalies, anal atresia, cardiac abnormalities, tracheoesophageal fistula, renal agenesis, and limb defects), and spinal anomalies (vertebral segmental deficits and scoliosis). As such, patients with radial deficiency should have screening tests for all these diseases, including an echocardiogram, renal ultrasound, complete blood count, spine radiographs, and chromosomal breakage analysis. We often find that a referral to a pediatric geneticist is helpful to coordinate and manage the testing for associated anomalies. Patients with ulnar longitudinal deficiency often have associated skeletal abnormalities, with fewer associated organ deficits. In these patients, a skeletal survey is often helpful in evaluating for spinal vertebral segmental anomalies and lower extremity deficiency such as fibular hemimelia and proximal focal femoral deficiency.

Developmental Deformities

Developmental deformities are diagnosed as the child ages. In most cases, such as in Madelung deformity or with multiple hereditary exostosis (MHE) syndrome (**Figure 19.15**), the deformity will progress slowly until skeletal maturity, at which point it will become stable. Appropriate diagnosis and treatment of these developmental deformities of the wrist rely on a thorough history and a careful physical examination. There is a positive family history associated with many patients that have Madelung deformity (female relatives) and autosomal dominant multiple hereditary exostosis (MHE), although spontaneous genetic mutations can occur. Additionally, the birth and perinatal history can be useful to diagnose postinfectious physeal arrest of the radius or ulna, or previous neonatal compartment syndrome, which can lead to progressive deformity due to decreased and asymmetric growth.

Patients with Madelung deformity are most commonly females who present between the ages of 10

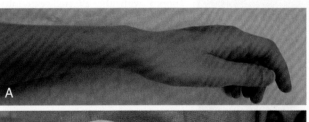
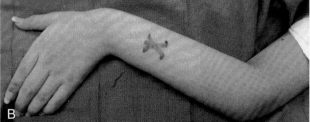

FIGURE 19.15 Developmental deformity of the wrist from (A) Madelung deformity with the typical volarly translated carpus and dorsally prominent ulna and (B) multiple hereditary exostosis syndrome causing impaired growth of the distal ulna and resulting radius deformity and severe ulnar deviation of the wrist.

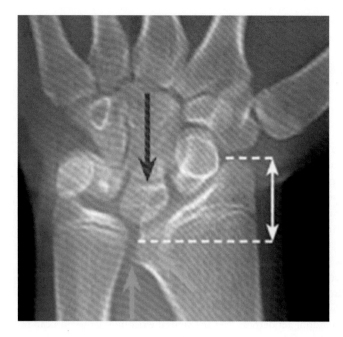

FIGURE 19.16 Madelung deformity. There is lucency and premature fusion (orange) at the locus of growth disturbance, triangular distortion of the distal epiphysis, and pyramidalization (red) of the wrist as it sinks into the defect, with the apex at the lunate. Distal radial height is increased (white) by retardation of ulnar growth (normal 12-15 mm). Interosseous space is widened, into which lunate may be displaced. Vickers ligament attaches immediately distal to the osteophyte arising from the ulnar aspect of the distal metaphysis of radius (green).
(From Diab M, Staheli LT. Practice of Paediatric Orthopaedics. 3rd ed. Philadelphia, PA: Wolters Kluwer, 2015.)

and 14 years of age with bowing of the radius and shortening of forearm length.[22] The wrist is typically volarly subluxated, leaving a prominent distal ulna with ulnar deviation of the hand. They typically have a loss of wrist extension and forearm supination and may have pain with weightbearing in wrist extension. Radiographs of the wrist reveal that the distal radius physis has a characteristic "flame" pattern along the volar/ulnar metaphysis due to the origin of a pathologically enlarged short radiolunate ligament (Vickers ligament), which tethers growth of the wrist (**Figure 19.16**). The carpal bones are pulled into a triangular pattern due to the increased radial inclination of the wrist and there is often significant ulnar positive variance with a dorsally prominent distal ulna. The forearm may be shortened with excessive bowing of the radius, with maintained radiocapitellar alignment at the elbow. MRI can be used to assess the distal radius physis and Vickers ligament, although this does not typically guide treatment, as the deformity is managed through radiographic measurements.

In patients with MHE, the physical examination reveals multiple prominent benign tumors (called exostoses or osteochondromas) about the hands, wrists, and other long bones in the body.[23] The tumors about the wrist can be prominent due to the lack of muscle at this level, and they may limit or block forearm rotation. The exostoses can be painful if bumped and may cause symptoms of nerve compression if the median and/or ulnar nerves are in close proximity. In some patients, the growth of the distal ulna is slowed leading to ulnar deviation of the hand. Over the long term, this growth discrepancy may tether and bow the radius, potentially leading to dislocation of the radial head at the elbow. Forearm, wrist, and hand radiographs are helpful in diagnosing and treating patients with MHE. Many exostoses can be characterized in one of two varieties; the pedunculated type look like cauliflower with a thin stalk whereas the sessile variety have a broad base connecting them to the affected bone.

Patients with wrist deformity due to infection or vascular compromise leading to growth arrest will have angular deviation of the wrist toward the affected bone. In patients with significant length discrepancy between the bones, limited forearm rotation will be present, although they typically maintain near normal wrist range of motion and finger function as long as the forearm muscles were not affected at the time of injury.

Most patients with developmental wrist deformity are treated based on symptoms and functional deficits. For Madelung patients near skeletal maturity, consideration for osteotomy of the distal radius and ulnar shortening osteotomy is given based on symptoms. Madelung patients with more than 2 to

3 years of skeletal growth remaining can undergo Vickers ligament excision along with physiolysis to halt progression of the deformity. Symptomatic treatment is also recommended for patients with MHE; large, symptomatic osteochondromas warrant surgical excision. Ulnar lengthening may be performed to decrease the tethering to growth caused by a shortened ulna and may prevent ultimate radiocapitellar dislocation.

Adolescent Onset Wrist Pain

Atraumatic wrist pain is common in females between the ages of 12 and 16 years[24] and physical examination can frequently provide the correct diagnosis and guide appropriate treatment. When evaluating these wrists, special attention should be given to inspection, palpation, range of motion, and provocative tests. Carpal ganglions are frequently associated with wrist pain and typically present with a large tender mass over the central dorsal wrist, accentuated by wrist flexion, or over the volar/radial wrist accentuated by wrist extension. Ganglions will transilluminate when light is shone through them in a darkened examination room.

Tenderness and swelling over the first dorsal synovial compartment of the wrist is a sign of DeQuervain tenosynovitis. In this disorder, the Finkelstein test will be positive as radial wrist pain is produced when patients grasp their thumb in their palm and ulnarly deviate their wrist. Other common sites of tendonitis will have tenderness over the extensor carpi ulnaris tendon (most ulnar dorsal tendon at the wrist level) or flexor carpi ulnaris tendon. Tenderness over the central wrist in wrist flexion can be a sign of Keinböck disease (avascular necrosis of the lunate) (**Figure 19.17**).

A midcarpal shift test can be used to diagnose symptomatic ligamentous laxity of the wrist. The examiner grasps the patient's hand and metacarpals with one hand and the distal radius with the other hand. A positive test is marked by a feeling of joint subluxation and relocation when the wrist is volarly flexed, then ulnary deviated while bringing the wrist back to neutral. The Watson test and TFCC provocative testing described above are also useful to help diagnose ligamentous injuries in the wrist.

When the diagnosis is not confirmed on physical examination, radiographs can be obtained to assess abnormal ulnar variance or signs of avascular necrosis of the lunate. Ultrasound can be used to diagnose ganglions that do not easily transilluminate. Tendinopathies are best treated with early immobilization and anti-inflammatory medications, followed by progressive motion and strengthening as tolerated. Wrist ganglions may be observed until they are large enough to cause significant discomfort or loss of motion, then may be aspirated (50%-60% or greater recurrence rate) or surgically removed (20% recurrence rate) depending on symptomatology.[25] Patients with ligamentous laxity and vague wrist pain frequently benefit from occupational therapy in 85% to 90% of cases. Referral is indicated in those patients that do not improve their pain or who do have a specific diagnosis.

● The Deformed Hand

Hand/finger deformities are the second most common congenital anomalies to cardiac deformities and are

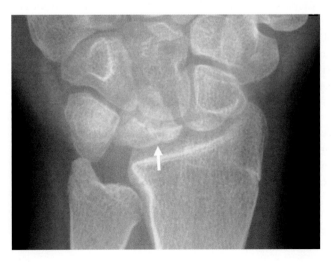

FIGURE 19.17 Posteroanterior radiographs demonstrating Kienbock disease or avascular necrosis of the lunate. Note sclerosis and collapse of the lunate (arrow).

commonly seen by pediatric upper extremity specialists. Post-traumatic deformity is also commonly seen. Many of deformities limit function of the hand and fingers and early evaluation and treatment are important in order to maximize use of the hand.

Post-Traumatic Hand Deformity

With hand and finger deformities in the setting of remote trauma, a careful history detailing the mechanism of injury, initial and subsequent treatment, and current symptomatology should be obtained. On examination, the skin and soft tissues should be assessed for scars from previous injuries or swelling and edema. The active and passive motion should be assessed and compared to the unaffected side. A large discrepancy between the active and passive motion of a digit implies that tendon adhesions or unrepaired tendon lacerations exist. For instance, patients with no active flexion of the DIP (distal interphalangeal) joint of a digit, but full passive motion, likely have a missed flexor digitorum profundus tendon injury. Deformity and malunion of the metacarpals and phalanges can also result in an extensor lag at a distal joint due to shortening of the bone, which relatively lengthens the tendon. Provocative testing for the digits (described above) should be performed as well to assess for specific injuries to the fingers that may have been undiagnosed. Dedicated radiographs of the affected digit are obtained for phalangeal deformity, and AP, lateral, and oblique radiographs are obtained for metacarpal or hand deformities. Ultrasound has been proven useful for the evaluation of flexor and extensor tendon injuries and does not typically require sedation in pediatric patients.

Treatment for malunion is indicated in patients with limited remodeling potential (coronal plane or malrotation deformity) and functional losses. Patients that meet criteria for surgical intervention from phalangeal or digital malunion most often benefit from corrective osteotomy. In the phalanges, this is complicated by the location of the deformity and the proximity of the tendons and neurovascular bundles to the site of potential osteotomy. Malunions of the phalangeal neck or condyles (**Figure 19.18**) should not have corrective osteotomy of the distal aspect of the phalanx, as this can lead to a loss of blood supply to the head of the phalanx and avascular necrosis. The difficulty in treating such deformities as established malunions underscores the importance of identifying and promptly treating acute injuries.

Congenital Hand Deformity

Congenital hand anomalies are found in approximately 2 per 1000 live births in the United States.[2]

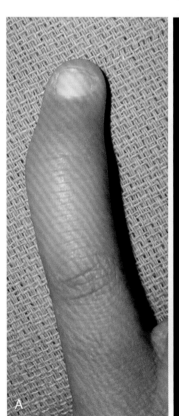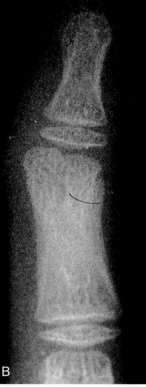

FIGURE 19.18 Permanent post-traumatic deformity resulting from untreated intra-articular fracture of the middle phalanx.

Additional morbidity can be seen in infants with congenital anomalies of the hand, due to systemic syndromes or associated malformation of the heart, kidney, or tracheoesophageal system. A family history of a similar malformation may be seen in many hand deformities and should be fully assessed. Although many hand deformities share common presumed underlying mechanisms of abnormal development, they have different physical examination findings. All patients with congenital hand anomalies should be referred to a pediatric upper extremity specialist for evaluation and possible surgical treatment.

Thumb Hypoplasia

Thumb hypoplasia occurs as a component of radial longitudinal deficiency and has similar syndromic associations that must be evaluated prior to any interventions.[26] These associations were highlighted earlier in the chapter in the section on wrist deformity. Half of children with thumb hypoplasia will have bilateral involvement, which may be asymmetric and even asymptomatic. Thumb hypoplasia can range from a small but normally functioning thumb, to severe deformity and instability of the CMC joint, to a floating thumb or complete thumb absence. Thumb function decreases with increasing severity of disease, and most patients without a stable CMC joint do not use their thumb for any function.

Determining the severity of thumb hypoplasia is the crux of the physical examination for these patients (**Figure 19.19**). Inspection of the hand should assess for thenar muscle bulk bilaterally and assess thumb/index web space pliability. Often, children with a narrowed web space will abduct their thumb through the unstable MCP joint in order to grasp larger objects. Collateral ligament stability should be assessed in radial and ulnar deviation, flexion and extension, and dorsal and volar translation. The function of the extensor and flexor pollicis longus muscles should be assessed as well, often using stickers or tenodesis for assistance in young children. The presence or absence of wrist deformity should be assessed as well. Children should be observed for using their hand for grasping and pinching simple objects such as a sticker or pen, to see if they have developed a cortical representation of their thumb as a useful digit. If not, most patients will use their index finger to grasp and pinch, which in turn, will pronate and diverge to give a better web space and function. This is termed autopollicization and is a sign that their thumb is unstable and not useful for reconstruction. In patients with an absent thumb, assessment of the index finger may reveal

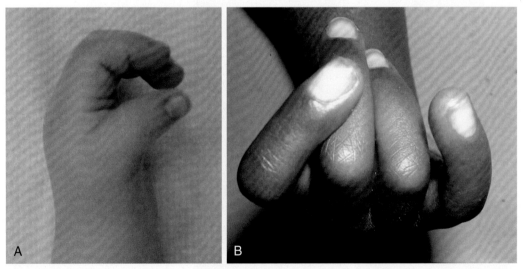

FIGURE 19.19 Thumb hypoplasia. A, Mild hypoplasia with underdeveloped thenar musculature and radial deviation of the unstable metacarpophalangeal joint. B, Congenital absence of the thumb and resulting autopollicization of the index finger and cortical recognition of the index finger in place of the thumb.

hypoplasia, stiffness, and even index/middle finger syndactyly. In these patients with limited radial finger function, the small finger may undergo autopollicization and is the patient's primary finger for pinching and grasping objects.

Radiographs of the hand including AP, lateral, and oblique views are useful to assess the underlying bone quality with particular focus on the CMC joint. Patients with hypoplastic thumbs may require reconstructive surgery to augment their thumb function. In mild cases with minimal hypoplasia, a stable MCP joint, normal first web space, and some thenar muscle function, reconstruction is not typically indicated. Patients that do not have a stable CMC joint and do not use their thumb for any function typically benefit from thumb ablation and pollicization of the index finger, wherein the index finger is surgically moved into the thumb position.

Syndactyly

Syndactyly, or fusion between adjacent fingers, occurs in two to three per 10,000 live births. Bilateral involvement is seen in 50% of patients, and many heritable forms are known, most of which are transmitted in an autosomal dominant fashion.[2,26] Syndactyly is associated with other skeletal abnormalities, including cleft hand, symbrachydactyly, synpolydactyly, and amniotic band syndrome, as well as with genetic syndromes. Acrocephalosyndactyly patients have craniosynostosis, midface hypoplasia, and a typical complex syndactyly that affects all five digits. Acrocephalopolysyndactyly syndrome patients have craniosynostosis, syndactyly, and preaxial polydactyly (detailed below). Patients with oculodentodigital dysplasia will have ring/small finger syndactyly as well as optic nerve hypoplasia, poor dentition with small teeth, and a narrow midface.

The physical examination aids in the classification of syndactyly (**Figure 19.20**). The normal web space runs halfway from the MCP joint to the PIP (proximal interphalangeal) joint on the volar surface of the hand. Any web space skin more distal than this, but less than the whole length of the finger is considered a partial syndactyly. A complete syndactyly has skin connection all the way to the tip of the fingers. Simple syndactyly has only skin and soft tissue connection between the digits, while a complex syndactyly has a bony connection. Patients with skeletal fusion at the distal phalanx often have a single nail plate over both fingers, known as a synonychia. More complicated bony fusion between fingers can limit finger motion. Over time, patients with syndactyly between digits of unequal length (thumb/index and ring/small fingers) may develop a deformity of the digits due to tethering of growth. Any patient with syndactyly and loss of digital motion or a synonychia should have a hand PA and lateral radiograph to evaluate for a complex syndactyly, synpolydactyly, or other skeletal manifestation. Advanced imaging is very rarely indicated.

Treatment in children with syndactyly is geared toward improving hand function by increasing independent finger function. Simple syndactyly release is commonly performed between 2 and 4 years of age, which decreases the risk of web space creep and complications from surgery. Early syndactyly release (<1 year of age) is performed in patients with a potential for tethered growth or to allow for independent thumb motion and function. Prompt referral to a specialist will help in appropriate timing of treatment and evaluation of other disorders.

Polydactyly

Another common congenital malformation of the hand is polydactyly, which is subdivided into preaxial (thumb), central, and postaxial (small finger) types.[26] Postaxial polydactyly is the most common subtype, being found in one in 300 patients of African descent where it is often seen in an autosomal dominant inheritance pattern (**Figure 19.21**). Preaxial polydactyly is less common and is frequently seen as an isolated genetic malformation. A better term for thumb polydactyly or thumb duplication is a split thumb, since the normal thumb is split into unequal parts, leaving neither thumb normal.

The classification and treatment protocols are guided by the physical examination and radiographic findings. For preaxial polydactyly, the level of the duplication should be assessed (**Figure 19.22**), as well as the active and passive joint motion of all the affected and unaffected joints. Typically, the radial digit

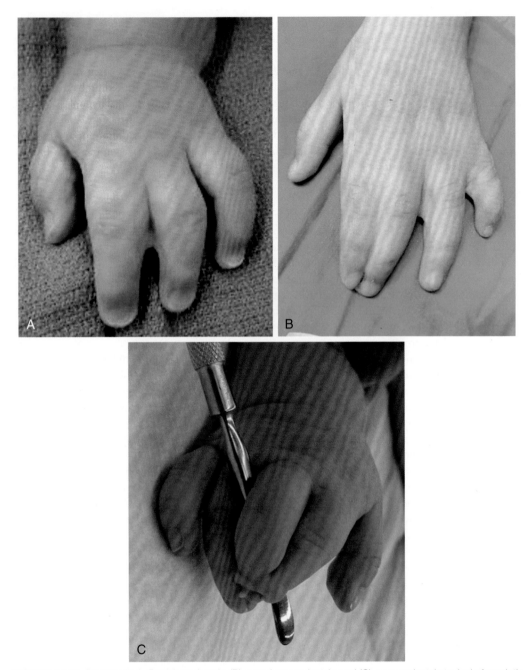

FIGURE 19.20 Syndactyly. A, Partial syndactyly, (B) complete syndactyly, and (C) acrosyndactyly typical of amniotic band syndrome.

is hypoplastic with limited function of any duplicated joints. Occasionally, duplications at the MCP joint will cause a diamond deformity of the thumb with divergent proximal phalanges and convergent distal phalanges. In postaxial polydactyly, the supernumerary digit is either well formed with a stable base (type A) or a small floating digit attached with a thin stalk of skin (type B). Finger radiographs should be obtained for all digits to fully evaluate the skeletal manifestations of the polydactyly and to guide treatment.

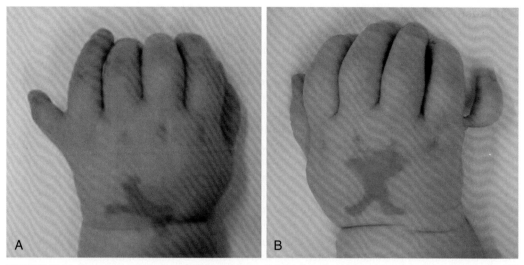

FIGURE 19.21 Postaxial polydactyly with (A) a well-formed digit articulating at the metacarpophalangeal joint and (B) a nubbin suspended only by a neurovascular pedicle and skin bridge.

Preaxial polydactyly is most often treated with ablation of the more hypoplastic thumb and reconstruction of the remaining thumb using skin, ligaments, and the nail fold from the hypoplastic digit. Osteotomies are performed to align the thumb joints perpendicular to the axis of the thumb, and the tendons are assessed to ensure that they are centrally located on the digit. In postaxial polydactyly type B, the radial digit may be amputated in the nursery using suture ligation, hemoclips, or bipolar electrocautery, although complications such as pain, neuroma formation, and cracked skin may develop. Surgical removal should be performed in patients with a type A postaxial polydactyly or a type B with a wide stalk.

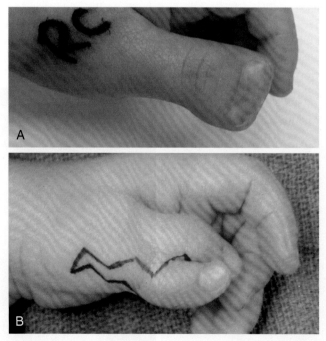

FIGURE 19.22 Preaxial polydactyly involving duplication of the distal phalanx (A) and duplication of the distal and proximal phalanges (B).

Symbrachydactyly/Cleft Hand

Central deficiency of the hand can present in two distinct patterns with different underlying mechanisms and presentations. Symbrachydactyly, which describes short, webbed fingers, presents as hypoplasia or absence of the central digits, often with preservation of one or both of the border digits. Symbrachydactyly is a sporadic anomaly thought to be caused by a vascular event during limb formation.[27] Cleft hand, also known as ectrodactyly, is a central deficiency of the hand, which can be associated with thumb/index syndactyly.[26] Bilateral cleft hand is often seen in association with bilateral cleft feet, which has autosomal dominant inheritance with variable penetrance.

The physical examination is used to differentiate between these two central deficiency syndromes (**Figure 19.23**). Patients with symbrachydactyly have a U-shaped or rounded central deficiency. In milder forms, they may have shortened central digits with absent middle phalanges and syndactyly between the digits. In more severe presentations, there may be hypoplasia or agenesis of all the digits, without any suitable finger function. Patients with cleft hand have a V-shaped or sharper central deficiency, often combined with thumb/index syndactyly or other digital malformations.

Most patients with symbrachydactyly function quite well and are, on average, happier than the average child. Surgical treatment is limited to syndactyly release to promote individual finger function or corrective surgery to allow for improved pinch or grasp. Cleft hand patients also function quite well, although surgical correction is indicated in certain patients. Prior to any surgical intervention, a thorough discussion with the family and occupational therapist should be undertaken to ensure that any intervention has sufficient benefit, either functionally or cosmetically, to be worth the risks of surgery.

Developmental Hand Deformity

Hand deformities may be acquired over time, typically from abnormal development or altered growth. Many of these conditions have a congenital basis of disease, but do not become apparent until the child grows and begins to learn hand function.

Trigger Thumb

While the exact cause of a trigger thumb is unclear, it is known that there is a size discrepancy between an enlarged flexor pollicis longus tendon and the first annular pulley of the thumb.[28] Occasionally, a trigger thumb is noticed when a mild injury occurs to the finger, and it is sometimes erroneously thought to be a dislocation of the IP joint. However, more frequently it is noticed as an asymptomatic deformity that presents sometime in the first 2 to 3 years of life.

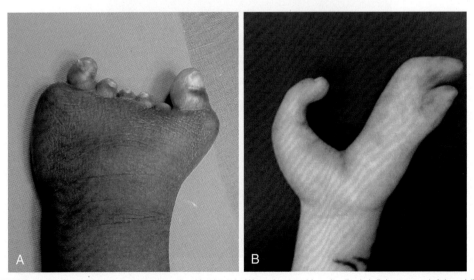

FIGURE 19.23 Typical appearance of symbrachydactyly (A) and central longitudinal deficiency or cleft hand (B).

The thumb is typically held in a flexed posture at the IP joint, with no active or passive extension noted and a palpable swelling of the tendon present at the level of the first annular pulley (Notta node) (**Figure 19.24**). On occasion, passive extension of the IP joint can be elicited with a pop, which typically pops back once the child flexes his or her thumb again. The contralateral

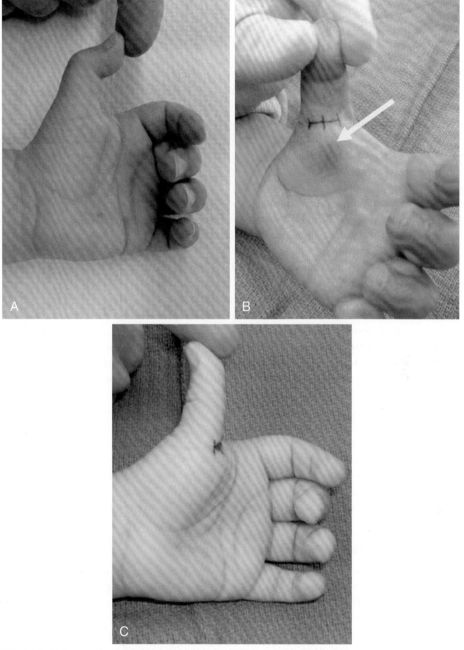

FIGURE 19.24 Clinical appearance of pediatric trigger thumb locked in flexion. Note the lack of passive interphalangeal joint extension (A) and the Notta node visible in the flexor pollicis longus tendon (arrow, B). After surgical release, full passive interphalangeal joint extension is restored (C).

thumb should always be examined, as it may be affected as well. Occasionally, the thumb will be locked in extension, which prevents active IP joint flexion, but leaves passive motion intact. The examination to assess for active IP flexion is sometimes difficult but can be assisted with wrist extension tenodesis and pressure along the volar forearm to induce motion of the flexor pollicis longus tendon.

Approximately one third of patients with pediatric trigger thumb will have complete resolution of symptoms with observation, and surgery is delayed until at least age 3 to see if the symptoms are resolving. If they do not resolve by age 3, surgical trigger thumb release may be performed. Therapy and splinting have not been demonstrated to improve the natural history of pediatric trigger thumb.

Clinodactyly/Camptodactyly

Coronal plane deformity of the small finger PIP joint is termed clinodactyly, while sagittal plane deformity is termed camptodactyly.[29] Clinodactyly is often inherited but is rarely associated with other syndromes. The deformity is occasionally progressive, but seldom limits function unless severe. Camptodactyly is present as two distinct types, the first being infantile, which presents at an early age. This type typically responds well to therapy and splinting with no long-term functional consequences. The adolescent type typically presents in the early teenage years and is typically more symptomatic and simultaneously less responsive to therapy.

On physical examination, the position and mobility of the finger should be assessed. In clinodactyly, there is an inward bend at the DIP joint with a shortened middle phalanx. The hand should be assessed in flexion to see if any digital crossover occurs, or if they have trouble grasping objects with their affected digits. In camptodactyly, the finger has a flexion contracture limiting passive PIP extension. Active PIP joint extension should be assessed, both with and without blocking MCP extension. By blocking MCP extension, the extrinsic finger extensors have increased pull and may correct the deformity. Additionally, there may be skin tightness on the volar surface of the proximal phalanx, which may limit passive extension of the digit. Radiographic evaluation of the finger with AP and lateral views is recommended to assess for middle phalanx pathology in clinodactyly and proximal phalanx head pathology in camptodactyly. In clinodactyly, there can be a trapezoidal middle phalanx with a proximal and distal physis, or a triangular middle phalanx with a bracket epiphysis (delta phalanx). In long-standing and severe camptodactyly, there may be flattening of the proximal phalanx head and incongruent joint surfaces.

Clinodactyly is treated conservatively in patients with minor deviation of the finger. Progressive deformity with a delta phalanx can be treated early (before age 6) with physiolysis, which untethers the epiphyseal bracket and allows for growth and deformity correction slowly over time. In older patients, the only correction is osteotomy of the middle phalanx, which requires a longer convalescence and potential risks of tendon adhesions and nonunion. Camptodactyly is most commonly treated with therapy and stretching exercises, which are maximized prior to any surgical intervention. The most serious complication from surgical correction of camptodactyly is loss of active finger flexion, which can severely limit hand function.

Multiple Hereditary Exostosis Syndrome

Patients with MHE occasionally have tumors arising in the phalanges that may cause deformity at the PIP joint.[30] These tumors may cause a mass effect around a joint and prevent full flexion or extension as they grow. Early identification of these problematic tumors is helpful to avoid more aggressive and potentially morbid treatments. Any patient with a developing deformity of the finger due to a tumor or mass should have dedicated radiographs of the finger involved. Surgical treatment is indicated for patients with developing deformity of the finger or mass effect blocking motion. Tumor excision is performed along with corrective osteotomy in the coronal plane, as this will not remodel over time.

● Conclusions

The hand and wrist are the most frequently injured parts of a child's body, and the hand is the second most common anatomic location for congenital anomalies. Therefore, any practitioner treating children and adolescents will be faced with the need to evaluate the injured or abnormal hand and wrist. The physical examination combined with a proper radiographic evaluation will allow for the appropriate diagnosis to be made, enabling prompt and proper treatment.

References

1. Valencia J, Leyva F, Gomez-Bajo GJ. Pediatric hand trauma. *Clin Orthop Relat Res.* 2005;(432):77-86.
2. Little KJ, Cornwall R. Congenital anomalies of the hand – principles of management. *Orthop Clin North Am.* 2016;47(1):153-168.
3. Pannu GS, Herman M. Distal radius-ulna fractures in children. *Orthop Clin North Am.* 2015;46(2):235-248.
4. Witney-Lagen C, Smith C, Walsh G. Soft cast versus rigid cast for treatment of distal radius buckle fractures in children. *Injury.* 2013;44(4):508-513.
5. Abzug JM, Little K, Kozin SH. Physeal arrest of the distal radius. *J Am Acad Orthop Surg.* 2014;22(6):381-389.
6. Bae DS, Gholson JJ, Zurakowski D, Waters PM. Functional outcomes after treatment of scaphoid fractures in children and adolescents. *J Pediatr Orthop.* 2016;36(1):13-18.
7. Bae DS, Waters PM. Pediatric distal radius fractures and triangular fibrocartilage complex injuries. *Hand Clin.* 2006;22(1):43-53.
8. Fishman FG, Barber J, Lourie GM, Peljovich AE. Outcomes of operative treatment of triangular fibrocartilage tears in pediatric and adolescent athletes. *J Pediatr Orthop.* 2018;38(10):e618-e622.
9. Earp BE, Waters PM, Wyzykowski RJ. Arthroscopic treatment of partial scapholunate ligament tears in children with chronic wrist pain. *J Bone Joint Surg Am.* 2006;88(11):2448-2455.
10. Kaawach W, Ecklund K, Di Canzio J, Zurakowski D, Waters PM. Normal ranges of scapholunate distance in children 6 to 14 years old. *J Pediatr Orthop.* 2001;21(4):464-467.
11. Godfrey J, Cornwall R. Pediatric metacarpal fractures. *Instr Course Lect.* 2017;66:437-445.
12. Abzug JM, Dua K, Bauer AS, Cornwall R, Wyrick TO. Pediatric phalanx fractures. *J Am Acad Orthop Surg.* 2016;24(11):e174-e183.
13. Lin JS, Popp JE, Balch Samora J. Treatment of acute Seymour fractures. *J Pediatr Orthop.* 2019;39(1):e23-e27.
14. Reyes BA, Ho CA. The high risk of infection with delayed treatment of open Seymour fractures: Salter-Harris I/II or juxta-epiphyseal fractures of the distal phalanx with associated nailbed laceration. *J Pediatr Orthop.* 2017;37(4):247-253.
15. Lankachandra M, Wells CR, Cheng CJ, Hutchison RL. Complications of distal phalanx fractures in children. *J Hand Surg Am.* 2017;42(7):574.e1-574.e6.
16. Miller A, Lightdale-Miric N, Eismann E, Carr P, Little KJ. Outcomes of isolated radial osteotomy for volar distal radioulnar joint instability following radial malunion in children. *J Hand Surg Am.* 2018;43(1):81.e1-81.e8.
17. Oda T, Wada T, Isogai S, Iba K, Aoki M, Yamashita T. Corrective osteotomy for volar instability of the distal radioulnar joint associated with radial shaft malunion. *J Hand Surg Eur Vol.* 2007;32(5):573-577.
18. De Smet L, Verhaegen F, Degreef I. Carpal malalignment in malunion of the distal radius and the effect of corrective osteotomy. *J Wrist Surg.* 2014;3(3):166-170.
19. Pryce JC. The wrist position between neutral and ulnar deviation that facilitates the maximum power grip strength. *J Biomech.* 1980;13(6):505-511.
20. Ekblom AG, Dahlin LB, Rosberg HE, et al. Hand function in children with radial longitudinal deficiency. *BMC Musculoskelet Disord.* 2013;14:116.
21. Cole RJ, Manske PR. Classification of ulnar deficiency according to the thumb and first web. *J Hand Surg Am.* 1997;22(3):479-488.
22. Kozin SH, Zlotolow DA. Madelung deformity. *J Hand Surg Am.* 2015;40(10):2090-2098.
23. Schmale GA, Conrad EU III, Raskind WH. The natural history of hereditary multiple exostoses. *J Bone Joint Surg Am.* 1994;76(7):986-992.
24. Ramavath AL, Unnikrishnan PN, George HL, Sathyamoorthy P, Bruce CE. Wrist arthroscopy in children and adolescent with chronic wrist pain: arthroscopic findings compared with MRI. *J Pediatr Orthop.* 2017;37(5):e321-e325.

25. Head L, Gencarelli JR, Allen M, Boyd KU, Wrist ganglion treatment: systematic review and meta-analysis. *J Hand Surg Am*. 2015;40(3):546-553.e8.

26. Kozin SH, Zlotolow DA. Common pediatric congenital conditions of the hand. *Plast Reconstr Surg*. 2015;136(2):241e-257e.

27. Woodside JC, Light TR. Symbrachydactyly-diagnosis, function, and treatment. *J Hand Surg Am*. 2016;41(1):135-143.

28. Kikuchi N, Ogino T. Incidence and development of trigger thumb in children. *J Hand Surg Am*. 2006;31(4):541-543.

29. Ty JM, James MA. Failure of differentiation: Part II (arthrogryposis, camptodactyly, clinodactyly, Madelung deformity, trigger finger, and trigger thumb). *Hand Clin*. 2009;25(2):195-213.

30. Woodside JC, Ganey T, Gaston RG. Multiple osteochondroma of the hand: initial and long-term follow-up study. *Hand (NY)*. 2015;10(4):616-620.

Note: Page numbers followed by "*f*" indicate figures and "*t*" indicate tables.